Neuroprotection and Regeneration of the Spinal Cord

Kenzo Uchida • Masaya Nakamura
Hiroshi Ozawa • Shinsuke Katoh
Editors

Yoshiaki Toyama
Honorary Editor

Neuroprotection and Regeneration of the Spinal Cord

Springer

Editors
Kenzo Uchida
Department of Orthopaedics
and Rehabilitation Medicine
Faculty of Medical Sciences
University of Fukui
Fukui, Japan

Hiroshi Ozawa
Department of Orthopaedic Surgery
Tohoku University Graduate School
of Medicine
Sendai, Japan

Masaya Nakamura
Department of Orthopaedic Surgery
Keio University School of Medicine
Tokyo, Japan

Shinsuke Katoh
Department of Orthopedic Surgery
School of Medicine
The University of Tokushima
Tokushima, Japan

Honorary Editor
Yoshiaki Toyama
Department of Orthopaedic Surgery
Keio University School of Medicine
Tokyo, Japan

ISBN 978-4-431-56150-7 ISBN 978-4-431-54502-6 (eBook)
DOI 10.1007/978-4-431-54502-6
Springer Tokyo Heidelberg New York Dordrecht London

Printed on acid-free paper

Springer is part of Springer Science+Business Media (www.springer.com)

Preface

During the last tens of years, we have witnessed major advances in the fields on molecular and cellular biologies, neurosciences around involving the spinal cord and nerve tissues, immunohistochemical neuropathology, and other relevant scientific technologies such as molecular neuroimaging. These advances in basic science areas have aided and facilitated neurosurgeons as well as spine surgeons in elaborate clinical studies, and, in turn, so many issues have once again prompted basic scientists to further investigate in the deepest areas of the spinal cord neuroscience and neuroimaging. So now, both basic scientists and neuro-orthopaedic surgeons have begun to mutually tightly communicate more closely for to enhance the basic neuropathology as well as neurosciences of the spinal cord. During these recent years, not only basic scientists but clinical physicians have been enthusiastically investigating understanding of spinal cord pathologies in order for to achieve better clinical treatments in the clinical areas. To enhancing enhance understanding of spinal cord neurosciences, it is essential to know be knowledgeable about the problems and difficulties in the clinical aspects of spinal cord diseases and then to communicate with basic scientists. This mutual communications will ultimately result in the best treatment for patients.

In this book, we have focused on recent outstanding records in neuroscience, cellular biology, neuropathology, and molecular neuroimaging. The contributors of the book's chapters are today's frontrunners in diverse fields of science in Japan, delivering outstanding lectures at medical conventions and publishing the highest-quality articles in top-ranking journals. Selected monographs are listed in this book for the readers in order to summarize the contemporary achievements in research into spinal cord neuroscience. Those who are new to the field are encouraged to enrich their work with the knowledge contained hereby and to enhance their creative research with these monographs. Clinicians and neurosurgeons will learn of new trends in neurochemistry and neuropathology as well as the study of practical applications for their work in clinical practice. The result will be a better understanding of works in basic neuroscience. Ultimately, it is believed that these works in neuroscience will bring about neurological improvements for patients and a better quality of life for them. We clinical neuro-orthopedic researchers hope that young practitioners can facilitate their outstanding work in the name of scientific advancement as well as patients' health care.

We thank the many outstanding authors who contributed to this volume in spite of their demanding clinical duties. Special thanks are given to the Governmental Committee on Ossification of Spinal Ligaments. We are also grateful to Springer Japan for the opportunity to share this knowledge and these monographs with others.

Fukui, Japan — Kenzo Uchida
Tokyo, Japan — Masaya Nakamura
Sendai, Japan — Hiroshi Ozawa
Tokushima, Japan — Shinsuke Katoh

Contents

Part I
Pathologies of Spinal Cord Injury

Chapter 1
The Mechanism Behind Functional Recovery After the Incomplete Spinal Cord Injury

Seiji Okada

Abstract Because the regenerative capability of the mammalian central nervous system (CNS) is poor, limited functional recovery occurs during the chronic phase of spinal cord injury (SCI). At the subacute phase of SCI, however, gradual functional recovery is observed to some extent in both rodents and humans in the incomplete SCI. Although the mechanism behind this functional recovery is not fully elucidated, considerable developments of knowledge in basic experimental research have resulted in an improved understanding of functional recovery after injury. In this review, we discuss the progress of research for the potential mechanisms underlying for spontaneous functional recovery, including healing process by reactive astrocytes and the propriospinal relay connections in the incomplete SCI.

Keywords Propriospinal relay connections • Reactive astrocytes • Spontaneous functional recovery • Stat3 (single transducer and activator of transcription 3)

1.1 Introduction

In the pathophysiology of SCI, it is generally accepted that SCI is a two-step process involving the primary mechanical injury and a following cascade of autodestructive injury [1]. Mechanical trauma rapidly leads to blood-spinal barrier disruption, neural cell death, axonal damage, and demyelination followed by a cascade of secondary injury that expands the additional inflammatory reaction at the

S. Okada (✉)
Department of Advance Medical Initiatives, Graduate school of Medical Sciences, Kyushu University, 3-1-1, Maidashi, Hikashi-ku, Fukuoka 812-8582, Japan

Department of Orthopedics, Graduate school of Medical Sciences, Kyushu University, 3-1-1, Maidashi, Hikashi-ku, Fukuoka 812-8582, Japan
e-mail: seokada@ortho.med.kyushu-u.ac.jp

K. Uchida et al. (eds.), *Neuroprotection and Regeneration of the Spinal Cord*,
DOI 10.1007/978-4-431-54502-6_1, © Springer Japan 2014

lesion site. The severity of secondary injury depends on the degree of the primary mechanical injury, and the neurological outcomes are affected by the combination of the primary and secondary injury. At the initial phase of SCI, any damage to the SCI usually causes immediate depression of all cord functions below the level of injury, and this serious transient breakdown of SCI function is called as the spinal shock. At the phase of spinal shock, the clinical paralysis of SCI patients as well as experimental SCI of rodents almost always exhibit severest state, and gradual functional improvements to some extent are observed with time course in case of the incomplete paralysis. Although the clinical time course of paralysis indicates that there is some sort of self-repair system after the CNS injury even in primates, the mechanisms underlying functional improvement in the incomplete SIC are poorly understood and referred to as withdrawal of the spinal shock. Understanding the self-repair mechanism inherent in mammals is surely to lead to novel therapeutic strategy for the treatment of CNS injury.

1.2 Reactive Astrocytes and Functional Recovery

To interpret the process of paralysis improvement in the subacute phase, we examined serial histological sections of contused spinal cord and followed motor function in the wild-type C57BL/6 mouse after produced contusion injury at the 12th thoracic levels (by IH impactor 70 Kdyn). In this model, complete paralysis was observed immediately after injury; however, gradual functional recovery was observed until the subacute phase of injury (–2 weeks after injury), followed by limited recovery afterwards. Firstly, we tried to confirm the secondary injury process in the acute phase by immunohistochemical analysis. Until several days after injury, the area of neural cells including neurons and oligodendrocytes gradually enlarged in a rostral-caudal direction, and some portions of neural cells were immune-positive for cleaved caspase 3, indicating that the secondary injury process lasted at this phase in this model during which we observed limited functional recovery. Meanwhile, astrocytes surrounding the lesion underwent a typical morphologic change of hypertrophy, process extension, and increased expression of intermediate filaments such as GFAP and Nestin by 7 days after SCI, characteristic of reactive astrocytes [2].

Notably, these responsive astrocytes eventually migrated centripetally to the lesion epicenter and gradually compacted the inflammatory cells, contracting the lesion area up until subacute phase after SCI (Fig. 1.1). During this process, gradual functional improvement as well as the repair of injured tissue was observed, and reactive astrocytes formed a physical barrier against inflammatory cells, commonly referred to as the glial scar [3]. After the migration of reactive astrocytes and completion of glial scar, functional improvement reached a plateau around 2 weeks after SCI.

The glial scar contains extracellular matrix molecules that chemically inhibit axonal regeneration and has been considered to definitely play a crucial part in CNS regeneration failure in the chronic phase of injury [4]. However, the process observed at subacute phase strongly suggests that the emergence and migration of reactive astrocytes have a prominent role in the repair of injured tissue and the restoration of motor function before the completion of the glial scar [3].

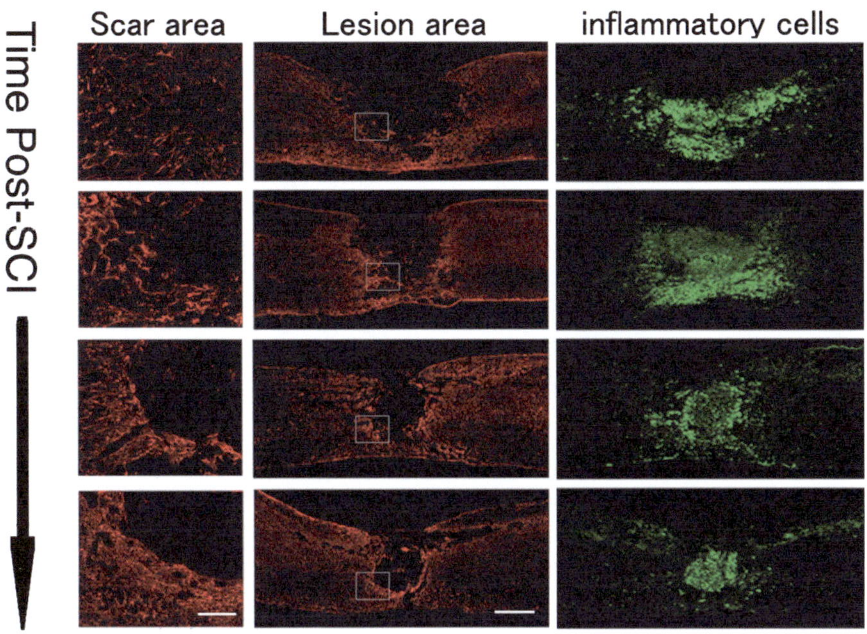

Fig. 1.1 Reactive astrocyte migration and the compaction of lesion area. At the subacute phase of SCI, reactive astrocytes gradually migrate centripetally to the lesion epicenter and gradually compact the CD11b-positive inflammatory cells. Scale bar: 100 μm (*left*) and 500 μm (*right*)

1.3 The Migration Mechanism of Reactive Astrocytes

The regulatory mechanisms behind the reactive response of astrocytes remain elusive. We investigated the role of signal transducer and activator of transcription 3 (Stat3) signaling since Stat3 is a principal mediator in a variety of biological processes including the wound healing and movement of various types of cells [3]. In addition, several reports suggested that Stat3 mediates certain aspects of astrogliosis downstream of the action of cytokines such as interleukin (IL)-6, leukemia inhibitory factor (LIF), and ciliary neurotrophic factor (CNTF) after CNS injury [5–8]. Actually, in the injured spinal cord, phosphorylated Stat3 prominently increased at 12 h after injury, which remained detectable with western blotting analysis for 2 weeks after SCI. We observed phosphorylation and nuclear translocation of Stat3 mainly in reactive astrocytes surrounding the lesion epicenter, but not in distant areas for several days after SCI [3].

To elucidate the role of Stat3 in reactive astrocytes, we performed experiments by using mice with a selective deletion of STAT3 under the control of Nestin gene promoter/enhancer ($STAT3^{N-/-}$), which is activated in reactive astrocytes after SCI. $STAT3^{N-/-}$ mice showed no apparent abnormalities in motor function and development, although they showed signs of hyperphagia and leptin resistance [9]. At 2 weeks after injury, widespread tissue damage, demyelination, and severe motor deficit were observed in this conditional STAT3 knockout mouse compared to the wild-type mouse. Interestingly, although the comparable tissue damage and reactive gliosis were observed around the lesion epicenter at acute phase of injury in both types of mice, the configuration of the gliosis remained relatively unchanged for the chronic phase of injury owing to their limited migration. As a result, the impaired contraction of inflammatory cells by reactive astrocytes brought about widespread damage and limited functional recovery in only $STAT3^{N-/-}$ mice [3]. To further investigate the relationship between STAT3 signaling and the function of reactive astrocytes, we analyzed pathophysiology after SCI in $SOCS3^{N-/-}$ mice [3]. SOCS3 is the protein suppressor of cytokine signaling 3, and negative feedback molecule of STAT3 and the bipolar relationship between STAT3 and SOCS3 has been noted in several deletion experiments [9]. In the injured spinal cord of $SOCS3^{N-/-}$ mice, rapid migration of reactive astrocytes to seclude inflammatory cells, enhanced contraction of lesion area, and dramatic improvement of functional recovery were observed [3]. These results suggest that STAT3 signaling associated with the migration of reactive astrocytes is a key regulator in the healing process after SCI.

Regarding the downstream of Stat3, several reports indicated a possible molecular link between Stat3-zinc signaling and cell movement [10–12]. The zinc transporter LIV1 was found to be the transcriptional downstream target of Stat3 and essential for the nuclear localization of Snail, a transcriptional repressor of the Cdh1 genes which encodes E-cadherin [10]. The absence of Stat3 therefore causes dysregulation of cell adhesion and impairs cell movements. In the SCI model, selective deletion of Stat3 in reactive astrocytes brought about their limited migration and impaired healing process after SCI. In addition, another study reported that zinc deficiency impaired compaction of inflammatory cells by reactive astrocytes after CNS injury similar to $STAT3^{N-/-}$ mice [11, 12]. On the other hand, astrocyte-targeted IL-6-expressing transgenic mice showed prompt migration of reactive astrocytes and compaction of inflammatory cells after CNS injury similar to $SOCS3^{N-/-}$ mice [13]. It stands to reason that enhanced phosphorylation of Stat3 in reactive astrocytes brought about the similar phenotype to $SOCS3^{N-/-}$ mice after SCI in this transgenic mice. We also confirmed the robust expression of LIV1 mRNA in reactive astrocytes of the wild-type mice but limited expression in $STAT3^{N-/-}$ mice after SCI [3]. Thus, Stat3-zinc signaling could be a radically new therapeutic target for the treatment of the CNS injury.

1.4 Therapeutic Strategy by GSK3 Inhibitor Stimulating Reactive Astrocyte Migration

Another therapeutic strategy stimulating the migration of reactive astrocytes using an inhibitor of glycogen synthase kinase-3 (GSK3) has also been suggested [14]. GSK3 is serine/threonine kinase originally identified as a regulator of glycogen synthase. Based on their involvement in several signaling pathways, GSK3 inhibition is considered to be a potential therapeutic target for several diseases [15, 16].

Actually, GSK3 inhibition was reported to be beneficial for SCI by reducing neural apoptosis and promoting axonal growth after injury [17]. In addition, considering that activation of the Wnt/beta-catenin pathway by this agent results in the increased migration of numerous cell types in a variety of pathophysiological contexts, inhibition of GSK3 leading to activation of beta-catenin was speculated to stimulate astrocytes migration. Renault-Mihara et al. reported that GSK3 inhibitor accelerated migration of reactive astrocytes after SIC by decreasing adhesive activity via reduced surface expression of beta1-integrin and promoted functional recovery [14]. They firstly performed experiments using a modified Boyden's chamber assay as well as transwell assay and demonstrated that GSK3 inhibitor significantly promoted astrocyte migration in vitro. Next, they examined in vivo effect of GSK3 inhibitor in mice SCI model. Intraperitoneal administration of GSK3 inhibitor for 5 days after SIC resulted in enhanced migration of reactive astrocytes, compaction of infiltrated inflammatory cells, and functional recovery. Reduced lesion volume, expression of chondroitin sulfate proteoglycans, and demyelination were also observed in the mice treated with GSK3 inhibitor. They also access the molecular mechanism underlying the pro-migratory effect of GSK3 inhibitor with DNA microarray analysis and in vitro membrane-coated transwell assay and demonstrated that pro-migratory effect of this agent relies on decreased adhesion strength especially through the reduced surface expression of beta1-integrin. Actually, the expression level of beta1-integrin at the lesion area of spinal cord was significantly decreased in the GSK3 inhibitor-treated mice. These results suggest that the pharmacological stimulation of reactive astrocytes migration is a feasible therapeutic strategy for the treatment of SCI.

1.5 Indirect Propriospinal Relay Contributes to Functional Recovery After SCI

Although the spontaneous functional recovery in the incomplete SCI is attributed to the spared axons, the propriospinal connections are also considered to be significant for the recovery for many years. Courtine et al. demonstrated that pronounced functional recovery can occur after severe SCI by the reorganization of descending and propriospinal connections [18]. They conducted a physiological and anatomical analysis of the basis for spontaneous recovery of hindlimb stepping after SCI in mice model with excitotoxic ablation of intrinsic spinal cord neurons. Firstly, they confirmed prominent functional recovery of hindlimb stepping after a single lateral (left) hemisection at thoracic segment 12 (T12). During the first week after injury, mice entirely lost the ability to step in the ipsilateral hindlimb, but retained the ability to step with the contralateral hindlimb. The steplike movements began to reappear on the ipsilateral side by 2 weeks after injury, and mice progressively recovered plantar stepping ability afterwards. By 7 weeks after injury, almost complete recovery in hindlimb stepping was observed in the ipsilateral side. Secondary, they placed a second lateral hemisection at 10 weeks after the first hemisection at the same level (T12) but on the contralateral side in mice that had recovered from the first lesion.

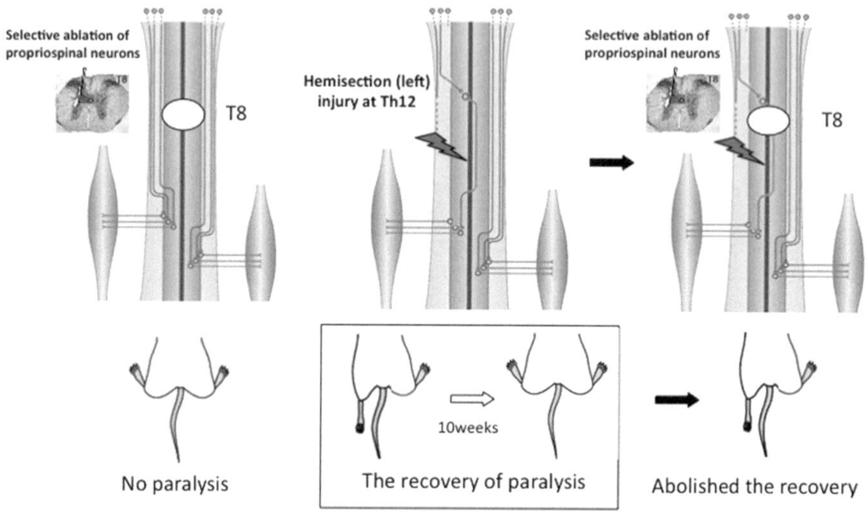

Fig. 1.2 Propriospinal relay connections after the hemisection injury. In the intact spinal cord, selective ablation of propriospinal neurons had only minor effect on hindlimb stepping (*left*), but completely abolished the spontaneously recovered stepping in mice with the hemisection injury that had recovered stepping function after 10 weeks

After this second lesion, mice showed complete paralysis of both hindlimbs with no signs of recovery of locomotor functions afterwards. This result suggests that recovery after the first hemisection was due to supraspinal information passing the injury site on the contralateral side, rather than to the sparing of fibers ipsilateral to the hemisection or to autonomous activity of lumbosacral locomotor circuits.

To examine further the role of thoracic propriospinal neurons in mediating the functional recovery observed after a hemisection, they ablated these neurons by infusing the axon-sparing excitotoxin *N*-methyl-D-aspartic acid (NMDA) into the gray matter. This NMDA infusion had only minor effects on stepping function in the uninjured mice because there was little effect on the major myelinated long descending fiber tracts (Fig. 1.2). However, in mice with a unilateral hemisection that had recovered stepping function after 10 weeks, infusions of NMDA completely abolished the spontaneously recovered stepping on the ipsilateral side, suggesting that local thoracic propriospinal neurons were essential for the spontaneous recovery of stepping observed after a hemisection injury (Fig. 1.2).

These findings show that the precise restoration of point-to-point connections made by long-tract descending axons from the brain to the lumbosacral locomotor circuits is not required to achieve meaningful functional recovery [18]. The reorganization of interactions between descending inputs and intrinsic spinal cord circuits that relay information past the lesion area is sufficient for the recovery of the motor function after severe/moderate SCI. Targeting interventions to augment the remodeling of relay connections is a feasible and easily achievable therapeutic strategy for the treatment of SCI.

1.6 Conclusions

To date, several kinds of cellular and molecular manipulations are suggested for the treatment of SCI, such as anti-inflammatory agents, neurotrophic factors, axonal regeneration promoter, re-myelination agents, and stem cell transplantations [19, 20]. However, little is known about which neural systems should be targeted and which strategy would be most effective. In addition, each strategy has both merits and demerits and is not always beneficial for the pathophysiology of SCI. Considering that innate physiological self-repair system after CNS injury is safest and most reasonable, understanding the mechanism behind a spontaneous functional recovery gives rise to a clue for novel, feasible, and potent therapeutic strategies for the treatment for SCI. Aside from reactive astrocytes and the propriospinal relay, substantial spontaneous recovery of functions may generally occur due to the activation of multiple compensatory mechanisms. Further basic scientific research should provide a rational basis for elucidation of the mechanisms underlying spontaneous functional recovery and establishment of a reliable therapy for the CNS injury.

Conflict of Interest The Author declares that he has no conflict of interest.

References

1. Beattie MS (2004) Inflammation and apoptosis: linked therapeutic targets in spinal cord injury. Trends Mol Med 10:580–583
2. Frisen J et al (1995) Rapid, widespread, and longlasting induction of nestin contributes to the generation of glial scar tissue after CNS injury. J Cell Biol 131:453–464
3. Okada S et al (2006) Conditional ablation of stat3 or socs3 discloses a dual role for reactive astrocytes after spinal cord injury. Nat Med 12:829–834
4. Silver J, Miller JH (2006) Regeneration beyond the glial scar. Nat Rev Neurosci 5:146–156
5. Sriram K et al (2004) Induction of gp130-related cytokines and activation of JAK2/STAT3 pathway in astrocytes precedes up-regulation of glial fibrillary acidic protein in the 1-methyl-4-phenyl-1,2,3,6-tetrahydropyridine model of neurodegeneration. J Biol Chem 279:19936–19947
6. Kerr BJ, Patterson PH (2004) Potent pro-inflammatory actions of leukemia inhibitory factor in the spinal cord of the adult mouse. Exp Neurol 188:391–407
7. Xia XG et al (2002) Induction of STAT3 signaling in activated astrocytes and sprouting septal neurons following entorhinal cortex lesion in adult rats. Mol Cell Neurosci 21:379–392
8. Klein MA et al (1997) Impaired neuroglial activation in interleukin-6 deficient mice. Glia 19:227–233
9. Mori H et al (2004) Socs3 deficiency in the brain elevates leptin sensitivity and confers resistance to diet-induced obesity. Nat Med 10:739–743
10. Yamashita S et al (2004) Zinc transporter LIVI controls epithelial mesenchymal transition in zebrafish gastrula organizer. Nature 429:298–302
11. Penkowa M et al (2001) Zinc or copper deficiency-induced impaired inflammatory response to brain trauma may be caused by the concomitant metallothionein changes. J Neurotrauma 18:447–463
12. Penkowa M et al (1999) CNS wound healing is severely depressed in metallothionein I- and II-deficient mice. J Neurosci 19:2535–2545

13. Penkowa M et al (2003) Astrocyte-targeted expression of IL-6 protects the CNS against a focal brain injury. Exp Neurol 181:130–148
14. Renault-Mihara F et al (2011) Beneficial compaction of spinal cord lesion by migrating astrocytes through glycogen synthase kinase-3 inhibition. EMBO Mol Med 3:682–696
15. Forde JE, Dale TC (2007) Glycogen synthase kinase 3: a key regulator of cellular fate. Cell Mol Life Sci 64:1930–1944
16. Chico LK, Van Eldik LJ, Watterson DM (2009) Targeting protein kinases in central nervous system disorders. Nat Rev Drug Discov 8:892–909
17. Dill J et al (2008) Inactivation of glycogen synthase kinase 3 promotes axonal growth and recovery in the CNS. J Neurosci 28:8914–8928
18. Courtine G et al (2008) Recovery of supraspinal control of stepping via indirect propriospinal relay connections after spinal cord injury. Nat Med 14:69–78
19. Harrop JS et al (2012) Evaluation of clinical experience using cell-based therapies in patients with spinal cord injury: a systematic review. J Neurosurg Spine 17:230–246
20. Grossman RG et al (2012) North American clinical trials network for the treatment of spinal cord injury: goals and progress. J Neurosurg Spine 17:6–10

Chapter 2
Microenvironment Within the Injured Spinal Cord Focusing on IL-6

Masaya Nakamura

Abstract In recent years, a variety of studies have been conducted towards the goal of achieving regeneration of the central nervous system using neural stem cells. However, various complex factors are involved in the regulation of neural stem cell differentiation, and many unresolved questions remain. It has been reported that after spinal cord injury, the intrinsic neural stem cells do not differentiate into neurons but into astrocytes, resulting in the formation of glial scars. Based on reports that the expression of IL-6 and the IL-6 receptor is sharply increased in the acute stages after spinal cord injury and that IL-6 may serve as a factor strongly inducing the differentiation of neural stem cells into astrocytes, we examined the effects of an antibody to the IL-6 receptor in cases of spinal cord injury and found that the antibody indeed suppressed secondary injury (caused by inflammatory reactions) and glial scar formation, facilitating functional recovery. In this paper, we present the data from this investigation and discuss the relationship between IL-6 signals and spinal cord injury.

Keywords Glial scar • IL-6 • Regeneration • Spinal cord injury

2.1 Introduction

The annual incidence of traumatic spinal cord injury (SCI) in Japan is about 40 per 1,000,000 population. Every year, about 5,000 individuals sustain SCI in this country. Recent advances in patient management during the acute stages of SCI have dramatically reduced the death rate from SCI. However, the total number of patients

M. Nakamura (✉)
Department of Orthopedic Surgery, Keio University School of Medicine,
35 Shinanomachi, Shinjuku, Tokyo 160-8582, Japan
e-mail: masa@a8.keio.jp

K. Uchida et al. (eds.), *Neuroprotection and Regeneration of the Spinal Cord*,
DOI 10.1007/978-4-431-54502-6_2, © Springer Japan 2014

with SCI suffering from complications, such as permanent paralysis of the extremities, sensory disturbances, bladder/bowel disturbances, and bedsores, is reported to be more than 100,000 in Japan. The treatments currently administered to patients with spinal cord injuries are not designed to cure paralysis but for control of systemic factors during the acute stages of injury, stabilization of dislocations and fractures by surgical decompression, reduction or fixation, and prevention of worsening of paralysis; none of these treatments affect the spinal cord itself. Of course, the number of patients who are able to resume social activities through rehabilitation beginning soon after injury has been increasing. On the other hand, there are many patients who are forced to be discharged severely paralyzed from the hospital. In the chronic stage, patient management is focused on rehabilitation, and no active treatment is provided other than expectant therapy for complications. In the 1990s, the effectiveness of massive doses of steroids in the acute stages of SCI was reported based on the results of animal studies and mass clinical studies. This therapy, however, was subsequently proven to be less effective than was initially reported. In recent years, several reports have been published describing adverse reactions to this therapy or casting doubts on the effectiveness of this therapy. At present, more than 10 years after it was first introduced, the need is felt for review of this steroid therapy [1].

Over the past decade, significant progress has been made in the field of stem cell biology pertaining to the central nervous system, and it has been revealed that neural stem cells are seen not only during the intrauterine period but also during adulthood. Furthermore, it is now possible to isolate and incubate these stem cells [2]. Neural stem cells are cells with self-copying potential and the capability of differentiation into diverse cell groups (neurons, astrocytes, oligodendrocytes, etc.). The mammalian central nervous system is an outcome of asymmetrical division of neural stem cells and sophisticated and complex interactions among these cells (involving secretory factors) during embryonic development. It has long been believed that the central nervous system can never regenerate after injury. However, there is now growing concern about regenerative medicine (tissue engineering) techniques aimed at inducing regeneration of the degenerated or injured central nervous system and restoration of its functions by reproducing the central nervous system generation process using intrinsic or extrinsic neural stem cells [3]. In this paper, we shall present our data and discuss the effects of IL-6 signals on the inflammatory reactions and intrinsic neural stem cells in the presence of SCI.

2.2 Neural Stem Cells and IL-6 Signals in Spinal Cord Injury

It has been shown that neural stem cells are also present in the spinal cord of mature mammals, but that in the event of injury, these neural stem cells do not differentiate into neurons but into astrocytes instead, to form glial scars [4]. Glial scars are primarily composed of activated astrocytes and express large amounts of chondroitin sulfate proteoglycan (CSPG) that suppresses the growth of axons. These scars are thus considered to be a great physical and chemical obstacle against axonal regeneration.

In a study using rat models with SCI, it was demonstrated that treatment with chondroitinase ABC, which can degrade CSPG, was useful in promoting axonal regeneration and functional recovery following SCI [5].

Based on the contention that changes in the microenvironment within the injured spinal cord could play an important role in the differentiation of neural stem cells exclusively into astrocytes, we examined the time-course of changes in the mRNA expression levels of various cytokines during the acute stages of SCI in rats, using RNase protection assays. This analysis revealed that while the expression of TGF-β (an anti-inflammatory cytokine) showed a subacute increase, reaching its peak 4–7 days after the injury, the expression of inflammatory cytokines (IL-1β, IL-6 and TNF-α) showed acute increase, reaching a peak within 12 h after the injury [6]. In particular, the SCI group exhibited an approximately 30-fold increase of IL-6 expression as compared to the sham-operated group. Regarding the signal transduction related to IL-6, it is known that while the expression of IL-6 activity is very weak in the presence of IL-6 alone, the complex formed by the binding of IL-6 to the IL-6 receptor serving as a ligand binds to gp130 (a membrane-bound receptor), leading to signal transduction to cells (trans-signaling) [7]. Because of this unique form of signal transduction, an increase in the expression of the IL-6 receptor is a key factor determining signal transduction related to IL-6. We quantified the expression of the IL-6 receptor by Western blotting in C57/B6 mice with SCI caused by compression at the level of the ninth thoracic vertebra and found that there was an approximately eightfold increase in the expression of this receptor within 12 h after the injury as compared to the level before the injury [8]. We paid close attention to this sharp increase of IL-6 and IL-6 receptor expression in the acute phase of SCI, based on the contention that this might be one of the factors responsible for the differentiation of neural stem cells into astrocytes and not neurons after SCI.

Neural stem cells are induced by interactions among various factors. In this connection, it has been found in vitro that IL-6 signals, including LIF and CNTF, act on neural stem cells to powerfully induce their differentiation into astrocytes [9]. This finding has also been endorsed in studies in vivo. In one such study, IL-6-knockout mice showed suppression of astrogliosis following SCI [10]; in another, mice showing excessive expression of IL-6 and the IL-6 receptor showed marked gliosis even after mild injury of the spinal cord [11]. It has also been shown that injury of the spinal cord resulted in a marked decrease of axonal growth in mice with excessive IL-6 signals as compared to that in intact mice [12]. On the basis of these previous findings, we contended that suppression of IL-6 signals in the acute stage of SCI might suppress the formation of glial scars. We, therefore, conducted a study in mice using a monoclonal antibody directed against the mouse IL-6 receptor (MR16-1), jointly with Chugai Pharmaceutical Co. Ltd [8].

First, we examined the effects of IL-6 signals on the differentiation of neural stem cells intrinsically present in the spinal cord. To this end, we collected neural stem cells from the spinal cords of 8-week-old mature mice and incubated them in vitro for 3 days to induce differentiation. In the control group, the cells showed scarcely any growth of cellular processes. In the group treated with IL-6 and the IL-6 receptor, however, marked growth of astroglial processes was noted. The percentage of cells differentiating into GFAP-positive astrocytes was also higher in the IL-6 + IL-6 receptor treatment group. This result can be interpreted as indicating that IL-6 signaling does indeed significantly stimulate the differentiation of neural stem cells into astrocytes, as reported previously. However, when the cells were incubated in the presence of both IL-6 and MR16-1 (an antibody directed against the IL-6 receptor), the effect of the IL-6 signals was attenuated. These results suggest that the blocking of the IL-6 signals with antibody directed against the IL-6 receptor can suppress the differentiation of intrinsic neural stem cells into astrocytes in vivo.

Then, we examined the effects of IL-6 signals on the formation of glial scars in vivo, using a mouse model of SCI. First, the spinal cord of the mouse was exposed at the level of the ninth thoracic vertebra; then, a 3-g weight was dropped from a height of 25 mm on to the exposed dura matter to induce contusion SCI. The mouse was given a single intraperitoneal injection of the IL-6 receptor antibody immediately after SCI. Two weeks later, specimens of spinal cord tissue were immunostained with various markers. In the mice with SCI, no softening or void formation was seen in the tissue specimens, unlike in rats and other models. Instead, large scars replacing the gray matter were found at the center of the injured spinal cord. In a previous study, this scar was characterized as being composed of connective tissue rich in type IV collagen and fibronectin [13]. When immunostained, the scar was found to contain no neurons, but groups of inflammatory cells. GFAP-positive glial scars were formed surrounding these scars composed of connective tissue. To mark the newly formed cells after SCI, we administered an intraperitoneal injection of bromodeoxyuridine (Brd-U), which is a substrate for DNA synthesis, to the animals for 14 consecutive days after the induction of SCI, and quantified the glial scars by using astrocyte formation as an indicator by double-staining with Brd-U and GFAP. This study revealed that the glial scar formation was suppressed at the center of the injured spinal cord. The number of double (Brd-U/GFAP)-positive cells was 25 % lower in the group treated with the IL-6 receptor antibody immediately after the injury than in the control group treated with IgG alone. To confirm that the IL-6 signals had actually been blocked, we examined the phosphorylation (activation) of STAT3 (a transcription factor acting in the IL-6/IL-6 receptor/gp130 signal pathway) by Western blotting and found a significant decrease of STAT3 phosphorylation in the IL-6 receptor antibody treatment group. This result endorses the proposition that the drug administered as a single intraperitoneal injection immediately after SCI acts on the injured spinal cord.

2.3 Inflammatory Cytokines in Spinal Cord Injury and Their Relationship to Secondary Injury

In addition to its effects on the neural stem cells, we shall also discuss the role of IL-6 as an inflammatory cytokine in cases of SCI. In regard to the pathogenesis of SCI, the concept of secondary injury was proposed many years ago. This concept proposes that self-destroying tissue damage occurs secondary to primary mechanical damage caused by the external force in cases of SCI. Histopathological examination has demonstrated that small bleeding spots due to enhanced vascular permeability are formed within 10 min after SCI and that edema, ischemia, and focal bleeding develop in the gray and white matter within a few hours after injury, causing progressive necrosis of the surrounding nerve cells due to the shortage of nutrients and oxygen. Clinically, paralysis associated with SCI is the most severe immediately after the injury. In cases where paresis develops following SCI, gradual recovery from paresis is seen for some period after the very acute phase. It is thus unknown to what precise extent secondary injury is involved in the paralysis seen after SCI. However, many reports of animal studies have demonstrated that suppression of secondary injury, for example, by the use of steroids, resulted in some alleviation of the paralysis. Therefore, reduction of secondary tissue damage is a major goal of treatment in cases of SCI [14, 15]. Factors known to stimulate the aforementioned self-destructive responses include NO, free radicals, glutamic acid, and MMP. In particular, the inflammatory cytokines seem to be closely involved in the secondary damage. Of course, increased or suppressed expression of a variety of cytokines has been demonstrated in the presence of SCI, and it is known that these cytokines have two distinctive effects (neurotoxic and neurotrophic effects). Although we need to be careful while interpreting the effects of these cytokines in cases of SCI, previous studies have suggested that the marked increase of IL-6 expression during the ultra-acute stage of SCI plays a central role in the inflammatory reactions and serves as a neurotoxic factor.

Therefore, to examine the effects of an antibody to the IL-6 receptor on the severity of these inflammatory reactions, we stained spinal cord tissue specimens (collected 2 weeks after injury) with Mac1 (CD11b), a marker of inflammatory cells, and quantified the degree of inflammatory cell infiltration. This analysis showed that the infiltration by Mac1-positive cells was decreased to 1/3 in the IL-6 receptor antibody treatment group as compared to that in the control group. This result endorses the reported finding that forced expression of IL-6 signals after SCI resulted in an approximately sixfold increase of neutrophil infiltration and twofold increase of macrophage infiltration [12]. Furthermore, the recent study demonstrated that temporal blockade of IL-6 signaling after SCI abrogates damaging inflammatory activity and promotes functional recovery by promoting the formation of alternatively activated M2 macrophages [16, 17]. In mice with SCI, connective tissue scars are formed, in contrast to the softening and void formation observed in the spinal cord tissue of rats and other animals. It has been shown that the size of such connective tissue scars is related to the severity of the SCI [13]. In our study also, the size of the connective tissue scars was quantified and compared between the control group and the IL-6 receptor antibody treatment group; the comparison revealed a significantly decreased size of the scars at the center of the injured spinal cord in the antibody-treated group. These results suggest that blocking of the IL-6 signals can suppress inflammatory reactions and secondary injury, thus attenuating injury of intact tissue.

On the basis of these findings, we examined the effects of IL-6 receptor antibody treatment on the functional recovery after SCI. The IL-6 receptor antibody treatment group showed significantly better recovery than the control group in terms of three different motor functions (spontaneous leg exercise, vertical standing, and continued exercise on a rotating rod). The possible reasons for this difference are: (1) suppression of glial scar formation suppressed the expression of axonal growth inhibitory factors present in the glial scars leading to stimulation of axonal regeneration, and (2) reduction of secondary damage allowed more intact cells to be protected from injury. Another possible mechanism is that suppression of the differentiation of neural stem cells into astrocytes leads to a relative increase in the efficiency of differentiation of these cells into neurons.

2.4 For Clinical Application

The relationship between IL-6 and SCI has been discussed above. IL-6 is a cytokine with diverse physiological activities. It is extensively involved in various phenomena occurring in vivo, including inflammation, immunity, and regulation of cell differentiation [7]. IL-6 was first identified as a factor involved in the differentiation of B cells into antibody-producing cells. Later, it was revealed that IL-6 is also involved in the differentiation and proliferation of not only B cells, T cells, and monocytes but also fibroblasts, osteoclasts, hematopoietic stem cells, and neural stem cells. It has also been shown that excessive IL-6 expression is involved in many diseases, such as rheumatoid arthritis, Crohn's disease, and Castleman's disease. A human-type monoclonal antibody to the IL-6 receptor has been developed jointly by Osaka University and Chugai Pharmaceutical Co. Ltd., for use in the treatment of rheumatoid arthritis. This antibody has exhibited excellent therapeutic efficacy in clinical trials [18]. This human-type monoclonal antibody (MRA, Atlizumab) has a potent inhibitory activity against IL-6 signals. Its safety profile and pharmacokinetic characteristics, such as its metabolism, distribution, and tolerance, have been evaluated in depth and already introduced clinically. This antibody is thus very close to the stage of clinical application for SCI.

The half-life of this human-type antibody in vivo is relatively short (about 7 days). This feature is ideal when considering the expression of IL-6 in cases of SCI. As illustrated above, IL-6 exerts both neurotrophic and neurotoxic effects, and it has been shown to protect nerve cells in vitro [19]. Considering the report that IL-6 treatment reduced the size of the cerebral infarct in cases of brain ischemia [20], it seems likely that IL-6 exerts variable activities depending on the condition, degree of IL-6 signal expression, and the timing of its administration. When excessive IL-6 was expressed after SCI, the activity of this cytokine as an inflammatory cytokine was much greater than its neurotrophic activity, leading to an increase in the area of injury and marked suppression of axonal regeneration [11]. This indicates that excessive IL-6 signals are neurotoxic, at least in the acute stages of SCI. However, we cannot rule out the possibility that it serves as a neurotrophic (neuroprotective) factor in the subacute to chronic stages of SCI. The IL-6 receptor antibody with a short half-life in vivo may be expected to block only the neurotoxic IL-6 signals in the acute stages of SCI and not to inhibit the neuroprotective signals during the subsequent phases of SCI. Therefore, this antibody offers promise as a means for suppressing the expression of neurotoxic IL-6 signals alone in cases of SCI.

2.5 Conclusions

Although various methods of treating central nervous system injury have been studied, no method for radical treatment of central nervous system injury has yet been established. Neural stem cells are receiving close attention as a tool for reconstruction of the injured neuronal network. However, there are many unresolved questions concerning the mechanism of regulation of their differentiation and functional recovery in cases of SCI. These issues need to be studied in further detail from various viewpoints. The IL-6 receptor antibody has been shown to modify the microenvironment around the injured spinal cord by alleviating the post-injury tissue destruction or secondary damage and glial scar formation. To achieve reconstruction of the injured neural network, the most practical method may be the combined use of such an environment-modifying factor and cell transplantation [3, 21–23]. We believe that an accumulation of basic studies in this field would allow regeneration and reconstruction of the spinal cord after injury in the near future.

Conflict of Interest The author declares that he has no conflict of interest.

References

1. Hugenholtz H (2003) Methylprednisolone for acute spinal cord injury: not a standard of care. Can Med Assoc J 168:1145–1146
2. Reynolds BA, Tetzlaff W, Weiss S (1992) A multipotent EGF-responsive striatal embryonic progenitor cell produces neurons and astrocytes. J Neurosci 12:4565–4574
3. Okano H (2002) The stem cell biology of the central nervous system. J Neurosci Res 69:698–707
4. Johansson CB, Momma S, Clarke DL et al (1999) Identification of a neural stem cell in the adult mammalian central nervous system. Cell 96:25–34
5. Bradbury EJ, Moon LD, Popat RJ et al (2002) Chondroitinase ABC promotes functional recovery after spinal cord injury. Nature 416:636–640
6. Nakamura M, Houghtling RA, MacArthur L, Bayer BM, Bregman BS (2003) Differences in cytokine gene expression profile between acute and secondary injury in adult rat spinal cord. Exp Neurol 184:313–325
7. Taga T, Kishimoto T (1997) Gp130 and the interleukin-6 family of cytokines. Annu Rev Immunol 15:797–819
8. Okada S, Nakamura M, Mikami Y et al (2004) Blockade of interleukin-6 receptor suppresses reactive astrogliosis and ameliorates functional recovery in experimental spinal cord injury. J Neurosci Res 76:265–276
9. Bonni A, Sun Y, Nadal-Vicens M et al (1997) Regulation of gliogenesis in the central nervous system by the JAK-STAT signaling pathway. Science 278:477–483

10. Klein MA, Moller JC, Jones LL et al (1997) Impaired neuroglial activation in interleukin-6 deficient mice. Glia 19:227–233
11. Brunello AG, Weissenberger J, Kappeler A et al (2000) Astrocytic alterations in interleukin-6/ Soluble interleukin-6 receptor alpha double-transgenic mice. Am J Pathol 157:1485–1493
12. Lacroix S, Chang L, Rose-John S, Tuszynski MH (2002) Delivery of hyper-interleukin-6 to the injured spinal cord increases neutrophil and macrophage infiltration and inhibits axonal growth. J Comp Neurol 454:213–228
13. Ma M, Basso DM, Walters P, Stokes BT, Jakeman LB (2001) Behavioral and histological outcomes following graded spinal cord contusion injury in the C57Bl/6 mouse. Exp Neurol 169:239–254
14. Dumont AS, Dumont RJ, Oskouian RJ (2002) Will improved understanding of the pathophysiological mechanisms involved in acute spinal cord injury improve the potential for therapeutic intervention? Curr Opin Neurol 15:713–720
15. Popovich PG, Jones TB (2003) Manipulating neuroinflammatory reactions in the injured spinal cord: back to basics. Trends Pharmacol Sci 24:13–17
16. Mukaino M, Nakamura M, Yamada O et al (2010) Anti-IL-6-receptor antibody promotes repair of spinal cord injury by inducing microglia-dominant inflammation. Exp Neurol 224: 403–414
17. Guerrero AR, Uchida K, Nakajima H et al (2012) Blockade of interleukin-6 signaling inhibits the classic pathway and promotes an alternative pathway of macrophage activation after spinal cord injury in mice. J Neuroinflammation 9:40
18. Choy EH, Isenberg DA, Garrood T et al (2002) Therapeutic benefit of blocking interleukin-6 activity with an anti-interleukin-6 receptor monoclonal antibody in rheumatoid arthritis: a randomized, double-blind, placebo-controlled, dose- escalation trial. Arthritis Rheum 46:3143–3150
19. Marz P, Cheng JG, Gadient RA et al (1998) Sympathetic neurons can produce and respond to interleukin 6. Proc Natl Acad Sci USA 95:3251–3256
20. Loddick SA, Turnbull AV, Rothwell NJ (1998) Cerebral interleukin-6 is neuroprotective during permanent focal cerebral ischemia in the rat. J Cereb Blood Flow Metab 18:176–179
21. Okano H, Ogawa Y, Nakamura M et al (2003) Transplantation of neural stem cells into the spinal cord after injury. Semin Cell Dev Biol 14:191–198
22. Okano H, Nakamura M, Yoshida K et al (2013) Steps toward safe cell therapy using induced pluripotent stem cells. Circ Res 112(3):523–533
23. Nakamura M, Okano H (2013) Cell transplantation therapies for spinal cord injury focusing on induced pluripotent stem cells. Cell Res 23(1):70–80

Chapter 3
Autophagy in Spinal Cord Injury: Pathogenic Roles and Therapeutic Implications

Autophagy in Spinal Cord Injury

Haruo Kanno and Hiroshi Ozawa

Abstract Autophagy is degradation of intracellular proteins and organelles to maintain cytoplasmic homeostasis, and it is also involved in various pathophysiological processes in many diseases. We previously investigated alternation of autophagic activity in damaged neural tissue after SCI. It was also examined whether administration of rapamycin to promote autophagy can induce neuroprotective effect in SCI. Our results of these studies demonstrated that molecular markers of autophagy such as Beclin 1 and LC3 were significantly upregulated in the injured spinal cord. The increased activity of autophagy was observed in neurons, astrocytes, and oligodendrocytes at the lesion site. Electron microscopy showed an increased formation of autophagic vacuoles in the damaged neural cells. In addition, the rapamycin administration in acute phase of SCI promoted autophagy in the injured spinal cord and reduced neural tissue damage and locomotor impairment. These findings indicated that autophagic activity is increased in damaged neural tissue after SCI. Furthermore the promotion of autophagy by rapamycin treatment can provide neuroprotective effect to improve locomotor function following SCI. Here, we summarize our previous studies and review the evidence in related articles regarding the role of autophagy in SCI.

Keywords Autophagy • Beclin 1 • LC3 • Rapamycin • Spinal cord injury

H. Kanno (✉) • H. Ozawa
Department of Orthopaedic Surgery, Tohoku University School of Medicine, 1-1 Seiryo-machi, Aoba-ku, Sendai 980-8574, Japan
e-mail: kanno-h@isis.ocn.ne.jp

K. Uchida et al. (eds.), *Neuroprotection and Regeneration of the Spinal Cord*,
DOI 10.1007/978-4-431-54502-6_3,

3.1 Introduction

Autophagy is degradation of intracellular proteins and organelles to maintain cytoplasmic homeostasis, and it is also involved in various pathophysiological processes in many diseases [1–4]. Autophagy works for the elimination and recycling of long-lived proteins and unwanted organelles in a cell during development and under stress conditions [1, 5, 6] (Fig. 3.1). Amino acid starvation is a well-known trigger for autophagy, which degrades proteins to free amino acids that help cell survival [2].

Previous studies suggested that autophagy has a cytoprotective function against cell death [7, 8]. Autophagy contributed to cytoprotection in neurodegenerative disease and traumatic brain injury [9–13]. On the contrary, previous studies suggested that autophagy also contributes to the induction of cell death [8, 14, 15]. Autophagy can lead to nonapoptotic programmed cell death, which is called autophagic cell death [3, 16]. Activation of autophagy can induce cell death in a myocardial ischemia and reperfusion model [17]. In addition, autophagy can lead to autophagic cell death in cerebral ischemia and in a renal ischemia and reperfusion injury [18, 19].

Beclin 1, a Bcl-2-interacting protein, is a mammalian ortholog of yeast Atg6/Vps30 and it is known to be a promoter of autophagy [20]. Beclin 1 is a component of the class III phosphatidylinositol-3-kinase (PI3K) complex that works for the formation of autophagosomes [21]. The Atg8 protein, known as microtubule-associated protein 1 light chain 3 (LC3), is essential for autophagy [22]. LC3 is bound to autophagosomal membrane and thus is considered a specific marker protein to monitor autophagy [23] (Fig. 3.1). Autophagy may be dysregulated in several disorders, including metabolic diseases, neurodegenerative disorders, infectious diseases, and cancer. Pharmacological approaches to upregulate or inhibit this pathway are currently receiving considerable attention [24]. The mammalian target of rapamycin (mTOR) signaling pathway is known as a main molecular mechanism to

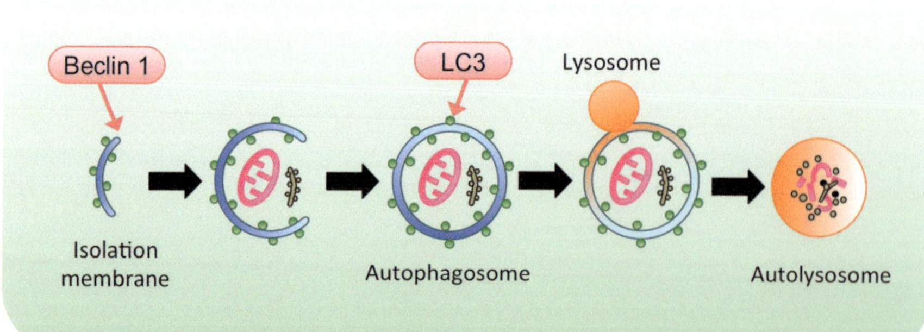

Fig. 3.1 Process of autophagy. A small volume of cytoplasm is enclosed by the isolation membrane, which results in the formation of an autophagosome. The autophagosome fuses with the lysosome where the cytoplasm is degraded. LC3 is bound to the autophagosomal membrane

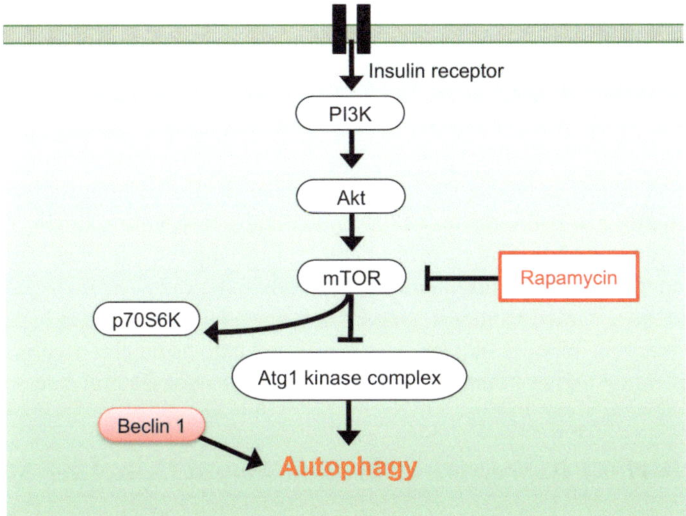

Fig. 3.2 Signaling pathway of autophagy regulation. mTOR pathway negatively regulates autophagy. Rapamycin, a specific inhibitor of mTOR, prevents phosphorylation of p70S6K and promotes autophagy. Beclin 1 protein promotes autophagy

regulate autophagic activity (Fig. 3.2). Recent studies revealed modulation of autophagy via mTOR signaling can be a therapeutic target for various diseases [24].

We previously reported that autophagic activity was upregulated in damaged neural tissue after SCI [25–27]. Furthermore our study demonstrated that pharmacological enhancement of autophagy provided neuroprotective effect following SCI [28, 29]. Here, we summarize our previous studies and review the evidence in related articles regarding the role of autophagy in SCI.

3.2 Upregulation of Beclin 1 Expression After Spinal Cord Injury

3.2.1 Summary

Beclin 1, a Bcl-2-interacting protein, is known to be a promoter of autophagy. We previously investigated the alterations in the Beclin 1 protein expression and the involvement of autophagy after SCI using a spinal cord hemisection model in mice [25]. In our results of immunohistochemistry and Western blot analysis, the Beclin 1 expression significantly increased at the lesion site after hemisection. The Beclin 1 expression was observed in neurons, astrocytes, and oligodendrocytes. These results suggested that autophagy can be activated in the injured spinal cord.

3.2.2 Increased Expression of Beclin 1 After SCI

To investigate an alteration of the Beclin 1 expression in the spinal cord, immunohistochemical staining of Beclin 1 was performed at 4 and 24 h and 3, 7, and 21 days after hemisection. The cells expressing Beclin 1 were increased in the injured side after hemisection (Fig. 3.3a). The cells expressing Beclin 1 were observed in both the gray matter and white matter of the injured side. In counting Beclin 1-positive cells, the number of Beclin 1-positive cells on the injured side was significantly higher than those on the contralateral side at each time point. The increased expression of Beclin 1 started from 4 h, peaked at 3 days, and lasted for at least 21 days after hemisection. Western blot analysis confirmed that the level of Beclin 1 protein was significantly higher in the injured side than in the contralateral side.

3.2.3 Beclin 1 Expression in Various Neural Cells After SCI

To investigate the Beclin 1 expression in a specific type of cells including neurons, astrocytes, and oligodendrocytes, the spinal cord sections at 3 days after hemisection were double stained for Beclin 1 and various cell type markers: NeuN for neurons, GFAP for astrocytes, and Olig2 for oligodendrocytes. In the double staining, the expression of Beclin 1 was observed in NeuN-, GFAP-, and Olig2-labeled cells. These results demonstrated the Beclin 1 expression to be observed in neurons, astrocytes, and oligodendrocytes.

3.2.4 Expression of Beclin 1 in Dying Cells

To detect Beclin 1 expression in dying cells, we performed double staining of Beclin 1 and TUNEL in the sections at 3 days after hemisection. The TUNEL-positive cells occasionally showed as Beclin 1 positive. Under higher magnification, most of the nuclei of the TUNEL-positive cells that did not show Beclin 1 positive were shrunken or fragmented, as is typical of apoptotic nuclei. On the other hand, most of the nuclei of the TUNEL-positive cells that were found to be Beclin 1 positive were round, as in autophagic cell death, and they had neither shrunken nor were fragmented.

3.3 Confirmation of Autophagy Induction After Spinal Cord Injury

3.3.1 Summary

To confirm induction of autophagy after SCI, we previously investigated expression of LC3, a characteristic marker of autophagy, in immunohistochemistry and Western blot using an SCI model in mice [26]. Electron microscopic analysis was

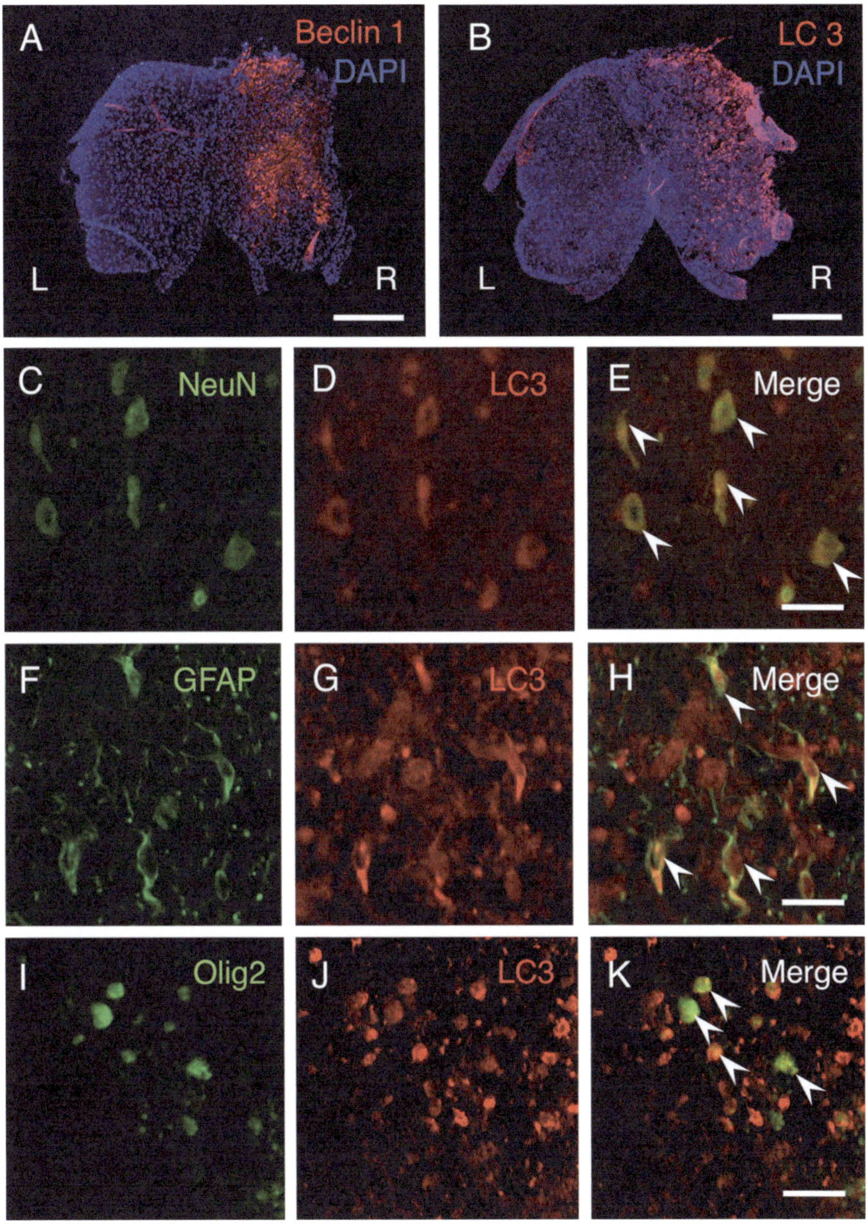

Fig. 3.3 Immunohistochemical staining of Beclin1 and LC3 in transverse sections at 3 days after hemisection. (**a**), (**b**) The cells expressing Beclin1 and LC3 were increased on the injured side (R) in comparison to the contralateral side (L). Scale bars = 500 μm. (**c**)–(**k**) In double staining of LC3 and cell type makers (*green*) on the injured side in transverse section at 3 days after hemisection, the LC3-positive cells were observed in the NeuN-, GFAP-, and Olig2-labeled cells (*arrowheads* in (**e**), (**h**), (**k**)). Scale bars = 50 μm

also performed to examine the formation of autophagy in the injured spinal cord. Immunohistochemistry showed that the number of the LC3-positive cells significantly increased at the lesion site after hemisection. The LC3-positive cells were observed in neurons, astrocytes, and oligodendrocytes. Western blot analysis demonstrated that the level of LC3-II protein expression significantly increased in the injured spinal cord. Electron microscopy showed an increased formation of autophagic vacuoles in the damaged neural cells. This study confirmed both biochemically and anatomically that autophagy was clearly activated in the damaged neural tissue after SCI.

3.3.2 Upregulation of Autophagy Marker, LC3 in Injured Spinal Cord

Immunohistochemical analysis showed that cells expressing LC3 were increased on the injured side in comparison to the contralateral side after hemisection. The cells expressing LC3 were observed in both the gray matter and the white matter of the injured side (Fig. 3.3b). In higher magnification on the injured side, the cells expressing LC3 displayed bright, punctate LC3 dots in the cytoplasm, indicating formation of autophagic vacuoles. The number of LC3-positive cells on the injured side was significantly higher than those on the contralateral side at 3 days. The increase of the LC3-positive cells commenced at 4 h and lasted for at least 21 days. The maximum number of LC3-positive cells on the injured side was observed at 3 days, and it thereafter decreased at 7 days after hemisection. Western blot analysis confirmed the level of LC3-II protein was significantly higher in the injured side than in uninjured spinal cord.

3.3.3 LC3 Expression in Various Neural Cells

Double staining of LC3 and various cell type markers revealed that the LC3-positive cells were observed in NeuN-, GFAP-, and Olig2-labeled cells on the injured side after hemisection (Fig. 3.3c–k).

3.3.4 Electron Microscopic Analysis for Autophagy Formation

Electron microscopic analysis after the hemisection demonstrated that the formations of numerous autophagic vacuoles including autophagosome with double-membrane structures (Fig. 3.1) were observed in the damaged cells on the injured side. A higher magnification showed that the autophagosomes were containing membranous structures and parts of the cytoplasm.

3.3.5 Expression of LC3 in Dying Cells

To confirm autophagy induction in dying cells, we performed double staining of LC3 and TUNEL using the spinal cord section at 3 days after hemisection. The double staining showed that the TUNEL-positive cells were occasionally LC3 positive. Higher magnification revealed that the nuclei of the TUNEL-positive cells that were not LC3 positive were shrunken or fragmented, typical of apoptotic nuclei. On the contrary, the nuclei of the TUNEL-positive cells that were found to be LC3 positive were round, as in autophagic cell death.

3.4 Autophagy Modulation as a Potential Therapeutic Target for Spinal Cord Injury

3.4.1 Summary

The mTOR is a serine/threonine kinase that negatively regulates autophagy (Fig. 3.2). Rapamycin, an inhibitor of mTOR signaling, can promote autophagy and exert neuroprotective effects in several diseases of the central nervous system. We previously investigated whether administration of rapamycin promotes autophagy and reduces neural tissue damage and locomotor impairment after spinal cord contusion injury in mice [28]. Our results demonstrated that the administration of rapamycin at 4 h after injury significantly promoted autophagic activity in the injured spinal cord. In addition, the rapamycin treatment significantly reduced neural tissue damage and locomotor impairment after SCI. These results indicate that rapamycin promoted autophagy by inhibiting the mTOR signaling pathway and induced neuroprotective effect after SCI (Fig. 3.4).

3.4.2 Inhibition of mTOR Promotes Autophagy After Spinal Cord Injury

To examine the effectiveness of the rapamycin treatment on the mTOR signaling pathway, the phosphorylation of p70S6K was evaluated by Western blot analysis. In our results, the phosphorylated p70S6K protein was significantly decreased after administration of rapamycin, indicating rapamycin actually inhibited mTOR after SCI (Fig. 3.4). We also investigated the activation of autophagy after rapamycin treatment, immunohistochemical staining, and Western blot analysis of LC3 were performed. Immunostaining of LC3 showed the number of LC3-positive cells was significantly increased in the rapamycin-treated mice compared with the vehicle-treated mice. In the Western blot analysis, the expression of LC3-II protein was significantly increased in the rapamycin-treated mice compared with the vehicle-treated mice.

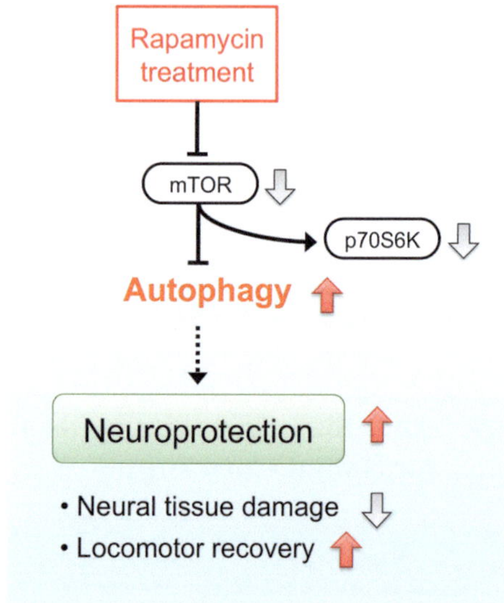

Fig. 3.4 Neuroprotective mechanism of rapamycin treatment in acute SCI. Rapamycin suppresses mTOR signaling pathway and promotes autophagy after SCI. The increased autophagic activity can produce neuroprotective effect and reduce neural tissue damage and locomotor impairment following SCI

3.4.3 Inhibition of mTOR Produces Neuroprotective Effect in Injured Spinal Cord

To investigate neural cell loss after injury, the number of NeuN-positive cells was compared between the vehicle and the rapamycin-treated mice by immunohistochemical staining. In our results, the number of NeuN-positive cells in the rapamycin-treated mice was significantly higher than those in the vehicle-treated mice at 42 days. Additionally, to investigate the effect of rapamycin on cell death after SCI, we performed TUNEL staining and compared the number of TUNEL-positive cells between the vehicle- and the rapamycin-treated mice at 3 days after injury. The number of TUNEL-positive cells was significantly lower in the rapamycin-treated mice compared to the vehicle-treated mice. These results indicated that rapamycin treatment can produce neuroprotective effect to reduce neuronal loss and cell death following SCI.

3.4.4 Inhibition of mTOR Improves Locomotor Recovery After Spinal Cord Injury

To evaluate the effect of rapamycin treatment on locomotor recovery after SCI, Basso mouse scale (BMS) was measured for 6 weeks [30]. In our result, the rapamycin-treated mice had significantly higher BMS scores than the vehicle-treated mice from 3 to 6 weeks. This data supports the neuroprotection produced by mTOR inhibition can improve locomotor function after SCI.

3.5 Discussion

3.5.1 Upregulation of Autophagy in CNS Injury

Previous studies demonstrated the expression of Beclin 1 to increase at lesion sites after traumatic brain injury and cerebral ischemia [9, 18, 31]. In such diseases, expression of LC3 increases at the lesion sites [18, 32–35]. These reports suggest that the autophagic activity increases in response to the neural tissue damage of the brain. Our previous studies first reported the increased expression of Beclin 1 and LC3 in the damaged neural tissue after SCI [25, 26]. Using electron microscopy, we also confirmed that the formation of autophagic vacuoles also increased in the damaged cells of the injured spinal cord [26]. Therefore, autophagy was activated in the damaged neural tissue after SCI.

3.5.2 Neuroprotective Function of Autophagy

Many studies reported that autophagy has a cytoprotective function against cell death. Autophagy has a cytoprotective function in neurodegenerative diseases [10–13]. Autophagy induced neuroprotection in traumatic brain injury and in neonatal hypoxia-ischemia induced brain injury [9, 36]. In models of Huntington disease, the stimulation of autophagy protects cells against apoptosis [37]. In addition, the inhibition of autophagy increases the apoptosis of neurons and also causes neurodegeneration in mice [10, 11]. One potential mechanism underlying these neuroprotective effects is the blocking of apoptosis by the activation of autophagy [12, 36, 38]. Interestingly, it has been suggested that mTOR inhibition enhances the clearance of mitochondria by inducing autophagy, thereby reducing cytosolic cytochrome c release and downstream caspase activation [24, 39]. Previous studies have demonstrated that inhibition of mTOR upregulates autophagy and shows cytoprotective functions by reducing apoptosis in various disease models, including the myocardial ischemia-reperfusion model [38] and neonatal hypoxia-ischemia-induced brain injury model [36]. In our results, rapamycin promoted autophagy by inhibiting the mTOR signaling and reduced neural tissue damage such as neuronal loss and cell death following SCI. These results suggested autophagy produced neuroprotective effect after SCI.

3.5.3 Autophagy Modulation as a Therapeutic Target for SCI

Autophagy may be dysregulated in various disorders, including metabolic diseases, neurodegenerative disorders, infectious diseases, and cancer. In several conditions, autophagy is inhibited and this can occur at different stages of the process to enhance disease, whereas in other cases autophagic activity may be permissive towards pathogenesis [24]. Recently, pharmacological approaches to upregulate or inhibit autophagy are receiving considerable attention. For example, autophagy upregulation may be of therapeutic benefit in certain neurodegenerative diseases and trauma [9, 36, 39]. Indeed, our study demonstrated that upregulation autophagy by mTOR inhibitor, rapamycin, resulted in reduction of neural tissue damage and locomotor impairment after SCI [28]. Therefore, the pharmacological modulation of autophagy may have clinical benefits for treatment of patients with SCI. Further studies to clarify the neuroprotective and neuroregenerative mechanisms regulated by autophagy are needed in order to approve the clinical use of pharmacological modulation of autophagy for patients with acute SCI.

3.5.4 Autophagic Cell Death

The autophagic process can lead to nonapoptotic programmed cell death, which is known as autophagic cell death [8]. Autophagic cell death is morphologically distinct from necrotic cell death and apoptotic cell death [14, 16]. The nucleus is shrunken and fragmented in apoptosis, but in autophagic cell death, the nucleus does not change [14, 18, 31]. Previous studies have shown autophagic cell death to be induced after brain trauma and cerebral ischemia and contributed to neural tissue damage [31, 33]. Our studies demonstrated that most of the nuclei in the TUNEL-positive cells expressed Beclin 1 or LC3 were round, which should normally be observed in autophagic cell death, and they were not either shrunken or fragmented as is observed in apoptotic nuclei [26, 40]. Therefore, these findings suggested autophagic cell death may occur in the injured spinal cord. However, the molecular mechanism defining the features of autophagic cell death is still unknown [8, 41, 42]. Further studies are needed to clarify the molecular mechanism of autophagic cell death in SCI.

3.6 Conclusion

Our previous studies demonstrated that molecular markers of autophagy such as Beclin 1 and LC3 were significantly upregulated in the injured spinal cord. The increased activity of autophagy was observed in neurons, astrocytes, and oligodendrocytes at the lesion site. Electron microscopy showed an increased formation of autophagic vacuoles in the damaged neural cells. In addition, the rapamycin administration in acute phase of SCI promoted autophagy in the injured spinal cord and reduced neural tissue damage and locomotor impairment. These findings indicated that autophagic activity is increased in damaged neural tissue after SCI. Furthermore the promotion of autophagy by rapamycin treatment can provide neuroprotective effect to improve locomotor function following SCI.

Conflict of Interest The authors declare that they have no conflict of interest.

References

1. Gozuacik D, Kimchi A (2004) Autophagy as a cell death and tumor suppressor mechanism. Oncogene 23:2891–2906
2. Klionsky D, Emr S (2000) Autophagy as a regulated pathway of cellular degradation. Science 290:1717–1721
3. Larsen K, Sulzer D (2002) Autophagy in neurons: a review. Histol Histopathol 17:897–908
4. Ogier-Denis E, Codogno P (2003) Autophagy: a barrier or an adaptive response to cancer. Biochim Biophys Acta 1603:113–128
5. Levine B, Klionsky D (2004) Development by self-digestion: molecular mechanisms and biological functions of autophagy. Dev Cell 6:463–477
6. Mele´ndez A, Tallo´czy Z, Seaman M et al (2003) Autophagy genes are essential for dauer development and life-span extension in *C. elegans*. Science 301:1387–1391
7. Rubinsztein DC, DiFiglia M, Heintz N et al (2005) Autophagy and its possible roles in nervous system diseases, damage and repair. Autophagy 1(1):11–22. doi:1513[pii]
8. Tsujimoto Y, Shimizu S (2005) Another way to die: autophagic programmed cell death. Cell Death Differ 12(Suppl 2):1528–1534. doi:10.1038/sj.cdd.4401777
9. Erlich S, Alexandrovich A, Shohami E et al (2007) Rapamycin is a neuroprotective treatment for traumatic brain injury. Neurobiol Dis 26:86–93
10. Hara T, Nakamura K, Matsui M et al (2006) Suppression of basal autophagy in neural cells causes neurodegenerative disease in mice. Nature 441(7095):885–889. doi:nature04724 [pii], 10.1038/nature04724
11. Komatsu M, Waguri S, Chiba T et al (2006) Loss of autophagy in the central nervous system causes neurodegeneration in mice. Nature 441(7095):880–884. doi:10.1038/nature04723
12. Pan T, Kondo S, Zhu W et al (2008) Neuroprotection of rapamycin in lactacystin-induced neurodegeneration via autophagy enhancement. Neurobiol Dis 32:16–25
13. Sarkar S, Ravikumar B, Floto RA et al (2009) Rapamycin and mTOR-independent autophagy inducers ameliorate toxicity of polyglutamine-expanded huntingtin and related proteinopathies. Cell Death Differ 16(1):46–56. doi:10.1038/cdd.2008.110
14. Kitanaka C, Kuchino Y (1999) Caspase-independent programmed cell death with necrotic morphology. Cell Death Differ 6(6):508–515. doi:10.1038/sj.cdd.4400526
15. Scarlatti F, Granata R, Meijer AJ et al (2009) Does autophagy have a license to kill mammalian cells? Cell Death Differ 16(1):12–20. doi:cdd2008101 [pii], 10.1038/cdd.2008.101
16. Clarke PG (1990) Developmental cell death: morphological diversity and multiple mechanisms. Anat Embryol 181(3):195–213
17. Matsui Y, Takagi H, Qu X et al (2007) Distinct roles of autophagy in the heart during ischemia and reperfusion: roles of AMP-activated protein kinase and Beclin 1 in mediating autophagy. Circ Res 100(6):914–922. doi:10.1161/01.RES.0000261924.76669.36
18. Rami A, Langhagen A, Steiger S (2008) Focal cerebral ischemia induces upregulation of Beclin 1 and autophagy-like cell death. Neurobiol Dis 29:132–141
19. Suzuki C, Isaka Y, Takabatake Y et al (2008) Participation of autophagy in renal ischemia/reperfusion injury. Biochem Biophys Res Commun 368(1):100–106. doi:10.1016/j.bbrc.2008.01.059
20. Liang XH, Jackson S, Seaman M et al (1999) Induction of autophagy and inhibition of tumorigenesis by Beclin 1. Nature 402(6762):672–676. doi:10.1038/45257
21. Kihara A, Kabeya Y, Ohsumi Y et al (2001) Beclin-phosphatidylinositol 3-kinase complex functions at the trans-Golgi network. EMBO Rep 2(4):330–335. doi:10.1093/embo-reports/kve061
22. Mizushima N (2004) Methods for monitoring autophagy. Int J Biochem Cell Biol 36:2491–2502
23. Kabeya Y, Mizushima N, Ueno T et al (2000) LC3, a mammalian homologue of yeast Apg8p, is localized in autophagosome membranes after processing. EMBO J 19:5720–5728
24. Rubinsztein DC, Codogno P, Levine B (2012) Autophagy modulation as a potential therapeutic target for diverse diseases. Nat Rev Drug Discov 11(9):709–730. doi:10.1038/nrd3802

25. Kanno H, Ozawa H, Sekiguchi A et al (2009) Spinal cord injury induces upregulation of Beclin 1 and promotes autophagic cell death. Neurobiol Dis 33:143–148
26. Kanno H, Ozawa H, Sekiguchi A et al (2011) Induction of autophagy and autophagic cell death in damaged neural tissue after acute spinal cord injury in mice. Spine (Phila Pa 1976) 36(22):E1427–E1434. doi:10.1097/BRS.0b013e3182028c3a
27. Kanno H, Ozawa H, Sekiguchi A et al (2009) The role of autophagy in spinal cord injury. Autophagy 5(3):390–392. doi:7724 [pii]
28. Sekiguchi A, Kanno H, Ozawa H et al (2012) Rapamycin promotes autophagy and reduces neural tissue damage and locomotor impairment after spinal cord injury in mice. J Neurotrauma 29(5):946–956. doi:10.1089/neu.2011.1919
29. Kanno H, Ozawa H, Sekiguchi A et al (2012) The role of mTOR signaling pathway in spinal cord injury. Cell Cycle 11(17):3175–3179. doi:10.4161/cc.21262
30. Basso DM, Fisher LC, Anderson AJ et al (2006) Basso Mouse Scale for locomotion detects differences in recovery after spinal cord injury in five common mouse strains. J Neurotrauma 23(5):635–659. doi:10.1089/neu.2006.23.635
31. Diskin T, Tal-Or P, Erlich S et al (2005) Closed head injury induces upregulation of Beclin 1 at the cortical site of injury. J Neurotrauma 22:750–762
32. Liu CL, Chen S, Dietrich D et al (2008) Changes in autophagy after traumatic brain injury. J Cereb Blood Flow Metab (Official J Int Soc Cereb Blood Flow Metab) 28(4):674–683. doi:10.1038/sj.jcbfm.9600587
33. Adhami F, Liao G, Morozov YM et al (2006) Cerebral ischemia-hypoxia induces intravascular coagulation and autophagy. Am J Pathol 169(2):566–583. doi:10.2353/ajpath.2006.051066
34. Uchiyama Y, Koike M, Shibata M (2008) Autophagic neuron death in neonatal brain ischemia/hypoxia. Autophagy 4(4):404–408
35. Wen YD, Sheng R, Zhang LS et al (2008) Neuronal injury in rat model of permanent focal cerebral ischemia is associated with activation of autophagic and lysosomal pathways. Autophagy 4(6):762–769
36. Carloni S, Buonocore G, Balduini W (2008) Protective role of autophagy in neonatal hypoxia-ischemia induced brain injury. Neurobiol Dis 32:329–339
37. Ravikumar B, Vacher C, Berger Z et al (2004) Inhibition of mTOR induces autophagy and reduces toxicity of polyglutamine expansions in fly and mouse models of Huntington disease. Nat Genet 36:585–595
38. Khan S, Salloum F, Das A et al (2006) Rapamycin confers preconditioning-like protection against ischemia-reperfusion injury in isolated mouse heart and cardiomyocytes. J Mol Cell Cardiol 41:256–264
39. Ravikumar B, Berger Z, Vacher C et al (2006) Rapamycin pre-treatment protects against apoptosis. Hum Mol Genet 15:1209–1216
40. Kanno H, Ozawa H, Sekiguchi A et al (2009) Spinal cord injury induces upregulation of Beclin 1 and promotes autophagic cell death. Neurobiol Dis 33(2):143–148. doi:S0969-9961(08)00217-9 [pii], 10.1016/j.nbd.2008.09.009
41. Kroemer G, Levine B (2008) Autophagic cell death: the story of a misnomer. Nat Rev Mol Cell Biol 9(12):1004–1010. doi:10.1038/nrm2529
42. Galluzzi L, Vitale I, Abrams JM et al (2012) Molecular definitions of cell death subroutines: recommendations of the Nomenclature Committee on Cell Death 2012. Cell Death Differ 19(1):107–120. doi:10.1038/cdd.2011.96

Chapter 4
The Role of the Endoplasmic Reticulum Stress Response in Neural Apoptosis of the Injured Spinal Cord

Masahiko Watanabe, Hiroyuki Katoh, Masahiro Kuroiwa, Takeshi Imai, Kaori Suyama, Daisuke Matsuyama, and Joji Mochida

Abstract Following spinal cord injury (SCI), oligodendrocyte progenitor cells (OPCs) that are abundantly present within the adult mammalian central nervous system proliferate around the lesion epicenter. However, most of these cells fail to differentiate into mature oligodendrocytes, hindering their potential for remyelination and functional recovery. One of the major inhibitory factors of OPC differentiation is apoptosis, which also leads to expansion of secondary injury and deterioration of neurological symptoms. There is a growing body of evidence linking the endoplasmic reticulum (ER) stress response to numerous neurodegenerative diseases. To investigate the role of ER stress response in apoptosis following SCI, we examined the in vitro and in vivo changes of ER stress effector proteins under stress conditions. Furthermore, the ER stress response was enhanced by gene transfection in vitro and the administration of amiloride in vivo, and their effect on apoptosis was studied. Amiloride is a Food and Drug Administration (FDA)-approved potassium-sparing diuretic used to treat hypertension, which has been reported to control ER stress and improve several neurological disorders in vivo. The 78 kDa glucose-regulated protein (GRP78), which is an ER chaperon that regulates protein folding in the ER and contributes to cell survival, was upregulated under stress conditions both in vitro and in vivo. However, when the stress became excessive, expression of GRP78 decreased and the expression of the pro-apoptotic factor C/EBP homologous transcription factor protein (CHOP) increased, leading to increased cell apoptosis. Overexpression of GRP78 by gene transfection protected cultured glial cells from ER stress-induced apoptosis. In the injured spinal cord of rats, amiloride treatment significantly reduced cellular apoptosis at the lesion epicenter and reduced the expansion of apoptosis caused by secondary injury.

M. Watanabe (✉) • H. Katoh • M. Kuroiwa • T. Imai • K. Suyama • D. Matsuyama • J. Mochida
Department of Orthopaedic Surgery, Surgical Science, Tokai University School of Medicine, 143 Shimokasuya, Isehara, Kanagawa 259-1193, Japan
e-mail: masahiko@is.icc.u-tokai.ac.jp

K. Uchida et al. (eds.), *Neuroprotection and Regeneration of the Spinal Cord*,
DOI 10.1007/978-4-431-54502-6_4, © Springer Japan 2014

Furthermore, the decrease in ER stress-induced apoptosis increased the number of OPCs in the injured spinal cord and brought about a significant improvement in hind limb function. These studies suggest that amiloride may be an effective treatment to reduce ER stress-induced apoptosis in the acute phase of SCI.

Keywords Apoptosis • Endoplasmic reticulum stress • Oligodendrocyte progenitor cell • Remyelination • Secondary injury

4.1 Introduction

There is an abundant population of oligodendrocyte progenitor cells (OPCs) in the adult mammalian central nervous system that proliferates in response to stress stimulations (e.g., demyelination, trauma). In a chemically induced demyelination model, OPCs proliferate, differentiate into oligodendrocytes, and remyelinate axons [1]. However, in a contusive spinal cord injury (SCI) model, OPCs proliferate but do not differentiate or remyelinate [2, 3]. Numerous factors direct the differentiation of OPCs, such as transcription factor Nkx2.2, which we previously demonstrated in a chemically induced demyelination model [4]. One of the major inhibitory factors of OPC differentiation and remyelination is apoptosis, because the majority of proliferated OPCs succumb to apoptosis. Recent reports focused on the endoplasmic reticulum (ER) stress response as one of the pathways that lead to delayed neural cell death in Alzheimer's disease and Parkinson's disease. Stress causes the misfolding of proteins in the ER, and their accumulation induces the synthesis of GRP 78, which eliminates unfolded proteins and maintains ER homeostasis. However, this unfolded protein response has its limitations; when the accumulation of unfolded proteins exceeds the processing capacity of GRP78, apoptosis is induced through caspase 12, Jun kinase, and CHOP [5]. In order to elucidate the involvement of the ER stress response in apoptosis after SCI, we examined the changes of GRP78 and CHOP under stress conditions in vitro and in vivo, especially focusing on OPC differentiation and expansion of secondary injury. We also investigated the effect of enhancing the ER stress response by performing gene transfection in vitro and by administrating the potassium-sparing diuretic amiloride in vivo and studying its effect on apoptosis.

4.2 In Vitro Evaluation of the ER Stress Response in Cultured Cells

The changes in GRP78 expression and apoptosis were investigated after administration of the ER stress inducers tunicamycin, which leads to accumulation of unfolded proteins in the ER, and the excitatory amino acid L-glutamate [6].

4.2.1 *The Response of GRP78 to ER Stress in C6 Glioma Cells*

4.2.1.1 Methods

Rat C6 glioma cells were plated onto 6-cm tissue culture dishes at a density of 2.0×10^6 cells/dish and maintained at 37 °C with 5 % CO_2 and 95 % air. The culture medium consisted of Dulbecco's modified eagle's medium (DMEM), 10 % (v/v) fetal bovine serum (FBS), and 1 % (v/v) penicillin–streptomycin. Cells were cultured for 24 h and then treated with either tunicamycin (3, 6, 12 μg/ml: T-group) or L-glutamate (10 and 40 mM: G-group) for 24, 48, and 72 h. C6 cells treated with tunicamycin or glutamate were washed once with phosphate-buffered saline (PBS) and stained for 15 min with allophycocyanin (APC)-conjugated Annexin V and propidium iodide (PI) according to the manufacturer's instructions. Quantification of apoptotic/necrotic cell death using APC-Annexin V and PI was performed using flow cytometry (FACSAria™ with FACSDiva™ software). In order to detect intracellular cytokines, treated cells were fixed and permeabilized using the IntraStain® reagent kit according to the manufacturer's instructions. For detection of cytoplasmic GRP78, cells were stained with rabbit polyclonal anti-GRP78 and the Alexa 488-conjugated anti-rabbit secondary antibody. Quantification of GRP78 expression under each condition was evaluated using flow cytometry.

4.2.1.2 Results

The number of Annexin V/PI-positive cells significantly increased in the T-group compared with the control in all conditions. The upregulation of GRP 78 was found at 48 and 72 h after treatment with 6 and 12 μg/ml, but not with 3 μg/ml tunicamycin (Fig. 4.1a–c). In the G-group, a significant increase of Annexin V/PI-positive cells was observed at 72 h after 10 mM treatment and at 48 and 72 h after 40 mM treatment, and the upregulation of GRP78 was found at 72 h after 40 mM treatment (Fig. 4.1d, e).

These results showed that the upregulation of GRP78 occurs when stress by tunicamycin and L-glutamate reaches a certain level.

4.2.2 *Overexpression of GRP78 Protects C6 Glioma Cells from ER Stress*

4.2.2.1 Methods

Using the Neon™ transfection system, C6 glioma cell line cells were transfected with a vector designed to induce transfected cells to transiently express green fluorescent protein (GFP) and GRP78. Twenty-four hours after transfection, GFP-positive and GFP-negative cells were sorted by fluorescence-activated cell sorting

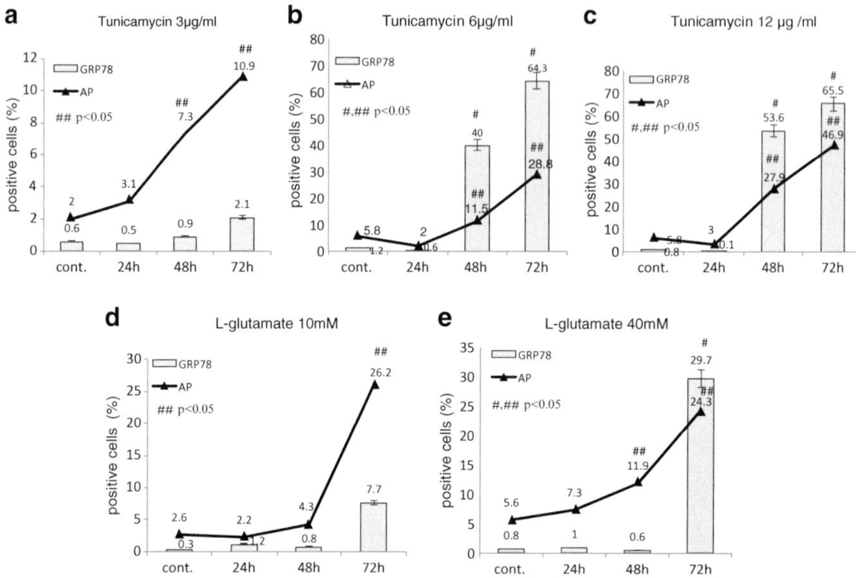

Fig. 4.1 In vitro evaluation of the ER stress response in cultured cells. The percentage of C6 glioma cells positive for GRP78 and Annexin V/PI (AP) after treatment with 24–72 h of the following: (**a**) 3 μg/ml, (**b**) 6 μg/ml, and (**c**) 12 μg/ml tunicamycin, (**d**) 10 mM L-glutamate, and (**e**) 40 mM L-glutamate. The number of AP-positive apoptotic cells increased significantly following treatment with 3, 6, and 12 μg/ml tunicamycin for 48–72 h, 10 mM L-glutamate for 72 h, and 40 mM L-glutamate for 48–72 h compared with control cells ($p<0.05$). The number of GRP78-positive cells increased significantly following treatment with 6 and 12 μg/ml tunicamycin for 48–72 h, and with 40 mM of L-glutamate for 72 h compared with control cells ($p<0.05$)

(FACS). Proteins were extracted from the sorted cells and GRP78 was detected using Immobilon Western Chemiluminescent HRP, which was quantified through densitometric scans of the films. In order to evaluate the cytoprotective characteristic of GFP78, GFP-positive and GFP-negative cells were cultured together and subjected to the same stress conditions as 4.2.1.1 and the number of Annexin V/PI-positive cells was quantified.

4.2.2.2 Results

Twenty-four hours after transfection, 41 % of the cells were positive for GFP. The level of GRP78 in GFP-positive cells was significantly higher than either GFP-negative cells or control cells without gene transfection (Fig. 4.2a). For the cells that received tunicamycin treatment, the number of Annexin V/PI-positive cells was significantly lower in the GFP-positive cells at 72 h after 3 μg/ml treatment and at 24–72 h after 6 and 12 μg/ml treatments when compared with GFP-negative cells (Fig. 4.2b–d). For the cells that received L-glutamate treatment, the number of

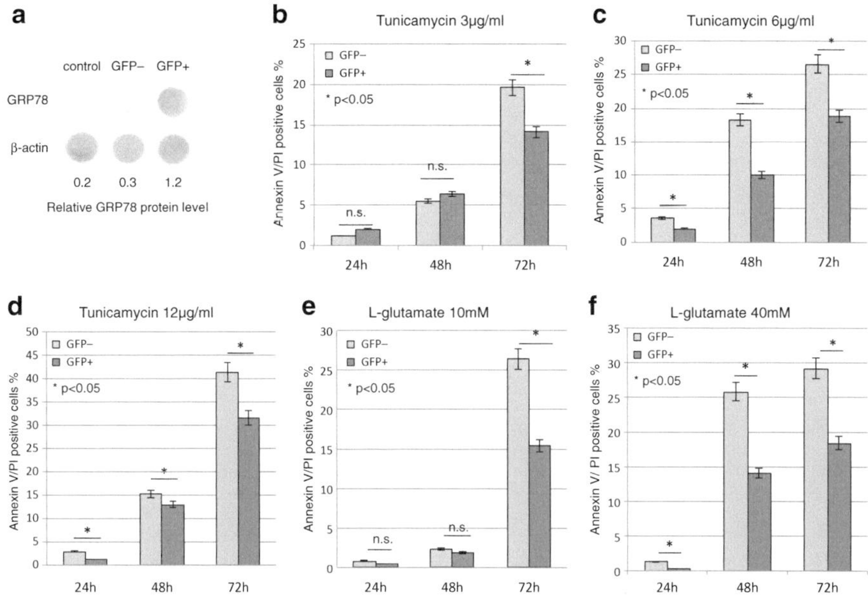

Fig. 4.2 Overexpression of GRP78 protects C6 glioma cells from ER stress. (**a**) Analysis of protein extracts from GFP-positive, GFP-negative, and untransfected control C6 cells confirms the expression of GRP78 in GFP-positive cells ($p<0.05$). (**b**)–(**f**) The percentage of GFP-negative and GFP-positive cells that labeled positive for AP. 24 h after transfection, the cells were treated with 24–72 h of the following: (**b**) 3 μg/ml, (**c**) 6 μg/ml, and (**d**) 12 μg/ml tunicamycin, (**e**) 10 mM L-glutamate, and (**f**) 40 mM L-glutamate. The survival rate of GFP-positive, GRP78-overexpressing cells was significantly higher than the GFP-negative cells following treatments with 3 μg/ml of tunicamycin for 72 h, 6 and 12 μg/ml tunicamycin for 24–72 h, 10 mM L-glutamate for 72 h, and 40 mM L-glutamate for 24–72 h ($p<0.05$)

Annexin V/PI-positive cells was significantly lower in the GFP-positive cells at 72 h after 10 mM treatment and at 24–72 h after 40 mM treatment (Fig. 4.2e, f).

The results show a higher survival rate under stress conditions for GFP-positive cells compared with GFP-negative cells, suggesting that overexpression of GRP78 protects cells from ER stress-induced apoptosis.

4.3 In Vivo Evaluation of the ER Stress Response in the Injured Spinal Cord and the Effect of Amiloride

The ER stress response of each cell type in the injured spinal cord (neurons, astrocytes, oligodendrocytes, and OPCs) was investigated. With the same SCI model, the effect of amiloride against SCI was investigated. Amiloride is a potassium-sparing diuretic used to treat hypertension in the United States that has recently been reported to have neuroprotective effects against multiple neurodegenerative diseases, such as Parkinson's disease and multiple sclerosis.

4.3.1 ER Stress Response in a Rat SCI Model

4.3.1.1 Methods

A moderate contusive SCI was induced in Sprague–Dawley rats using an IH impactor. The sham group received a laminectomy without SCI.

Rats were sacrificed at 1, 3, 5, 7, and 14 days post injury ($n=5$ for each group). Using five adjacent spinal cord sections 8 mm distal from the lesion epicenter, the expression ratio of GRP78 and CHOP was evaluated in neurons, astrocytes, oligodendrocytes, and OPCs using double immunohistochemical staining. Quantitative evaluation of GRP78 and CHOP expression was performed in the anterior horn area for neurons and in the dorsal column white matter for the remaining cell types.

4.3.1.2 Results

Compared with the sham group, significantly higher GRP78 expression was observed in the contused spinal cord at 5 days after injury, followed by a gradual decrease in expression. GRP78 expression was highest in astrocytes and lowest in OPCs. In contrast, CHOP expression within the damaged spinal cord gradually increased over time and showed a significantly higher expression compared with the sham group at 7 days after injury. CHOP expression was significantly higher in OPCs compared to astrocytes at 5, 7, and 14 days after injury. These results showed that the ER response varies according to cell type, with the greatest response in astrocytes and the lowest in OPCs.

4.3.2 Amiloride Reduces Apoptosis and Expansion of Secondary Injury After SCI

A moderate contusive SCI was induced in Sprague–Dawley rats using an IH impactor. Daily intraperitoneal injections of amiloride (10 mg/Kg body weight) or PBS were performed for 28 days ($n=6$ for each group), during which hind limb locomotor function was assessed using the Basso, Beattie, and Bresnahan (BBB) scale. At 3, 7, and 14 days after injury, the rats were anesthetized, and a sample of the injured spinal cord was resected for western blot analysis of GRP 78 and CHOP expression. For histological analysis, the spinal cords were resected from another group of rats, and apoptosis was assessed using the TUNEL assay. Immunostaining for GRP78, NG2 for OPCs, and GFAP for astrocytes was also performed, and the percentages of positive cells in the dorsal funiculus were assessed.

4.3.2.1 Results

BBB scores were significantly higher in the amiloride group after 11 days after injury (Fig. 4.3a). Western blot analyses revealed that GRP78 expression was

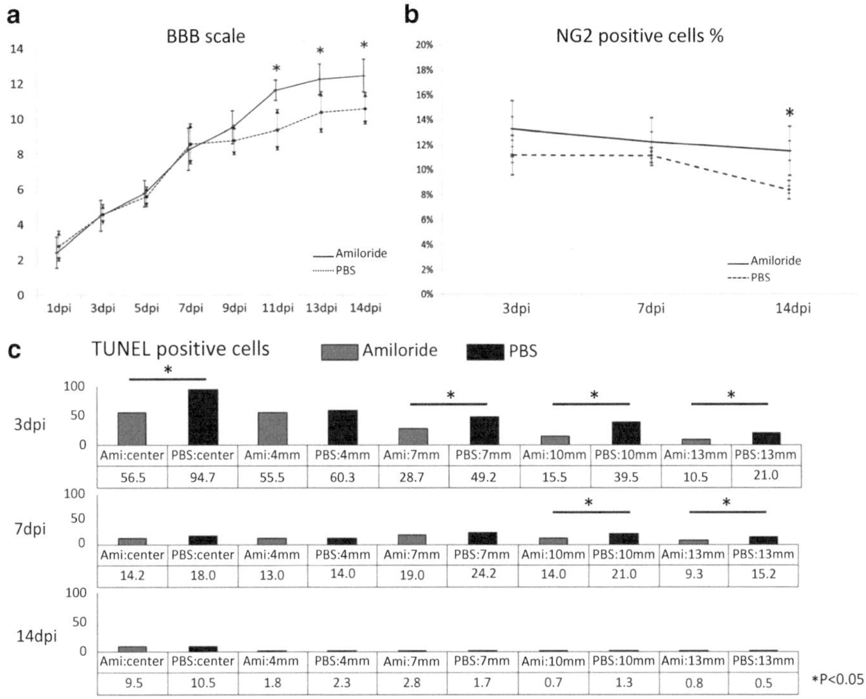

Fig. 4.3 In vivo evaluation of the ER stress response in the injured spinal cord and the effect of amiloride. (**a**) BBB hind limb motor function scores were significantly higher in the amiloride group compared to the PBS group after post injury day 11 ($p<0.05$). (**b**) Although the percentage of NG2-positive cells gradually decreased in both groups, the amiloride group had a significantly higher rate compared to the PBS group on post injury day 14 ($p<0.05$), suggesting that the NG2-positive cells were preferentially spared by amiloride treatment. (**c**) The percentage of TUNEL-positive apoptotic cells was significantly lower on post injury day 3 and the expansion of TUNEL-positive area was significantly reduced in the amiloride group on post injury day 7 ($p<0.05$)

highest at 3 days after injury in both groups but subsequently showed a declining trend. Compared with the PBS group, GRP78 expression was significantly higher at 3 days after injury, while CHOP expression was significantly lower at 7 days after injury in the amiloride group. A decrease in apoptosis was observed in the amiloride group, with significantly fewer TUNEL-positive cells at 3 days after injury and significantly smaller TUNEL-positive area at 7 days after injury (Fig. 4.3b). Quantification of all cell types in the dorsal funiculus revealed that the ratio of NG2-positive OPCs gradually decreased over time in both groups with higher values in the amiloride group at all time points. In particular, at 14 days after injury, the ratio of OPCs was significantly higher in the amiloride group (Fig. 4.3c). In contrast, while the ratio of GFAP-positive astrocytes gradually increased, there was no significant difference observed between the two groups. These results indicate that amiloride treatment reduces apoptosis and expansion of secondary injury after SCI, leading to improved survival of OPCs.

4.4 Discussion

The severity of neural damage resulting from SCI depends on the combination of the initial mechanical damage and the subsequent secondary damage caused by a self-destructive mechanism, which enlarges the damaged area. During this process, the damage which begins predominantly in the gray matter expands to the white matter, and the segmental palsy deteriorates to a transverse palsy [7]. Since the primary pathology of white matter injury is the destruction of myelin sheaths of the long tracts, remyelination has the potential to restore long-tract function, making it extremely important in the functional prognosis of an SCI patient. Although stem cells, including neural stem cells, exist in the adult mammalian central nervous system, their numbers are severely limited. On the other hand, OPCs that have the capacity to differentiate into mature oligodendrocytes are abundantly present in the adult mammalian brain and spinal cord. We previously reported on the proliferation and differentiation of OPCs and the subsequent remyelination observed in a chemically induced demyelination model of the adult rat spinal cord [1]. The remyelination and recovery of neurological deficits often seen in the initial stages of multiple sclerosis is believed to arise from a similar process. However, in a contusive SCI, OPCs proliferate but often do not differentiate into oligodendrocytes [2, 3]. There are a number of factors that direct the differentiation of OPCs [8], such as the transcription factor Nkx2.2, which we demonstrated in the chemically induced demyelination model [4]. When we investigated the expression levels of Nkx2.2 in a contusive SCI model, we found that Nkx2.2 is also upregulated, but to a much smaller degree when compared to the chemically induced demyelination model [9]. Although there may be other factors that need to be studied, the fact that a majority of the proliferated OPCs succumb to apoptosis indicates that apoptosis is a major inhibitory factor of OPC differentiation and remyelination. There are three major pathways that bring about apoptosis to cells of the central nervous system: the extrinsic pathway via Fas ligand, the intrinsic pathway via mitochondrial failure, and the ER stress pathway that has been shown to cause delayed neural cell death. The traumatic stress generated by SCI causes structurally abnormal unfolded proteins to accumulate in the ER, triggering the ER stress pathway that leads to cellular apoptosis.

The accumulation of unfolded proteins in the ER induces the dissociation of the ER chaperone GRP78 from three ER transmembrane effector proteins: activating transcription factor 6 (ATF6), inositol requiring kinase 1 (IRE1), and RNA-activated protein kinase-like ER resident kinase (PERK) [10–13]. GRP78 facilitates the refolding of unfolded proteins and exhibits cytoprotective effects against ER stress. Activated ATF6 is proteolytically cleaved at the Golgi apparatus and promotes transcription of ER chaperones at the nucleus [14]. Activated IRE1 promotes the transcription of ER chaperones by splicing X-box binding protein 1 (XBP1) mRNA to induce XBP1 protein synthesis [12, 15]. PERK inhibits protein synthesis via phosphorylation of the α-subunit of eukaryotic initiation factor-2 (eIF2α) [15, 16]. Activated eIF2α induces the translation of activating transcription factor 4 (ATF4), which promotes GRP78 gene transcription and concurrently induces the expression of CHOP, a pro-apoptotic transcription factor that is a crucial mediator of ER stress-induced apoptosis [17–19]. Thus, the PERK-eIF2α pathway elicits two opposing effects: a cytoprotective effect by inhibiting mRNA translation and inducing GRP78 transcription and a cytotoxic effect via CHOP expression.

When the accumulation of unfolded proteins exceeds the processing capacity of GRP78, high concentrations of ionized calcium (5 mM) are released from the ER into the cytoplasm, which contains only 0.1 μM of ionized calcium [20]. This increase of ionized calcium in the cytoplasm activates Jun kinase and Caspase 12, triggering a cascade leading to apoptosis. Overexpression of GRP78 using gene transfection alleviated the tunicamycin- and L-glutamate-induced apoptosis in cultured cells.

Our in vivo results reveal an increase of GRP78 in the acute phase after SCI, followed by an increase of CHOP at 5–7 days post injury, which is in accordance with the timing of apoptosis. Regarding the change in GRP78 among cell types, the ER response was highest in astrocytes and lowest in OPCs. The high capacity of astrocytes to deal with ER stress may be correlated with the survival of astrocytes and the formation of the glial scar after SCI, while the limited capacity of OPCs to deal with ER stress explains the susceptibility of OPCs to apoptosis. Therefore, if it were possible to regulate ER stress, it may be possible to inhibit apoptosis and reduce the spread of secondary injury, while increasing the survival of OPCs and inducing remyelination.

The enhancement of the ER stress response using amiloride reduced the expansion of secondary injury and contributed to OPC survival. Amiloride is a potassium-sparing diuretic approved by the FDA to treat hypertension, and its neuroprotective effects against SCI [21] and neurodegenerative diseases, such as Parkinson's disease [22] and multiple sclerosis [23], have been reported. This increase in GRP78 expression and the decrease in CHOP expression suggest that the reduction in apoptosis observed after amiloride is due to either the enhanced response to ER stress or a reduction in ER stress. In addition to the reduction of secondary injury, the improvement in functional recovery observed with amiloride treatment may also be a result of remyelination by the OPCs that were spared from apoptosis. Although we consider amiloride a promising therapeutic agent for treating SCI by targeting the ER stress pathways, we also believe that it is necessary to confirm the enhancement of remyelination in the chronic phase of SCI.

4.5 Conclusion

The ER stress response, which greatly affects the prognosis of SCI patients, was investigated in vitro and in vivo. GRP78 is expressed in response to stress and refolds the accumulated unfolded protein in the ER, but excessive stress induces expression of CHOP and leads to ER destruction and apoptosis. The ability to cope with ER stress varied between cell types, with the highest in astrocytes and the lowest in OPCs. The enhancement of the ER stress response with amiloride resulted not only in a reduction of the secondary injury process but also in an increase of OPC survival and differentiation, raising the possibility of eventual remyelination and recovery of neurological deficits in SCI patients.

Acknowledgments We thank our staff at the Teaching and Research Support Center, Tokai University, for their advice and technical assistance. All animal experiments were conducted in accordance with the protocol approved by the Animal Experimentation Committee at our institution. This work was supported in part by Grant-in-Aid for Scientific Research from the Ministry of Education, Culture, Sports, Science and Technology, Japan (21591907).

Disclaimer We report no conflict of interest concerning the materials or methods used in this study or the findings specified in this paper.

References

1. Watanabe M, Toyama Y, Nishiyama A (2002) Differentiation of proliferated NG2-positive glial progenitor cells in a remyelination lesion. J Neurosci Res 69:826–36
2. McTigue DM, Wei P, Stokes BT (2001) Proliferation of NG2-positive cells and altered oligodendrocyte numbers in the contused rat spinal cord. J Neurosci 21:3392–3400
3. Ishii K, Toda M, Nakai Y et al (2001) Increase of oligodendrocyte progenitor cells after spinal cord injury. J Neurosci Res 65:500–507
4. Watanabe M, Hadzic T, Nishiyama A (2004) Transient upregulation of Nkx2.2 expression in oligodendrocyte lineage cells during remyelination. Glia 46:311–322
5. Larner SF, Hayes RL, Wang KK (2006) Unfolded protein response after neurotrauma. J Neurotrauma 23:807–829
6. Suyama K, Watanabe M, Sakabe K et al (2011) Overexpression of GRP78 protects glial cells from endoplasmic reticulum stress. Neurosci Lett 504:271–276
7. Watanabe M, Fujimura Y, Nakamura M et al (1998) Changes of amino acid levels and aspartate distribution in the cervical spinal cord after traumatic spinal cord injury. J Neurotrauma 15:285–293
8. Schonberg DL, McTigue DM (2009) Iron is essential for oligodendrocyte genesis following intraspinal macrophage activation. Exp Neurol 218:64–74
9. Suyama K, Watanabe M, Sakai D et al (2007) Nkx2.2 expression in differentiation of oligodendrocyte precursor cells and inhibitory factors for differentiation of oligodendrocyte after traumatic spinal cord injury. J Neurotrauma 24:1013–1025
10. Bertolotti A, Zhang Y, Hendershot LM et al (2000) Dynamic interaction of BiP and ER stress transducers in the unfolded-protein response. Nat Cell Biol 2:326–332
11. Shen J, Chen X, Hendershot L et al (2002) ER stress regulation of ATF6 localization by dissociation of BiP/GRP78 binding and unmasking of Golgi localization signals. Dev Cell 3:99–111
12. Ron D, Walter P (2007) Signal integration in the endoplasmic reticulum unfolded protein response. Nat Rev Mol Cell Biol 8:519–529
13. Schröder M (2008) Endoplasmic reticulum stress response. Cell Mol Life Sci 65:862–894
14. Haze K, Yoshida H, Yanagi H et al (1999) Mammalian transcription factor ATF6 is synthesized as a transmembrane protein and activated by proteolysis in response to endoplasmic reticulum stress. Mol Biol Cell 10:3787–3799
15. Yoshida H, Matsui T, Yamamoto A et al (2001) XBP1 mRNA is induced by ATF6 and spliced by IRE1 in response to ER stress to produce a highly active transcription factor. Cell 107:881–891

16. Harding HP, Zhang Y, Ron D (1999) Protein translation and folding are coupled by an endoplasmic-reticulum-resident kinase. Nature 21:271–274
17. Zinszner H, Kuroda M, Wang X et al (1998) CHOP is implicated in programmed cell death in response to impaired function of the endoplasmic reticulum. Genes Dev 12:982–995
18. Oyadomari S, Mori M (2004) Roles of CHOP/GADD153 in endoplasmic reticulum stress. Cell Death Differ 11:381–389
19. Woehlbier U, Hetz C (2011) Modulating stress responses by the UPRosome: a matter of life and death. Trends Biochem Sci 36:329–337
20. Schroder M, Kaufman RJ (2005) The mammalian unfolded protein response. Annu Rev Biochem 74:739–789
21. Durham-Lee JC, Mokkapati VU, Johnson KM et al (2011) Amiloride improves locomotor recovery after spinal cord injury. J Neurotrauma 28:1319–1326
22. Arias RL, Sung ML, Vasylyev D et al (2008) Amiloride is neuroprotective in an MPTP model of Parkinson's disease. Neurobiol Dis 31:334–341
23. Friese MA, Craner MJ, Etzensperger R et al (2007) Acid-sensing ion channel-1 contributes to axonal degeneration in autoimmune inflammation of the central nervous system. Nat Med 13:1483–1489

Chapter 5
Roles of Microglia in Spinal Cord Injury

Tadanori Ogata, Tadao Morino, Hideki Horiuchi, and Hiromasa Miura

Abstract Microglia, immune cells in the central nervous system, have been reported to proliferate and become activated in damaged neuronal tissue. After experimental spinal cord injuries, proliferation of microglia in the injured site has been detected. Activated microglia release many substances which modulate secondary neuronal degeneration and regeneration after spinal cord injury. However, whether microglia are good or bad is under debate. In the acute phase of spinal cord injury, several papers suggested detrimental effects of activated microglia. Released glutamate and oxygen free radicals and cytokines, including TNF-α and interleukins, may directly induce damage of neurons and oligodendrocytes. On the other hand, activated microglia shows a neuroprotective effect via the production of neurotrophic factors.

Some experimental trials have proposed candidates of therapeutic modules for the treatment of spinal cord injury by controlling microglia functions. Here, we review experimental works, both in vivo and in vitro, on the complex and varied responses of microglia in terms of both detrimental and beneficial effects.

Keywords Cytokine • Microglia • Neuronal death • Spinal cord injury

5.1 Introduction

Spinal cord injury (SCI) is one of the most serious conditions in the field of orthopedic surgery. Spinal cords in mammals do not demonstrate marked regeneration following injury. It is necessary to develop an effective treatment to inhibit

T. Ogata (✉) • T. Morino • H. Horiuchi
Spine Center, Ehime University Hospital, Tohon-City, Ehime 791-0295, Japan
e-mail: ogata@m.ehime-u.ac.jp

H. Miura
Department of Orthopedic Surgery, Ehime University Graduate School of Medicine, Tohon-City, Ehime 791-0295, Japan

K. Uchida et al. (eds.), *Neuroprotection and Regeneration of the Spinal Cord*,
DOI 10.1007/978-4-431-54502-6_5, © Springer Japan 2014

secondary neuronal damage and to promote neuronal regeneration after SCI. Several pharmacological trials have been performed for the treatment of traumatic SCI. However, only high-dose steroid therapy has been established as an effective treatment for this condition. After trauma-induced SCI, direct damage, including axonal tears and mechanical cell damage, is followed by secondary neurodegeneration processes such as tissue swelling, energy failure by ischemia, and the toxic reaction of hyperexcitability [1, 2]. Suppression of the secondary neurodegeneration processes is a possible target for the treatment of SCI.

Microglia were first described by del Rio-Hortega [3] in the early part of the twentieth century. Postnatally, microglia are present in all regions of the central nervous system (CNS) in a nonoverlapping territorial manner and comprise a large proportion of the total cellular makeup of the CNS, which is estimated to be as high as 12 % [4].

Microglia, the resident immune cells in the CNS, have been reported to proliferate after ischemic brain damage [5]. Proliferated microglia after CNS injury may play a pivotal role in the processes of secondary neurodegeneration. Whether microglia are good or bad is under debate, with strong support for a dual role or differential activation of microglia. In this chapter, we comment on the roles of microglia after SCI.

5.2 Microglia Proliferation After SCI

Microglia have been reported to proliferate in many neurodegenerative diseases such as Alzheimer's disease [6], Parkinson's disease [7, 8], and HIV encephalopathy [9, 10]. In experimental SCI models, proliferation and activation of microglia in the injured spinal cord has been proven [11–13]. In order to observe secondary degenerating processes, including immune reactions, after SCI, we developed a rat spinal cord mild compression model [14]. When the rat thoracic (T11 level) spinal cord was gently compressed by a 20-g weight, complete ischemia was achieved without any destructive damage such as bleeding or axonal tears [15]. Using this model, microglia proliferation was observed in the spinal cord tissue after compression-ischemic injury [14]. When the spinal cord was compressed for 10 and 20 min, an enormous amount of microglia was observed mainly in the gray matter at 48 and 72 h after compression, although only a small amount of microglia proliferation was observed at 24 h after the compression (Fig. 5.1). Microglia proliferation was mainly observed in the gray matter. In the white matter, there was some proliferation of microglia due to compression; however, the number was usually less than in gray matter. Microglia proliferation was remarkable only in the compressed part of the thoracic spinal cord. There were few microglia in the cervical and lumbar spinal cord in this model.

The proliferated microglia (positive to OX42 staining) strongly expressed TNF-α and iNOS proteins (Fig. 5.2). These results suggest that microglia proliferated for several days after the spinal cord ischemic injury, and activated microglia modified neurodegenerative processes by secreting cytokines and nitric oxide. Microglia

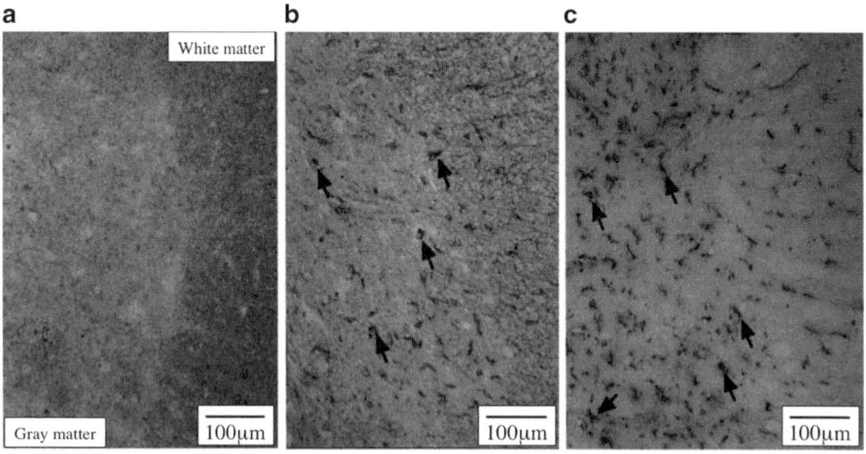

Fig. 5.1 Histological changes in spinal cord tissue 48 h after the compression injury. Rats were treated with thoracic cord compression by a 20-g weight for 20 min (**b**, **c**) or laminectomy alone (a; sham). Compressed part of the cords were subjected to lectin staining (**a**, **b**) or OX-42 staining (**c**). Only a few lectin-positive cells were observed in the thoracic cord of the sham animals (**a**). On the other hand, lectin-positive cells (*arrows*) were remarkably increased in the compressed cords (**b**). OX-42-positive cells (*arrows*) were also observed in the compressed cord (**c**). (From [14] with permission)

proliferation in the spinal cord was also observed in the model of peripheral nerve injury. Mika et al. reported that microglia proliferation was strongly observed in the dorsal lumbar spinal cord after peripheral nerve injury [16].

5.3 Detrimental Effects of Microglia in the Degeneration Processes of SCI

Although microglia may play an important role against infection in the CNS, overstimulation of this immune reaction may accelerate neuronal damage after SCI. Figure 5.3 shows a schema of the detrimental effects of microglia in the central and peripheral nervous systems.

Pathologically activated microglial cells release various harmful components such as nitric oxide (NO), superoxide (O_2^-), and several kinds of cytokines including interleukin (IL)-1 and IL-6 and tumor necrosis factor-α (TNF-α), which can directly or indirectly affect biological functions of neurons, aggravate neurotoxicity, and may even eventuate downstream in exacerbating neurodegeneration and the pathway of cell death [17–22]. Zhang and Fedoroff [23] reported that neurons in mixed neuron-microglia cultures survived longer than those in pure neuron cultures; however, when they treated the mixed culture by lipopolysaccharide (LPS), microglia impeded neuronal survival. These papers indicate that substances (cytokines and nitric oxide) released from activated microglia is possibly toxic to neurons.

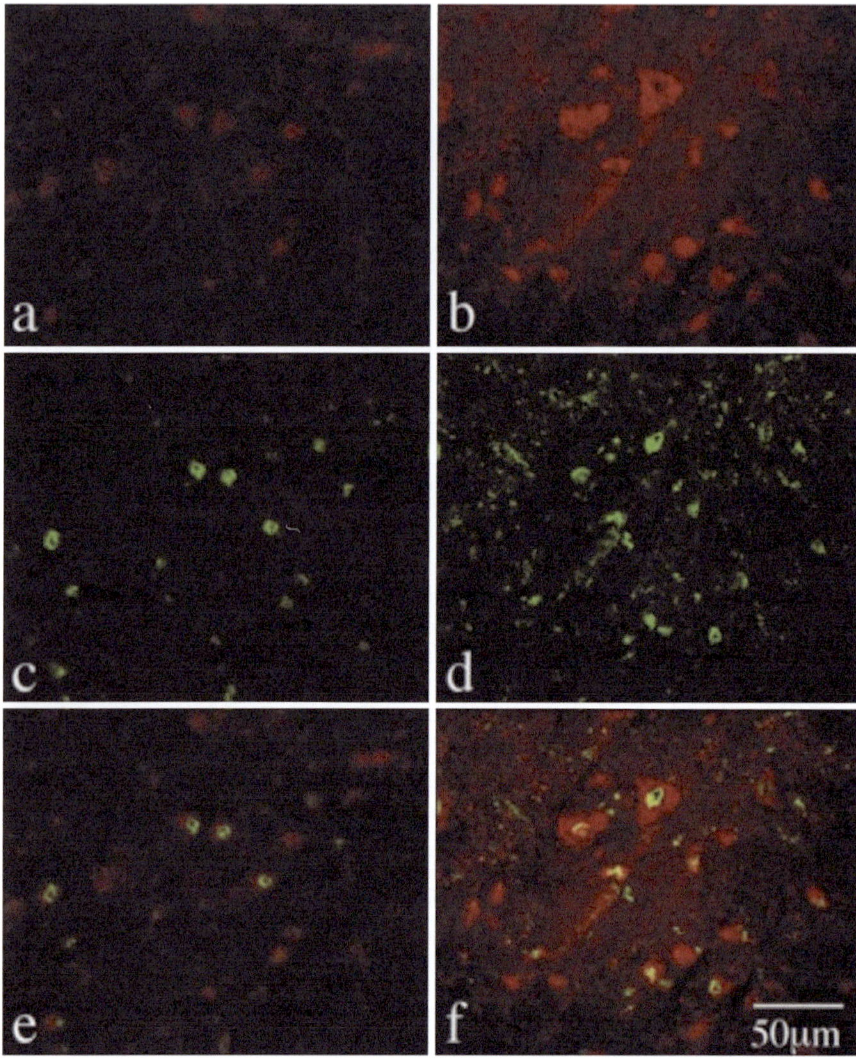

Fig. 5.2 Double staining of OX-42/TNF-α and OX-42/iNOS. Freezing sections were exposed to anti-TNF-α antibody (**a**, **c**, **e**) or anti-iNOS antibody (**b**, **d**, **f**) in the presence of anti-OX42 antibody. (**a**) TNF-α positive cells, (**b**) iNOS positive cells, (**c**) and (**d**) OX-42 positive cells, (**e**) double staining of OX-42/TNF-α, and (**f**) double staining of OX-42/*i*NOS. (From [14] with permission)

Neumann et al. [24] reported that application of recombinant TNF inhibited neurite outgrowth and branching of cultured hippocampal neurons. This effect was absent in the neurons of TNF receptor-deficient animals. Westmoreland et al. [25] reported that the addition of TNF-α induced cell death in cultured human neuronal cell lines and pentoxifylline, which inhibits the effects of TNF-α, had a significant protective effect in this assay. Viviani et al. [26] reported that activation of TNF-α release from

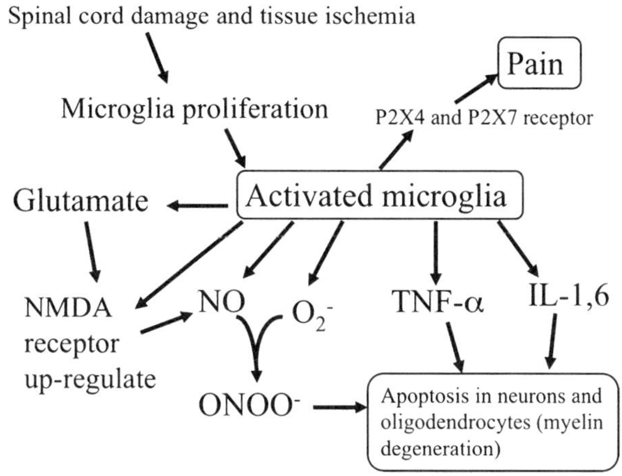

Fig. 5.3 Schema of the detrimental effects of activated microglia after injury of the nervous system

glial cells induced neuronal death, which was inhibited by the addition of TNF-α antibody in a glia-neuron co-culture. Other cytokines, released from activated microglia, also influence the progress of secondary neuronal damage. Interlrukin-1 (IL-1) has been reported to induce neuronal damage in both acute and chronic neurodegenerative disease [27] and cell death caused by ischemia, brain injury, or excitotoxins [28]. Interleukin 6 (IL-6) has also been reported to be toxic to neurons. Chronic exposure to IL-6 during neuronal development induced cell damage and death in a subpopulation of developing granule neurons, and increased the susceptibility of the granule neurons to a toxic insult produced by excessive activation of NMDA receptors [29]. In addition, IL-6-deficient mice showed an increased resistance to glutamate toxicity [30].

Nitric oxide (NO) and superoxide (O_2^-), which are released by activated microglia, are also reported to be toxic to the neuronal system due to production of peroxynitrite ($ONOO^-$) during degeneration [31]. There is evidence that the concomitant production of superoxide, required for the generation of peroxynitrite by NO, is provided by pathologically activated microglia [32]. The particularly high neurotoxicity of $ONOO^-$, which destroys neuronal cell membranes, has been shown in previous studies [33, 34].

The possible contribution of microglia by glutamate signaling has been reported. The activation of ionotropic glutamate receptors in microglia has deleterious consequences to neurons and oligodendrocytes. NMDA receptor expression was upregulated in activated microglia following ischemia [35, 36]. The activation of NMDA receptors in microglia leads to NO release. Pharmacological blockade of NMDA receptors and inhibition of iNOS prevents oligodendrocyte cell death [37]. Thus, NMDA receptor blockade protects oligodendrocytes by reducing the release of NO from microglia [37, 38]. Activated microglia itself can release glutamate which directly induces damage of neurons and oligodendrocytes. Both resting and activated microglia release glutamate through the cystine/glutamate antiporter [39]. However, glutamate released through resting microglia is rapidly and efficiently removed by glutamate transporters in other glial cells, mainly astrocytes. In contrast, the activation of microglia induces the release of factors, such as reactive oxygen species, TNF-α, and IL-1β that impair the function of glutamate transporters, resulting in an increase in extracellular levels of glutamate [39].

Peripheral nerve injury (neuropathic pain) and peripheral tissue injury (inflammation) induce abnormal pain sensation such as hyperalgesia and allodynia. Central sensitization, which is an enhanced responsiveness of nociceptive neurons in the CNS, is thought to be a mechanism for hyperalgesia and allodynia. Recent studies revealed that microglia in the spinal dorsal horn are activated in response to peripheral nerve or tissue injury and are involved in persistent pain sensation [40–43]. Inhibition of microglia proliferation and activation in spinal cord with minocycline [16, 44, 45] and propentofylline [46] ameliorated allodynia and hyperalgesia after peripheral nerve injuries. These results strongly indicate that the activation of microglia directly induced neuropathic and inflammatory pain.

The key mechanism of microglia-related pain is mediated via purinergic ionotropic receptors, such as P2X4 and P2X7, in activated microglia [47]. Tsuda et al. [48] reported that P2X4 receptor expression increased strikingly in the ipsilateral spinal cord after peripheral nerve injury, and P2X4 receptors were induced in hyperactive microglia but not in neurons or astrocytes. Pharmacological blockade of spinal P2X4 receptors reversed tactile allodynia caused by peripheral nerve injury without affecting acute pain behaviors in naive animals. Kobayashi et al. [49] reported that both P2X7 mRNA and protein increased in the spinal cord after peripheral nerve injury. Double-labeling studies revealed that cells expressing increased P2X7 mRNA and protein after nerve injury were predominantly microglia in the dorsal horn. Intrathecal application of a P2X7 antagonist suppressed mechanical hypersensitivity after the peripheral injury.

5.4 Beneficial Effects of Microglia After SCI

The effects of activated microglia on SCI are not limited to the harmful side. Activated astrocytes and microglial cells also confer beneficial effects on injured neurons and interfere with neurogenesis [50–52]. Prewit et al. [53] reported that increasing the presence of activated macrophage/microglial cells at a SCI site can provide an environment beneficial to the promotion of regeneration of sensory axons. Rabchevsky et al. [54] reported that implantation of cultured microglia promote neural regeneration after SCI.

Well-controlled inflammation, depending on the timing and amount, may possibly lessen and/or repair CNS damage. Nakanishi et al. [55] reported that cultured microglia released leukemia inhibitory factor (LIF), which promotes the differentiation of neural stem/progenitor cells. Kerr and Patterson [56] showed that LIF overexpression also causes the development of severe hindlimb motor dysfunction, an effect mediated by the enhanced activation of microglia/macrophages. To the contrary, they also reported that daily administration of LIF (25 mg/kg/day) promotes oligodendrocyte survival after SCI [57].

Growing evidence showed that microglial cells, under certain circumstances, can exert neuroprotective and supportive effects and enhance synthesis of neurotrophic factors.

Kerr and Patterson [57] reported that insulin-like growth factor-1(IGF-1) released from microglia promoted neuronal regeneration. Lehrmann et al. [58] reported that microglia is a major source of transforming growth factor (TGF)-β1 production after CNS injury. Application of TGF-β1 decreased infarct size after focal cerebral ischemia [59] and protected hippocampal neurons after global cerebral ischemia [60].

Nerve growth factor (NGF), a typical neuroregenerative protein, has also been reported to release from microglia in several CNS damage conditions [61, 62]. Other neuroprotective factors, such as brain-derived neurotrophic factor (BDNF) and glial cell line-derived neurotrophic factor (GDNF), have been reported to release from microglia in some pathological conditions of the CNS [63, 64]. Yang et al. [65] reported that mechanically injured astrocyte-conditioned medium (ACM) could provoke beneficial activation of microglial cells. Microglial cells released BDNF through the exposure of ACM, and the neurons cocultured with microglia showed the promotion of neurite outgrowth, which was suppressed by the addition of BDNF neutralizing antibody. Specific inhibition of the p38 mitogen-activated protein kinase inhibited the effects of ACM, including BDNF promotion and subsequent neurite outgrowth.

As mentioned above, microglia also contribute to the regeneration and preservation of damaged neurons and oligodendrocytes via the releasing of some trophic substances. However, it is still uncertain what causes the beneficial activation of microglial cells after CNS injury.

5.5 Possible Therapeutic Modules by Modification of Microglial Function for the Treatment of SCI

To summarize so far, microglia have two faces on the processes of neuronal degeneration after SCI. It has been suggested that the level of the inflammatory stimulus regulates the level of the microglial response. For example, Li et al. [66] demonstrated that, although high levels of LPS (>1 μg/mL) induced proinflammatory cytokine expression and neurotoxicity, lower concentrations (<500 ng/mL) increased neuronal cell viability and promoted neurite extension.

In recent years, a new classification of microglia has entered the literature. Described as an alternatively activated subset of microglia (M2), these cells have markers that can differentiate them from classically activated microglia (M1) [67, 68]. The M2 microglia are typically considered to be less inflammatory than M1 microglia; they are characterized by reduced NO production and increased anti-inflammatory cytokine production. The M2 microglia are involved in tissue repair, wound healing, and extracellular matrix remodeling [67]. After injury or in vitro following exposure to IL-4 or IL-13, microglia develop this nontoxic M2 phenotype, resulting in extensive neurite elongation and outgrowth across inhibitory surfaces [68, 69]. Therefore, control of microglia function may become a novel therapeutic strategy for the treatment of SCI.

The inhibition of pathological immune reactions by classically activated microglia (M1) may ameliorate secondary neurodegeneration in the acute stage after SCI. Several substances have been reported to inhibit microglial proliferation or functions (Table 5.1).

Microglia proliferation/activation can be controlled by some substances. Cl-adenosine, an unselective agonist of adenosine receptors, induced apoptosis of rat-cultured microglia [70]. Nakamura et al. [71] reported that an adenosine receptor analog and propentofylline, a xanthine derivative, inhibited microglia proliferation and phagocytosis activity of microglia. Minocycline, a second-generation tetracycline, has been reported to decrease microglia/macrophage activation and proliferation [72–74]. Application of minocycline reduced delayed oligodendrocyte death, attenuated axonal degeneration, and improved functional outcome after SCI [75, 76]. Tawfik et al. [46] reported that propentofylline treatment to nerve injured rats resulted in significantly decreased microglia proliferation in the spinal cord tissue and reversal of nerve injury-induced allodynia. Mika et al. [16] also found that chronic intraperitoneal injection of minocycline and pentoxifylline (cytokine inhibitor) inhibited activation of microglia and diminished neuropathic pain symptoms after peripheral nerve injury.

Pharmacological control of toxic substances release from microglia has been attempted using cultured microglia. Si et al. [21] reported that propentofylline inhibited cytokine release from cultured microglia by cAMP elevation. Adenosine induces adenylate cyclase activation via adenosine receptors, which provides intracellular cAMP elevation. Propentofylline increases cAMP as phosphodiesterase inhibition. Thus, the inhibitory effect of adenosine and propentofylline on microglia function is mediated by a common intracellular mechanism, such as cAMP-dependent kinase.

We have reported that alprostadil alfadex, a prostaglandin E1 (PGE1) analog, showed inhibition of LPS-induced release of TNF-α and NO from rat-cultured spinal cord microglia [77]. The inhibitory effects of the PGE1 analog may be mediated by EP1 and EP2 receptor subtypes. Caggiano and Kraig [78] demonstrated that EP1 and EP2 receptor subtypes were present in rat-cultured microglia. The EP1 receptor is related to intracellular calcium elevation, and adenylate cyclase activity is increased by EP2 receptor stimulation [79]. In our data [77], inhibition of protein kinase A by H89 inhibited the PGE1 action on LPS-induced TNF-α release, but showed no effect on NO release. The working mechanism of PGE1 on TNF-α release may involve the EP2 receptor-adenylate cyclase-cyclic AMP-protein kinase A pathway. On the other hand, the protein kinase C inhibition by staurosporine blocked the PGE1 action on LPS-induced NO release. These results suggest that PGE1 inhibited the TNF-α (cytokine) release and NO release by different mechanisms, such as activation of protein kinase A and protein kinase C.

Adenosine triphosphate (ATP) is also a strong inhibitor of microglia action [80]. We have tested the effects of endogenous purines (ATP, ADP, CTP, UDP, UTP) and P_2y receptor agonists (ADPβS and 2-methylthio-ATP) on LPS-induced cytokine (TNF-α, IL-1β and IL-6) release from cultured spinal cord microglia. The rank order of inhibitory potency of endogenous purines on TNF-α release was: ATP > ADP >>

Table 5.1 Candidates of therapeutic modalities for SCI by inhibition of microglial reaction

Year	Authors	Candidates (substances or treatments)	Experimental methods	Findings	Reference no.
1996	Ogata and Schubert	Adenosine receptor analog	Microglia culture	Induction of microglia apoptosis	[70]
1997	Nakamura et al.	Adenosine receptor analog propentofylline	Microglia culture	Inhibition of microglial proliferation and phagocytosis ability	[71]
1998	Si et al.	Propentofylline cAMP analog	Microglia culture	Inhibition of microglia proliferation and release of cytokines, NO, and O_2^-	[21]
2002	Chuai et al.	Prostaglandin E1 analog	Microglia culture	Inhibition of TNF-α and NO release	[77]
2003	Ogata et al.	ATP and selective P2y-receptor analog	Microglia culture	Inhibition of cytokines (TNF-α, IL-1β, IL-6) and NO release	[80]
2007	Yune et al.	Minocycline	SCI contusion model	Improvement of motor function and inhibition of pro-nerve growth factor production in microglia	[72]
2007	Tawfik et al.	Propentofylline	Peripheral nerve injury	Inhibition of microglia proliferation and induction of pain relief	[46]
2008	Morino et al.	Systemic hypothermia	SCI compression model	Improvement of motor function and inhibition of microglia proliferation	[86]
2009	Mika et al.	Minocycline, pentoxifylline	Peripheral nerve injury	Inhibition of microglia proliferation and induction of pain relief	[16]
2012	Morizane et al.	Local hypothermia	SCI contusion model	Improvement of motor function and inhibition of microglia proliferation and TNF-α production	[87]

The substances or treatments mentioned above were shown experimentally to inhibit microglia proliferation and/or inhibit toxic substances from activated microglia. Application of these substances, or introduction of hypothermic treatments, possibly inhibits neuronal damage through the activation of microglia after SCI

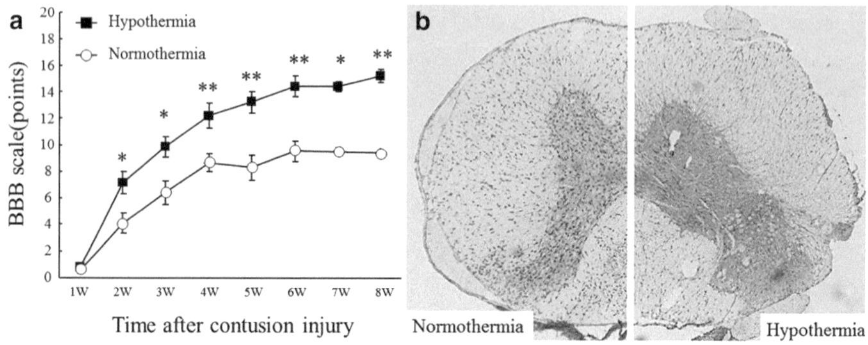

Fig. 5.4 Effect of local hypothermic treatment for SCI. Spinal cord contusion injuries were performed, and temperature control devices were operatively placed in the rats. The local temperature of the injured spinal cord was controlled at 33 °C (*closed circles*) and 37 °C (*open circles*) for 48 h after the injury. (**a**) Rat hindlimb functions were evaluated using the BBB scale. Data are the means ± SEM ($n = 9$ to 10). Significant differences between the two groups were shown as *asterisks* ($^*P < 0.05$, $^{**}P < 0.01$). (**b**) Microglia proliferation after spinal cord injury. The spinal cords were taken out of the animals at 72 h after the spinal cord injury. The axial slices were stained by an anti-OX-42 antibody. (From [87] with permission)

UTP>UDP>CTP. The addition of 10 μM 2-methylthio-ATP showed a similar potency as 100 μM ATP. The addition of ADPβS, however, showed less effect. These endogenous purines and selective ATP receptor agonists showed a similar inhibitory effect in their rank order on LPS-induced IL-6 release. The application of P_2y receptor agonists might be considered as a pharmacological treatment for several pathological conditions of the spinal cord, including toxic immunoreactions.

Cooling the damaged tissue should be a powerful module on inflammatory responses after SCI. Systemic cooling has been reported to protect neurons after traumatic or ischemic brain damage [81, 82]. Using several SCI models, systemic hypothermic treatment under general anesthesia also showed successful neuroprotection after CNS injury [83–85]. The target of hypothermic treatments may be, at least in part, somewhat delayed in response after injury. Using the thoracic (T11) spinal cord mild compression model [14], we performed systemic mild hypothermia treatment (33 °C) under general anesthesia for 1 h after the injury [86]. Compared with normothermic animals (37 °C), remarkable inhibition of microglia proliferation and tissue TNF-α content were observed in parallel with recovery of motor activity in the hindlimbs. However, longer hypothermic treatment should be necessary for more severe injuries, such as the spinal cord contusion model. In order to achieve more stable and effective spinal cord cooling for the treatment of severe SCI, we developed a novel thermoelectric cooling device using Peltier modules [87]. Using this device, we performed local mild hypothermia (33 °C) for 48 h. During the hypothermic treatment, rats were awake and could move in the cage. Hindlimb motor function, evaluated using a BBB scale [88], in the hypothermic animals was significantly higher than that in the normothermic animals from 2 to 8 weeks after the injury (Fig. 5.4a). Compared with normothermic animals, the hypothermic treatment significantly reduced the number of OX42-positive cells (microglia; Fig. 5.4b) and TNF-α-positive cells. The TNF-α content in the injured spinal cord tissue was also significantly inhibited by hypothermic treatment. These results suggest that inhibition of microglia proliferation and activation by hypothermia is a reasonable therapeutic module for the treatment of acute SCI.

5.6 Conclusion

We have not fully understood the roles of microglia in the pathophysiology of SCI. Microglia have an unreasonable attitude, like a "difficult child," in spite of their excellent ability to protect the nervous system (against infection or the release of neurotrophic factors). However, growing evidence has brought us some method to control microglial functions. We hope that we will obtain a way to adequately control microglial function during the progress of degeneration and regeneration processes after SCI. Future research is needed to focus on clarifying the signals and mechanisms by which microglia can be guided to promote optimal functional recovery.

Conflict of Interest The authors declare that they have no conflict of interest.

References

1. Benveniste H, Drejer J, Schousboe A et al (1984) Elevation of the extracellular concentration of glutamate and aspartate in rat hippocampus during transient cerebral ischemia monitored by intracerebral microdialysis. J Neurochem 43:1369–1374
2. Choi DW, Rothman SM (1990) The role of glutamate neurotoxicity in hypoxic-ischemic neuronal death. Annu Rev Neurosci 13:171–182
3. del Rio-Hortega P (1932) Microglia. In: Penfield W (ed) Cytology and cellular pathology of the nervous system. P.B. Hoeber, New York, pp 483–534
4. Lawson LJ, Perry VH, Dri P et al (1990) Heterogeneity in the distribution and morphology of microglia in the normal adult mouse brain. Neuroscience 39:151–170
5. Morioka T, Kalehua AN, Streit WJ (1991) The microglial reaction in the rat dorsal hippocampus following transient forebrain ischemia. J Cereb Blood Flow Metab 11:966–973
6. Banati RB, Schubert P, Rothe G et al (1994) Modulation of intracellular formation of reactive oxygen intermediate in peritoneal macrophages and microglia/brain macrophages by propentofylline. J Cereb Blood Flow Metab 14:145–149
7. Czlonkowska A, Kurkowska-Jastrzebska I, Czlonkowski A et al (2002) Immune processes in the pathogenesis of Parkinson's disease D a potential role for microglia and nitric oxide. Med Sci Monit 8:RA165–RA177
8. Perry V, Gordon S (1988) Macrophages and microglia in the nervous system. Trends Neurosci 11:273–277
9. Antinori A, Giancola ML, Alba L et al (2001) Cardiomyopathy and encephalopathy in AIDS. Ann N Y Acad Sci 946:121–129
10. Diesing TS, Swindells S, Gelbard H et al (2002) HIV-1-associated dementia: a basic science and clinical perspective. AIDS Read 12:358–368

11. Carlson SL, Parrish ME, Springer JE et al (1998) Acute inflammatory response in spinal cord following impact injury. Exp Neurol 151:77–88
12. Isaksson J, Farooque M, Holtz A et al (1999) Expression of ICAM-1 and CD11b after experimental spinal cord injury in rats. J Neurotrauma 16:165–173
13. Watanabe T, Yamamoto T, Abe Y et al (1999) Differential activation of microglia after experimental spinal cord injury. J Neurotrauma 16:255–265
14. Morino T, Ogata T, Horiuchi H et al (2003) Delayed neuronal damage related to microglia proliferation after mild spinal cord compression injury. Neurosci Res 46:309–318
15. Hamamoto Y, Ogata T, Morino T et al (2007) Real-time direct measurement of spinal cord blood flow at the site of compression: relationship between blood flow recovery and motor deficiency in spinal cord injury. Spine 32:1955–1962
16. Mika J, Osikowicz M, Rojewska E et al (2009) Differential activation of spinal microglial and astroglial cells in a mouse model of peripheral neuropathic pain. Eur J Pharmacol 623:65–72
17. Chao CC, Hu S, Molitor TW et al (1992) Activated microglia mediated neuronal cell injury via nitric oxide mechanism. J Immunol 149:2736–2741
18. Dawson VL, Dawson TM, Barteley DA et al (1993) Mechanism of nitric oxide mediated neurotoxicity in primary brain cultures. J Neurosci 13:2651–2661
19. Hanisch UK (2002) Microglia as a source and target of cytokines. Glia 40:140–155
20. Meda L, Cassatella MA, Szendrei GI et al (1995) Activation of microglial cells by beta-amyloid protein and interferon-gamma. Nature 374:647–650
21. Si Q, Nakamura Y, Ogata T et al (1998) Differential regulation of microglial activation by propentofylline via cAMP signalling. Brain Res 812:97–104
22. Tanaka M, Sotomatsu A, Yoshida T et al (1994) Detection of superoxide production activated microglia using sensitive and specific chemiluminescence assay and microglia-mediated PC 12h cell death. J Neurochem 63:266–270
23. Zhang SC, Fedoroff S (1996) Neuron-microglia interactions in vitro. Acta Neuropathol 91:385–395
24. Neumann H, Schweigreiter R, Yamashita T et al (2002) Tumor necrosis factor inhibits neurite outgrowth and branching of hippocampal neurons by a rho-dependent mechanism. J Neurosci 22:854–862
25. Westmoreland SV, Kolson D, Gonzalez-Scarano F (1996) Toxicity of TNF alpha and platelet activating factor for human NT2N neurons: a tissue culture model for human immunodeficiency virus dementia. J Neurovirol 2:118–126
26. Viviani B, Corsini E, Galli CL et al (1998) Glia increase degeneration of hippocampal neurons through release of tumor necrosis factor-alpha. Toxicol Appl Pharmacol 150:271–276
27. Allan SM, Tyrrell PJ, Rothwell NJ (2005) Interleukin-1 and neuronal injury. Nat Rev Immunol 5:629–640
28. Patel HC, Boutin H, Allan SM (2003) Interleukin-1 in the brain: mechanisms of action in acute neurodegeneration. Ann N Y Acad Sci 992:39–47
29. Conroy SM, Nguyen V, Quina LA et al (2004) Interleukin-6 produces neuronal loss in developing cerebellar granule neuron cultures. J Neuroimmunol 155:43–54
30. Fisher J, Mizrahi T, Schori H et al (2001) Increased post-traumatic survival of neurons in IL-6-knockout mice on a background of EAE susceptibility. J Neuroimmunol 119:1–9
31. Xia Y, Dawson VL, Dawson TM et al (1996) Nitric oxide synthase generates superoxide and nitric oxide in arginine-depleted cells leading to peroxynitrite-mediated cellular injury. Proc Natl Acad Sci USA 93:6770–6774
32. Boje KM, Arora PK (1992) Microglial-produced nitric oxide and reactive nitrogen oxides mediate neuronal cell death. Brain Res 587:250–256
33. Dalloz F, Maupoil V, Lecour S et al (1997) In vitro studies of interactions of NO donor drugs with superoxide and hydroxyl radicals. Mol Cell Biochem 177:193–200
34. Eliasson MJ, Huang Z, Ferrante RJ, Moskowitz MA et al (1999) Neuronal nitric oxide synthase activation and peroxynitrite formation in ischemic stroke linked to neural damage. J Neurosci 19:5910–5918

35. Gottlieb M, Matute C (1997) Expression of ionotropic glutamate receptor subunits in glial cells of the hippocampal CA1 area following transient forebrain ischemia. J Cereb Blood Flow Metab 17:290–300
36. Kaur C, Sivakumar V, Ang LS et al (2006) Hypoxic damage to the periventricular white matter in neonatal brain: role of vascular endothelial growth factor, nitric oxide and excitotoxicity. J Neurochem 98:1200–1216
37. Murugan M, Sivakumar V, Lu J et al (2011) Expression of N-methyl-D-aspartate receptor subunits in amoeboid microglia mediates production of nitric oxide via NF-κB signaling pathway and oligodendrocyte cell death in hypoxic postnatal rats. Glia 59:521–539
38. Tahraoui SL, Marret S, Bodénant C et al (2001) Centralrole of microglia in neonatal excitotoxic lesions of the murine periventricular white matter. Brain Pathol 11:56–71
39. Domercq M, Sánchez-Gómez MV, Sherwin C et al (2007) System xc- and glutamate transporter inhibition mediates microglial toxicity to oligodendrocytes. J Immunol 178:6549–6556
40. McMahon SB, Malcangio M (2009) Current challenges in glia-pain biology. Neuron 64:46–54
41. Milligan ED, Watkins LR (2009) Pathological and protective roles of glia in chronic pain. Nat Rev Neurosci 10:23–36
42. Scholz J, Woolf CJ (2007) The neuropathic pain triad: neurons, immune cells and glia. Nat Neurosci 10:1361–1368
43. Schomberg D, Olson JK (2012) Immune responses of microglia in the spinal cord: contribution to pain states. Exp Neurol 234:262–270
44. Ledeboer A, Sloane EM, Milligan ED et al (2005) Minocycline attenuates mechanical allodynia and proinflammatory cytokine expression in rat models of pain facilitation. Pain 15:71–83
45. Raghavendra V, Tanga F, DeLeo JA (2003) Inhibition of microglial activation attenuates the development but not existing hypersensitivity in a rat model of neuropathy. J Pharmacol Exp Ther 306:624–630
46. Tawfik VL, Nutile-McMenemy N, Lacroix-Fralish ML et al (2007) Efficacy of propentofylline, a glial modulating agent, on existing mechanical allodynia following peripheral nerve injury. Brain Behav Immun 21:238–246
47. Inoue K, Tsuda M (2012) Purinergic systems, neuropathic pain and the role of microglia. Exp Neurol 234:293–301
48. Tsuda M, Shigemoto-Mogami Y, Koizumi S et al (2003) P2X4 receptors induced in spinal microglia gate tactile allodynia after nerve injury. Nature 424:778–783
49. Kobayashi K, Takahashi E, Miyagawa Y et al (2011) Induction of the P2X7 receptor in spinal microglia in a neuropathic pain model. Neurosci Lett 504:57–61
50. Gras G, Chrétien F, Vallat-Decouvelaere AV et al (2003) Regulated expression of sodium-dependent glutamate transporters and synthetase: a neuroprotective role for activated microglia and macrophages in HIV infection? Brain Pathol 13:211–222
51. Buisson A, Lesne S, Docagne F et al (2003) Transforming growth factor-beta and ischemic brain injury. Cell Mol Neurobiol 23:539–550
52. Zadran S, Jourdi H, Rostamiani K et al (2010) Brain-derived neurotrophic factor and epidermal growth factor activate neuronal m-calpain via mitogen-activated protein kinase-dependent phosphorylation. J Neurosci 30:1086–1095
53. Prewitt CM, Niesman IR, Kane CJ et al (1997) Activated macrophage/microglial cells can promote the regeneration of sensory axons into the injured spinal cord. Exp Neurol 148:33–443
54. Rabchevsky AG, Streit WJ (1997) Grafting of cultured microglial cells into the lesioned spinal cord of adult rats enhances neurite outgrowth. J Neurosci Res 47:34–48
55. Nakanishi M, Niidome T, Matsuda S et al (2007) Microglia-derived interleukin-6 and leukaemia inhibitory factor promote astrocytic differentiation of neural stem/progenitor cells. Eur J Neurosci 25:649–658

56. Kerr BJ, Patterson PH (2004) Potent pro-inflammatory actions of leukemia inhibitory factor in the spinal cord of the adult mouse. Exp Neurol 188:391–407
57. Kerr BJ, Patterson PH (2005) Leukemia inhibitory factor promotes oligodendrocyte survival after spinal cord injury. Glia 51:73–79
58. Lehrmann E, Kiefer R, Christensen T et al (1998) Microglia and macrophages are major sources of locally produced transforming growth factor-β1 after transient middle cerebral artery occlusion in rats. Glia 24:437–448
59. Henrich-Noack P, Prehn JH, Krieglstein J (1994) Neuroprotective effect of TGF-β1. J Neural Transm Suppl 43:33–45
60. Henrich-Noack P, Prehn JH, Krieglstein J (1996) TGF-β1 protects hippocampal neurons against degeneration caused by transient global ischemia. Dose–response relationship and potential neuroprotective mechanisms. Stroke 27:1609–1615
61. Heese K, Fiebich BL, Bauer J et al (1997) Nerve growth factor (NGF) expression in rat microglia is induced by adenosine A2a-receptors. Neurosci Lett 231:83–86
62. Heese K, Hock C, Otten U (1998) Inflammatory signals induce neurotrophin expression in human microglial cells. J Neurochem 70:699–707
63. Batchelor PE, Liberatore GT, Wong JY et al (1999) Activated macrophages and microglia induce dopaminergic sprouting in the injured striatum and express brain-derived neurotrophic factor and glial cell line-derived neurotrophic factor. J Neurosci 19:1708–1716
64. Suzuki H, Imai F, Kanno T et al (2001) Preservation of neurotrophin expression in microglia that migrate into the gerbil's brain across the blood brain barrier. Neurosci Lett 312:95–98
65. Yang H, Feng GD, Liang Z et al (2012) In vitro beneficial activation of microglial cells by mechanically-injured astrocytes enhances the synthesis and secretion of BDNF through p38MAPK. Neurochem Int 61:175–186
66. Li L, Lu J, Tay SS et al (2007) The function of microglia, either neuroprotection or neurotoxicity, is determined by the equilibrium among factors released from activated microglia in vitro. Brain Res 1159:8–17
67. Colton CA (2009) Heterogeneity of microglial activation in the innate immune response in the brain. J Neuroimmune Pharmacol 4:399–418
68. Kigerl KA, Gensel JC, Ankeny DP et al (2009) Identification of two distinct macrophage subsets with divergent effects causing either neurotoxicity or regeneration in the injured mouse spinal cord. J Neurosci 29:13435–13444
69. Butovsky O, Talpalar AE, Ben-Yaakov K et al (2005) Activation of microglia by aggregated β-amyloid or lipopolysaccharide impairs MHC-II expression and renders them cytotoxic whereas IFN-γ and IL-4 render them protective. Mol Cell Neurosci 29:381–393
70. Ogata T, Schubert P (1996) Programmed cell death in rat microglia is controlled by extracellular adenosine. Neurosci Lett 218:91–94
71. Nakamura Y, Si QS, Kataoka K (1997) Inhibitory effect of adenosine agonists and propentofylline on the proliferation and transformation of cultured microglia. In: Okada Y (ed) The role of adenosine in the nervous system. Elsevier, Amsterdam, pp 97–102
72. Yune TY, Lee JY, Jung GY et al (2007) Minocycline alleviates death of oligodendrocytes by inhibiting pro-nerve growth factor production in microglia after spinal cord injury. J Neurosci 27:7751–7761
73. Tikka TM, Koistinaho JE (2001) Minocycline provides neuroprotection against N-methyl-D-aspartate neurotoxicity by inhibiting microglia. J Immunol 166:7527–7533
74. Wells JE, Hurlbert RJ, Fehlings MG et al (2003) Neuroprotection by minocycline facilitates significant recovery from spinal cord injury in mice. Brain 126:1628–1637
75. Lee SM, Yune TY, Kim SJ et al (2003) Minocycline reduces cell death and improves functional recovery after traumatic spinal cord injury in the rat. J Neurotrauma 20:1017–1027
76. Stirling DP, Khodarahmi K, Liu J et al (2004) Minocycline treatment reduces delayed oligodendrocyte death, attenuates axonal dieback, and improves functional outcome after spinal cord injury. J Neurosci 24:2182–2190
77. Chuai M, Ogata T, Morino T et al (2002) Prostaglandin E1 analog inhibits the microglia function: suppression of lipopolysaccharide-induced nitric oxide and TNF-α release. J Orthop Res 20:1246–1252

78. Caggiano AO, Kraig RP (1999) Prostaglandin E receptor subtypes in cultured rat microglia and their role in reducing lipopolysaccharide-induced interleukin-1beta production. J Neurochem 72:565–575
79. Minghetti L, Nicolini A, Polazzi E et al (1997) Prostaglandin E2 downregulates inducible nitric oxide synthase expression in microglia by increasing cAMP levels. Adv Exp Med Biol 433:181–184
80. Ogata T, Chuai M, Morino T et al (2003) Adenosine triphosphate inhibits cytokine release from lipopolysaccharide-activated microglia via P2y receptors. Brain Res 981:174–183
81. Busto R, Dietrich WD, Globus MY et al (1989) Postischemic moderate hypothermia inhibits CA1 hippocampal ischemic neuronal injury. Neurosci Lett 101:299–304
82. Colbourne F, Corbett D (1994) Delayed and prolonged post-ischemic hypothermia is neuroprotective in the gerbil. Brain Res 654:265–272
83. Yu CG, Jimenez O, Marcillo AE et al (2000) Beneficial effects of modest systemic hypothermia on locomotor function and histopathological damage following contusion-induced spinal cord injury in rats. J Neurosurg 93:85–93
84. Low TP Jr, Cho KS, Carg MS et al (2009) Systemic hypothermia improves histological and functional outcome after cervical spinal cord contusion in rats. J Comp Neurol 514:433–448
85. Dimar JR, Shields CB, Zhang YP et al (2000) The role of directly applied hypothermia in spinal cord injury. Spine 25:2294–2302
86. Morino T, Ogata T, Takeba J et al (2008) Microglia inhibition is a target of mild hypothermic treatment after the spinal cord injury. Spinal Cord 46:425–431
87. Morizane K, Ogata T, Morino T et al (2012) A novel thermoelectric cooling device using Peltier modules for inducing local hypothermia of the spinal cord: the effect of local electrically-controlled cooling for the treatment of spinal cord injuries in conscious rats. Neurosci Res 72:279–282
88. Basso DM, Beattie MS, Bresnahan JC (1995) A sensitive and reliable locomotor rating scale for open field testing in rats. J Neurotrauma 12:1–21

Part II
Pathologies of Chronic Compressive Spinal Cord

Chapter 6
Biomechanics of the Spinal Cord and the Pia Mater

Hiroshi Ozawa, Takeo Matsumoto, Toshiro Ohashi, and Masaaki Sato

Abstract Biomechanical analysis of the spinal cord is important to clarify the morphological plasticity of the spinal cord. In the present study, the elastic moduli of the gray and white matter were measured in situ by using a pipette aspiration method. The mechanical properties and function of the pia mater were investigated. Furthermore, the effect of the tensile stress on the morphology of the spinal cord was investigated. No significant difference in elastic moduli was observed between the gray and white matter of spinal cord. The elastic modulus of the pia mater was 2,300 kPa, which was 460 times higher than that of the spinal cord parenchyma. The pia mater triples the elastic modulus of the spinal cord covered by it compared with the parenchyma and increases the overall stiffness of the spinal cord. As a result of being tightly covered by the pia mater, the compressed spinal cord contains a large amount of strain energy, which enables shape restoration after decompression. The length of the spinal cord was decreased by 9.7 % after the separation to remove longitudinal tensile stress. The tensile stress along the craniocaudal axis in the spinal cord did not affect the spinal cord deformation in response to the compression, but it did affect the shape recoverability after the decompression.

Keywords Biomechanics • Elastic modulus • Pia mater • Spinal cord

H. Ozawa (✉)
Department of Orthopaedic Surgery, Tohoku University School of Medicine,
1-1 Seiryomachi, Aobaku, Sendai 980-8574, Japan
e-mail: hozawa@med.tohoku.ac.jp

T. Matsumoto
Department of Mechanical Engineering, Nagoya Institute of Technology, Nagoya, Japan

T. Ohashi
Faculty of Engineering, Hokkaido University, Sapporo, Japan

M. Sato
Graduate School of Biomedical Engineering, Tohoku University, Sendai 980-8574, Japan

K. Uchida et al. (eds.), *Neuroprotection and Regeneration of the Spinal Cord*,
DOI 10.1007/978-4-431-54502-6_6, © Springer Japan 2014

6.1 Introduction

Biomechanical analysis of the spinal cord is important to clarify the morphological plasticity of the spinal cord. The spinal cord is deformed in response to compression, and as a result, its cross-sectional area is reduced as observed on CT myelograms and axial MR images obtained in patients with cervical compressive myelopathy. Several factors regulate the deformation of the spinal cord. The elastic modulus of the parenchyma and the Poisson ratio are physical factors inherent in the spinal cord. The pia mater and the dentate ligament are factors that may affect the physical attributes of the spinal cord. The spinal cord is physiologically stretched along the craniocaudal axis and is subjected to tensile stress.

In the present study, the elastic moduli of the gray and white matter were measured in situ by using a pipette aspiration method. The mechanical properties and function of the pia mater were investigated. Furthermore, the effect of the tensile stress on the morphology of the spinal cord was investigated.

6.2 Elastic Moduli of the Gray and White Matter of the Spinal Cord

The gray matter of the spinal cord mainly consists of nerve cells, whereas the white matter consists of dendrites and axons. The gray matter has been thought to be softer than the white matter [1, 2], although no definite evidence to this effect has been published. In the present study, the elastic moduli of the gray and white matter were measured in situ by using a pipette aspiration method, which we have developed for the assessment of soft biological tissue.

6.2.1 Materials and Methods

6.2.1.1 Specimen Preparation

Eight Japanese white rabbits weighing an average of 2,600 g (range 2,400–2,800 g) were killed by intravenous injection of a high dose of pentobarbiturate. The C4–6 spinal column containing the spinal cord was excised from each rabbit. Using an osteotome, each column was transversely cut at the level of the intervertebral discs. Three spinal cord specimens were removed from their respective vertebral canals, and they were immediately placed in physiological saline at room temperature (16 °C) until mechanical testing.

Each of the three-dimensional cross sections (axial, frontal, and sagittal) was displayed as follows by using a microslicer: a specimen was cut transversely for the axial section; the second specimen from the same rabbit was vertically cut anterior

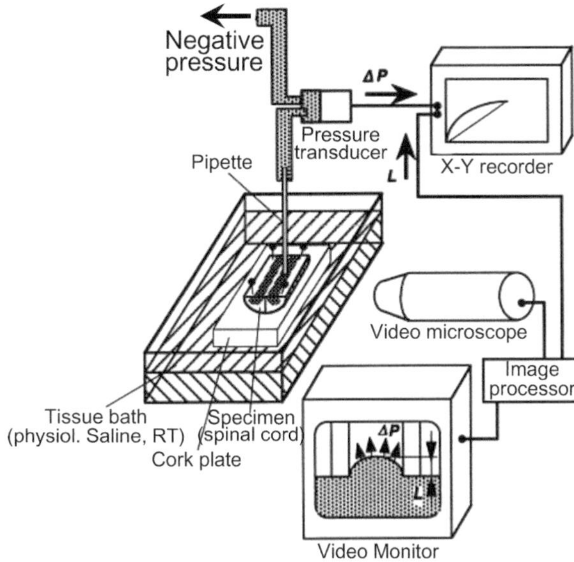

Fig. 6.1 Schematic diagram of the experimental setup

to the central canal for the frontal section; and the last specimen was cut in the middle of the right half of the spinal cord for the sagittal section. The gray and white matter were distinguished by their colors on the surface of each cross section.

The specimens were treated carefully and quickly so that testing was completed within 15 min after cutting with the microslicer. As long as each specimen was only visually inspected, the surface of the specimens did not begin dissolving into the physiological saline within 30 min after the cutting. All experiments were finished within 1 h after the rabbit was killed.

6.2.1.2 Experimental Apparatus and Procedure

The experimental setup used in the present study was similar to that used by Ohashi et al. [2] except for the apparatus used to apply negative pressure to the specimens (Fig. 6.1). As a substitute, we used a small vacuum pump with a large reservoir (20 L) to control the negative pressure precisely.

Each specimen was fixed on a cork plate by pins with the cut surface to be measured facing upward. Care was taken not to apply any external load. A glass pipette (0.8 mm in inner and 1.09 mm in outer diameter) was connected to a reservoir and a pressure transducer with silicone tubing. All of the tubing was filled with physiological saline. The transducer was calibrated with a mercury manometer before each experiment. The color was noticeably different between the white and gray matter on the cut surface. After a micromanipulator was used to set the tip of the pipette perpendicular to the gray or white matter appearing on the cut surface of the specimen, negative pressure was applied at a rate of −1 cm H_2O/s (range 0 to −5 cm H_2O).

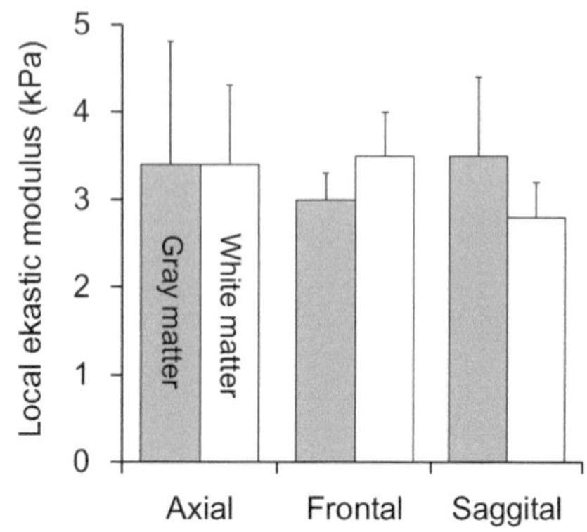

Fig. 6.2 Elastic moduli of *gray* and *white* matter of the spinal cord ($n=8$, mean ± SD). The difference between the *gray* and *white* matter was significant neither in each section nor among all cross sections

To measure the elastic moduli of the gray and white matter separately, the pipette was applied to areas at least 1 mm apart from the boundary between the two types of matter. The deformation process of the aspirated tissue into the pipette was observed on a video monitor through a video microscope. The aspirated length was measured with a video dimension analyzer, and the pressure–deformation curve was continuously recorded on an X–Y recorder.

6.2.1.3 Determination of Local Modulus of Elasticity

In a separate study [3], finite element analysis of the pipette aspiration method was performed. The initial value of the modulus of elasticity (i.e., the Young modulus) was calculated by comparing the pressure–deformation curve obtained in the experiment with that in the finite element analysis.

6.2.2 Results

The pressure–deformation curves revealed typical hysteresis. Accordingly, the pressure–deformation relationship during aspiration was different from that during unloading, indicating that the spinal cord has marked viscoelasticity.

The elastic moduli of the gray and white matter were 3.4 ± 1.4 (mean ± SD) and 3.4 ± 0.9 kPa in the axial section, 3.0 ± 0.3 and 3.5 ± 0.5 kPa in the frontal section, and 3.5 ± 0.9 and 2.8 ± 0.4 kPa in the sagittal section, respectively. The difference between the elastic moduli of the gray and white matter was significant neither in each section nor among all sections using the Kruskal–Wallis test (Fig. 6.2).

6.2.3 *Discussion*

The pipette aspiration technique was originally applied to the measurement of the mechanical properties of red cells and endothelial cell membranes of vessels [4]. By changing the diameter of the pipette, any size of soft tissue can be tested [5]. One of the advantages of this method is that different areas in a specimen can be measured in situ. The computer simulation has indicated that the modulus of elasticity obtained by this method is an averaged one of the hemispheric area with the diameter corresponding to the pipette diameter at its tip [3]. When using this method, the prerequisite condition of specimens is that they are soft enough to deform under the aspiration pressure applied through the pipette. In the present study, by using a thin pipette of 0.8 mm in diameter, the elastic moduli of the gray and the white matter could be measured separately in situ.

One of the limitations of this study is that we had to cut specimens to display the surface to be aspirated. Because nerve cells connect with their axons and dendrites in the gray matter and dendrites and axons adhere to each other in the white matter, cutting of the specimen would break such connections, and the tissue adjacent to the cut surface may become loose. The Young modulus measured on the surface of the gray and white matter may thus be a little lower than that measured in vivo. Nevertheless, at present there is no experimental evidence to refute the absence of significant difference in elastic moduli found between the gray and white matter in the present study.

6.3 Mechanical Properties and Function of the Spinal Pia Mater

Little attention has been paid to the function of the pia mater. In current accounts the function of the pia mater is described as that of a scaffold for the vasculature of the spinal cord parenchyma such as the anterior and posterior spinal arteries [6, 7]. There have been several articles concerning the mechanical properties of the pia mater [8, 9]; although its elasticity has been described, the elastic modulus of the pia mater has not been measured.

In the present study, the mechanical properties and function of the pia mater were investigated using the following methods: (1) a tensile test of the rabbit spinal cord with and without the pia mater to measure its elastic modulus and (2) a compression test of the rabbit spinal cord to clarify the effect of the pia mater on spinal cord stiffness.

6.3.1 *Measurement of the Elastic Modulus of the Pia Mater*

6.3.1.1 Specimen Preparation

Nine Japanese white rabbits were killed by intravenous injection of a high dose of pentobarbital. The cervical spinal column and cord from C5 through C6 were excised from each rabbit. Spinal cord segments were removed from the excised

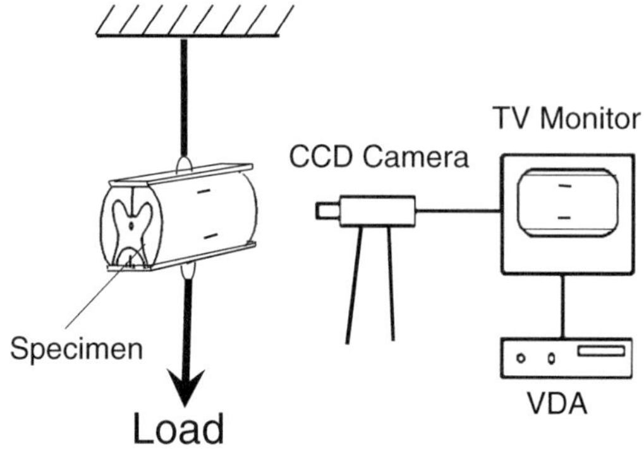

Fig. 6.3 Tensile test of the spinal cord. A specimen was hung up with the ventral plate and slightly elongated with a small load hooked on the dorsal plate. The image of the specimen was continuously taken with a CCD camera and displayed on a TV monitor. The load was increased at 60 s intervals, and the vertical distance between two predetermined marks on the specimen surface was measured

spinal columns taking care to keep the pia mater intact. The specimens were immediately placed in a physiological saline solution at room temperature (16 °C) until mechanical testing. All tests were accomplished within 30 min after the excision.

6.3.1.2 Tensile Test

For the tensile test, each spinal cord segment was cut into two pieces whose axial lengths were about 10 mm. One was the piece with the pia mater, and the other was the one whose pia mater had been carefully stripped off circumferentially under a microscope. Two small plastic plates (3 × 10 mm), each with a hook, were attached to the ventral and dorsal sides of the specimen with cyanoacrylate adhesive. Each specimen was then hung up with the hook of the ventral plate and was slightly elongated with a small load (0.32 g) on the dorsal plate. The image of the specimen was taken continuously with a CCD camera [OVM1000NM, Olympus, Japan] and displayed on a TV monitor (Fig. 6.3). The axial length (*lo*) and width (*wo*) of the specimen and vertical distance (*do*) between two predetermined marks on the specimen surface were measured on the TV monitor at the initial load. The load (*F*) was increased with 1.23 g (specimens with pia) or 0.49 g (specimens without pia), each at 60 s intervals, and the vertical distance between the marks (*d*) was measured at each loading immediately before the increment.

6.3.1.3 Calculation of the Elastic Modulus of the Pia Mater

The load–elongation (*F*–*d*) relationship of each specimen was converted into the stress–strain relationship using *lo, wo*, and *do*. Strain (λ) was calculated as the form of the stretch ratio:

$$\lambda = d / do.$$

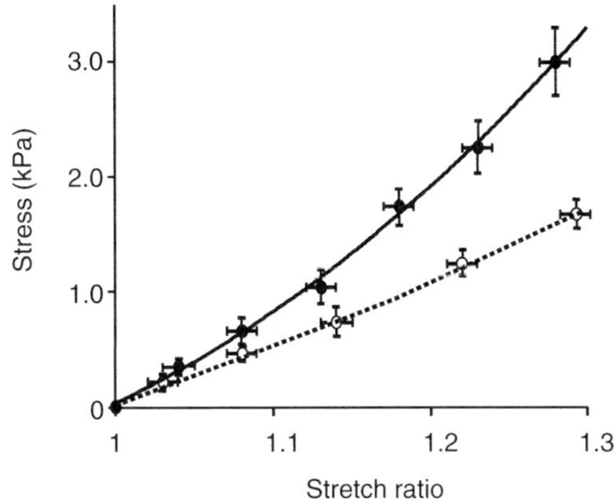

Fig. 6.4 Stress–strain curve was linear in the spinal cord without the pia mater. In contrast, the stress–strain relationship was nonlinear in the spinal cord with the pia mater, showing a concave upward curve that is commonly observed in connective tissue (*open circle*, spinal cord without pia; *filled circle*, spinal cord with pia; mean ± SEM)

Stress (σ) was obtained assuming incompressibility as follows:

$$\sigma = F\lambda / (wo\,lo).$$

Elastic moduli of specimens with the pia mater (*Eall*) and those of specimens without the pia mater (*Emed*) were obtained from the slope of the stress–strain curve. The mean thickness of the pia mater (*wpia*) was measured in histological sections of intact spinal cords.

The spinal cord parenchyma and pia mater were regarded as a composite material of the Voigt model. The elastic modulus of the composite material is a summation of the values of multiplication of the elastic moduli and volume ratio of each material. In other words, the elastic modulus of the whole spinal cord including the pia mater (*Eall*) depends on the elastic moduli of the pia mater and the spinal cord parenchyma and the ratio of their thickness. The apparent elastic modulus (*Eall*) can be expressed as follows according to the rule of mixtures:

$$Eall = Epia \cdot 2wpia / wo + Emed\left(1 - 2wpia / wo\right).$$

The elastic modulus of the pia mater (*Epia*), therefore, is given by the following equation:

$$Epia = \left\{Eall \cdot wo - Emed\left(wo - 2wpia\right)\right\} / \left(2wpia\right).$$

6.3.1.4 Results

The stress–strain relationship was approximately linear in spinal cord specimens without the pia mater. In contrast, this relationship was nonlinear in specimens containing the pia mater, demonstrating a concave upward curve similar to that commonly observed in connective tissue (Fig. 6.4).

The elastic moduli of spinal cords with and without the pia mater were 16 ± 5 and 5 ± 2 kPa, respectively. The presence of the pia mater increased the elastic modulus of the spinal cord threefold. The width of the spinal cord cross section was 5 ± 0.5 mm

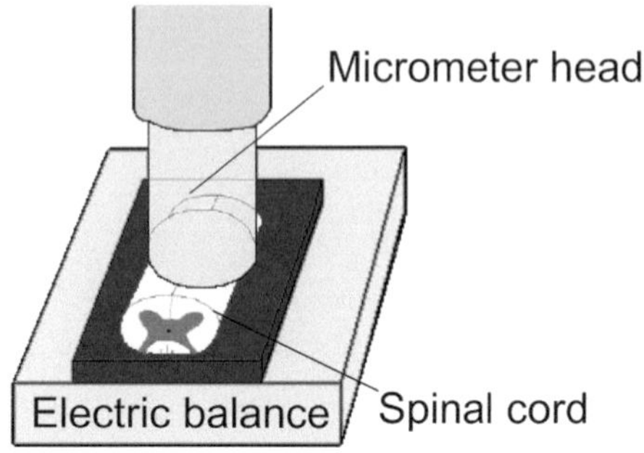

Fig. 6.5 Compression test of the spinal cord. A micrometer head compressed the specimen placed on an electric balance with a 50 μm increase at 60 s intervals. The load applied to the specimen was measured 30 s after every increase in compression

and the thickness of the pia mater was 12 ± 3 μm (five specimens). The elastic modulus of the pia mater was calculated to be 2,300 kPa, which was 460 times greater than that of the spinal cord without the pia mater.

6.3.2 Compression Test of the Spinal Cord with an Intact or Incised Pia Mater Stiffness of the Spinal Cord

6.3.2.1 Materials and Methods

Four Japanese white rabbits were used in this test. The method of specimen preparation was the same as that used for the tensile test. Each spinal cord segment was divided into two pieces for the compression test. In one piece, the pia mater was kept intact, and in the other it was incised longitudinally at both sides while viewed with a microscope. Each specimen was transferred into a Petri dish filled with physiological saline solution, which was then placed on an electrical balance (model AEG-220; Shimadzu Corp., Kyoto, Japan). The specimen was compressed using a micrometer head (model MHK-25V; Mitutoyo Corp., Kanagawa, Japan) with a 50 μm increase in compression at 60 s intervals (Fig. 6.5). The original measurement was obtained at the point at which the micrometer head touched the surface of the specimen. The load applied to the specimen was measured 30 s after every increase in compression. Stiffness, a parameter indicating the amount of mechanical resistance against a unit deformation, was calculated as the ratio of the load increment to the 50 μm increase in compression.

Specimens were fixed in 10 % neutral buffered formalin after the compression test. They were then dehydrated and embedded in paraffin. Sections 5 μm thick were obtained and stained with H&E. The morphological characteristics of the specimens were observed.

6.3.2.2 Results

There was no significant difference in stiffness between specimens with an intact pia mater and those with an incised pia at a compression less than 1 mm.

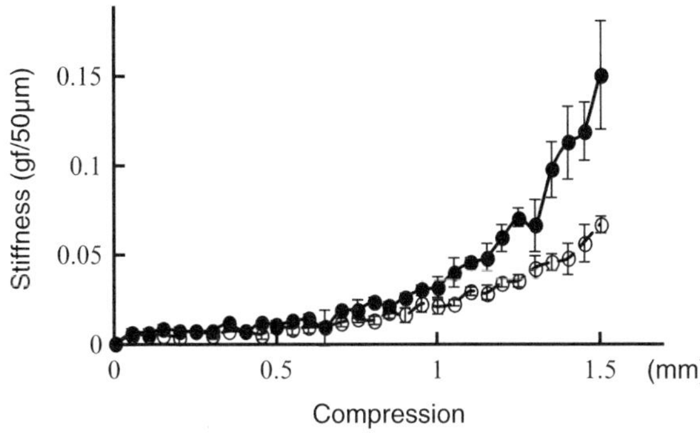

Fig. 6.6 The stiffness is shown as the ratio of the load increment to the increase of 50 μm deformation. No significant difference between the stiffness of specimens with the intact and incised pia mater was found at compression less than 1.00 mm. With an increase in the compression over 1.00 mm, the stiffness of the specimen with the intact pia mater increased significantly more than that of the one with the incised pia mater ($p<0.05$) (*open circle*, spinal cord with incised pia; *filled circle*, spinal cord with intact pia; mean ± SD)

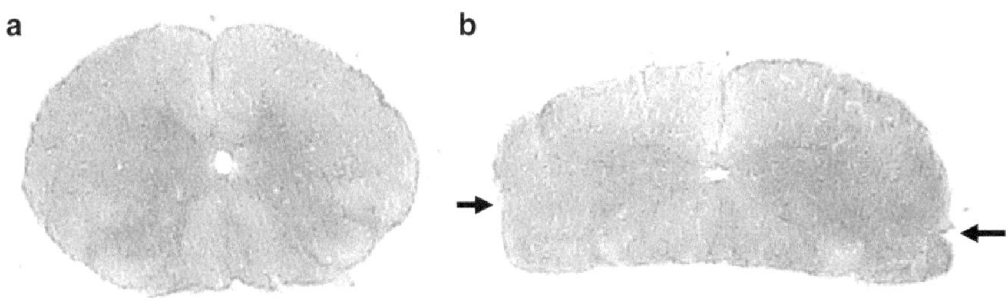

Fig. 6.7 The shape of the specimen with the intact pia mater was well restored after the removal of the compression on H&E-stained section (**a**), while the specimen with the incised pia mater remained in a deformed state (**b**). *Arrows* indicate places where the pia mater was cut at both sides of the specimen (×10)

At a compression greater than 1 mm, however, the stiffness of the specimen with the intact pia mater increased significantly more than the one with the incised pia mater ($p<0.05$) (Fig. 6.6).

A histological investigation revealed that the shapes of specimens with an intact pia mater were well restored after removal of the compression. In contrast, specimens with an incised pia mater remained deformed (Fig. 6.7).

6.3.3 *Discussion*

Our results demonstrated the following. The pia mater had an elastic modulus of 2,300 kPa, which was 460 times greater than that of the spinal cord parenchyma. By covering the parenchyma, it tripled the elastic modulus of the spinal cord as a whole.

The pia mater increased the stiffness of the spinal cord and enhanced its recovery of shape after removal of the compression.

Spinal pia mater consists of two layers: the intima pia (inner layer) and the epipial tissue (outer layer). The inner layer is a network of fine elastic fibers closely attached to spinal cord parenchyma. The outer layer is relatively thick and formed by a loose mesh of collagen fiber bundles that partially extends into the arachnoid trabeculae [10]. The elastic moduli of elastic and collagen fibers have been reported to be approximately 600 kPa and 1,000 MPa, respectively [11]. Accordingly, the elastic modulus of the pia mater, which measured 2,300 kPa in the present study, seems to depend mainly on the elasticity of the elastic fibers and partly on that of the collagen fibers.

Stiffness indicates the inflexibility of the spinal cord against compression; this is expressed as the ratio of the increment of the load to an increase in compression. When tissue is resistant to deformation, which is referred to as high stiffness, the load sharply increases as the compression increases. On the other hand, when tissue is easily deformed, referred to as low stiffness, the load gradually increases. The results of the present study verified that spinal cord containing an intact pia mater had greater stiffness. Thus, the pia mater is rigid enough to increase the overall stiffness of the spinal cord.

After the compression test, the shape of the spinal cord with an intact pia mater was well restored; however, the shape of the spinal cord with an incised pia mater scarcely recovered. This indicates that, as a result of being tightly covered by the pia mater, the compressed spinal cord contains a large amount of strain energy, which enables shape restoration after decompression.

6.4 Effect of the Tensile Stress on the Morphology of the Spinal Cord

The spinal cord is physiologically stretched along the craniocaudal axis and is subjected to tensile stress. Breig and el-Nadi [12] reported that the spinal canal decreases in length when the spine is extended and increases in length when the spine is flexed in human cadavers. The spinal cord adapts to these changes of length by elongating and shortening itself. Tensile stress in the spinal cord is produced by the stretching of the spinal cord.

In cervical myelopathy, the spinal cord is deformed according to compression as observed on CT myelograms and axial MR images. The cross-sectional area of the spinal cord decreases in response to compression and increases after surgery [13]. Although various mechanical factors regulating the morphology of the spinal cord have been studied, the influence of physiological tensile stress in the spinal cord has not been studied from the viewpoint of the morphological plasticity. The purpose of this study was to investigate the effect of the tensile stress on the morphology of the spinal cord under compression and decompression in rabbits.

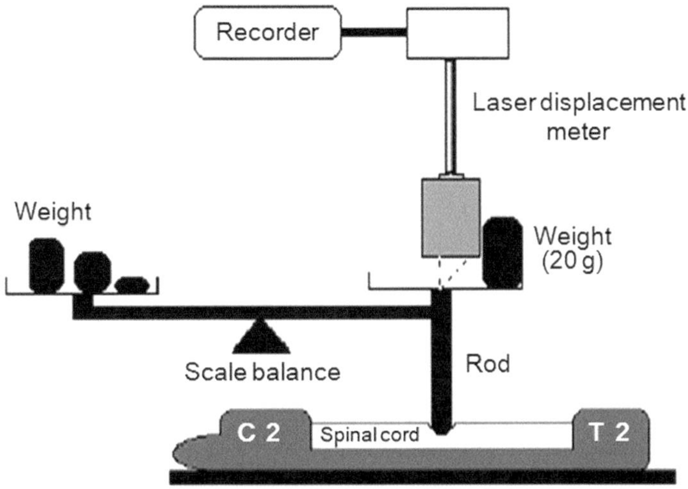

Fig. 6.8 Schematic drawing of the indentation test of the spinal cord. A rod of 5 mm in diameter was placed on the spinal cord. The rod was connected with a pan of a scale balance. Varying the weight on the other scalepan, the indentation of the rod on the spinal cord was measured with a laser displacement meter as a vertical displacement of the pan

6.4.1 Materials and Methods

Four Japanese rabbits were killed by intravenous injection of a high-dose pentobarbital. The spinal column and cord from C1 to T2 were excised from each rabbit. The specimens were maintained moist with a physiological saline solution during testing. Room temperature was kept at 18 °C.

All tests were accomplished within 40 min after the excision. The laminae and lateral masses between C3 and C7 were removed, and the specimen was put on the flat test table with the vertebral body down. After removal of the posterior half of the dura mater and the arachnoid membrane, the dentate ligaments and anterior and posterior rootlets were carefully dissected between C3 and C7. It was confirmed that the spinal cord on the spinal column did not adhere to the surrounding structure. A rod of 5 mm in diameter was placed on the midline of the spinal cord. The rod was connected with a pan of a scale balance (Fig. 6.8). Varying the weight on the other scalepan, the indentation of the rod on the spinal cord was measured as a vertical displacement of the pan using a laser displacement meter (LD-1100S-005, Ono Sokki, Tokyo, Japan) at C3/4 and C5 levels (2 points). The origin of the measurement was taken as the point before applying the load. The load on the spinal cord was increased from 0 to 1, 3, 5, 10, and 20 g and then decreased to 10, 5, 3, 1, and 0 g at 60 s intervals. The displacement was measured just before the load change. Then, the spinal cord was cut transversely and separated at C2/3 and C7/T1, and the

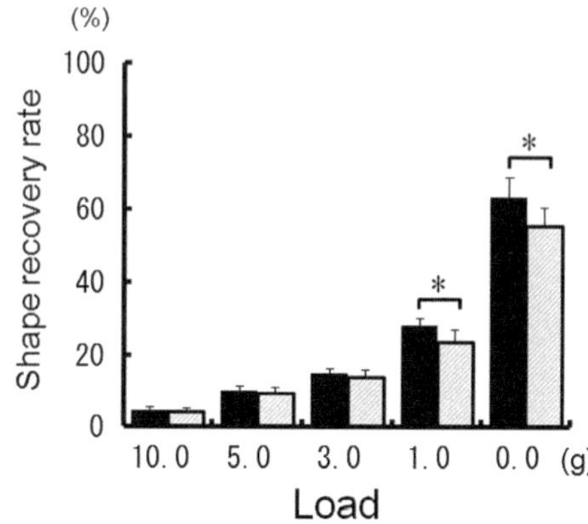

Fig. 6.9 Shape recovery rate after the separation (*shaded bar*) was significantly lower than that before the separation (*black bar*) at both 1 and 0 g ($n = 8$, mean ± SD, $*p < 0.05$)

longitudinal tensile stress was removed. The samples were measured again with the same protocol at 2 points 10 mm caudal to each premeasured point on the spinal cord so that the residual indentation of the spinal cord caused by the previous measurement did not affect the new measurement. The shape recovery rate was defined as the proportion of elastic recovery under unloaded condition to the maximum deformation as follows: a shape recovery rate (%) = (maximum indentation − residual indentation)/maximum indentation × 100.

The shape recovery rate of 100 % indicated a complete recovery to the original condition.

6.4.2 Results

The craniocaudal length of the spinal cord between C2/3 and C7/T1 was 55.5 ± 3.9 mm before the separation and 50.1 ± 3.8 mm after the separation. The spinal cord was shortened by 9.7 % after the separation ($p < 0.01$).

The recovery rate was not significantly different between the separated and unseparated cords until 3 g (Fig. 6.9). At the load of 1 g, the recovery rate was 28.0 ± 2.2 % before the separation and 23.6 ± 3.5 % after the separation. At the load of 0 g, the recovery rate was 63.1 ± 5.9 % before the separation and 55.5 ± 5.3 % after the separation. The recovery rate after the separation was significantly lower than that before the separation at both 1 and 0 g ($p < 0.05$).

6.4.3 Discussion

Reid [14] described that the length of the spinal dura mater and spinal cord was increased in flexion and that the average stretching between C2 and C5 was approximately 10 %. Kuwazawa et al. [15] reported that the mean elongation of the length of the cervical cord from extension to flexion was 11.7 mm in recumbent volunteers and 9.5 mm in erect volunteers on T2WI sagittal MR images. These values corresponded to 10.9 % and 8.9 % of the length in the extension position, respectively. In the present study, the spinal cord was placed in the straight position, and it was shortened by 10 % after the separation. This value was in agreement with the aforementioned studies.

We described the factors causing shape recoverability of the spinal cord after decompression in cervical myelopathy [16]. Shape recovery at an early stage after decompression may result from the movement of interstitial fluid from the periphery of the compressed site to the decompressed site. The spinal cord parenchyma exhibited viscoelasticity and an extremely low limit of elasticity [17]. This indicates that the shape recovery of the spinal cord after decompression cannot occur by itself. The shape recovery must thus be induced by the strain energy in the spinal cord, that is, the intramedullary pressure [18]. Iida and Tachibana [19] demonstrated that the spinal cord intramedullary pressure is increased by mechanical compression on the anterior structure of the spinal canal and stretching of the cord in canine studies. Therefore, the tensile stress in the spinal cord can increase the intramedullary pressure and enhance the shape recoverability of the spinal cord [20].

Conflict of Interest The authors declare that they have no conflict of interest.

References

1. Levine DN (1997) Pathogenesis of cervical spondylotic myelopathy. J Neurol Neurosurg Psychiatry 62:334–340
2. Ohashi T, Matsumoto T, Abe H et al (1997) Intramural distribution of local elastic moduli in bovine thoracic aorta measured by pipette aspiration method. Cellular Eng 2:12–18
3. Aoki T, Ohashi T, Matsumoto T et al (1997) The pipette aspiration applied to the local stiffness measurement of soft tissue. Ann Biomed Eng 25:581–587
4. Evans EA (1973) New membrane concept applied to the analysis of fluid shear and micropipette-deformed red cells. Biophys J 13:941–954
5. Sato M, Levesque MJ, Nerem RM (1987) An application of the micropipette technique to the measurement of the mechanical properties of cultured bovine aortic endothelial cells. J Biomech Eng 109:27–34
6. Kokubun S, Tanaka Y (1995) Type of cervical disc herniation and relation to myelopathy and radiculopathy. J Back Musculoskelet Rehabil 5:145–154
7. Panjabi MM, White AAШ (1988) Biomechanics of nonacute cervical spinal cord trauma. Spine 13:838–842
8. Breig A (1960) Biomechanics of the central nervous system: some basic normal and pathologic phenomena. Year Book Publishing, Chicago
9. Tunturi AR (1978) Elasticity of the spinal cord, pia, and denticulate ligament in the dog. J Neurosurg 48:975–979
10. Millen JW, Woollam DHM (1961) On the nature of the pia mater. Brain 84:514–520
11. Fung YC (1993) Biomechanics: mechanical properties of living tissues, 2nd edn. Springer, New York
12. Breig A, el-Nadi AF (1966) Biomechanics of the cervical spinal cord. Relief of contact pressure on and overstretching of the spinal cord. Acta Radiol Diagn 4:602–624

13. Ozawa H, Matsumoto T, Ohashi T et al (2004) Mechanical properties and function of the spinal pia mater. J Neurosurg Spine 1:122–127
14. Reid JD (1960) Effects of flexion-extension movements of the head and spine upon the spinal cord and nerve roots. J Neurol Neurosurg Psychiatry 23:214–221
15. Kuwazawa Y, Pope MH, Bashir W et al (2006) The length of the cervical cord: effects of postural changes in healthy volunteers using positional magnetic resonance imaging. Spine 31:E579–583
16. Bilston LE, Thibault LE (1996) The mechanical properties of the human cervical spinal cord in vitro. Ann Biomed Eng 24:67–74
17. Ozawa H, Matsumoto T, Ohashi T et al (2001) Comparison of spinal cord gray matter and white matter softness: measurement by pipette aspiration method. J Neurosurg 95(2 Suppl):221–224
18. Tachibana S, Kitahara Y, Iida H et al (1994) Spinal cord intramedullary pressure. A possible factor in syrinx growth. Spine 19:2174–2178
19. Iida H, Tachibana S (1995) Spinal cord intramedullary pressure: direct cord traction test. Neurol Med Chir (Tokyo) 35:75–77
20. Ozawa H, Matsumoto T, Ohashi T et al (2011) Stretch along the craniocaudal axis improves shape recoverability of the spinal cord. J Biomech 44:2313–2315

Chapter 7
Biomechanical Analysis of Compressive Myelopathy: The Influence of Morthometry of the Spinal Cord

Norihiro Nishida, Tsukasa Kanchiku, and Toshihiko Taguchi

Abstract Patients with cervical spondylotic myelopathy (CSM) vary according to the degree of spinal cord compression and the cross-sectional cord shape. We used a three-dimensional finite element method (3D-FEM) to analyze the stress distributions of the spinal cord under three cross-sectional cord morphometry. Experimental condition for the 3D-FEM spinal cord, anterior compression shape (central, lateral, and diffuse types), and invagination of the ligamentum flavum was established. The stress distribution in the spinal cord was increased by the pincer movement of ligamentum flavum and by the anterior compression of the spinal cord. The range of stress distribution observed for the diffuse type was also wider than for the central and lateral types. This simulation model showed that the clinical symptoms of CSM due to compression of the diffuse type may be stronger than for the central and lateral types. Therefore, careful follow-up is needed when there is anterior compression of the spinal cord with diffuse type.

Keywords Cervical spondylotic myelopathy • Dynamic factor • Finite element method • Pincer mechanism • Spinal cord morphometry

7.1 Introduction

Cervical spondylotic myelopathy (CSM) is spinal paralysis for cervical canal stenosis and instability or trauma. The neurologic dysfunction may initially be mild and associated with minimal disability; however, progressive spinal cord compression can lead to severe neurologic deterioration major disability. CSM manifests itself following static or dynamic compression of the spinal cord. Static factors include

N. Nishida (✉) • T. Kanchiku • T. Taguchi
Department of Orthopaedic Surgery, Yamaguchi University Graduate School of Medicine, 1-1-1 Minami-Kogushi, Ube, Yamaguchi 755-8505, Japan
e-mail: nishida3@yamaguchi-u.ac.jp

K. Uchida et al. (eds.), *Neuroprotection and Regeneration of the Spinal Cord*,
DOI 10.1007/978-4-431-54502-6_7,

developmental canal stenosis, bulging of the intervertebral disc posterior margin, and hypertrophy of the ligamentum flavum. Dynamic factors include invagination of the ligamentum flavum (buckling) and a pincer effect (anterior and posterior cord impingement) [1, 2] during neck extension. CSM is divided into tract symptoms due to white matter disorder and segmental failure by the gray matter disorder. These differ according to the degree of spinal cord compression and the cross-sectional cord shape [3, 4]. The latter factor was the basis of a study on myelopathy patients that classified cord morphology according to the deformity.

There have been several reports on the relationship between cross-sectional cord shapes and prognosis [3–7]. The spinal cord shape was classified into three general morphological types (central, lateral, and diffuse) by Fujiwara et al. [8].

The prognosis of CSM patients varies according to the morphometry of spinal cord compression. Nishida et al. used a three-dimensional finite element method (3D-FEM) to analyze the stress distribution in the spinal cord with neck extension and under three anterior compression shapes [9].

7.2 Analysis Using FEM of CSM

7.2.1 Spinal Cord Model and Extension Model

The 3D-FEM spinal cord model consisted of gray matter, white matter, and pia mater (Fig. 7.1). In order to simplify calculation in the model, the denticulate ligament, dura, nerve root, and blood were not included. The ligamentum flavum model also was established (Fig. 7.2). The shapes resulting from anterior compression on the spinal cord were classified as central type, lateral type, and diffuse type (Fig. 7.3).

The model simulated CSM under three shapes of anterior compression of the spinal cord, as well as dynamic compression under neck extension of the cervical spinal cord. The ligamentum flavum was located at the anterior surface of the cephalad lamina and at the superior margin of the caudal lamina.

The spinal cord consists of three distinctive materials referred to as white matter, gray matter, and pia mater. The mechanical properties (Young's modulus and Poisson's ratio) of the gray and white matter were determined using data obtained by the tensile stress strain curve and stress relaxation under various strain rates [10, 11]. The mechanical properties of pia mater and the ligamentum flavum were obtained from the literature [12, 13].

For the simulation of CSM under neck extension, the extension angle of the superior margin of spinal cord was 20°. Based on the assumption that the caudal vertebral body of the responsible lesion in CSM patients was stable, the bottom of the ligamentum flavum was constrained in all directions. The superior margin of the ligamentum flavum shifted distally according to the movement of cephalad lamina. The angle of neck extension and the direction in which the ligamentum flavum moved were obtained from each angle of C3–C4 kinematic MRI published by Iwabuchi et al. [14] (Fig. 7.4).

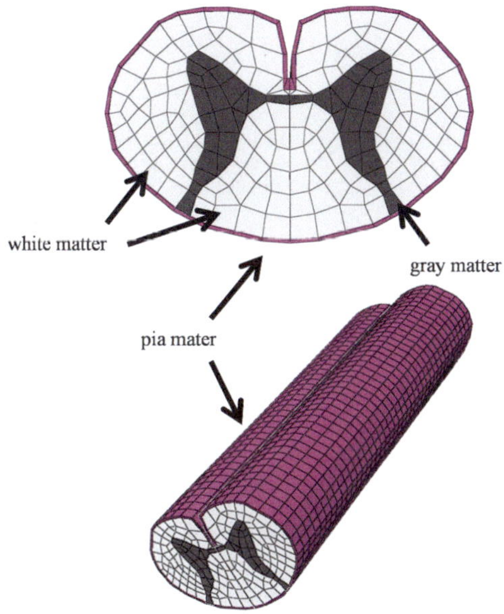

Fig. 7.1 The three-dimensional finite element method (3D-FEM) model of the spinal cord consisted of *gray* matter, *white* matter, and pia mater

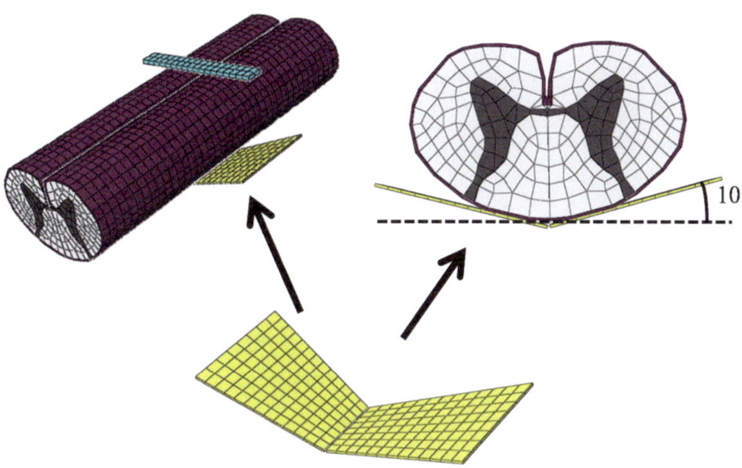

Fig. 7.2 The ligamentum flavum model was established using the rear of the spinal cord

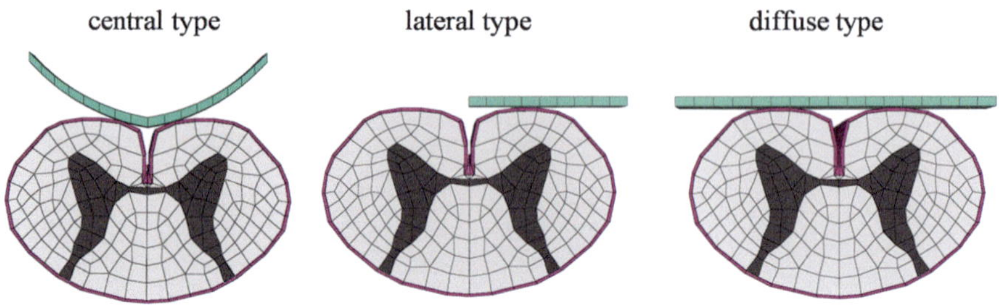

Fig. 7.3 The shapes for anterior compression of the spinal cord were central type, lateral type, and diffuse type

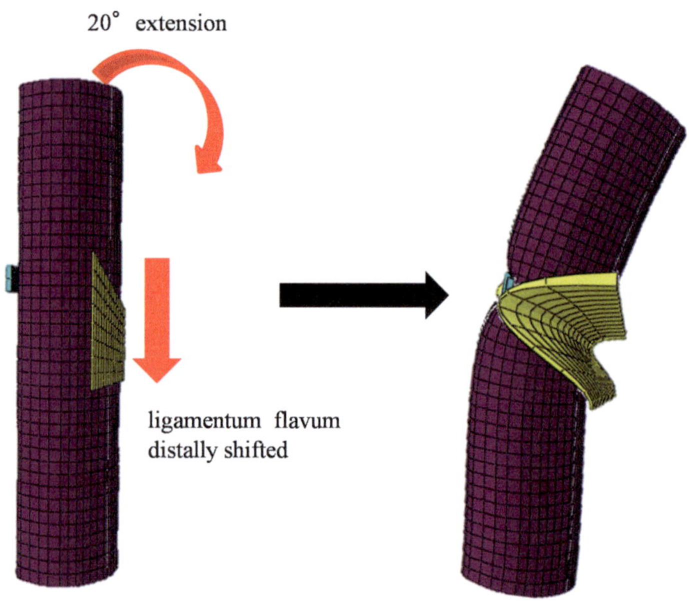

Fig. 7.4 For the simulation of neck extension, an extension of 20° was applied to the spinal cord. The ligamentum flavum moved distally in accordance with movement of the cephalad lamina

FEM analysis was conducted under each of the above conditions and in duplicate to test the reproducibility of results with this model.

7.2.2 Stress Distribution

When the shape of the spinal cord resulting from anterior compression was the central type, stress distributions were observed in the posterior horn and in parts of the posterior funiculus, lateral funiculus, and anterior horn beneath the invagination by ligamentum flavum. Under anteroposterior compression, high stress distributions were observed in the gray matter, anterior funiculus, and part of the lateral funiculus (Fig. 7.5a).

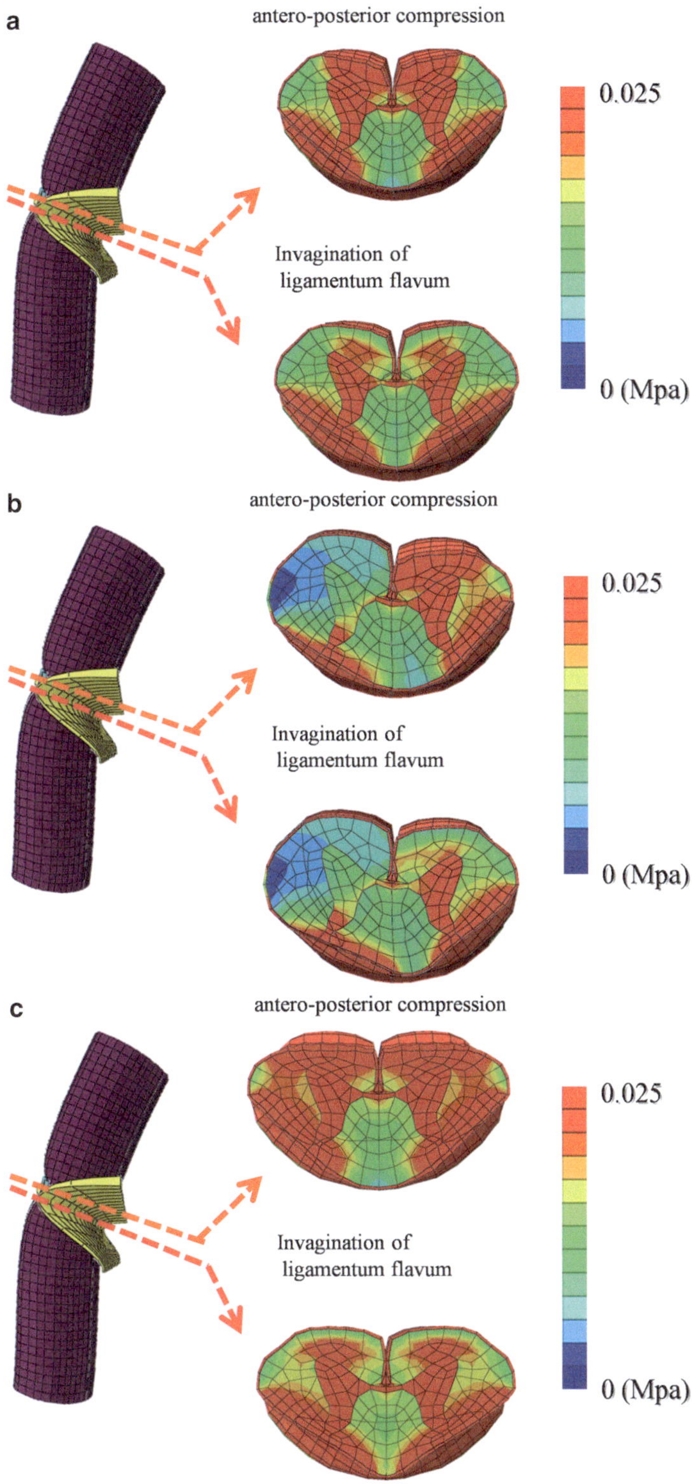

Fig. 7.5 Stress distributions under invagination of the ligamentum flavum and under anteroposterior compression are shown for the central-, lateral-, and diffuse-type shapes following anterior compression of the spinal cord (**a**–**c**)

When the shape of the spinal cord resulting from anterior compression was the lateral type, stress distributions were observed in the gray matter and lateral funiculus on the compression side, as well as parts of the posterior funiculus and posterior horn on the non-compression side beneath the invagination by ligamentum flavum. Under anteroposterior compression, high stress distributions were observed in the gray matter, anterior funiculus, and lateral funiculus on the compression side (Fig. 7.5b).

When the shape of the spinal cord resulting from anterior compression was the diffuse type, stress distributions were observed in the gray matter, lateral funiculus, and posterior funiculus beneath the invagination by ligamentum flavum. Under anteroposterior compression, high stress distributions were observed in the gray matter, anterior funiculus, lateral funiculus, and part of the posterior funiculus (Fig. 7.5c).

7.3 Discussion

Although it is the most common reason for spinal cord dysfunction in the elderly, CSM has no pathognomonic symptoms or physical signs. Because no single neurologic feature is unique to cervical myelopathy, diagnosis must be established by the affirmation of associated clinical signs and symptoms, in parallel with the exclusion of other clinical entities that may also show these signs.

CSM is a well-described clinical syndrome that can arise due to a combination of etiological factors. This clinical entity manifests itself following static or dynamic compression of the spinal cord, causing compression of the enclosed cord and leading to local tissue ischemia, injury, and neurologic impairment. Static factors include developmental canal stenosis, bulging of the intervertebral disc posterior margin, and hypertrophy of the ligamentum flavum. With regard to dynamic factors, the spinal cord of CSM patients is likely to be compressed during neck extension because of the protrusion of ligamentum flavum and intervertebral discs into the spinal canal (pincer mechanism) [2]. Recent developments in imaging have enabled closer examination of the cervical spine through improved CT and MRI. Using multidetector-row CT, Machino et al. reported narrowing of the spinal cord cross-sectional area during neck extension in patients with CSM [7]. In healthy individuals, Muhle et al. found that the subarachnoid space was smallest at extension compared to its size at mid-position and at flexion of the cervical spine. These workers also showed an increasing prevalence of functional cord impingement from the posterior aspect and from both the anterior and posterior aspects during neck extension in patients with advancing stages of degenerative disease of the cervical spine [15, 16].

With regard to morphological changes in the spinal cord, the symptoms of CSM patients differ according to the degree of spinal cord compression and the cross-sectional cord shape. Yu et al. reported that the severity of symptoms correlated with the degree of spinal cord deformity [5]. Kameyama et al. reported that a triangular-shaped spinal cord was associated with severe and irreversible pathological changes [3], while Shimomura et al. found this shape was associated with a more severe prognosis compared to oval-shaped or boomerang-shaped spinal cords [4]. The spinal cord shape was classified into three general morphological types (central, lateral, and diffuse) by Fujiwara et al. [8]. These authors reported that the prognosis of CSM patients with the diffuse-type shape was poorer than those with the central or lateral types.

In pathology-based studies, Ono et al. [17] and Ogino et al. [18] described how patients with severe myelopathy had spinal cord atrophy and also presented with extensive degeneration and infarction of the entire gray matter and white columns, except for the anterior funiculus. In the present analysis, stress distributions in the anterior funiculus were also increased. However, since this increase is not associated with any clinical symptoms or with apoptosis, the current results merely provide an estimate for the possible range of increased stress distribution at this site. Nevertheless, the observed morphometric pattern was similar to a prior clinical report, and hence these results may still be applicable to the clinical situation.

In the present study, stress distribution in the spinal cord was increased by the invagination of ligamentum flavum during neck extension. However, the range of stress distributions for the three types of anterior compression of spinal cord was not uniform (Fig. 7.5a–c). The range of stress distribution observed for the diffuse type was wider than for the central and lateral types.

In addition, stress distribution in the spinal cord was increased by the pincer movement of ligamentum flavum and by anterior compression of the spinal cord. However, in this situation, the range of stress distribution for the three types of anterior compression of the spinal cord was not uniform. The range of stress distribution under anteroposterior compression was also wider for the diffuse type compared to the central and lateral types. Moreover, the compressed spinal cord shape with diffuse type was a triangular shape and was supposed to be a severe prognosis.

7.4 Conclusion

The symptoms of CSM associated with diffuse type may therefore be stronger than for CSM with the central or lateral types. More careful follow-up is needed when the shape resulting from anterior compression of the spinal cord is the diffuse type.

References

1. Taylor AR (1953) Mechanism and treatment of spinal-cord disorders associated with cervical spondylosis. Lancet 1:717–720
2. Penning L (1961) Some aspects of plain radiography of the cervical spine in chronic myelopathy. Neurology 12:513–19
3. Kameyama T, Hashizume Y, Ando T et al (1995) Spinal cord morphology and pathology in ossification of the posterior longitudinal ligament. Brain 118:263–278

4. Shimomura T, Washimi M (2004) The natural course of cervical spondylotic myelopathy: follow-up of conservative treatment after admission. Rinsho-Seikeigeka 39(4):439–444
5. Yu YL, Stevens JM, Kandall B et al (1983) Cord shape and measurements in cervical spondylotic myelopathy and radiculopathy. Am J Neuroradiol 4:839–842
6. Hayashi H, Okada K, Hashimoto J et al (1988) Cervical spondylotic myelopathy in the aged patient. A radiographic evaluation of the aging changes in the cervical spine and etiologic factors of myelopathy. Spine 13:619–625
7. Machino M, Yukawa Y, Ito K et al (2011) Dynamic changes in dural sac and spinal cord cross-sectional area in patients with cervical spondylotic myelopathy. Spine 36(5):399–403
8. Fijiwara K, Yonenobu K, Hiroshima K et al (1986) The evaluation of viability of the spinal cord by CT myelography. Rinsho Seikei Geka 21:355–361 (Japan)
9. Nishida N, Kato Y, Imajo Y et al (2012) Biomechanical analysis of cervical spondylotic myelopathy: the influence of dynamic factors and morphometry of the spinal cord. J Spinal Cord Med 35(4):256–261
10. Ichihara K, Taguchi T, Yoshinori S et al (2001) Gray matter of the bovine cervical spinal cord is mechanically more rigid and fragile than the white matter. J Neurotrauma 18(3):361–367
11. Ichihara K, Taguchi T, Sakuramoto I et al (2003) Mechanism of the spinal cord injury and the cervical spondylotic myelopathy: new approach based on the mechanical features of the spinal cord white and gray matter. J Neurosurg 99(3 suppl):278–285
12. Tunturi AR (1978) Elasticity of the spinal cord, pia and denticulate ligament in the dog. J Neurosurg 48:975–979
13. Ueno H, Taguchi T, Toyoda K, Ichihara K, Kawai S, Kawano K (2002) Mechanical characteristic with the aging of the lumbar vertebrae ligamentum flavum. Seikeigeka to saigaigeka 51(4):367–369 (Japan)
14. Iwabuchi M, Kikuchi S, Yabuki S (2005) Kinematic MRI and preoperative evaluation in cervical spondylotic myelopathy. Rinsyo Seikeigeka 40(1):13–17 (Japan)
15. Muhle C, Wiskirchen J, Weinert D et al (1998) Biomechanical aspects of the subarachnoid space and cervical cord in healthy individuals examined with kinematic magnetic resonance imaging. Spine 23:556–567
16. Muhle C, Metzner J, Weinert D et al (1998) Classification system based on kinematic MR imaging in cervical spondylotic myelopathy. Am J Neuroradiol 19:1763–1771
17. Ono K, Ota H, Tada K et al (1977) Cervical myelopathy secondary to multiple spondylotic protrusions. A clinicopathologic study. Spine 2:109–125
18. Ogino H, Tada K, Okada K et al (1983) Canal diameter, anteroposterior compression ratio, and spondylotic myelopathy of the cervical spine. Spine 8:1–15

Chapter 8
Morphologic Change and Glial Response to Unilateral Spinal Cord Compression

Hiroshi Ozawa and Jianwu Zhao

Abstract In cervical myelopathy, unilateral compression of the spinal cord would be expected to produce Brown-Séquard syndrome. However, transverse lesion syndrome occurs in most clinical cases. In order to reveal the mechanism by which unilateral compression induces transverse damage to the spinal cord, damage of the gray and white matter in each half of the spinal cord was examined precisely using the density of reactive glial cells. The cervical spinal cord in rabbits was unilaterally compressed with a small screw. The area of each half of the damaged cord and the densities of GFAP-positive astrocytes and reactive microglias of the compressed and contralateral halves were investigated. As the compression increased, the area of the compressed half of the spinal cord decreased significantly compared to the contralateral half. The densities of GFAP-positive astrocytes in the gray matter and the anterior funiculus significantly increased in the compressed half. There were no significant differences in the densities at the lateral and dorsal funiculi between the compressed and contralateral halves. The tissue damage in the gray matter of the compressed half was markedly higher. These findings provide evidence for the mechanistic basis of spinal cord damage that leads to transverse lesion syndrome in unilateral compression myelopathy.

Keywords Astrocyte • Microglia • Transverse lesion syndrome • Unilateral spinal cord compression

H. Ozawa (✉)
Department of Orthopaedic Surgery, Tohoku University School of Medicine, 1-1 Seiryomachi, Aobaku, Sendai 980-8574, Japan
e-mail: hozawa@med.tohoku.ac.jp

J. Zhao
Department of Orthopaedics, Chian-Japan Union Hospital, Jilin University, Changchun 130033, China

K. Uchida et al. (eds.), *Neuroprotection and Regeneration of the Spinal Cord*, DOI 10.1007/978-4-431-54502-6_8, © Springer Japan 2014

8.1 Introduction

In cervical myelopathy due to chronic compression, the spinal cord is compressed either locally in cases of spondylosis and disc herniation or over its entire width in the cases of ossification of the posterior longitudinal ligament (OPLL) and spinal canal stenosis. The former type of compression is classified into median and unilateral compression [1–3]. Theoretically, unilateral compression of the spinal cord should produce a Brown-Séquard syndrome consisting of ipsilateral motor dysfunction and contralateral sensory disturbances below the level of the lesion. However, it clinically produces transverse lesion syndrome consisting of bilateral motor and sensory deficits of the lower limbs with almost equal severity in most cases [4–7]. This suggests that the unilateral compression exerts some mechanical effects on the contralateral side of the spinal cord as well as the compressed side.

The pathomechanisms of spinal cord injury and myelopathy have been investigated. Numerous pathophysiologies of myelopathy resulting from either compression of the entire width or the median compression of the spinal cord have been reported [8–10]. In these experiments, however, the full width of the spinal cord was compressed or, if locally compressed, the compression site was not controlled. There have been no models reported in which the spinal cord is compressed unilaterally with control of the site and severity. Further the pathophysiology of the contralateral side compared to the compressed side has not been described in a unilateral compression model [11].

In order to reveal the mechanism by which the unilateral compression induced the transverse damage to the spinal cord, damage of the gray and white matter in each half of the spinal cord was examined via quantitative assessment of the glial cells.

8.2 Materials and Methods

8.2.1 Spinal Cord Compression Model

The experiments were conducted on Japanese white rabbits weighing approximately 3,000 g (range 2,800–3,200 g). The rabbits were anesthetized with intravenous pentobarbiturate (25 mg/kg). Following exposure of the anterior aspect of C5 body, the body was perforated to the epidural space using a high-speed drill (2 mm in diameter) under a microscope. The hole was localized 2 mm to the right of the midline. A screw (2.1 mm in diameter) with a round tip was gradually driven through the hole to compress the spinal cord. For the appropriate evaluation of the proliferating glial cells, the screw was placed to protrude 2 mm into the spinal canal as mild compression and 3 mm as moderate compression. Three rabbits served as sham controls. They were examined for motor functions using Tarlov's rate of functional recovery [12] the next day and 1 week after the surgery.

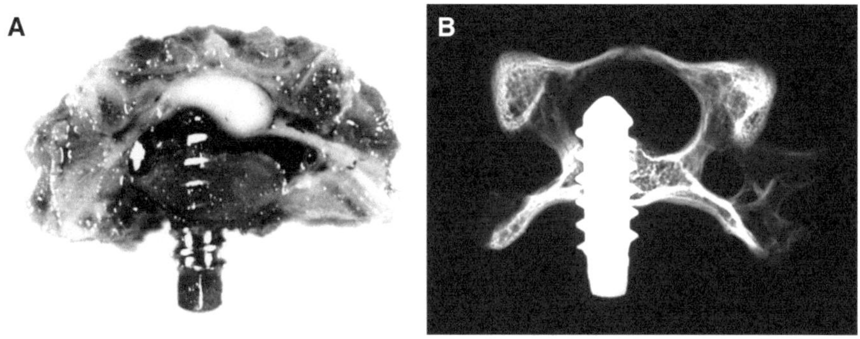

Fig. 8.1 (**a**) Transverse slab of the C5 vertebra and the spinal cord with the screw cut 3 mm in thickness, showing the deformation of the spinal cord by the unilateral compression. (**b**) Softex radiograph showing the position of the screw and the extent of compression

8.2.2 Tissue Preparation and Staining

Rabbits were sacrificed by the intravenous injection of a high dose of pentobarbiturate 1 week after the surgery for hematoxylin and eosins (HE), Kluver-Barrera (KB) medullary sheath staining, and GFAP immunohistostaining and 48 h after the surgery for RCA-1 immunohistostaining. The cervical spine and spinal cord were removed together with the screw in situ. The specimen was fixed in 10 % neutral-buffered formalin. The C5 vertebra was transversely cut above and below the screw with a diamond band saw to obtain a 3-mm-thick slab (Fig. 8.1a). A Softex radiograph of the slab was taken for the assessment of the position of the screw (Fig. 8.1b). The screw was then removed from the slab. Spinal cord specimens were taken out of the slabs and fixed in the same fixative, and sections 5 μm thick were obtained. The sections were stained by HE and KB medullary sheath staining for the observation of the axons and myelins and for the measurement of the area.

8.2.3 Measurement of Compression Rate

On the Softex radiographs of the transverse slabs of the C5 vertebrae with the screws, the areas of the protruding screws in the spinal canal and the areas of the spinal canals were measured using an image scanner and a personal computer with the software of the NIH image version 1.6. The ratio of the former to the latter was defined as "the compression rate."

8.2.4 Measurement of Gray and White Matter Area in Each Half of the Spinal Cord

On the slide of the KB medullary sheath staining, the spinal cord was divided into the compressed half and the contralateral half by the line of anterior median fissure and the posterior median sulcus through the central canal. The areas of the gray and white matter in each half of the spinal cord were measured using the image scanner interfaced with a computer.

8.2.5 Immunohistochemistry

Immunohistostaining of the astrocyte was carried out using an antibody to GFAP (polyclonal antibody; Dako, Glostrup, Denmark). Microglia were stained with an immunoperoxidase method using a lectin Ricinus communis agglutinin (RCA-1; Vector Laboratories, Burlingame, CA, USA) according to the method described by He and colleagues [13].

8.2.6 Count of Glial Cells

To count the GFAP-positive astrocytes, ten selected sections of the anterior and dorsal horns in the gray matter and the anterior, lateral, and dorsal funiculi in the white matter on the compressed and contralateral halves were determined on the GFAP staining slide; the center of each anterior and posterior horn section was defined as the midpoint of the line between the central canal and the tip of the anterior and dorsal horns. The center of each funiculus section was defined as the midpoint of the thickness of the funiculus. The section covered an area measuring 0.21×0.32 mm. The density of GFAP-positive astrocytes was calculated from the number of the cells in each section. The density of GFAP-positive astrocytes in the gray matter was defined as the average of the densities in the anterior and dorsal horns. The density of GFAP-positive astrocytes in the white matter was defined as the average of the densities in the anterior, lateral, and dorsal funiculi.

8.3 Results

The compression rate was defined by the ratio of the area of the protruding screw in the spinal canal to the area of the spinal canal. The compression rate was 17.1 ± 3.7 % (mean ± SD) in the mild compression group and 31.8 ± 3.2 % in the moderate compression group. The difference in the rate between the mild compression and moderate compression was considered extremely significant by unpaired *t*-test ($p < 0.0001$).

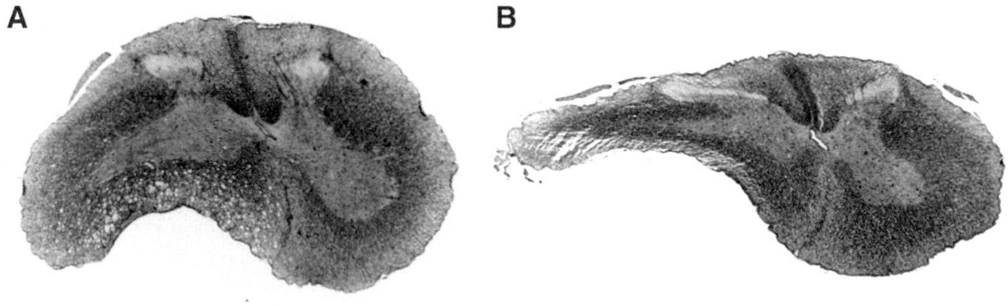

Fig. 8.2 The spinal cord was deformed into the shape of a reversed comma. The compressed half of the spinal cord was shaped like a boomerang and the contralateral half like a semicircle. The midline of the spinal cord, connecting the anterior median fissure to the posterior median sulcus through the central canal, was curved convexly to the contralateral half. (**a**) Under mild compression and (**b**) under moderate compression (Kluver-Barrera, ×10)

No apparent abnormal walking or movements of the upper and lower limbs were observed during the observation period of 1 week after surgery in rabbit (Tarlov rate 4).

8.3.1 Morphologic Change

In these animals, the spinal cord was deformed into the shape of a reversed comma. The compressed half of the spinal cord was shaped like a boomerang and the contralateral half like a semicircle. The midline of the spinal cord, connecting the anterior median fissure to the posterior median sulcus through the central canal, was curved convexly to the contralateral half. The anterior funiculus and the anterior horn were flattened in the compressed half (Fig. 8.2).

8.3.2 Area of Gray Matter and White Matter in Compressed Half and Contralateral Half

The area of each half of the spinal cord is shown in Table 8.1. The areas of both halves with moderate compression were significantly smaller than those in the sham animals ($p<0.001$), as were those associated with mild compression ($p<0.01$). Comparisons between the compressed and contralateral halves revealed no significant differences in surface areas following mild compression, whereas there were significant differences with moderate compression ($p<0.05$).

To analyze the reductions in the gray vs. white matter, the ratio of the gray matter to the white matter (gray/white matter) was calculated. However, via this approach, no significant differences in the ratios between the compressed and contralateral halves were found.

Table 8.1 Area and ratio of the gray matter to the white matter area (gray/white matter) under the compression (mean ± SEM)

	Compressed half		Contralateral half	
	Area	Gray/white matter	Area	Gray/white matter
Sham[a]	5.89 ± 0.17	0.30 ± 0.02		
Mild compression	5.06 ± 0.22	0.27 ± 0.02	5.29 ± 0.21	0.25 ± 0.01
Moderate compression	3.75 ± 0.31[b, c, e]	0.23 ± 0.03	4.32 ± 0.24[b, d]	0.24 ± 0.01

[a]Average of both halves of the spinal cord
[b]Significantly lower than sham ($p<0.001$)
[c]Significantly lower than the compressed half in mild compression ($p<0.001$)
[d]Significantly lower than the contralateral half in mild compression ($p<0.01$)
[e]Significantly lower than the contralateral half in moderate compression ($p<0.05$)

8.3.3 Astrocyte Response

The densities of GFAP-positive astrocytes of both halves under the moderate compression were significantly higher than those in sham animals ($p<0.001$ in the compressed half, $p<0.05$ in the contralateral half) (Fig. 8.3). The GFAP-positive glial density in the compressed half with moderate compression was significantly higher than seen with mild compression ($p<0.01$). Comparisons between the compressed and contralateral halves revealed that compressed half contained significantly higher GFAP-positive glial density than the contralateral half following either mild or moderate compression ($p<0.05$, $p<0.01$, respectively). As the compression increased, the density of GFAP-positive astrocytes increased markedly in the anterior horn of the compressed half (Fig. 8.4a).

In the dorsal horn, the density of the GFAP-positive glia of both halves with moderate compression was significantly higher than those in sham animals ($p<0.01$, $p<0.05$, respectively). Comparison of the two halves demonstrated no significant difference with mild compression; however, the glial density of the compressed half was significantly higher than that of the contralateral side under moderate compression ($p<0.01$) (Fig. 8.4b).

In the anterior funiculus, the GFAP-positive glial density in the two halves of the cord under mild and moderate compression was significantly higher than in the shams (each $p<0.01$). The glial density within the compressed half under the moderate compression was significantly higher than seen with mild compression ($p<0.01$). In contrast, the glial density within the contralateral half following moderate compression did not increase significantly compared to mild compression. Comparison of both halves of the spinal cord revealed no significant difference with mild compression; however, the glial density of the compressed half was markedly increased in comparison to the contralateral half following moderate compression ($p<0.05$) (Fig. 8.4c).

In the lateral funiculus, the GFAP-positive glial density within both halves of the spinal cord following mild and moderate compressions was significantly higher

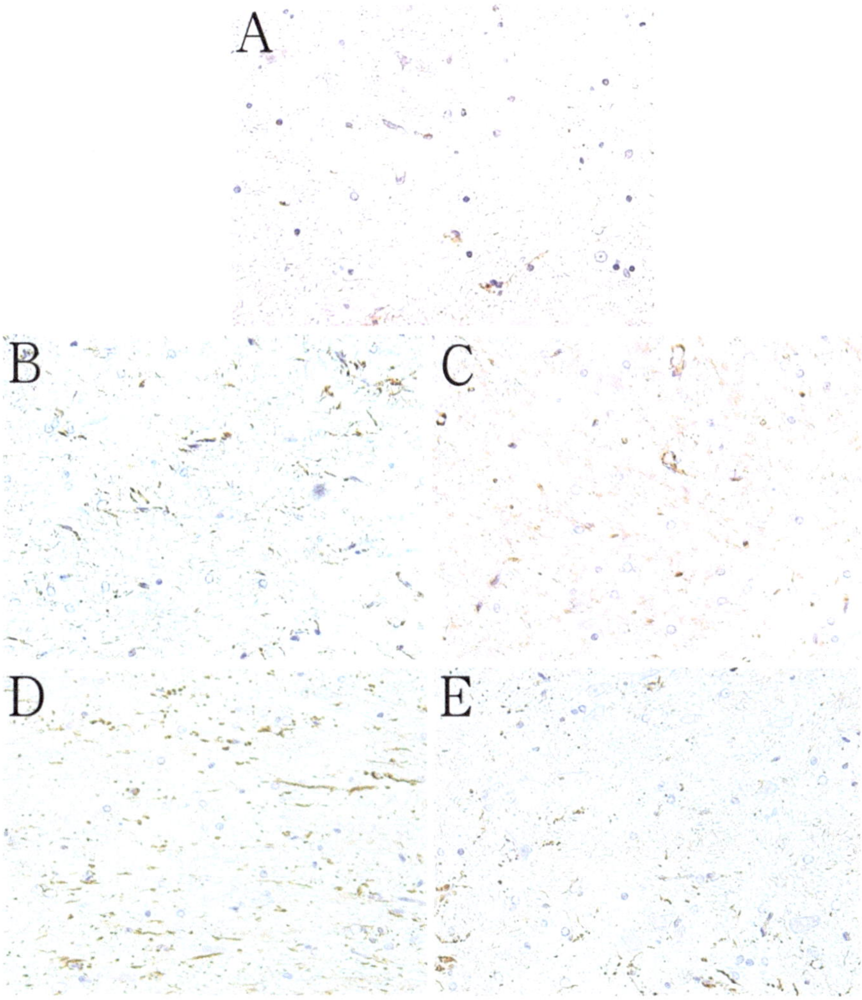

Fig. 8.3 Compared with the sham animals (**a**), extensive proliferation of GFAP-positive astrocytes in the anterior horn was seen in the compressed half (**b**) and the contralateral half (**c**) with mild compression and in the compressed half (**d**) and contralateral half (**e**) under moderate compression (GFAP stain, ×80)

than those in the sham animals (each $p<0.005$) (Fig. 8.5). Comparison of both halves of the spinal cord revealed no significant differences with the mild and moderate compression (Fig. 8.4d).

In the dorsal funiculus, the glial density in both halves under mild and moderate compression was significantly higher than in the shams (each $p<0.005$). There were no significant differences between either half of the cord following either mild or moderate compression (Fig. 8.4e).

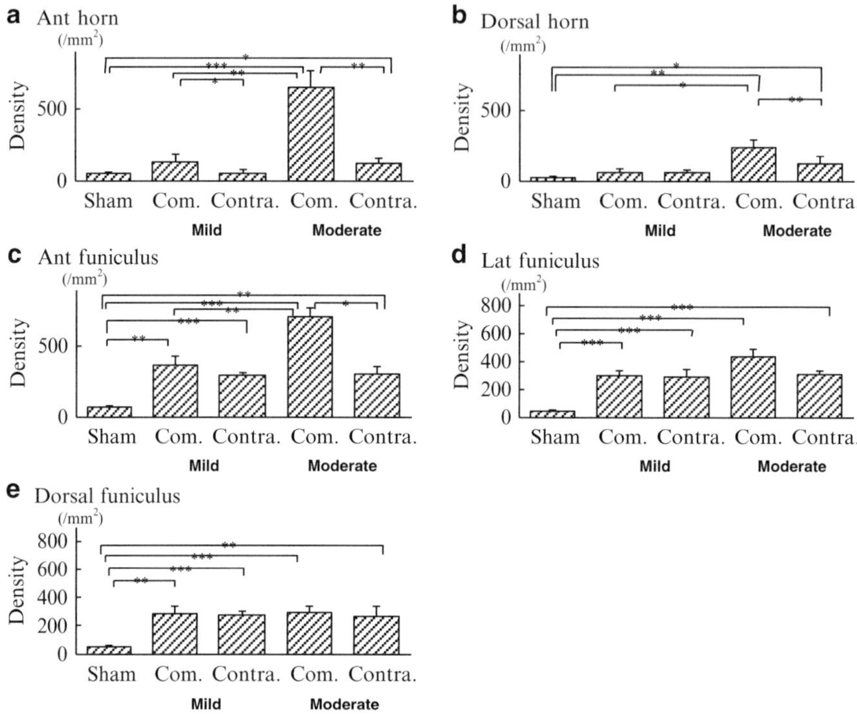

Fig. 8.4 The densities of GFAP-positive astrocytes increased in the two halves of the unilaterally compressed spinal cord. The density markedly increased in the *gray* matter and the anterior funiculus in the compressed half (Com.) compared with the contralateral half (Contra.) according to the increase in the compression. The differences in densities at the lateral and dorsal funiculi were not significant between the two halves of the spinal cord. (**a**) Anterior horn. (**b**) Dorsal horn. (**c**) Anterior funiculus. (**d**) Lateral funiculus. (**e**) Posterior funiculus (***$p<0.001$, **$p<0.01$, *$p<0.05$)

8.3.4 Relationship Between Area and Density of GFAP-Positive Astrocytes

The relationship between the area and the density of GFAP-positive astrocytes in the gray and white matter is shown in Fig. 8.6. Based upon the area reduction, the density of the compressed half increased more than that of the contralateral half in both the gray and white matter. Analyses of covariance (ANCOVA) were carried out to evaluate the influence of the compression on the variable density of GFAP-positive astrocytes in the gray and white matter independently of the area reduction. The densities of GFAP-positive astrocytes in the gray and white matter were entered as a dependent measure. The side of compressed or contralateral in the spinal cord

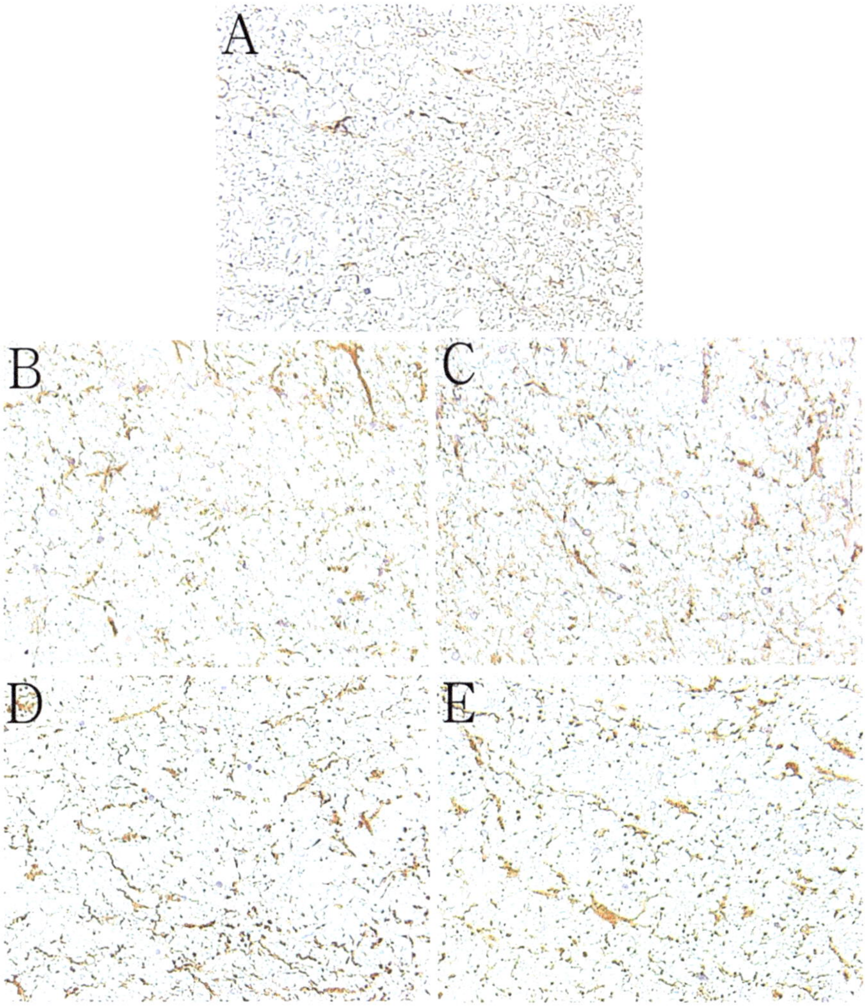

Fig. 8.5 Compared with the sham animals (**a**), extensive proliferations of GFAP-positive astrocytes at the lateral funiculus were seen in the compressed half (**b**) and the contralateral half (**c**) under mild compression and in the compressed half (**d**) and contralateral half (**e**) under moderate compression (GFAP stain, ×80)

was entered as a fixed variable, and the areas of gray and white matter were entered as covariate. The density of GFAP-positive astrocytes in the compressed half was significantly higher than that of the contralateral half in both the gray ($p<0.05$) and white matter ($p<0.05$). GFAP-positive astrocytes proliferated in the compressed half more than in the contralateral half of the unilaterally compressed spinal cord independent of the area reduction.

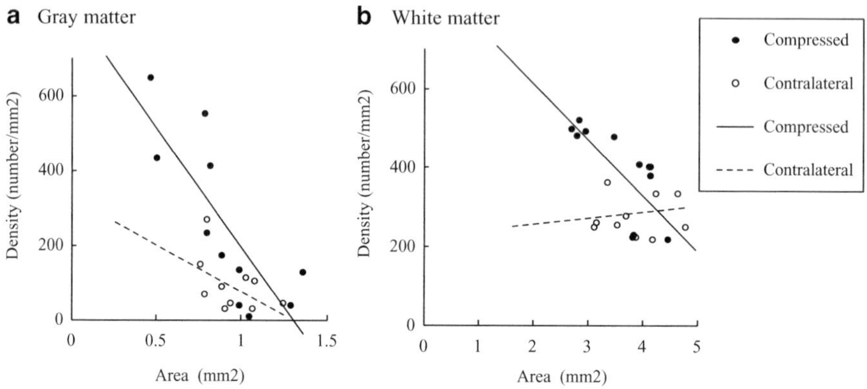

Fig. 8.6 Relationship between the area and the density of GFAP-positive astrocytes in the *gray* and *white* matter. Based on the area of reduction, the density of the compressed half increased more than that of the contralateral half in the gray and white matter. The density of GFAP-positive astrocytes in the compressed half was significantly higher than that of the contralateral half in the *gray* ($p<0.05$) and *white* matter ($p<0.05$) independently of the area reduction by ANCOVA. (**a**) *Gray* matter, (**b**) *white* matter

8.3.5 *Microglia Response*

Microglia were classified morphologically into resting and reactive microglia based on the RCA-1-positive structures observed by a light microscopy. The resting microglia have long finely branched processes from mainly opposite poles of the perinuclear cytoplasm. The reactive microglia have shortened and thickened processes that extend in all directions from enlarged cytoplasms.

In the sham group, resting microglia with long finely branched processes from perinuclear cytoplasms were observed adjacent to neurons in the gray matter more than in the white matter in the lectin RCA-1 immunostaining. No reactive microglia was found in both gray and white matters.

In the mild compression group, the mild proliferation of reactive microglia, which have shortened and thickened processes that extend in all directions from enlarged cytoplasms, was observed in the anterior horn of the compressed half of the spinal cord. In contrast, only a few reactive microglia were observed in the anterior horn of the contralateral half. No reactive microglia was found in the white matters on both halves (Fig. 8.7).

The numbers of resting and reactive microglia in the sham and mild compression groups are shown in Table 8.2. There was no significant difference in the total numbers of resting and reactive microglia in the gray and the white matters between the sham and mild compression groups 48 h after the surgery. Reactive microglia in the anterior horn of the compressed half, however, increased significantly compared to the other areas and it was not observed in the white matter.

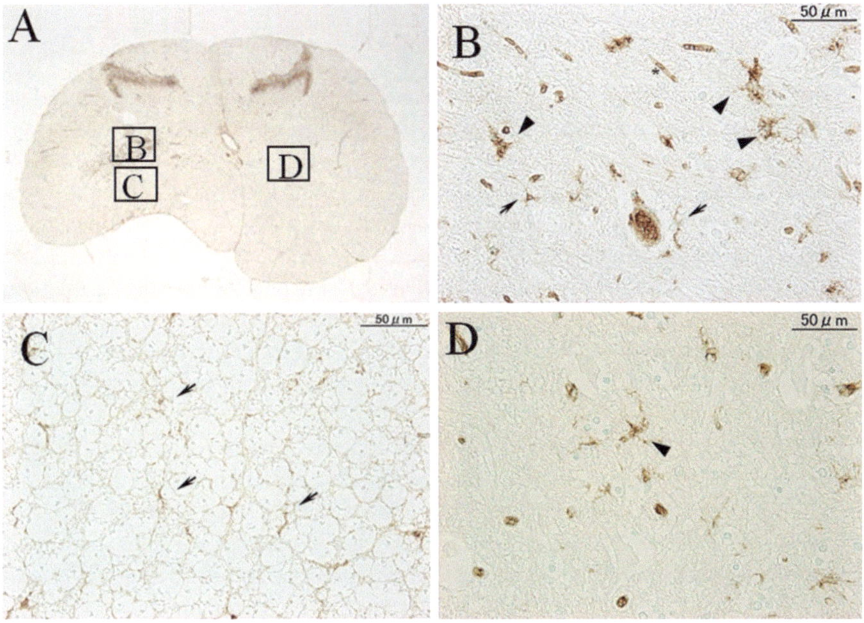

Fig. 8.7 In the deformed spinal cord under mild compression (**a**), reactive microglias (*arrowhead*) and resting microglias (*arrow*) were observed in the anterior horn of the compressed half (**b**). *Asterisks* show some of RCA-positive vascular vessels. No reactive microglia was found in the white matter of the compressed half (**c**). A few reactive microglias (*arrowhead*) were observed in the anterior horn of the contralateral half (**d**) (RCA-1 stain, ×200)

Table 8.2 The numbers of resting and reactive microglia in the mild compression and sham groups (mean ± SD)

		Mild compression			Sham[a]
		Resting	Reactive	Total	Resting
Compression side (right side)	Anterior horn	18.8 ± 5.9	10.8 ± 3.3[b]	29.6 ± 3.3	31.0 ± 2.8
	Dorsal horn	25.2 ± 4.9	3.8 ± 3.8	29.0 ± 1.9	32.5 ± 3.5
	Anterior funiculus	14.6 ± 0.5	0 ± 0	14.6 ± 0.5	17.5 ± 0.7
	Lateral funiculus	14.8 ± 0.8	0 ± 0	14.8 ± 0.8	16.0 ± 1.4
	Dorsal funiculus	15.8 ± 2.0	0 ± 0	15.8 ± 2.0	14.5 ± 0.7
Contralateral side (left side)	Anterior horn	26.8 ± 4.8	2.6 ± 2.2	29.4 ± 3.1	31.0 ± 4.2
	Dorsal horn	29.2 ± 2.0	0.2 ± 0.4	29.4 ± 2.1	29.5 ± 0.7
	Anterior funiculus	14.8 ± 1.3	0 ± 0	14.8 ± 1.3	17.0 ± 1.4
	Lateral funiculus	16.6 ± 1.8	0 ± 0	16.6 ± 1.8	16.6 ± 0.0
	Dorsal funiculus	15.8 ± 1.1	0 ± 0	15.8 ± 1.1	16.0 ± 1.4

[a]No reactive microglia was found in any area in the sham group

[b]Significantly higher than the dorsal horn of the compression side and anterior and dorsal horn of contralateral side ($p < 0.01$)

8.4 Discussion

To date, there have been several pathologic studies of cervical spondylotic myelopathy. Ito and colleagues have described neuropathologies of seven patients with various degrees of severity of cervical spondylotic myelopathy who were autopsied [14]. They concluded that there was a common pattern of lesion progression in cervical spondylotic myelopathy with atrophy and neuronal loss in the anterior horn and intermediate zones developing first, followed by degeneration of the lateral and posterior funiculi. Extensive destructive change such as axonal loss, myelin destruction, and cavity formation in the degenerating spinal cord was observed in the terminal stages of this progression. Our model most likely corresponds to the latent stage of paralysis and reveals the histological changes that are associated with myelopathy in patients with unilateral compression of the cervical spinal cord.

Proliferation of GFAP-positive astrocytes is considered as the hallmark of the CNS response to neural injury. GFAP is useful to detect the gliotic response in ischemic brain injury [15, 16] and assess the damage in neurotoxic brain injury [17]. In this study, the intensity of GFAP immunoreactivity was correlated with the severity of the compression not only at the site of compression but also at rostral and caudal points [18]. It is therefore reasonable to assume that increased numbers of GFAP-positive astrocytes can serve as an indicator of tissue injury in CNS. This assumption, however, must be evaluated in relation to any potential reduction in the issue area. The results of ANCOVA performed to evaluate the GFAP-positive astrocyte proliferation independent of the area reduction clearly demonstrated that GFAP-positive astrocytes proliferated in the compressed half more than in the contralateral half of the unilateral compressed spinal cord.

Microglias, one of the inflammatory cells in the CNS, are rapidly activated in response to any CNS insult. Microglial activation occurs as a graded response, characterized by their transformation into phagocytic cells with macrophage-like morphology (reactive microglia) and proliferation [19]. In the present study, the distribution of GFAP-positive astrocytes in the unilateral spinal compression corresponded to that of reactive microglia. Microglia respond more rapidly than any other cells to a variety of injuries in the CNS [20]. The microglial reaction precedes the astroglial reaction by release of astroglia-stimulating factors [21] and macrophage migration inhibitory factor [22], which increase astrocytic glutamine synthetase and GFAP immunoreactivity and promote reactive astrocytosis. These studies account for the analogy between the distributions of the reactive microglia and the GFAP-positive astrocytes in the present study.

In the present study, damage occurred even in the contralateral half of the unilaterally compressed spinal cord due to the mechanical stress exerted from the compressed half of the spinal cord. Using a finite element analysis model (FEM) of unilateral spinal cord compression, the stress concentration at the gray matter of the compressed half was markedly higher than that of the contralateral half. In contrast, equivalent stress concentrations were shown in the lateral funiculus of both halves [23]. The density of GFAP-positive astrocytes reported in the present study was compatible with the stress distributions predicted from the FEM. The observed discrepancy in the histological reaction between the anterior horn and the lateral funiculus of the two halves is most likely linked to differences in the stress concentration.

In compression myelopathy, neurological symptoms and signs theoretically depend on the site and severity of the compression. The compression of only a half of the spinal cord should present a pure Brown-Séquard syndrome. However, only 23 % of 129 paramedian herniation cases with cervical myelopathy presented Brown-Séquard syndrome, whereas the remaining 77 % presented transverse lesion syndrome. The majority of patients with transverse lesion syndrome revealed the ipsilateral predominant palsy of the same upper limb as the compressed side of the spinal cord and bilateral motor and sensory deficits of the lower limbs that were equivalent [7]. Based on the density of GFAP-positive astrocytes in the unilateral compressed spinal cord, the damage in the gray matter of the compressed half was significantly higher than that of the contralateral half, whereas the damage at the lateral funiculus, where the lateral pyramidal and the dorsal spinocerebellar tracts are located, and the dorsal funiculus did not show significant differences between the compressed and contralateral halves. These findings provide evidence for the mechanistic basis of spinal cord damage that leads to transverse lesion syndrome in unilateral compression myelopathy.

8.5 Conclusion

Under the unilateral compression, the density of GFAP-positive astrocytes in the gray matter and the anterior funiculus increased significantly in the compressed half compared to the contralateral half of the spinal cord. The densities in the lateral and dorsal funiculi, however, were not significant differences between the both halves. The distribution of GFAP-positive astrocytes in the unilateral spinal compression corresponded to that of reactive microglia. These findings provide evidence for the mechanistic basis by which unilateral compression induces transverse damage to the spinal cord.

Conflict of Interest The authors declare that they have no conflict of interest.

References

1. Brain W, Northfield D, Wilkinson M (1952) The neurological manifestations of cervical spondylosis. Brain 75:187–225
2. Hinck VC, Sachdev NS (1966) Developmental stenosis of the cervical spinal canal. Brain 89:27–36
3. Fujiwara K, Yonenobu K, Ebara S et al (1989) The prognosis of surgery for cervical compression myelopathy. An analysis of the factors involved. J Bone Joint Surg Br 71:393–398
4. Crandall PH, Batzdorf U (1966) Cervical spondylotic myelopathy. J Neurosurg 25:57–66

5. Jabbari B, Pierce JF, Boston S et al (1977) Brown-Séquard syndrome and cervical spondylosis. J Neurosurg 47:556–560
6. Finelli PF, Leopold N, Tarras S (1992) Brown-Séquard syndrome and herniated cervical disc. Spine 17:598–600
7. Kokubun S, Tanaka Y (1995) Type of cervical disc herniation and relation to myelopathy and radiculopathy. J Back Musculoskelet Rehabil 5:145–154
8. Hashizume Y, Iijima S, Kishimoto H et al (1984) Pathology of spinal cord lesions caused by ossification of the posterior longitudinal ligament. Acta Neuropathol (Berl) 63:123–130
9. Harkey HL, Al-Mefty O, Marawi I et al (1995) Experimental chronic compressive cervical myelopathy: effects of decompression. J Neurosurg 83:336–341
10. Uchida K, Baba H, Maezawa Y et al (1998) Histological investigation of spinal cord lesions in the spinal hyperostotic mouse (twy/twy): morphological changes in anterior horn cells and immunoreactivity to neurotropic factors. J Neurol 245:781–793
11. Ozawa H, Wu ZJ, Tanaka Y et al (2004) Morphologic change and astrocyte response to unilateral spinal cord compression in rabbits. J Neurotrauma 21:944–955
12. Tarlov I, Klinger H (1954) Spinal cord compression studies 2. Time limits for recovery after acute compression in dogs. AMA Arch Neurol Psych 71:271–290
13. He BP, Strong MJ (2000) A morphological analysis of the motor neuron degeneration and microglial reaction in acute and chronic in vivo aluminum chloride neurotoxicity. J Chem Neuroanat 17:207–215
14. Ito T, Oyanagi K, Takahashi H et al (1996) Cervical spondylotic myelopathy. Clinicopathologic study on the progression pattern and thin myelinated fibers of the lesions of seven patients examined during complete autopsy. Spine 21:827–833
15. Schmidt-Kastner R, Szymas J, Hossmann KA (1990) Immunohistochemical study of glial reaction and serum-protein extravasation in relation to neuronal damage in rat hippocampus after ischemia. Neuroscience 38:527–540
16. Norenberg MD (1994) Astrocyte responses to CNS injury. J Neuropathol Exp Neurol 53:213–220
17. O'callaghan JP (1991) Assessment of neurotoxicity: use of glial fibrillary acidic protein as a biomarker. Biomed Environ Sci 4:197–206
18. Farooque M, Badonic T, Olsson Y et al (1995) Astrocytic reaction after graded spinal cord compression in rats: immunohistochemical studies on glial fibrillary acidic protein and vimentin. J Neurotrauma 12:41–52
19. Kreutzberg GW (1996) Microglia: a sensor for pathological events in the CNS. Trends Neurosci 19:312–318
20. Gehrmann J, Matsumoto Y, Kreutzberg GW (1995) Microglia: intrinsic immuneffector cell of the brain. Brain Res Brain Res Rev 20:269–287
21. Giulian D, Young DG (1986) Brain peptides and glial growth II. Identification of cells that secrete glia-promoting factors. J Cell Biol 102:812–820
22. Koda M, Nishio Y, Hashimoto M et al (2004) Up-regulation of macrophage migration-inhibitory factor expression after compression-induced spinal cord injury in rats. Acta Neuropathol 108:31–36
23. Ozawa H, Kokubun S, Ohashi T et al (2002) Biological and biomechanical analysis of the response to unilateral spinal cord compression. J Jpn Orthop Assoc 76:S940 (In Japanese)

Chapter 9
Morphological Changes in Anterior Horn Cells, Immunoreactivity to Neurotrophic Factors, and Neuronal Cell Death of Spinal Cord Lesions in the Spinal Hyperostotic Mouse (*twy/twy*) with Chronic Mechanical Cord Compression

Kenzo Uchida, Hideaki Nakajima, Shoei Furukawa, Tomoo Inukai, Yasuhisa Maezawa, and Hisatoshi Baba

Abstract We examined the morphology of spinal accessory motoneurons, immunoreactivity to brain-derived neurotrophic factor (BDNF) and neurotrophin (NT)-3, and reactive astrocytosis in 70 tiptoe-walking Yoshimura (*twy/twy*) mice that develop calcification at C1–C2 vertebral level compressing the spinal cord. At the level of compression, the area of neuronal soma, total length of dendrites, and numbers of wheat germ agglutinin-horseradish peroxidase (WGA-HRP)-labeled accessory motoneurons decreased significantly. Rostral to the compressive lesion, opposite findings were evidenced; enhanced BDNF and NT-3 immunoreactivities were evident in the anterior horn cells, increasing in response to a more severe degree of compression, with larger population of BDNF-positive astrocyte-like cells.

Our results suggest increased functional activity of anterior horn cells at levels rostral to the site of compression. We speculate that the presence of BDNF and NT-3 in neurons and astrocyte-like cells is proportionate to the severity of chronic mechanical compression and may contribute to the heterotropic neuronal reserve and survival. The numbers of TUNEL-positive neurons in the gray matter and oligodendrocytes in the white matter of the spinal cord of the *twy/twy* mouse increased with progressive mechanical compression.

K. Uchida (✉) • H. Nakajima • T. Inukai • Y. Maezawa • H. Baba
Department of Orthopaedics and Rehabilitation Medicine, Faculty of Medical Sciences, University of Fukui, Matsuoka Shimoaizuki 23-3, Eiheiji, Fukui 910-1193, Japan
e-mail: kuchida@u-fukui.ac.jp

S. Furukawa
Laboratory of Molecular Biology, Gifu Pharmaceutical University, Mitahora-higashi, Gifu 502-0002, Japan

K. Uchida et al. (eds.), *Neuroprotection and Regeneration of the Spinal Cord*, DOI 10.1007/978-4-431-54502-6_9, © Springer Japan 2014

Keywords Anterior horn cell • Apoptosis • Neurotrophins • Spinal accessory motoneuron • Tiptoe-walking Yoshimura (*twy/twy*) mouse

9.1 Introduction

We have previously documented that a 40–50 % reduction in the transverse area of the cervical cord represents the critical threshold for favorable postoperative neurological recovery [1, 2]. Chronic compression of the spinal cord results in atrophy and loss of anterior horn cells associated with irreversible spinal cord damage [3–5]. Clinically, however, even in cases with severe compression detected on radiological examination, decompression may result in favorable recovery from a profound paresis. This unexpected outcome may be explained by the survival of a group of motoneurons even in the presence of considerable mechanical compression [1, 2].

In order to elucidate the mechanisms of neuronal reserve and survival of anterior horn cells, we used the tiptoe-walking Yoshimura (*twy/twy*) mouse, a model of spinal cord compression [6]. We examined morphological changes in spinal accessory motoneurons, expression of brain-derived neurotropic factor (BDNF) and neurotrophin (NT)-3 [7], and neuronal cell death [8], which have been used as markers of motoneuron survival and neuronal plasticity [9–11].

9.1.1 Topographic Morphology of Wheat Germ Agglutinin-Horseradish Peroxidase-Labeled Spinal Accessory Motoneurons

Representative photomicrographs showing WGA-HRP-labeled accessory motoneurons in the medial cell pool of the ICR and *twy* mice are shown in Fig. 9.1, and results of morphological analysis of these motoneurons are summarized in Table 9.1. At sites A and B of the *twy* mice, the mean area of the neuron soma was significantly larger than in ICR mice ($P<0.05$), where the proportion of the number of WGA-HRP-labeled motoneurons at site C, the compression level, was significantly lower. The total length of dendrites at sites A and B was significantly longer than in the corresponding levels of ICR mice ($P<0.05$).

9.1.2 Three-Dimensional Computerized Display of Spinal Accessory Motoneurons

In the *twy* mice, at site B, the level immediately rostral to the compressive lesion, the elongated dendrites extended rostrally and ventrally as if the motoneuron avoided posterior compression (*arrow*, Fig. 9.2c). At site C dendrites were shorter (Fig. 9.2d)

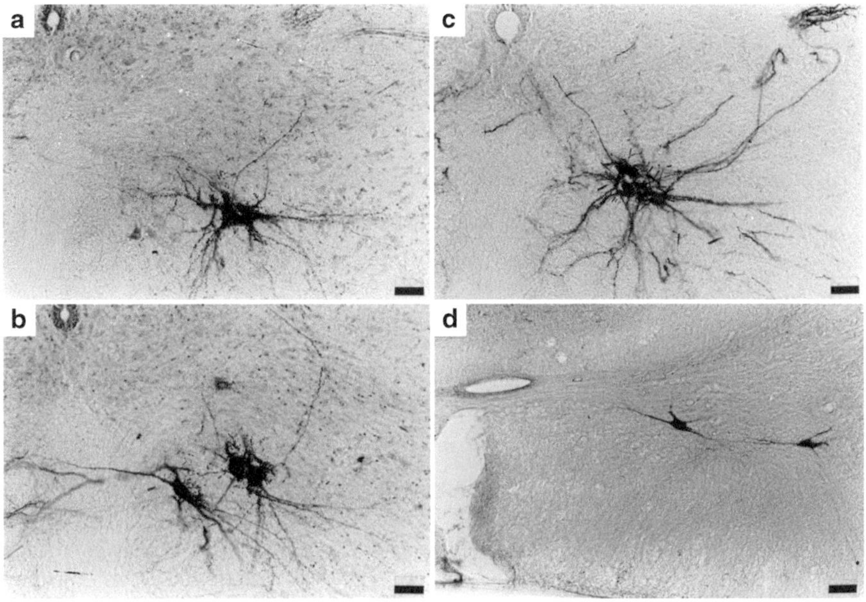

Fig. 9.1 Photomicrographs showing wheat germ agglutinin-horseradish peroxidase-labeled spinal accessory motoneurons. (**a**) A motoneuron at C2–C3 segments in a representative control ICR mouse; (**b**) site A in the *twy* mouse, the most rostral level; (**c**) site B, the level immediately rostral to the compressive lesion; (**d**) site C, the site of mechanical compression at C2–C3 cord segments. The *top side* in each panel represents the dorsal aspect of the cord. Scale bar = 50 μm (Reprinted, with permission, from [7])

9.1.3 Localization of Brain-Derived Neurotropic Factor Immunoreactivity in the Anterior Gray Matter and Its Relationship to the Magnitude of Compression

At site B, BDNF immunoreactivity in the anterior horn cells of *twy* mice was significantly higher than in ICR and site A in *twy* mice (Fig. 9.3c). More severe compression at site C (TRAS < 50 %; $n = 8$) correlated with increased BDNF immunoreactivity in anterior horn cells at site B. Also, more labeled non-neuronal astroglia- and microglia-like cells were detected at sites B and C.

9.1.4 Localization of Neurotrophin-3 Immunoreactivity in the Anterior Gray Horn and Its Relationship to the Magnitude of Compression

At site B in *twy* mice, immunostaining for NT-3 V4 antibody was significant in the anterior horn cells, with enhanced immunoreactivity in the neuron soma and dendrites (Fig. 9.4c) compared with those seen at site A in *twy* and ICR mice.

Table 9.1 Results of morphological measurements of neuronal soma and dendrites of the wheat germ agglutinin-horseradish peroxidase-labeled spinal accessory motoneurons in the medial cell pool of the *twy* and control ICR mice

	Spinal cord level				
	Site A[a]	Site B[b]	Site C[c]	Mean (SD)	Total number (SD)
twy mouse (*n*=30)					
1. Neuron					
Number	34.7 (10.1)	67.9 (10.5)*	3.7 (3.2)**		106.3 (18.1)*
Area of soma (μm2)	574.0 (138.4)*	565.9 (98.9)*	324.4 (170.7)	488.0 (180.2)**	
Number of segments	7.4 (1.1)	7.6 (1.0)	5.7 (1.1)	6.9 (1.4)	
Maximum branch order	3.0 (0.8)	3.1 (0.7)	2.8 (0.7)	3.0 (0.7)	
Total length (μm)	577.0 (142.5)*	523.8 (157.8)*	242.6 (150.8)	242.6 (150.8)	
Maximum branch length (μm)	190.6 (61.5)	183.1 (61.1)	96.9 (50.1)	156.9 (71.4)*	
ICR mouse (*n*=6)					
1. Neuron					
Number	29.5 (12.1)	93.7 (10.0)	24.3 (5.5)		145.8 (17.0)
Area of soma (μm2)	529.2 (44.1)	519.4 (46.9)	526.3 (83.8)	524.8 (57.5)	
2. Dendrite					
Number of segments	7.5 (1.0)	8.3 (0.5)	6.2 (1.2)	7.3 (1.3)	
Maximum branch order	3.2 (0.8)	3.2 (0.8)	3.0 (0.9)	3.1 (0.8)	
Total length (μm)	531.8 (79.2)	418.3 (1.3)	435.6 (169.4)	461.9 (134.0)	
Maximum branch length (μm)	169.3 (28.7)	123.0 (40.7)	118.6 (38.2)	137.0 (41.4)	

$^{*}P<0.05$, $^{**}P<0.01$ (Wilcoxon's signed-ranks test), compared with the corresponding data of ICR mice

[a]Site A: the level most rostral to C1 ventral root. Values are mean (SD)

[b]Site B: the level immediately rostral to the compression lesion between C1 ventral and C2 dorsal roots

[c]Site C: compression site between C2 and C3 dorsal roots (Reprinted, with permission, from [7])

9.1.5 Topographic and Quantitative Analysis of Brain-Derived Neurotropic Factor and Neurotrophin-3 Immunoreactivity

BDNF was detected as a band with a molecular weight of 17–19 kDa (Fig. 9.5a) and NT-3 as a 30 kDa band (Fig. 9.5b). At site B in *twy* mice, BDNF and NT-3 expression was 70.7 % (*lane 6* in Fig. 9.5a) and 72.7 % (*lane 6* in Fig. 9.5b), respectively ($P<0.05$) when compared with that at site C. Immunoreactivity of both neurotrophins increased significantly at the level distal to the compressed segment (*lane 8*).

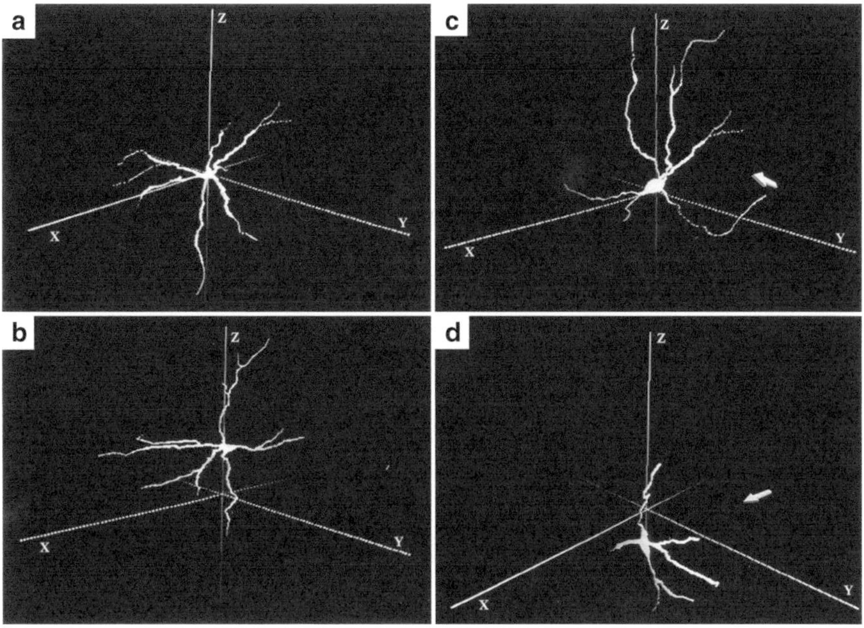

Fig. 9.2 Three-dimensional computer display of the dendritic arborization of the wheat germ agglutinin-horseradish peroxidase-labeled spinal accessory motoneurons (*abscissa* lateral direction, *ordinate* anteroposterior direction, and z-axis longitudinal direction). The compression force is applied in the x–y plane marked by *arrows* in (**c**) and (**d**). (**a**) Motoneuron at C2–C3 segment in the control ICR mouse; (**b**) site A in the *twy* mouse, the most rostral level; (**c**) site B, the level immediately rostral to the compressive lesion; (**d**) site C, the compression level at the C2–C3 cord segments (Reprinted, with permission, from [7])

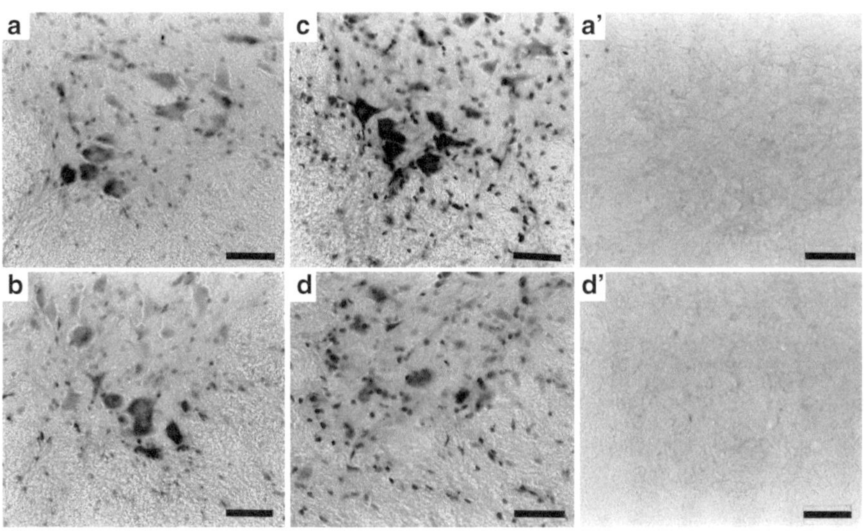

Fig. 9.3 Photomicrographs showing localization of immunoreactivity of brain-derived neurotropic factor in the anterior gray horn of a representative ICR mouse (**a**) and *twy* mouse (**b**–**d**) with a transverse remnant area of 60 %. (**b**) Site A; (**c**) site B; (**d**) site C. (**a′**, **d′**) Negative controls for ICR and *twy* mice, respectively. *Top* posterior aspect of the spinal cord. Scale bars = 50 μm (Reprinted, with permission, from [7])

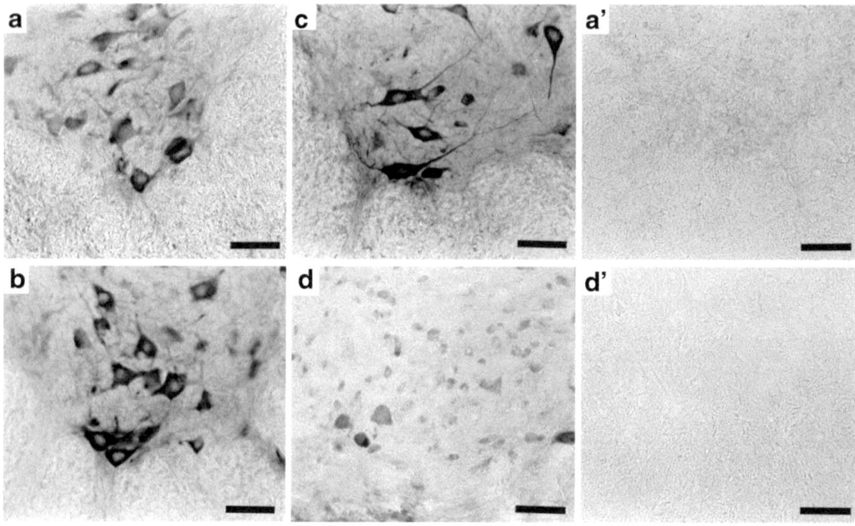

Fig. 9.4 Photomicrographs showing localization of immunoreactivity of neurotrophin-3 in a representative control ICR mouse (**a**) and *twy* mouse with a transverse remnant area of 55 % (**b**–**d**). (**b**) Site A; (**c**) site B; (**d**) site C. (**a**′, **d**′) Negative controls for ICR and *twy* mice, respectively. *Top,* dorsal aspect of the cord. Scale bars = 50 μm (Reprinted, with permission, from [7])

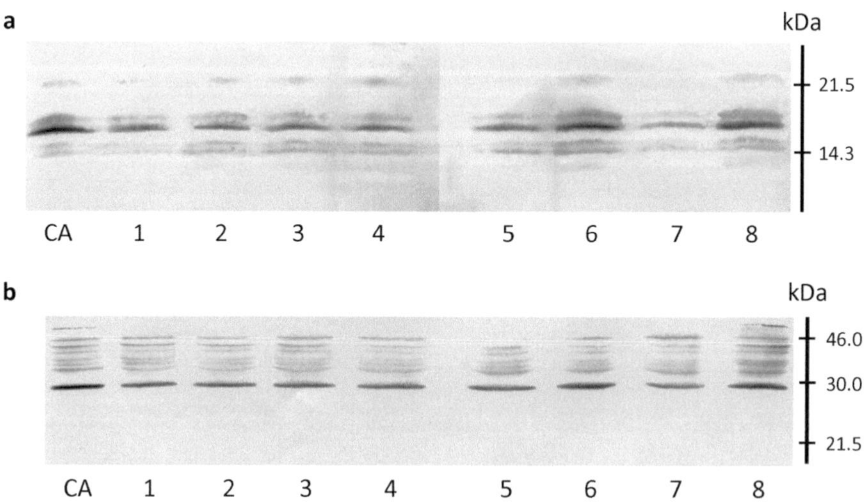

Fig. 9.5 Photomicrograph showing the expression of brain-derived neurotropic factor (**a**) and neurotrophin-3 (**b**) by Western blot analysis. The lane number shows each level of the spinal cord in the ICR (*lanes 1–4*) and *twy* (*lanes 5–8*) mice; *CA* refers to the hippocampus. *Lanes 1* and *5* in site A, the level most rostral to the C1 ventral root; *lanes 2* and *6* in site B, the level immediately rostral to compression between C1 ventral and C2 dorsal roots; *lanes 3* and *7* site C, between C2 and C3 dorsal roots (the compressed level in the *twy* mouse); *lanes 4* and *8*, the level between C3 and C4 dorsal roots (Reprinted, with permission, from [7])

9.1.6 *TUNEL Staining in the* twy/twy *Mouse Spinal Cord*

Figure 9.6 shows the topographic distribution of TUNEL-positive cells in the chronically compressed spinal cord of moderately and severely compressed *twy/twy* mouse examined by the TUNEL method. No TUNEL-positive cells were identified in both the gray and white matters of the control ICR mouse spinal cord. In contrast, TUNEL-positive cells were found in the gray and white matter in the *twy/twy* mouse with moderate compression. In comparison, fewer TUNEL-positive cells are found in the severe compression group particularly in the anterior horn, though these cells were abundant particularly in the anterior columns.

9.2 Discussion

Using the *twy* mice, we have previously demonstrated a significant reduction in the number of anterior horn cells at the level of mechanical compression [6, 7]. A progressively smaller number of these cells was noted when TRAS was 70 % of the normal value, reaching an asymptote approximately below 50 %. Interestingly, we also found increased population of spinal accessory motoneurons at levels rostral to the C1 vertebra (sites free of direct mechanical compression) [12]. The latter finding led us to speculate that a group of motoneurons may translocate rostrally to avoid chronic mechanical compression. Rostral to the site of mechanical compression (site B), we found enlargement of neuron soma and dendritic elongation of the WGA-HRP-labeled accessory motoneurons, which correlated significantly with deterioration of TRAS values measured at the site of compression. Somal size and dendritic arborization increase in order to facilitate synaptic connection [13] representing enhanced synaptic circuits [14, 15] to compensate the compromised function of spinal cord motoneurons.

Nerve growth factors, such as BDNF and NT-3, promote development of neurite outgrowth, growth, and differentiation of neurons, as well as their survival [16]. Our study found increased BDNF and NT-3 immunoreactivities in anterior horn cells, in close association with increased neuronal density of spinal accessory motoneurons when TRAS ranged between 50 % and 70 %. We postulate that considerable amounts of neuropeptides are transported retrogradely [17–19] and/or from the brain [20] in order to increase neuronal activity as well as axonal transport. It is known that astroglial cells produce BDNF [21] and other nerve growth factors [22]. In *twy* mice, when TRAS was 55 % of the control, a number of infiltrated astroglial cells, positive for BDNF immunostaining, were detected at sites rostral to the site of compression, related to increased number of motoneurons: another possible mechanism to enhance neuronal repair and regeneration. The present study demonstrated increased numbers of TUNEL-positive neurons in the gray matter and oligodendrocytes in the white matter of the spinal cord of the *twy/twy* mouse with progressive mechanical compression, which probably contributes to axonal degeneration and demyelination in the *twy/twy* mouse spinal cord with severe compression [8].

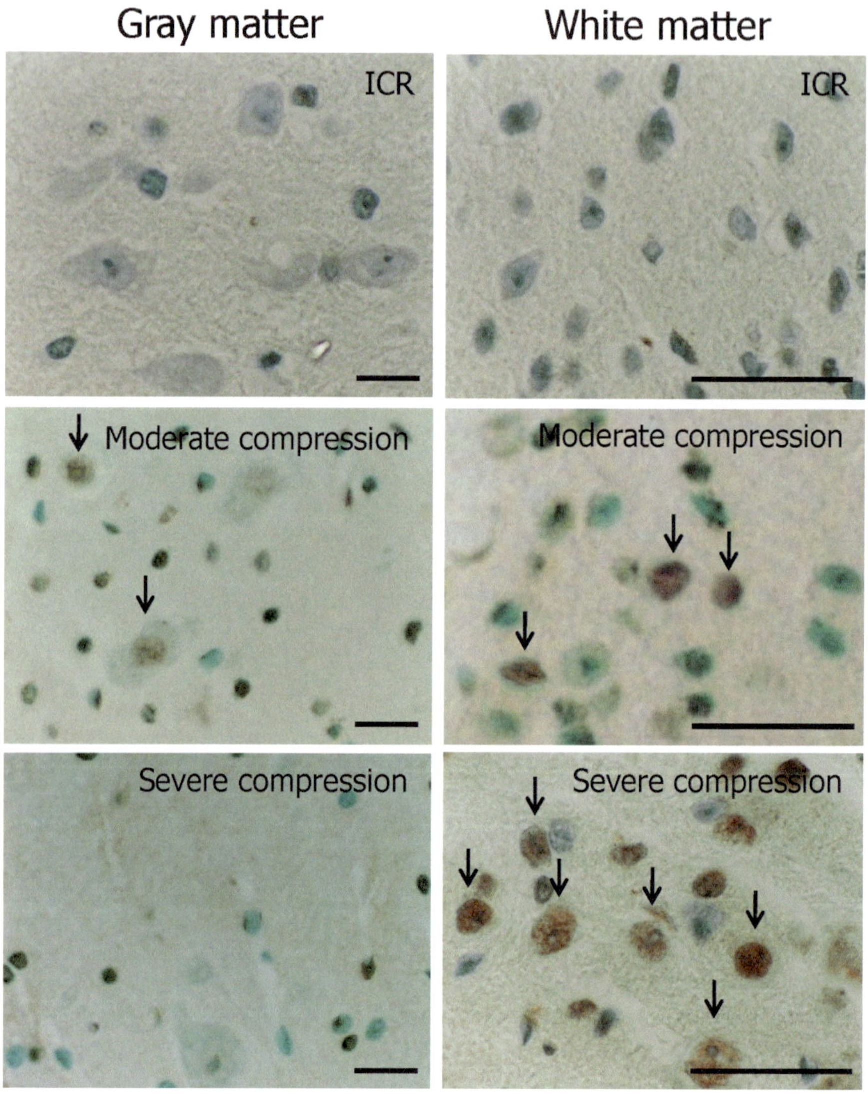

Fig. 9.6 Photomicrographs of terminal deoxynucleotidyl transferase (TdT)-mediated dUTP nick-end labeling (TUNEL) staining in representative control ICR mice (*upper photos*) and *twy/twy* mice with moderate compression (*middle photos*) or severe compression (*lower photos*). *Left column*: photomicrographs taken by a roupe (×3). The *white rectangular area* (anterior horn of the gray matter) and *black rectangular area* (anterior column of the white matter) are enlarged in the same row in the *middle* and *right columns*, respectively. *Black arrows*: representative TUNEL-positive cells. TUNEL-positive cells in the gray and white matter are noted in *twy/twy* mouse. Scale bars = 50 μm

9.3 Conclusion

WGA-HRP-labeled accessory motoneurons expressed significant BDNF and NT-3 immunoreactivities that correlated with enlargement of neuronal soma and extensive dendritic arborization at levels rostral to the site of mechanical compression. Astroglial cells at these levels may play a role in neuronal reserve and survival. There is a significant correlation between the proportion of apoptotic neurons and oligodendrocytes in the compressed area of the spinal cord and the magnitude of cord compression.

Acknowledgment This work was supported in part by Grants-in-Aid for General Scientific Research of the Ministry of Education, Science and Culture of Japan (grants numbers 09671480, C15591571, B16390435, B18390413, and B19791023). This work was also supported in part by grants from the Investigation Committee on Ossification of the Spinal Ligaments, Public Health Bureau of the Japanese Ministry of Health and Welfare.

Conflict of Interest All authors declare that they have no conflict of interest.

References

1. Baba H, Uchida K, Maezawa Y et al (1996) Lordotic alignment and posterior migration of the spinal cord following en bloc open-door laminoplasty for cervical myelopathy: a magnetic resonance imaging study. J Neurol 243:626–632
2. Baba H, Maezawa Y, Uchida K et al (1997) Plasticity of the spinal cord contributes to neurological improvement after treatment by cervical decompression. A magnetic resonance imaging study. J Neurol 244:455–460
3. Mizuno J, Nakagawa H, Iwata K et al (1992) Pathology of spinal cord lesions caused by ossification of the posterior longitudinal ligament, with special reference to reversibility of the spinal cord lesion. Neurol Res 14:312–314
4. al-Mefty O, Harkey HL, Marawi I et al (1993) Experimental chronic compressive cervical myelopathy. J Neurosurg 79:550–561
5. Martin D, Schoenen J, Delree P et al (1992) Experimental acute traumatic injury of the adult rat spinal cord by a subdural inflatable balloon: methodology, behavioral analysis, and histopathology. J Neurosci Res 32:539–550
6. Baba H, Maezawa Y, Imura S et al (1996) Quantitative analysis of the spinal cord motoneuron under chronic compression: an experimental observation in the mouse. J Neurol 243:109–116
7. Uchida K, Baba H, Maezawa Y et al (1998) Histological investigation of spinal cord lesions in the spinal hyperostotic mouse (*twy/twy*): morphological changes in anterior horn cells and immunoreactivity to neurotropic factors. J Neurol 245:781–93
8. Inukai T, Uchida K, Nakajima H et al (2009) Tumor necrosis factor-alpha and its receptors contribute to apoptosis of oligodendrocytes in the spinal cord of spinal hyperostotic mouse (*twy/twy*) sustaining chronic mechanical compression. Spine 34:2848–57
9. Henderson CE, Camu W, Mettling C et al (1993) Neurotrophins promote motor neuron survival and are present in embryonic limb bud. Nature 363:266–270
10. Sendtner M, Holtmann B, Kolbeck R et al (1992) Brain-derived neurotrophic factor prevents the death of motoneurons in newborn rats after nerve section. Nature 360:757–759

11. Yan Q, Elliott JL, Matheson C et al (1993) Influences of neurotrophins on mammalian motoneurons in vivo. J Neurobiol 24:1555–1577
12. Baba H, Maezawa Y, Uchida K et al (1997) Three-dimensional topographic analysis of spinal accessory motoneurons under chronic mechanical compression: an experimental study in the mouse. J Neurol 244:222–229
13. Koziol JA, Tuckwell HC (1978) Analysis and estimation of synaptic densities and their spatial variation on the motoneuron surface. Brain Res 150:617–624
14. Purves D, Lichtman JW (1985) Geometrical differences among homologous neurons in mammals. Science 228:298–302
15. Turner AM, Greenough WT (1985) Differential rearing effects on rat visual cortex synapses. Synaptic and neuronal density and synapses per neuron. Brain Res 329:195–203
16. Funakoshi H, Frisen J, Barbany G et al (1993) Differential expression of mRNAs for neurotrophins and their receptors after axotomy of the sciatic nerve. J Cell Biol 123:455–465
17. DiStefano PS, Friedman B, Radziejewski C et al (1992) The neurotrophins BDNF, NT-3, and NGF display distinct patterns of retrograde axonal transport in peripheral and central neurons. Neuron 8:983–993
18. Maisonpierre PC, Belluscio L, Friedman B et al (1990) NT-3, BDNF, and NGF in the developing rat nervous system: parallel as well as reciprocal patterns of expression. Neuron 5:501–509
19. Zhou XF, Rush RA (1993) Localization of neurotrophin-3-like immunoreactivity in peripheral tissues of the rat. Brain Res 621:189–199
20. Ernfors P, Persson H (1991) Developmentally regulated expression of HDNF/NT-3 mRNA in rat spinal cord motoneurons and expression of BDNF mRNA in embryonic dorsal root ganglion. Eur J Neurosci 3:953–961
21. Barde YA, Edgar D, Thoenen H (1982) Purification of a new neurotrophic factor from mammalian brain. EMBO J 1:549–553
22. Lu B, Yokoyama M, Dreyfus CF et al (1991) NGF gene expression in actively growing brain glia. J Neurosci 11:318–326

Chapter 10
In Vivo Tracing of Neural Tracts in Tiptoe-Walking Yoshimura Mice by Diffusion Tensor Tractography

Morito Takano, Yuji Komaki, Keigo Hikishima, Tsunehiko Konomi, Kanehiro Fujiyoshi, Osahiko Tsuji, Hideyuki Okano, Yoshiaki Toyama, and Masaya Nakamura

Abstract In ossification of the posterior longitudinal ligaments (OPLL), axonal disruption results in motor and sensory function impairment. *Twy* (tiptoe-walking Yoshimura) mice develop spontaneous calcification in the cervical ligaments, thereby causing chronic compression of the spinal cords. To determine whether in vivo diffusion tensor tractography (DTT) can evaluate the axonal disruption of the chronic compressive spinal cords in *twy* mice, 6-, 15-, and 20-week-old *twy* mice were chronologically subjected to DTT. MRI was performed using a 7.0-Tesla magnet with a surface coil (CryoProbe). Diffusion tensor images were analyzed using TrackVis (Massachusetts General Hospital, MA, USA). We succeeded in depicting in vivo high-resolution DTT of the *twy* mice. The progress of the ligamentous calcification was observed at C2–3 level in each *twy* mouse, and the number of RT-97 or SMI31 positive fibers was decreased depending on the severity of the compression of the spinal cord. Quantitative analysis of sequential DTT enabled to detect subtle damage of the compressed spinal cord prior to the deterioration of neurological function in *twy* mice. Thus, in a clinical setting, DTT could be a new effective imaging modality in patients with cervical OPLL.

M. Takano • Y. Toyama • M. Nakamura (✉)
Department of Orthopaedic Surgery, Keio University,
Shinanomachi35, Shinjuku-Ku, Tokyo 160-8582, Japan
e-mail: masa@a8.keio.jp

Y. Komaki • K. Hikishima
Department of Physiology, Keio University, Tokyo, Japan

Central Institute for Experimental Animals, Kanagawa, Japan

T. Konomi • K. Fujiyoshi
National Hospital Organization Murayama Medical Center, Tokyo, Japan

O. Tsuji
Saitama Social Insurance Hospital, Saitama, Japan

H. Okano
Department of Physiology, Keio University, Tokyo, Japan

K. Uchida et al. (eds.), *Neuroprotection and Regeneration of the Spinal Cord*,
DOI 10.1007/978-4-431-54502-6_10, © Springer Japan 2014

Keywords Diffusion tensor tractography • Ossification of the posterior longitudinal ligament • *twy* mouse

10.1 Introduction

Ossification of the posterior longitudinal ligament (OPLL) of the cervical spine compresses the spinal cord and causes myelopathy. Surgical treatment for OPLL is clearly indicated when the patient shows severe or progressive cervical myelopathy, and the surgery should be performed as soon as possible. However, for patients without any symptoms or with only mild myelopathy in spite of evident OPLL on plain radiography of the cervical spine, the indication for and timing of surgical treatment remain controversial. Although conventional magnetic resonance imaging (MRI) provides useful information about the compressed spinal cord [1], a discrepancy is sometimes seen between the degree of spinal cord compression and the clinical symptoms.

Diffusion tensor imaging (DTI) is an MRI technique that evaluates the diffusion of extracellular water molecules within white matter fibers. The DTI parameters are described as disclosing subtle pathological changes in white matter integrity, and they have been useful for analyzing various central nervous system disorders [2, 3]. Diffusion tensor tractography (DTT) refers to the analysis and reconstruction of the DTI data, by which the orientation of nerve fibers can be followed to trace specific neural pathways [4]. The applications of DTT were recently reported to include cases of spinal cord compression in humans [5, 6]. DTT is useful for grading the neurological severity in cervical spondylotic myelopathy, because it provides objective measures in terms of microstructural changes. However, to the best of our knowledge, there are no reports on the chronological changes in this disease, including comparisons between DTT findings and histological/functional analyses in animal models.

Tiptoe-walking Yoshimura (*twy*) mice are reported to be a good in vivo model for the pathological changes underlying spinal cord dysfunction related to chronic compression [7, 8]. This mouse develops spontaneous spinal cord compression, so it is suitable for investigating the effects of chronic mechanical compression of the spinal cord without any artificial manipulation. The purpose of this study is to determine the relevance of DTT for evaluating the tract fibers of the compressed spinal cord by comparing the chronological in vivo DTT findings with histological findings and motor performance in *twy* mice.

10.2 Comparisons of MR Images with Histology

In *twy* mice, the conventional MRI were chronologically performed at 6, 15, and 20 weeks of age using a 7.0-Tesla magnet (BioSpec 70/16; Bruker BioSpin, Ettlingen, Germany) with a cryogenic quadrature RF surface probe (CryoProbe;

Bruker BioSpin AG, Fällanden, Switzerland) to improve the sensitivity [9]. Conventional and diffusion tensor MRI were performed under general anesthesia induced by intramuscular injection of ketamine (50 mg/kg; Sankyo, Tokyo, Japan) and xylazine (5 mg/kg; Bayer, Leverkusen, Germany) and maintained by isoflurane (Foren; Abbott, Tokyo, Japan). In 20-week-old *twy* mice, severe spinal cord compression was observed at the C2–3 level due to calcification of the atlantoaxial membrane (Fig. 10.1a). Consistent with the histological findings, the MR images precisely depicted severe spinal cord compression (Fig. 10.1b, c). To examine the effect of ectopic calcification on the spinal cord in 20-week-old *twy* mice, we measured the transverse area of the spinal cord histologically and compared it with the canal stenosis ratio (Table 10.1) (Fig. 10.1d, e). There was a significant negative correlation between the transverse area of the spinal cord and the canal stenosis ratio ($r=-0.7840$, $p=0.0457$, Fig. 10.1f).

10.3 Sequential Changes in Diffusion Tensor Tractography

Chronological T2-weighted images (T2WI) of the upper cervical spinal cord enabled the progression of spinal cord compression due to ectopic calcification to be depicted in the same *twy* mouse (Fig. 10.2a). DTI data sets were acquired with a spin-echo sequence based on the Stejskal-Tanner diffusion preparation. Mild and moderate spinal cord compression caused the tract fibers in DTI to detour around the ectopic calcification at 6 and 15 weeks of age, whereas the tract fibers were interrupted by severe spinal cord compression at 20 weeks of age (Fig. 10.2b).

Diffusion tensor tractography images were computed using the Diffusion Toolkit and TrackVis software (Massachusetts General Hospital, MA, USA). The diffusion tensor can be represented as an ellipsoid, where a proton at the center of the voxel has an equal probability of diffusing to any point in that ellipsoid. Fiber tracking was initiated from a manually selected region of interest (ROI), from which tracking lines were propagated bidirectionally according to the principal eigenvector in each voxel. For the tractography, an ROI was placed at the C2–3 level as the epicenter ROI and at the C0–1 level as the control ROI. We determined the number of tract fibers in each specimen at the C2–3 level (epicenter site) and the C0–1 level (control/rostral site). To analyze the sequential changes in the tract fibers of the compressed spinal cords quantitatively, we determined the canal stenosis ratios and configured tract fiber (TF) ratios (Fig. 10.3a, Table 10.1) in 6-, 15-, and 20-week-old *twy* mice. The TF ratio did not significantly change in the 15-week-olds, but decreased sharply in the 20-week-olds (Fig. 10.3b). To examine the significance of the depicted tract fibers, we compared the tract fibers depicted by DTT with the RT-97- and SMI31-positive fibers in the 20-week-old *twy* mice (Fig. 10.3c, e). The tissue sections were stained with the following primary antibodies: anti-RT-97 (mouse IgG_1, 1:200, Millipore, MA, USA) for normal neurofilaments and anti-SMI31 (mouse IgG_1, 1:200, Covance) for hyperphosphorylated normal axons. There was a positive correlation between the TF ratio and the RT-97-positive area ($r=0.7865$, $p=0.0449$, Fig. 10.3d) and SMI31-positive area ($r=0.7746$, $p=0.0489$, Fig. 10.3f).

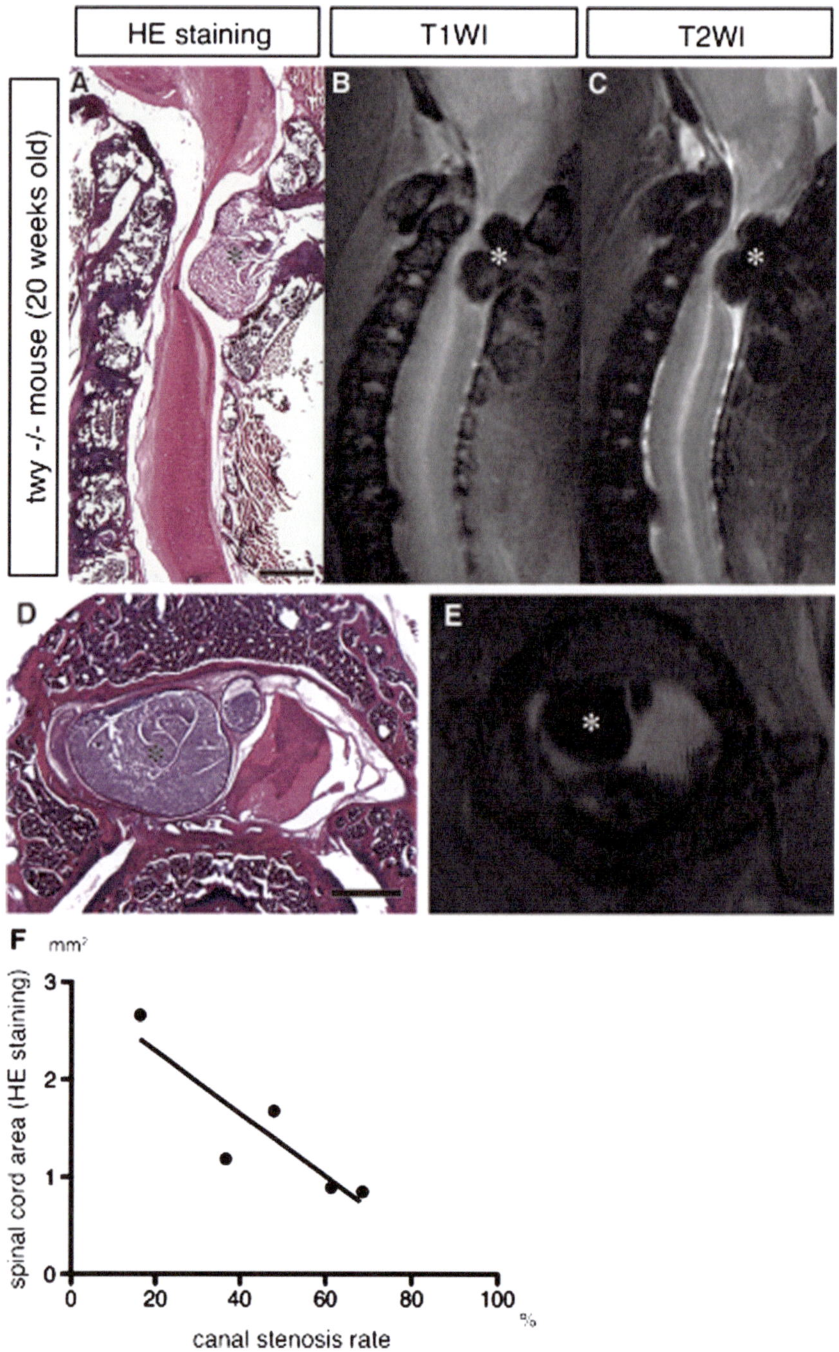

Fig. 10.1 Representative HE-stained sagittal and axial images of the *twy* mice. Scale bar: 1 mm (**a**), 500 μm (**d**). Sagittal and axial MRI (**b**, **c**, **e**) showed notable cervical spinal cord compression resulting from ectopic calcification (*). The spinal cord area was correlated with the canal stenosis ratio (**f**, $r = -0.7840$)

Table 10.1 Definition of the canal stenosis ratio and tract fiber (TF) ratio

Canal stenosis ratio = 100 − (spinal cord area/spinal canal area) × 100	
TF ratio = number of tract fibers at the C2–3 level/ number of tract fibers at the C0–1 level	

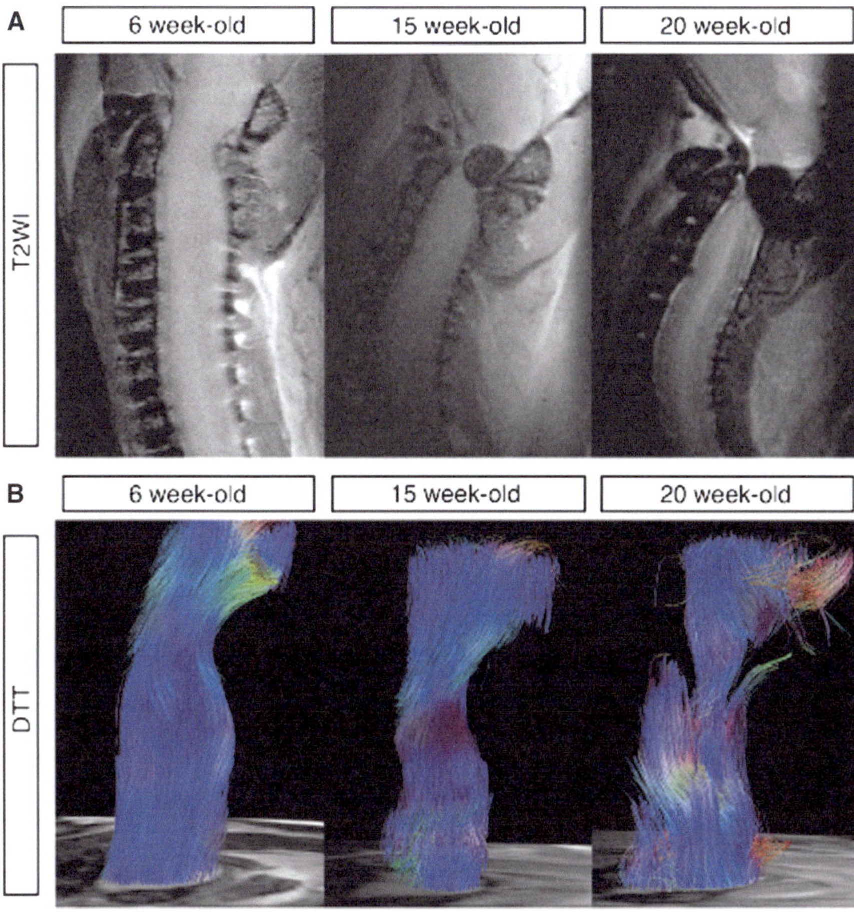

Fig. 10.2 Sagittal T2-weighted image (**a**) and diffusion tensor tractography (**b**) of the *twy* mice observed chronologically (at 6, 15, and 20 weeks of age). The results showed that calcification in the atlantoaxial membrane gradually progressed, while the number of tract fibers gradually decreased

10.4 Correlations Among the TF Ratio, Canal Stenosis Rate, and Motor Performance

The canal stenosis progressed with the age of the *twy* mice. To examine the chronological relationship between the TF ratio and canal stenosis ratio, we analyzed their correlation in five *twy* mice at 6, 15, and 20 weeks of age (Fig. 10.4a). As the *twy*

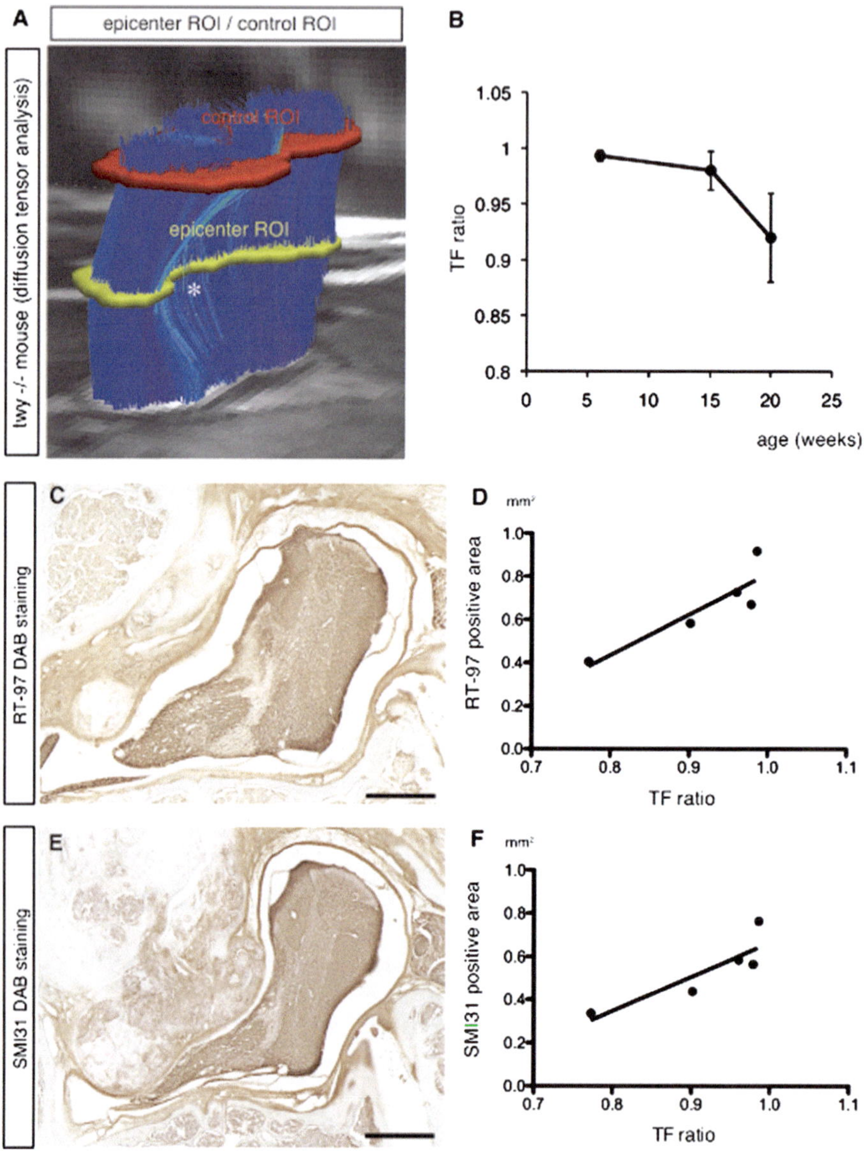

Fig. 10.3 The tract fibers were generated by placing the ROIs at the C0–1 and C2–3 levels (**a**). The TF ratio tended to decrease with the animal's age (**b**). Correlations between the TF ratio and the area of neurofilament staining for RT-97 (**c**) and SMI31 (**e**). Scale bar: 500 μm (**d**, $r = 0.7865$: **f**, $r = 0.7746$)

mice became older, the canal stenosis became more prominent, causing a decrease in the TF ratio. Interestingly, two-part linear regression analysis [10] revealed that canal stenosis over 50 % caused a sharp decrease in the TF ratio (intersection point: 52 %, Fig. 10.4b).

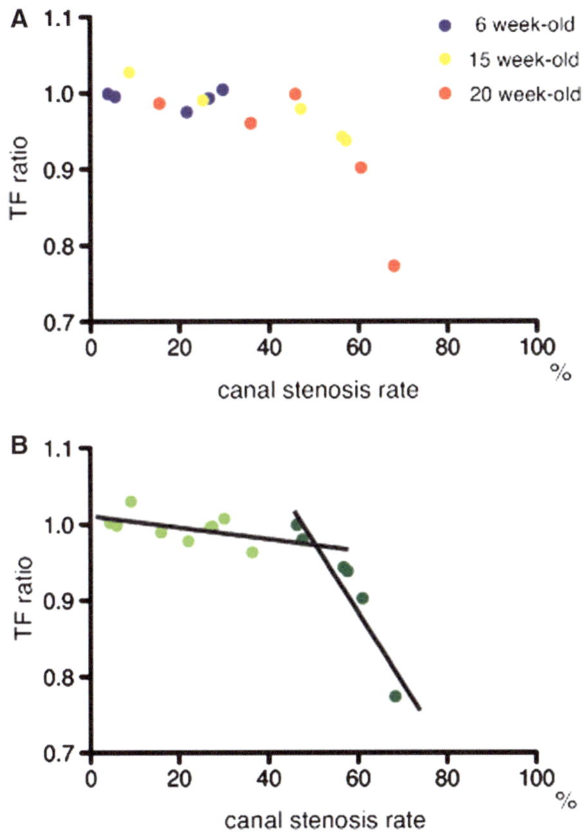

Fig. 10.4 Correlations between the TF ratio and canal stenosis ratio (**a**, *blue dots*, 6-week-olds; *yellow dots*, 15-week-olds; *red dots*, 20-week-olds). Two-part linear regression analysis showed that canal stenosis over 50 % caused a sharp decrease in the TF ratio (**b**, *light green*, $r=-0.2827$; *dark green*, $r=-0.8705$)

Since *twy* mice show progressive paralysis due to the chronic spinal cord compression, we examined the motor function in the mice by the Rota-Rod treadmill test (Muromachi Kikai Co., Ltd., Tokyo, Japan) and DigiGait analysis (Mouse Specifics, Quincy, MA, USA) and compared the results with the TF ratio and canal stenosis ratio in the 20-week-old *twy* mice. Both the Rota-Rod treadmill latency and stride length sharply decreased when the TF ratio was below 0.9 (Fig. 10.5a, b) and canal stenosis ratio was over 60 % (Fig. 10.5c, d). Consistent with the Rota-Rod treadmill analysis, the DigiGait analysis revealed that two *twy* mice with severe spinal cord compression (canal stenosis ratio >60 %) could not walk on the treadmill, whereas the other *twy* mice with mild or moderate spinal cord compression (canal stenosis ratio <50 %) could walk on the treadmill at a speed of 8 cm/s.

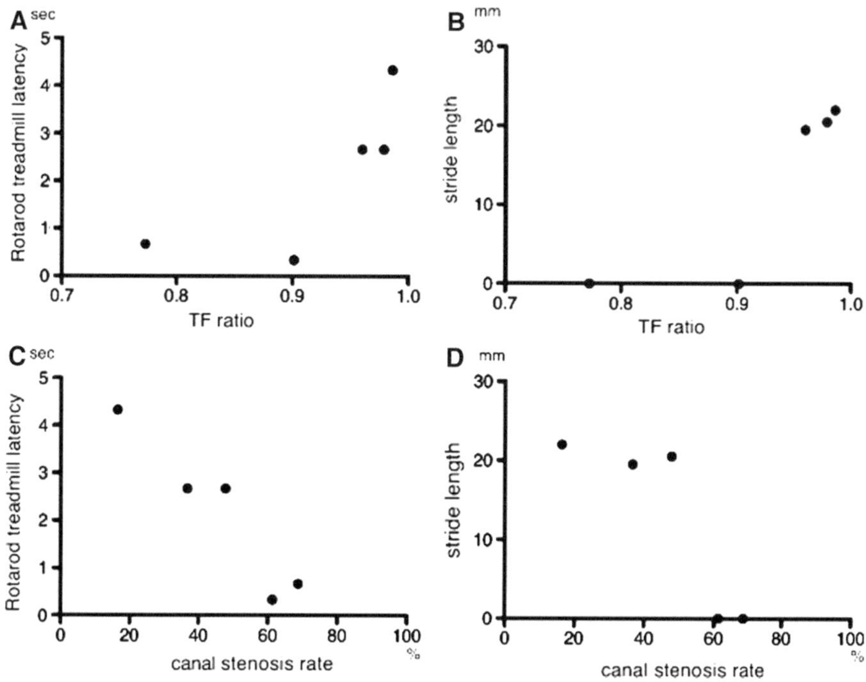

Fig. 10.5 Correlations among the TF ratio, canal stenosis ratio, and functional parameters. (**a**) TF ratio and Rota-Rod treadmill latency; (**b**) TF ratio and stride length; (**c**) canal stenosis rate and Rota-Rod treadmill latency; (**d**) canal stenosis rate and stride length

10.5 Discussion

In the present study, we show that in vivo DTT could depict the chronological changes in the tract fibers of the chronic progressive spinal cord compression in *twy* mice. The number of tract fibers depicted by DTT was significantly correlated with the areas of RT-97^{+} and SMI-31^{+} neurofilaments and the results of motor function analyses. In addition, our results suggest that, in particular, over 50 % spinal canal stenosis causes a sharp decrease in the tract fibers even before a prominent neurological deficit is seen.

Previous studies on the surgical outcomes of OPLL patients demonstrated that the postoperative recovery is poor in those with a greater than 50–60 % compromise of the spinal canal by the ossified lesion [11, 12]. Recent reports examining the surgical option for treating patients with cervical myelopathy caused by OPLL [13, 14] suggested that the surgical results depend on the severity of the preoperative neurological deficit, and, therefore, the cervical myelopathy must be diagnosed as early as possible. However, there are no reports describing a useful and objective tool for determining the surgical indication for cervical myelopathy. Conventional MRI undoubtedly provides useful information about the compressed spinal cord. However, sometimes there is a discrepancy between the degree of spinal cord compression and the clinical symptoms.

We previously demonstrated that DTT is very useful for examining spinal cord injuries and peripheral nerve injuries in experimental animal models [15–17]. In the clinic, Kara et al. suggested that DTT can show abnormalities in the compressive spinal cord before the development of T2 hyperintensity on conventional MRI sequences in patients with cervical spondylotic myelopathy [18]. Although DTT is thought to have great potential for detecting cervical myelopathy, it is unclear how DTT would show the pathological changes of the compressed spinal cord. Accordingly, we focused on *twy* mice, which develop spontaneous cervical myelopathy due to ectopic ossified ligaments.

Baba et al. previously reported that the chronic compression of the cervical spinal cord of *twy* mice causes the loss of motor neurons at the injury epicenter [19]. Yato et al. also reported that spinal motor neuron atrophy and loss in the gray matter of *twy* mice were observed when the severity of spinal canal stenosis was 30 % or more [20]. Given the variation in the severity of spinal cord compression due to ligamentous calcification in these mice, it is important to observe the chronological changes in the spinal cord of live *twy* mice, which has never been reported previously.

In the present study, we performed in vivo imaging of *twy* mice with a 7T MRI and CryoProbe and examined the chronological changes in their compressed spinal cords. To the best of our knowledge, this is the first study to show the chronological changes of DTT parameters in *twy* mice using high-resolution MRI. We demonstrated that the TF ratio decreased sharply at around 50 % spinal canal stenosis. Our results resemble clinical evidence and suggest that irreversible changes in neurofilaments increase dramatically at over 50 % spinal canal stenosis. It is noteworthy that the decrease in TF ratio preceded the functional deterioration, which occurred at around 60 % spinal canal stenosis.

10.6 Conclusion

In conclusion, DTT could be a new effective imaging modality in patients with cervical myelopathy due to ligamentous calcifications. In this study, subtle damage visible in the neurofilaments could be quantitatively analyzed at each stage of disease by measuring the tract fibers. Thus, in a clinical setting, the TF ratio could be a useful parameter for making decisions about the indications and timing of surgical treatment for cervical myelopathy due to OPLL.

Acknowledgement Ministry of Health, Labor and Welfare Sciences Research Grant funds were received to support this work.

References

1. Vedantam A, Jonathan A, Rajshekhar V (2011) Association of magnetic resonance imaging signal changes and outcome prediction after surgery for cervical spondylotic myelopathy. J Neurosurg Spine 15(6):660–666. doi:10.3171/2011.8.SPINE11452
2. Assaf Y, Pasternak O (2008) Diffusion tensor imaging (DTI)-based white matter mapping in brain research: a review. J Mol Neurosci 34(1):51–61. doi:10.1007/s12031-007-0029-0
3. Chang Y, Jung TD, Yoo DS, Hyun JK (2010) Diffusion tensor imaging and fiber tractography of patients with cervical spinal cord injury. J Neurotrauma 27(11):2033–2040. doi:10.1089/neu.2009.1265
4. Mori S, Zhang J (2006) Principles of diffusion tensor imaging and its applications to basic neuroscience research. Neuron 51(5):527–539. doi:10.1016/j.neuron.2006.08.012
5. Demir A, Ries M, Moonen CT, Vital JM, Dehais J, Arne P, Caille JM, Dousset V (2003) Diffusion-weighted MR imaging with apparent diffusion coefficient and apparent diffusion tensor maps in cervical spondylotic myelopathy. Radiology 229(1):37–43. doi:10.1148/radiol.2291020658
6. Facon D, Ozanne A, Fillard P, Lepeintre JF, Tournoux-Facon C, Ducreux D (2005) MR diffusion tensor imaging and fiber tracking in spinal cord compression. AJNR Am J Neuroradiol 26(6):1587–1594
7. Okawa A, Nakamura I, Goto S, Moriya H, Nakamura Y, Ikegawa S (1998) Mutation in Npps in a mouse model of ossification of the posterior longitudinal ligament of the spine. Nat Genet 19(3):271–273. doi:10.1038/956
8. Uchida K, Baba H, Maezawa Y, Kubota C (2002) Progressive changes in neurofilament proteins and growth-associated protein-43 immunoreactivities at the site of cervical spinal cord compression in spinal hyperostotic mice. Spine 27(5):480–486
9. Baltes C, Radzwill N, Bosshard S, Marek D, Rudin M (2009) Micro MRI of the mouse brain using a novel 400 MHz cryogenic quadrature RF probe. NMR Biomed 22(8):834–842. doi:10.1002/nbm.1396
10. Kouda K, Iki M, Fujita Y, Tamaki J, Yura A, Kadowaki E, Sato Y, Moon JS, Morikawa M, Tomioka K, Okamoto N, Kurumatani N (2011) Alcohol intake and bone status in elderly Japanese men: baseline data from the Fujiwara-kyo osteoporosis risk in men (FORMEN) study. Bone 49(2):275–280. doi:10.1016/j.bone.2011.04.010
11. Baba H, Imura S, Kawahara N, Nagata S, Tomita K (1995) Osteoplastic laminoplasty for cervical myeloradiculopathy secondary to ossification of the posterior longitudinal ligament. Int Orthop 19(1):40–45
12. Iwasaki M, Okuda S, Miyauchi A, Sakaura H, Mukai Y, Yonenobu K, Yoshikawa H (2007) Surgical strategy for cervical myelopathy due to ossification of the posterior longitudinal ligament, Part 1: clinical results and limitations of laminoplasty. Spine 32(6):647 653. doi:10.1097/01.brs.0000257560.91147.86
13. Sakai K, Okawa A, Takahashi M, Arai Y, Kawabata S, Enomoto M, Kato T, Hirai T, Shinomiya K (2011) Five-year follow-up evaluation of surgical treatment for cervical myelopathy caused by ossification of the posterior longitudinal ligament: a prospective comparative study of anterior decompression and fusion with floating method versus laminoplasty. Spine. doi:10.1097/BRS.0b013e31821f4a51
14. Tani T, Ushida T, Ishida K, Iai H, Noguchi T, Yamamoto H (2002) Relative safety of anterior microsurgical decompression versus laminoplasty for cervical myelopathy with a massive ossified posterior longitudinal ligament. Spine 27(22):2491–2498. doi:10.1097/01.BRS.0000031270.69596.4E
15. Fujiyoshi K, Yamada M, Nakamura M, Yamane J, Katoh H, Kitamura K, Kawai K, Okada S, Momoshima S, Toyama Y, Okano H (2007) In vivo tracing of neural tracts in the intact and injured spinal cord of marmosets by diffusion tensor tractography. J Neurosci 27(44):11991–11998. doi:10.1523/JNEUROSCI.3354-07.2007

16. Takagi T, Nakamura M, Yamada M, Hikishima K, Momoshima S, Fujiyoshi K, Shibata S, Okano HJ, Toyama Y, Okano H (2009) Visualization of peripheral nerve degeneration and regeneration: monitoring with diffusion tensor tractography. Neuroimage 44(3):884–892. doi:10.1016/j.neuroimage.2008.09.022
17. Konomi T, Fujiyoshi K, Hikishima K, Komaki Y, Tsuji O, Okano HJ, Toyama Y, Okano H, Nakamura M (2012) Conditions for quantitative evaluation of injured spinal cord by in vivo diffusion tensor imaging and tractography: preclinical longitudinal study in common marmosets. Neuroimage 63(4):1841–1853. doi:10.1016/j.neuroimage.2012.08.040
18. Kara B, Celik A, Karadereler S, Ulusoy L, Ganiyusufoglu K, Onat L, Mutlu A, Ornek I, Sirvanci M, Hamzaoglu A (2011) The role of DTI in early detection of cervical spondylotic myelopathy: a preliminary study with 3-T MRI. Neuroradiology 53(8):609–616. doi:10.1007/s00234-011-0844-4
19. Baba H, Maezawa Y, Imura S, Kawahara N, Nakahashi K, Tomita K (1996) Quantitative analysis of the spinal cord motor neuron under chronic compression: an experimental observation in the mouse. J Neurol 243(2):109–116
20. Yato Y, Fujimura Y, Nakamura M, Watanabe M, Yabe Y (1997) Decreased choline acetyltransferase activity in the murine spinal cord motor neurons under chronic mechanical compression. Spinal Cord 35(11):729–734

Chapter 11
Microarray Analysis of Expression of Cell Death-Associated Genes in Spinal Cord Cells with Cyclic Tensile Strain

Kenzo Uchida, Hideaki Nakajima, Takayuki Hirai, Sally Roberts, William E.B. Johnson, and Hisatoshi Baba

Abstract Previous studies have described alterations in gene expression following spinal cord injury, but this response to mechanical stimuli is difficult to investigate in vivo. Therefore, we have investigated the effect of cyclic tensile strain on cultured spinal cord cells from E15 Sprague–Dawley rats. Microarray analysis of gene expression and categorization of identified genes were performed using Gene Ontology (GO) and Kyoto Encyclopedia of Genes and Genomes (KEGG) systems.

The application of cyclic tensile strain reduced the viability of cultured spinal cord cells significantly in a dose- and time-dependent manner. GO analysis identified candidate genes related to "apoptosis" (44) and to "response to stimulus" (17). KEGG analysis identified changes in the expression levels of 12 genes of the mitogen-activated protein kinase (MAPK) signaling pathway, which were confirmed to be upregulated and validated by RT-PCR analysis. Spinal cord cells undergo cell death in response to cyclic tensile strain, which were dose- and time-dependent, with upregulation of various genes, in particular of the MAPK pathway.

Keywords Cultured cell • Cyclic tensile strain • Microarray • Mitogen-activated protein kinase (MAPK) signaling pathway • Spinal cord

K. Uchida (✉) • H. Nakajima • T. Hirai • H. Baba
Department of Orthopaedics and Rehabilitation Medicine, Faculty of Medical Sciences, University of Fukui, Matsuoka Shimoaizuki 23-3, Eiheiji, Fukui 910-1193, Japan
e-mail: kuchida@u-fukui.ac.jp

S. Roberts
Institute for Science and Technology in Medicine, Keele University at the RJAH Orthopaedic Hospital, Oswestry, Shropshire SY10 7AG, UK

W.E.B. Johnson
Life and Health Sciences, Aston University, Aston Triangle, Birmingham B4 7ET, UK

K. Uchida et al. (eds.), *Neuroprotection and Regeneration of the Spinal Cord*,
DOI 10.1007/978-4-431-54502-6_11,

11.1 Introduction

Mechanical stresses applied to the spinal cord can potentially induce profound and irreversible paresis, secondary to induced neuronal cell necrosis and apoptosis [1, 2]. Examples of such mechanically induced spinal cord damage include not only spinal cord compression but also distraction insult [3, 4], where tensile strain forms an important part of the injury mechanism. The primary mechanical event can initiate a cascade of molecular and cellular events such as changes in gene expression levels that are necessary for cell recovery or cell death [5–8].

Such changes have been documented in various in vivo models of spinal cord injury using microarray analysis [9–11], in an attempt to stabilize, both biologically and functionally, the spinal cord once injured [12, 13]. However, these in vivo experimental settings suffer from several disadvantages over in vitro experimentation, such as activation of resident inflammatory cells or invasion of foreign cells from the periphery [14]. The complexity of the in vivo situation limits the access to specific areas of tissue or cell type of interest, preventing real-time and spatial measurement of biological or mechanical parameters [15]. Thus, the importance of in vitro models becomes evident.

The use of neuronal cell culture models allows for better control of the extracellular environment, cell specificity while being relatively easy to manipulate. The Flexercell Strain Unit (FX3000®, Flexercell International, Hillsborough, NC) is a cell-stretching apparatus that allows application of cyclic tensile force to cultured cells [16–18]. In our previous study using this equipment [19], cyclic tensile strain on cultured spinal cord cells increased the expression levels of nerve growth factor, brain-derived neurotrophic factor, trkB, p75 neurotrophin receptor (p75NTR), glial cell line-derived neurotrophic factor, and caspase-9 mRNAs in the acute phase, followed by increased lactate dehydrogenase release and induction of necrotic cell death.

The present study was thus designed to examine further the molecular changes and gene expression profiles in cultured spinal cord cells using the above cell-stretching apparatus and DNA microarray technology.

11.1.1 Cyclic Tensile Stress-Induced Spinal Cord Cell Death

Under the condition of 10 % tensile strain (typically found in spinal cord injuries [19]) at a frequency of 0.5 Hz (Fig. 11.1a, b), the proportion of living green-stained spinal cord cells decreased in a time-dependent manner, whereas that of dead red-stained cells increased simultaneously. Transmission electron microscopy (TEM) examination showed that all cells at 0 h appeared viable, with large nuclei, and dotted with chromatin. When subjected to tensile strain, some cells showed deformity of the nuclei and cytoplasm at 6 h, and chromatin condensation and fragmentation were observed at 24 h; morphological changes indicative of early apoptosis (Fig. 11.1c).

The cell survival rate of cultures under cyclic strain decreased from 83 ± 24 % at 2 h to 40 ± 11 % at 72 h (Fig. 11.2a), becoming significant after 6 h. Figure 11.2b shows that increasing the strain rate independently of the strain level was associated

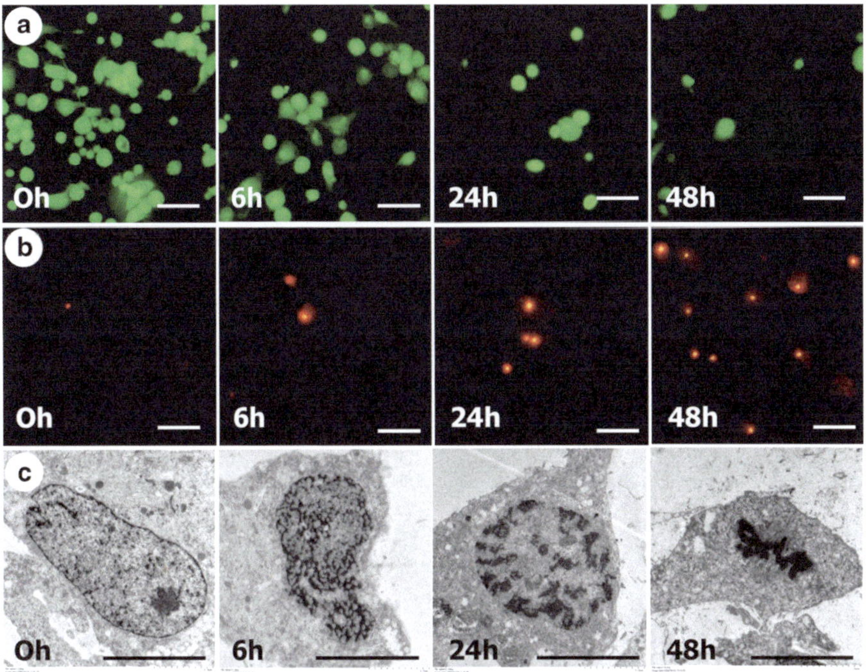

Fig. 11.1 The application of cyclic tensile strain induced apoptotic cell death in spinal cord cells. Representative serial photomicrographs are shown of cells exposed to a tensile strain of 10 % strain at 0.5 Hz at 0, 6, 24, and 48 h (**a**, **b**). The number of *green-stained living cells* decreased (**a**: *top row*) while the number of *red-strained dead cells* increased (**b**: *middle row*) in a time-dependent manner during cyclic tensile strain application. Transmission electron microscopy (TEM) examination (**c**: *bottom row*): all cells at 0 h appeared viable, with large nuclei, and *dotted* with chromatin and abundant rough endoplasmic reticulum; some cells at 6 h showed deformity of nuclei and cytoplasm. TEM at 24 h showed some cells with condensed and fragmented nuclei and condensed chromatin, and the change progressed at 48 h (**c**: *bottom row*). Bar = 100 μm (**a**, **b**), 50 μm (**c**) (Reprinted, with permission, from [20])

with increased spinal cord cell death. Conversely, the cell survival rate in cultures subjected to a 15 % strain level at a frequency of 0.5 Hz was also significantly lower than that seen at the standard level. Therefore, increasing the strain level independently of the strain rate was also associated with increased spinal cord cell death.

11.1.2 Cluster Analysis of Gene Expression Profiles

There was altered expression of 3,412 genes after the application of a cyclic tensile strain of 10 % at 0.5 Hz during 72 h, which were profiled using hierarchical cluster analysis in a time course manner and divided into six clusters (Fig. 11.3). Genes of clusters 1, 2, and 3 were upregulated in a time-dependent manner; those of cluster 4 were upregulated in a time-independent manner. Genes of clusters 5 and 6 were downregulated in a time-dependent manner.

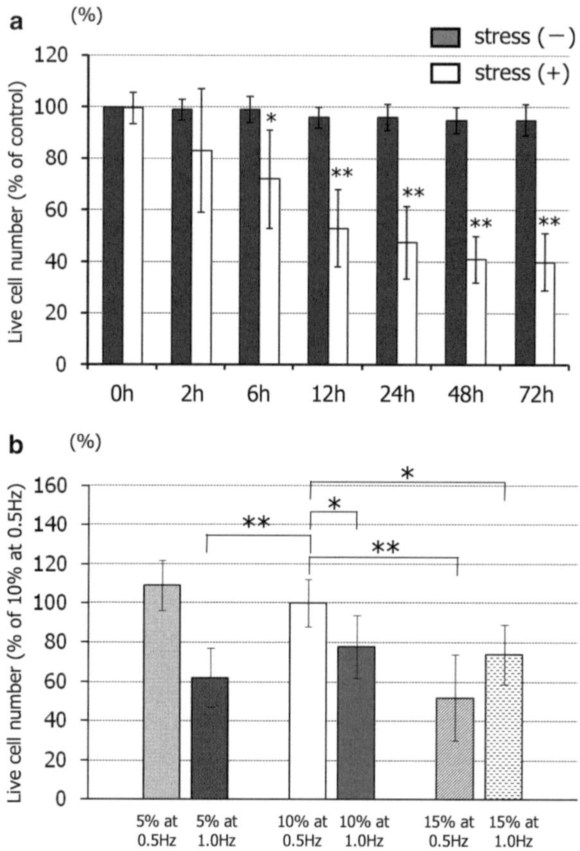

Fig. 11.2 The survival rate of spinal cord cells was dependent on the level, frequency, and duration of the applied tensile strain. The survival rate (%) of living cells during the application of a standardized cyclic tensile strain (10 %, 0.5 Hz) compared with stress-free baseline (**a**). *Gray bar*, stress-free condition; *white bar*, cyclic tensile strain condition. The survival rate (%) of living cells after 6 h at three different strain levels of 5 %, 10 %, and 15 % and two different strain frequencies of 0.5 and 1 Hz compared with that at the standardized strain level of 10 % at 0.5 Hz frequency (**b**). Data are expressed as mean ± SEM of six experiments. *$P<0.05$, **$P<0.01$ (Reprinted, with permission, from [20])

11.1.3 Identification of Upregulated Genes Through Gene Ontology Analysis

Based on the results of clustering analysis, we tested the genes by all GO terms and identified the upregulated genes related to cyclic tensile strain among clusters 1, 2, and 3. Forty-four genes related to "apoptosis" were expressed in the early phase (cluster 3), whereas 17 genes related to "response to stimulus" were expressed in the late phase (cluster 1).

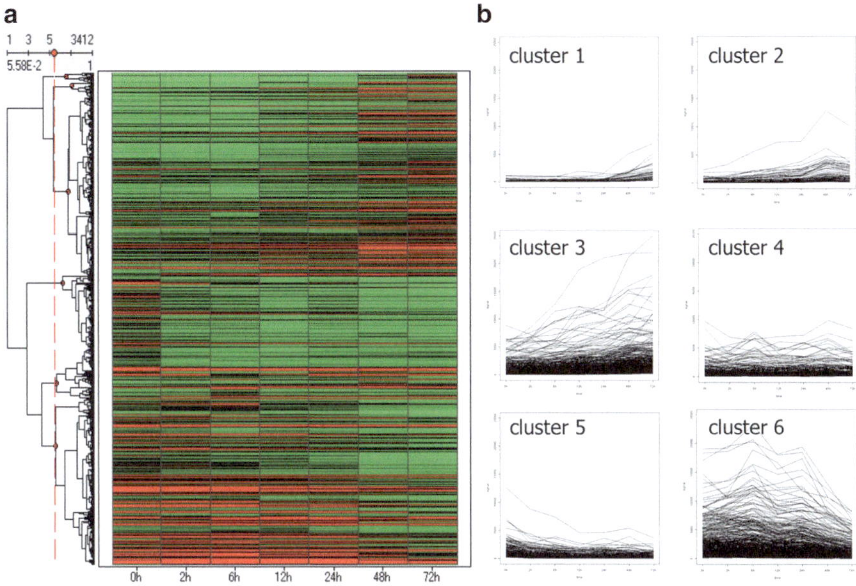

Fig. 11.3 Gene expression profiles in spinal cord cells after the application of cyclic tensile stress. The hierarchical clustering data are presented graphically as a heatmap (**a**). These genes were subsequently grouped into six subclusters (clusters 1–6) according to the time course of gene expression pattern (**b**) (Reprinted, with permission, from [20])

11.1.4 Identification of Upregulated Genes Using Kyoto Encyclopedia of Genes and Genomes Analysis

We tested the genes by all Kyoto Encyclopedia of Genes and Genomes (KEGG) terms in clusters 1, 2, and 3 including those upregulated in a time-dependent manner. Four pathways were significantly included in cluster 1, 3 pathways in cluster 2, and 24 pathways in cluster 3.

11.1.5 Gene-Specific Real-Time Reverse Transcription Polymerase Chain Reaction (Rt-Pcr) in Mapk Signaling Pathway

In further examination of KEGG analysis of cluster 3, which included many of the upregulated genes, we found that the MAPK signaling pathway contained 12 candidate genes among the 15 genes that were significantly upregulated. These genes were calcium channel voltage-dependent L-type alpha-1F subunit (Cacnalf or CACN), neurotrophic tyrosine kinase receptor type 2 (Ntrk2 or trkA/B), fibroblast

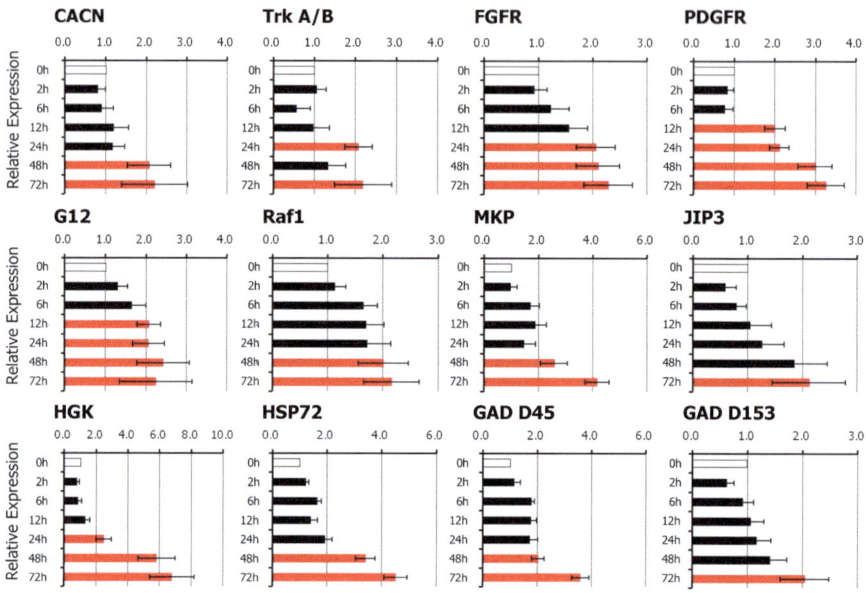

Fig. 11.4 The effects of cyclic tensile stress on gene expression levels analyzed by real-time RT-PCR. Application of cyclic tensile stress resulted in significant increases in mRNA expression levels of platelet-derived growth factor receptor (PDGFR), guanine nucleotide binding protein gamma 12 (G12) at 12 h, neurotrophic tyrosine kinase receptor type 2 (trkA/B), fibroblast growth factor receptor (FGFR), mitogen-activated protein kinase kinase kinase kinase 4 (HGK) at 24 h, and calcium channel voltage-dependent L-type alpha-1F subunit (CACN), v-raf-leukemia viral oncogene 1 (Raf1), dual-specificity phosphatase 1 (MKP), mitogen-activated protein kinase 8 interacting protein 3 (JIP3), heat shock protein 72 (HSP72), DNA-damage-inducible alpha (GAD D45), and DNA-damage-inducible transcript 3 (GAD D153) at 48–72 h. *Red bars* indicate significant differences ($P<0.05$) in upregulation at least twofold in comparison to controls. Data are mean ± SEM of three experiments (Reprinted, with permission, from [20])

growth factor receptor 2 (Fgfr2 or FGFR), platelet-derived growth factor receptor, beta polypeptide (Pdgfrb or PDGFR), v-raf-leukemia viral oncogene 1 (Raf1 or Raf), guanine nucleotide binding protein (G protein) gamma 12 (Gng12 or G12), dual-specificity phosphatase 1 (Dusp1 or MKP), mitogen-activated protein kinase kinase kinase kinase 4 (Map4k4 or HGK), mitogen-activated protein kinase 8 interacting protein 3 (Mapk8ip3 or JIP3), heat shock protein 72 (Hspa 72 or HSP72), growth arrest and DNA-damage-inducible alpha (Gadd45a or GAD D45), and DNA-damage-inducible transcript 3 (Ddit3 or GAD D153). These 12 genes were identified to test differential expression using real-time RT-PCR analysis. The mRNA expression levels of PDGFR and G12 significantly increased from the mid period of application of cyclic tensile stress (12-h stress duration), while CACN, trkA/B, FGFR, Raf1, MKP, HGK, JIP3, HSP72, GAD D45, and GAD D153 mRNA expression levels increased during the late phase of cyclic tensile strain (24–72 h duration) (Fig. 11.4).

11.2 Discussion

In vitro systems offer several advantages over in vivo systems in the analysis of cellular responses to their mechanical environment. By precisely controlling the loading conditions, the quantitative relationship between the severity of mechanical injury and response to the injury can be evaluated [21]. The physiological strain conditions of neuronal cells are not as high as other cells [22], showing ischemic changes at 11 % strain [23], but not at a 6 % strain level [24]. PC12 cells were subjected to cyclic tensile strain levels ranging from 4 to 16 % at strain frequencies of 1–2 Hz as physiological mechanical conditions [22]. Based on these reports and considering primary cultured spinal cord cells [19], we selected the range of cyclic tensile strain most appropriate to our culture system in the present study. Our results suggest that both the level of strain applied and frequency of its application influence cell viability. Furthermore, the results demonstrate that a higher strain level at a lower strain rate can have a similar effect as a lower strain level at a higher strain rate in neuron-rich spinal cord cells.

DNA microarray was used to understand the molecular mechanism of neuronal responses to cyclic tensile strain. Forty-four progressively upregulated genes related to "apoptosis" among cluster 3 and 17 late phase upregulated genes related to "response to stimulus" among cluster 1 were identified using the GO system. Furthermore, the KEGG/pathway analysis identified different pathways in the upregulated genes in a time-dependent manner in the clusters 1, 2, and 3. Indeed, the MAPK kinase pathway was identified by KEGG analysis of the alterations in gene expression seen in the mechanically loaded spinal cord cells. MAPKs are a family of related serine/threonine protein kinases that transduce several signals responsible for cell proliferation or cellular stress and are also intracellular signaling systems that induce optimal stress responses. In KEGG analysis, the MAPK signaling pathway can be classified into three main groups [25]: the classical MAP pathway, the c-Jun N-terminal kinase or stress-activated protein kinase (JNK), the p38 MAPK signaling pathway, and the ERK pathway. In the present study, the mRNA expression levels of PDGFR and G12 significantly increased during the mid period of cyclic tensile strain application, while CACN, Raf1, MKP, JIP3, HSP72, GAD D45, and GAD D153 mRNA levels increased during the late phase of the cyclic tensile strain application. These genes, which were further identified by real-time RT-PCR analysis, may play an important role in the response of spinal cord cells to neuronal injury. Gene expression of trkA/B, FGFR, PDGFR, and Raf1 could facilitate neuronal survival, while gene expression of G12, HSP72, GAD D45, and GAD D153 could be involved in DNA damage.

Considered together with our previous findings [19], we can conclude that certain apoptosis-specific genes are activated in neuronal cell-rich cultures during the application of cyclic tensile stress [20]. The clinical relevance of tensile strain may specifically include the tethering effect with the developmental ascensus medullaris [19], cervical myelopathy in association with kyphotic deformity [4], and complicated spinal cord distraction injury.

11.3 Conclusion

Cultured spinal cord cell death was induced depending on the level and duration of cyclic tensile strain applied with alterations in gene expression and particular upregulation of members of the MAPK pathway.

Acknowledgment This work was supported in part by Grants-in-Aid for General Scientific Research of the Ministry of Education, Science and Culture of Japan (grants numbers 16390435, 18390411, 19791023, 21591895, and 21791389). This study was also supported by grants from Research Program of Spinal Cord Intractable Pain (2009), The Public Health Bureau of the Japanese Ministry of Health and Welfare.

Conflict of Interest All authors declare that they have no conflict of interest.

References

1. Baptiste DC, Fehlings MG (2006) Pathophysiology of cervical myelopathy. Spine J 6:190S–197S
2. Uchida K, Baba H, Maezawa Y et al (2003) Increased expression of neurotrophins and their receptors in the mechanically compressed spinal cord of the spinal hyperostotic mouse (*twy/twy*). Acta Neuropathol 106:29–36
3. Ghafoor AU, Martin TW, Gopalakrishnan S et al (2005) Caring for the patients with cervical spine injuries: what have we learned? J Clin Anesth 17:640–649
4. Uchida K, Nakajima H, Sato R et al (2009) Cervical spondylotic myelopathy associated with kyphosis or sagittal sigmoid alignment: outcome after anterior or posterior decompression. J Neurosurg Spine 11:521–528
5. Hayes RL, Yang K, Raghupathi R et al (1995) Changes in gene expression following traumatic brain injury in the rat. J Neurotrauma 12:779–790
6. Raghupathi R, McIntosh TK (1996) Regionally and temporally distinct patterns of induction of c-fos, c-jun and junB mRNAs following experimental brain injury in the rat. Brain Res Mol Brain Res 37:134–144
7. Sall JM, Morehead M, Murphy S et al (1996) Alterations in CNS gene expression in a rodent model of moderate traumatic brain injury complicated by acute alcohol intoxication. Exp Neurol 139:257–268
8. Yakovlev AG, Faden AI (1995) Molecular biology of CNS injury. J Neurotrauma 12:767–777
9. Carmel JB, Galante A, Soteropoulos P et al (2001) Gene expression profiling of acute spinal cord injury reveals spreading inflammatory signals and neuron loss. Physiol Genomics 7:201–213
10. Song G, Cechvala C, Resnick DK et al (2001) GeneChip analysis after acute spinal cord injury in rat. J Neurochem 79:804–815
11. Tachibana T, Noguchi K, Ruda MA (2002) Analysis of gene expression following spinal cord injury in rat using complementary DNA microarray. Neurosci Lett 327:133–137
12. Aimone JB, Leasure JL, Perreau VM et al (2004) Spatial and temporal gene expression profiling of the contused rat spinal cord. Exp Neurol 189:204–221
13. Di Giovanni S, Knoblach SM, Brandoli C et al (2003) Gene profiling in spinal cord injury shows role of cell cycle in neuronal death. Ann Neurol 53:454–468
14. Popovich PG, Stokes BT, Whitacre CC (1996) Concept of autoimmunity following spinal cord injury: possible roles for T lymphocytes in the traumatized central nervous system. J Neurosci Res 45:349–363

15. Morrison B 3rd, Saatman KE, Meaney DF et al (1998) In vitro central nervous system models of mechanically induced trauma: a review. J Neurotrauma 15:911–928
16. Gilbert JA, Weinhold PS, Banes AJ et al (1994) Strain profiles for circular cell culture plates containing flexible surfaces employed to mechanically deform cells in vitro. J Biomech 27:1169–1177
17. Matsumoto T, Kawakami M, Kuribayashi K et al (1999) Cyclic mechanical stretch stress increases the growth rate and collagen synthesis of nucleus pulposus cells in vitro. Spine (Phila Pa 1976) 24:315–319
18. Nakatani T, Marui T, Hitora T et al (2002) Mechanical stretching force promotes collagen synthesis by cultured cells from human ligamentum flavum via transforming growth factor-beta1. J Orthop Res 20:1380–1386
19. Uchida K, Nakajima H, Takamura T et al (2008) Gene expression profiles of neurotrophic factors in rat cultured spinal cord cells under cyclic tensile stress. Spine (Phila Pa 1976) 33:2596–2604
20. Uchida K, Nakajima H, Hirai T et al (2010) Microarray analysis of expression of cell death-associated genes in rat spinal cord cells exposed to cyclic tensile stresses in vitro. BMC Neurosci 11:84
21. Morrison B 3rd, Meaney DF, Margulies SS et al (2000) Dynamic mechanical stretch of organotypic brain slice cultures induces differential genomic expression: relationship to mechanical parameters. J Biomech Eng 122:224–230
22. Haq F, Keith C, Zhang G (2006) Neurite development in PC12 cells on flexible micro-textured substrates under cyclic stretch. Biotechnol Prog 22:133–140
23. Morrison B 3rd, Cater HL, Wang CC et al (2003) A tissue level tolerance criterion for living brain developed with an in vitro model of traumatic mechanical loading. Stapp Car Crash J 47:93–105
24. Tanoue M, Yamaga M, Ide J et al (1996) Acute stretching of peripheral nerves inhibits retrograde axonal transport. J Hand Surg Br 21:358–363
25. Davis RJ (1993) The mitogen-activated protein kinase signal transduction pathway. J Biol Chem 268:14553–14556

Chapter 12
Spinal Kyphosis Causes Demyelination and Neuronal Loss in the Spinal Cord

Masaya Nakamura, Kentaro Shimizu, and Yoshiaki Toyama

Abstract The spinal cord has remarkable ability to resist chronic compression; however, delayed paralysis is sometimes seen following the development of spinal kyphosis. In the past, no animal model to clarify the mechanism of spinal cord damage due to spinal kyphotic deformity has been available. We developed a new experimental model of chronic spinal cord compression using a bird, to evaluate the effects of chronic compression associated with kyphotic deformity of the cervical spine on the spinal cord.

As kyphosis progressed, the spinal cord flattening became more marked, causing histopathological changes, including demyelination and neuronal loss. Demyelination of the axons progressed in the order of the anterior, lateral, and then posterior funiculus. Furthermore, microangiography suggested that vascular disturbance in addition to mechanical compression may have contributed to the development of histological changes. In conclusion, progressive kyphosis of the cervical spine resulted in demyelination of nerve fibers in the funiculi and neuronal loss in the anterior horn due to chronic compression of the spinal cord. These histological changes seem to be associated with both continuous mechanical compression and vascular changes in the spinal cord.

Keywords Cervical spine • Chronic compression • Kyphotic deformity

12.1 Introduction

Delayed spinal cord paralysis due to spinal deformity, in particular, local kyphosis, is often observed clinically in patients with neurofibromatosis, spinal caries, and congenital spinal kyphosis and in those after radiotherapy, trauma, or osteoporotic

M. Nakamura (✉) • K. Shimizu • Y. Toyama
Department of Orthopaedic Surgery, School of Medicine, Keio University, Shinanomachi 35, Tokyo, Shinjuku-Ku 160-8582, Japan
e-mail: masa@a8.keio.jp

K. Uchida et al. (eds.), *Neuroprotection and Regeneration of the Spinal Cord*,
DOI 10.1007/978-4-431-54502-6_12, © Springer Japan 2014

fracture. However, because of the lack of an appropriate animal model of spinal kyphosis, it still remains unclear how spinal kyphosis causes dysfunction of the spinal cord, resulting in such delayed paralysis. In our previous study, local kyphotic deformity of the cervical spine was produced by laminectomy of the cervical spine in juvenile animals, and histological and vascular changes in the spinal cord compressed by the kyphotic deformity were investigated.

12.2 Spinal Kyphotic Deformity Model

Several animal models of spinal cord compression have been reported. Although mice with hereditary osteocartilaginous abnormalities (twy mice) are well known as a model of spontaneous chronic spinal cord compression, there are several problems such as reproducibility of the degree and direction of compression [1]. Other animal models include gradual compression with screws [2–6] or balloons [7]; these models, which involve artificial compression in a stepwise manner, require frequent operative manipulations and the results obtained from these models are difficult to translate directly into clinical cases. Most of the other animal models of spinal cord compression reported previously were models of acute compression.

We used seventy-five 5-week-old Japanese small game fowls weighing approximately 200–300 g. Under general anesthesia induced by intraperitoneal injection of sodium pentobarbital (30 mg/kg body weight), a median incision was placed on the posterior neck of the animal. The paravertebral muscles were dissected and cut horizontally between C4 and C6. Then, using a high-speed drill, laminectomy and bilateral facetectomy at the C4–5 level were performed to induce local instability between C4 and 5 (Fig. 12.1). Only the skin was sutured with an uninterrupted suture without repairing the transected muscles (operated group). In the control group, only the skin incision was made. At different time points after surgery, the spine and spinal cord were removed en bloc after transcardial perfusion. Then, plain lateral-view x-rays of the cervical spine were obtained. The angle formed by the major axes of C4 and 5 vertebral bodies at the apex of kyphosis was measured to yield the kyphotic angle (Fig. 12.2).

12.3 Progressive Kyphosis of the Cervical Spine Caused Compression of the Cervical Spinal Cord

While the control animals maintained straight alignment of the middle cervical spine (Fig. 12.3a), the animals in the operated group developed severe kyphotic deformity in the middle cervical spine with hyper lordosis of the lower cervical spine to keep their head upright (Fig. 12.3b–f). Their kyphotic deformity progressed intensively with time until 3 weeks after the surgery and stabilized thereafter. The mean kyphotic angle was $51.6 \pm 5.0°$ in the operated group at 8 weeks after

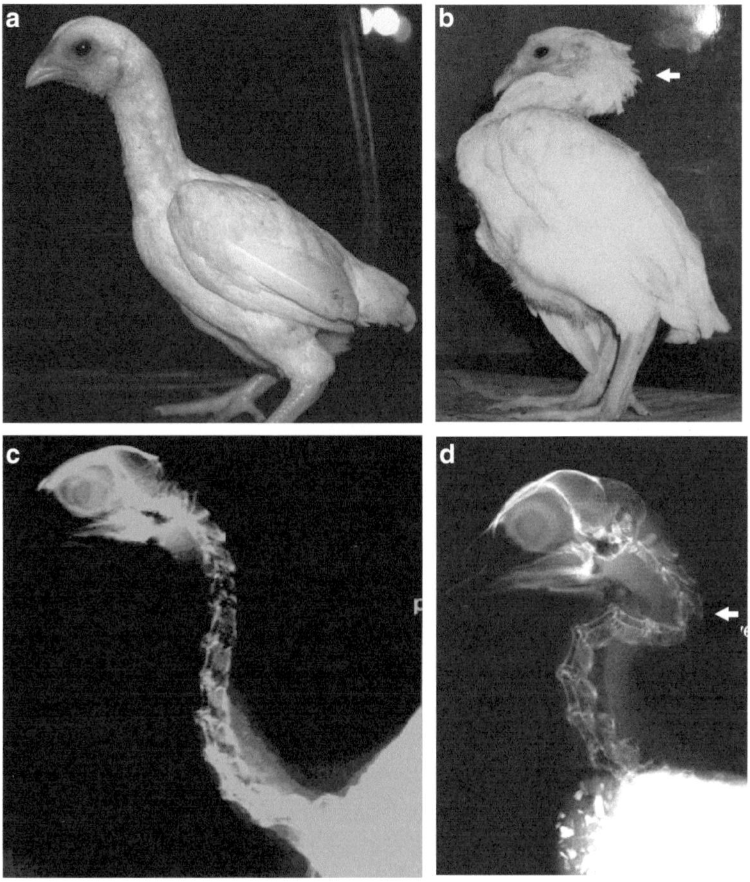

Fig. 12.1 Photographs of Japanese small game fowl in the control (**a**) and the operated group (**b**). Roentgenograms of its cervical lateral views in the control (**c**) and operated group (**d**). Severe kyphotic deformity was observed at the mid-cervical lesions in the operated group (*arrow head*) because the animals tries to keep their heads upright and parallel to the ground

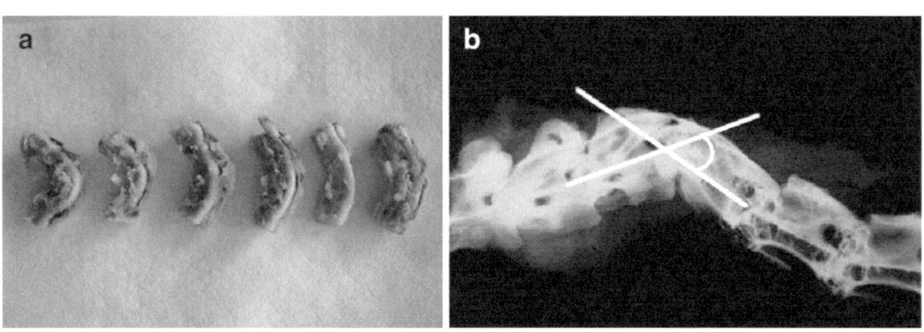

Fig. 12.2 (**a**) Photograph of the dissected spine and spinal cord tissues. (**b**) Measurement of kyphotic angle

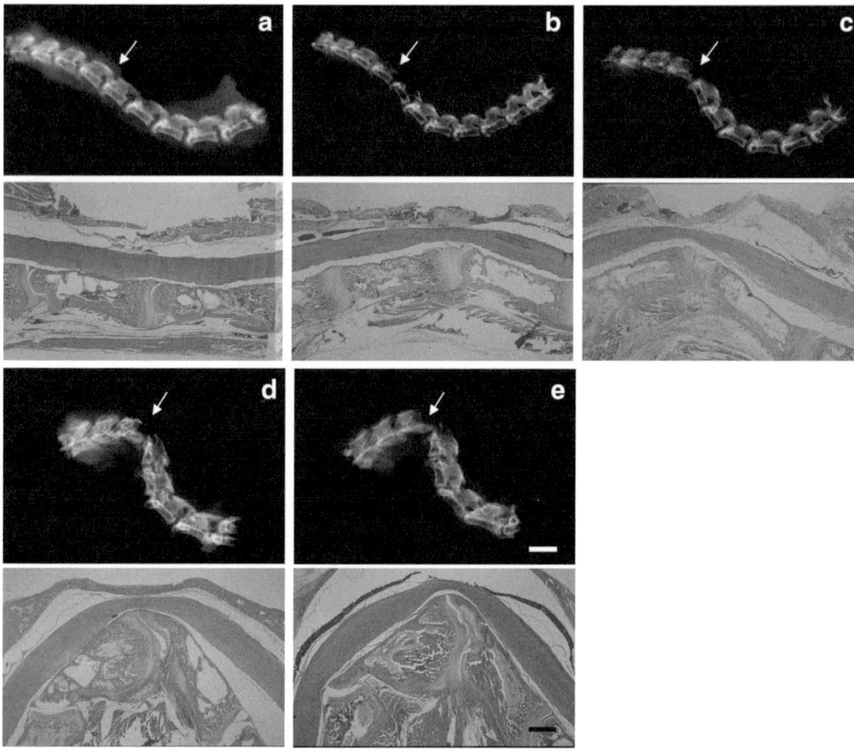

Fig. 12.3 Changes in kyphotic deformities of cervical spine after surgery. As the birds grew, kyphotic deformity progressed until 3 weeks, which were maintained thereafter. (**a**) 1 day, (**b**) 3 days, (**c**) 1 week, (**d**) 3 weeks, and (**e**) 8 weeks after the surgery (*arrows*: C4–5 level). The spinal cord was compressed ventrally due to vertebral deformity. Bar in (**e**) is 2.5 mm in the *upper row* of (**e**), 1 mm in the *lower row* of (**e**)

surgery and 14.2 ± 2.8° in the control group. Intramedullary hemorrhage and giant cavities, which are characteristics of acute compression, were not observed in this model. At the apex of the kyphosis, the spinal cord was compressed severely, and spinal cord flattening was most evident. There was a strong negative correlation between the kyphotic angle of the cervical spine and the spinal cord flattening ratio ($r = -0.913$) (Fig. 12.4). None of the animals, however, developed apparent motor paralysis during the postoperative observation period. In the previous animal studies, the reproducibility of the occurrence of delayed paralysis was poor, and it has been shown that delayed paralysis developed only after spinal cord compression became very severe, that is, compression due to stenosis of 50 % or more of the spinal canal [5, 6]. This finding is consistent with the finding in patients with OPLL or neurofibromatosis (which causes very severe spinal cord compression due to kyphosis) and patients with cervical spondylotic myelopathy [8]. On the other hand, kyphosis, in general, is more likely to cause paralysis than scoliosis [9–12]. However, it is still unknown to date as to what severity of kyphosis may be associated with delayed

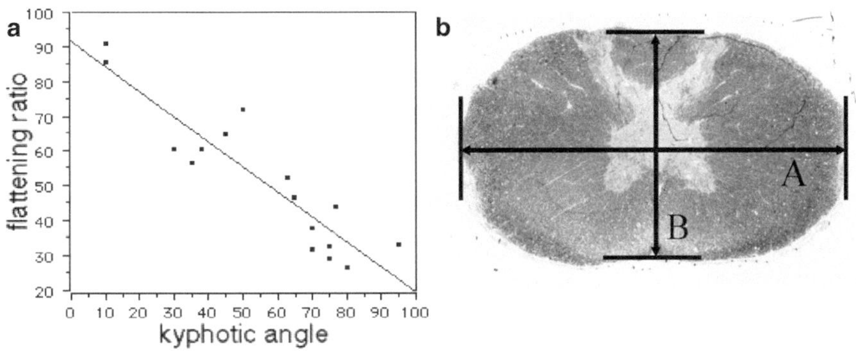

Fig. 12.4 (**a**) Flattening ratio (%) was calculated by $B/A \times 100$ (%) (A: transverse diameter, B: anteroposterior diameter). (**b**) Correlation between the kyphotic angle and the spinal cord flattening ratio. There was a strong negative correlation between kyphotic deformity and spinal cord flattening ratio ($r = -0.913$)

spinal cord paralysis. Several investigators have reported that the critical kyphotic angle at which paralysis is likely to occur was between 80° and 90° [13, 14]. This issue remains to be addressed in the future.

12.4 Progressive Kyphotic Deformity Caused a Loss of Motor Neurons and Demyelination

In some animals, spine and spinal cord tissues were embedded in paraffin, cut into sagittal sections together after rapid demineralization, and stained with hematoxylin and eosin (HE). While there were abundant motor neurons with large soma at the lamina IX in the control group (Fig. 12.5a, b), their number decreased in the operated group and the spared motor neurons showed severe atrophy (Fig. 12.5c, d: arrows). In the operated group, severe demyelination was observed in the anterior funiculus (Fig. 12.6a), and no such changes were found in the control groups (Fig. 12.6b). Demyelination in the posterior funiculus of the operated group was mild and difference between the two groups was less obvious (Fig. 12.6c, d). Myelin area ratio (MAR), which indicates the percent of the area of the myelin sheath relative to the total area of each captured image, was calculated. The average MAR in the anterior funiculus were 27.6 ± 5.2 % and 24.5 ± 4.7 % at 4 and 8 weeks after the surgery, respectively. There was a negative correlation between the kyphotic angle and the MAR of the anterior funiculus at both 4 week ($r = -0.881$) and 8 week ($r = -0.883$) after the surgery. The average MARs the lateral funiculus were 32.3 ± 4.7 % and 30.2 ± 3.6 % at 4 and 8 week after the surgery, respectively. There was a week negative correlation between the kyphotic angle and the MARs of the lateral funiculus at both 4 week ($r = -0.884$) and 8 week ($r = -0.897$) after the surgery. In contrast, the average MARs of the posterior funiculus were 40.4 ± 3.0

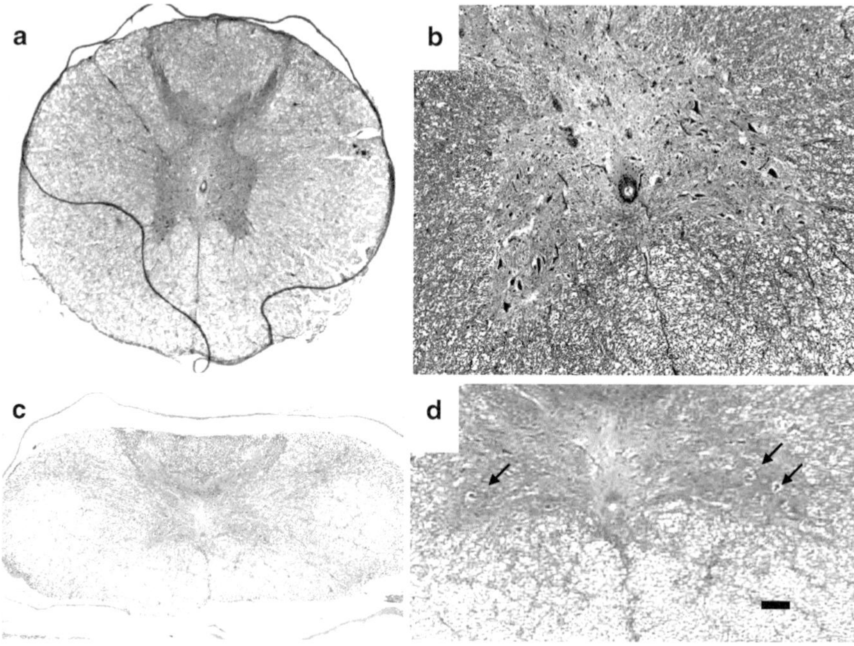

Fig. 12.5 Photomicrographs of anterior horn in the control (**a**) and the operated groups (**b**: kyphotic angle 95°). Fewer motor neurons in lamina IX at the anterior horn were observed in the operated group compared to the control group (hematoxylin and eosin staining). Bar is 200 μm in (**a**, **c**) and 100 μm in (**b**, **d**)

and 35.4 ± 3.0 at 4 and 8 week after the surgery, respectively. There was no significant correlation between the kyphotic angle and MARs of the posterior funiculus at either 4 week ($r=-0.587$) or 8 week ($r=-0.444$) after the surgery. Taking these results together, demyelination of the compressed white matter due to kyphotic deformity progressed in the order of anterior, lateral, and posterior funiculus; the posterior funiculus tended to be preserved even in the cases of severe compression (Fig. 12.7). The anterior funiculus in the operated group, which was the most extensively compressed, showed most marked histological changes such as demyelination and irregularity of the spared myelin sheath. The loss of the axons and vacuole formation were also apparent (Fig. 12.8a, b) compared to the control animals (Fig. 12.8c, d). Deformation of the myelin sheath surrounding the spared axons and recruitment of reactive astrocytes and macrophages were also observed (Fig. 12.8b)

Previous studies using various models of spinal cord compression revealed that severe compression could cause histological changes in the spinal cord [15]. The present study was designed to examine the histological changes in the spinal cord caused by progressive spinal kyphosis. As the kyphosis progressed, an increase in the degree of flattening of the spinal cord and histological changes, including the loss

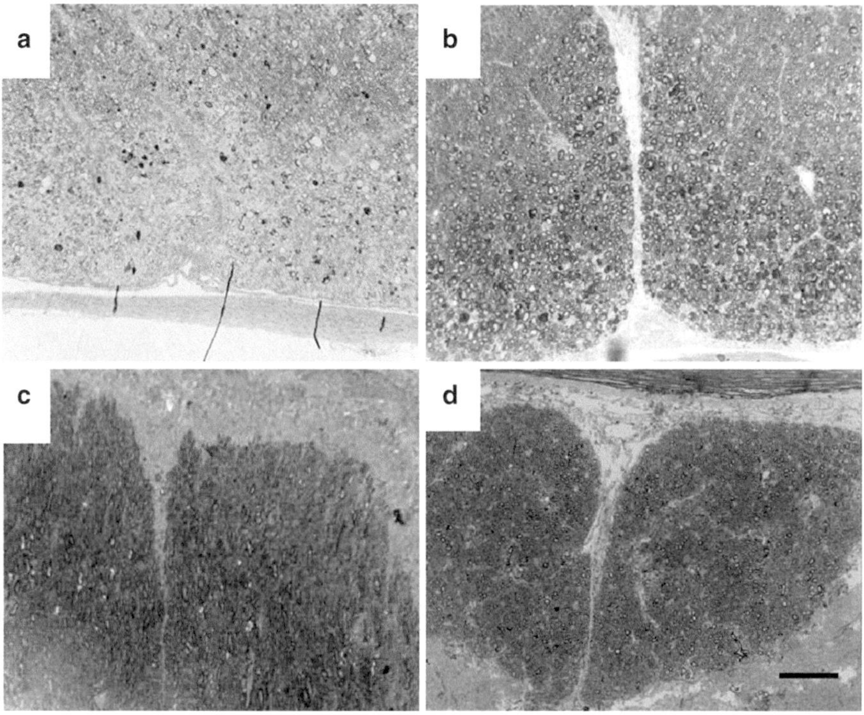

Fig. 12.6 Sections of the spinal cord at the level of maximum compression (toluidine blue staining). Severe demyelination of the axons in the anterior funiculus was observed in the operated group (**a**) compared to the control group (**b**). Myelin sheath in the posterior funiculus was preserved in the operated group (**c**) despite the severe kyphosis of 75°. The difference in the histology was less obvious between the operated group (**c**) and the control group (**d**). Bar is 100 μm in (**a**–**d**)

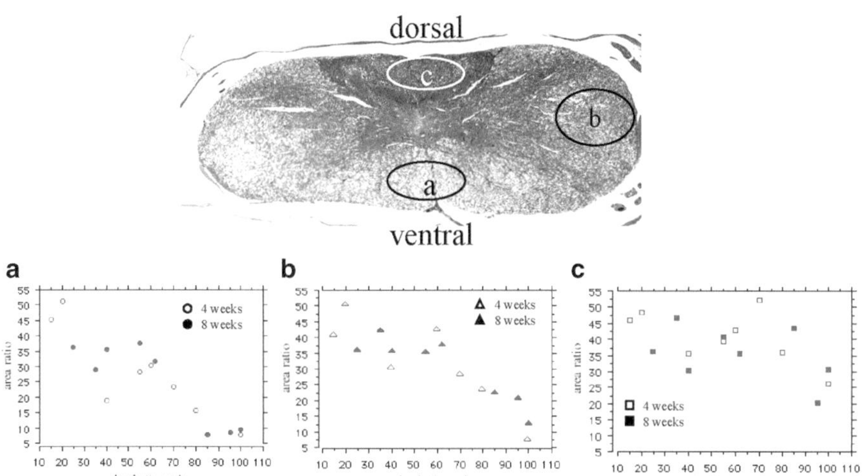

Fig. 12.7 Correlation between kyphotic angles and myelin sheath ratios (at 4 and 8 weeks after surgery. (4 weeks, *white point*; 8 weeks, *black point*). (**a**) Anterior funiculus (4w; $r=-0.881$, 8w; $r=-0.883$), (**b**) lateral funiculus (4w; $r=-0.884$, 8w; $r=-0.897$), and (**c**) posterior funiculus (4w; $r=-0.587$, 8w; $r=-0.444$)

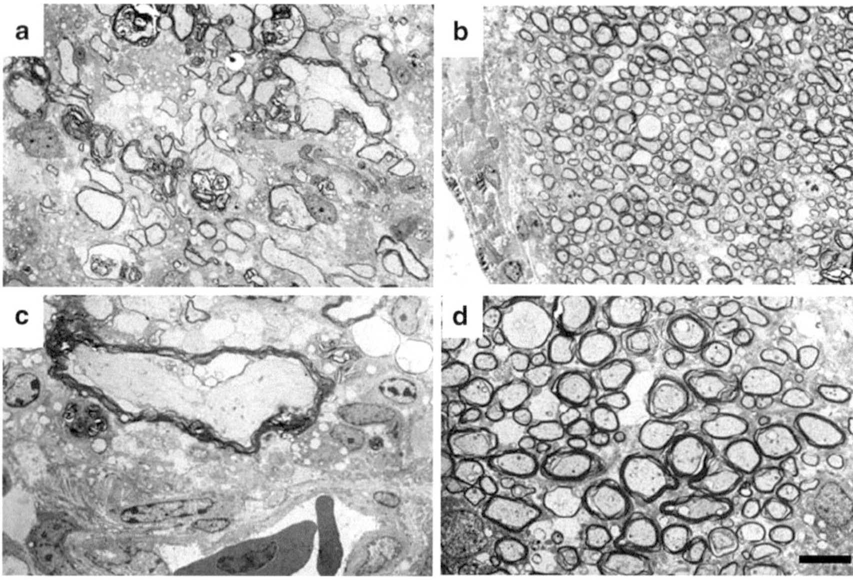

Fig. 12.8 An electron micrograph of the anterior funiculus. In the operated group (**a**, **b**), the axons were relatively preserved, but thinning and deformity of the myelin sheath were observed at the level of the most intensive compression. The change such as focal vacuolation and gliosis was seen among axons. In the control group (**c**, **d**), the structure of axons and myelin sheath were normal. Bar is 5 μm in (**a**, **c**), 10 μm in (**b**, **d**). (**a**, **c**) 1,000× (**b**, **d**) 2,000×

of anterior horn cells and demyelination of the anterior funiculus, were observed. As kyphosis progressed further, the demyelination of the axon spread to the lateral funiculus and then to the posterior funiculus. Marked histological changes were seen on the ventral side of the spinal cord, probably due to continued mechanical stress caused by the kyphotic deformity.

12.5 Kyphotic Deformity of the Cervical Spine Causing Loss of Intramedullary Blood Vessels

Eight weeks after the surgery, transcardiac systemic angiography was performed in both the operated and control groups using India ink to examine the distribution of the blood vessels in the spinal cord at the area of spinal kyphosis [16]. India ink (0.5 ml/body weight, 40 °C) containing 10 % gelatin was perfused transcardially for 10 min. The spinal cord were dissected from the animals and were stored frozen for 24 h to induce coagulation of gelatin, fixed in 10 % formalin for 7 days, and then cut into transverse and sagittal sections for the observation under the microscope.

It is known that the spinal cord vascular system of birds resembles that of humans [16]. In the control group, there was a dense distribution of blood vessels supplied

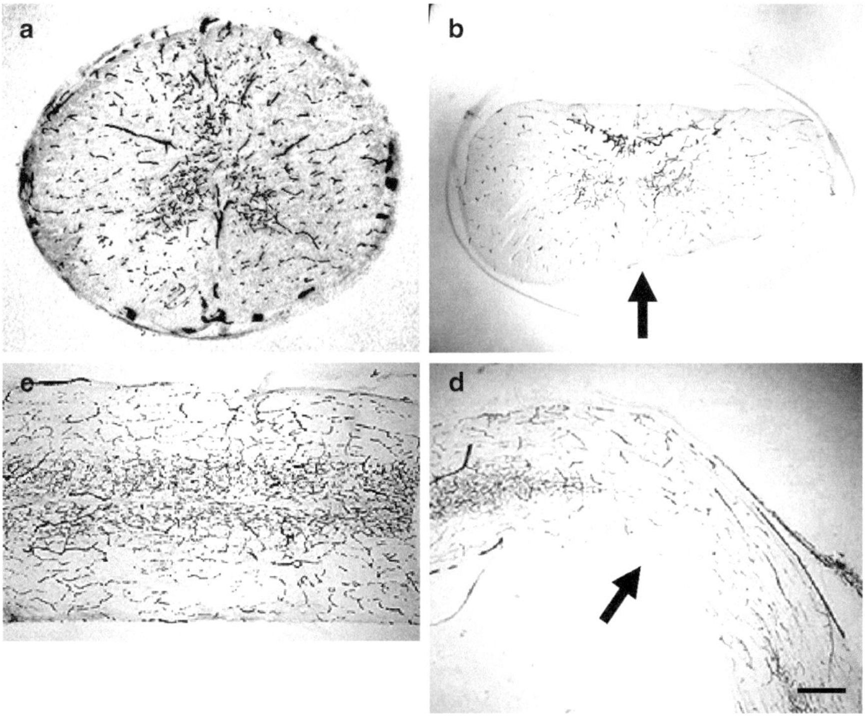

Fig. 12.9 Microangiogram. In the control group (**a**, **c**) normal intramedullary vasculatures are observed. Distributions of the capillary vessels at the ventral part of spinal cord were poor at the level of the most intensive compression in the operated group (**b**, **d**). (**a**, **b**) were transverse, (**c**, **d**) were sagittal sections. Bar is 50 μm in (**a**, **b**), 40 μm in (**c**, **d**)

by the anterior, posterior, and coronal arteries. The central artery branching from the anterior spinal artery leads through the anteromedial fissure toward the central canal and supplies blood to two-third of ventral part of spinal cord [16]. Density of blood vessels in the gray matter was higher than that in the white matter (Fig. 12.9a, c).

In the operated group, the small blood vessels in the compressed spinal cord showed a marked reduction in the network size, a decrease in number, interruption, and abnormal arrangement, of the blood vessels. As the kyphotic angle increased, these changes became more marked especially in the ventral side of the spinal cord that was directly exposed to mechanical compression (Fig. 12.9b, d). Breig [17] and Turnbull [18] reported that spinal cord flattening led to deformation of the intramedullary blood vessels, such as twisting and extension. It is known that the incidence of paraplegia associated with congenital kyphosis is highest in patients whose apex of kyphosis is located between T4 and T9 (the watershed area for the spinal cord blood supply) [19]. These findings suggest that the histological abnormalities associated with spinal cord flattening may be related, at least, in part, to ischemia. In the present study, angiography revealed a reduction in the density of capillary networks and interruption of capillaries at the compressed spinal cord. Considering the facts that changes in the capillary networks were more marked on the ventral side and that the number of blood vessels filled with the contrast material decreased as the kyphosis progressed, histological changes of the spinal cord, such as demyelination and neuronal loss may be due to the vascular changes in addition to mechanical compression.

Conflict of Interest The authors declare that they have no conflict of interest.

References

1. Hosoda Y, Yoshimura Y, Higaki S (1981) A new breed of mouse showing multiple osteochondral lesions-twy mouse. Ryumachi 21:157–164 (in Japanese)
2. Al-Mefty O, Harkey HL, Marawi I et al (1993) Experimental chronic compressive cervical myelopathy. J Neurosurg 79:550–561
3. Gooding MR, Wilson CB, Hoff JT (1975) Experimental cervical myelopathy. Effects of ischemia and compression of the canine cervical spinal cord. J Neurosurg 43:9–17
4. Hoff J, Nishimura M, Pitts L et al (1977) The role of ischemia in the pathogenesis of cervical spondylotic myelopathy. Spine 2:100–108
5. Kurokawa T, Tanaka H, Seki H et al (1975) Study about the origin of cervical spondylotic myelopathy: a preliminary report - animal experiment about the spinal cord compression which gradually increases. J Jpn Orthop Assoc 49:769–771 (in Japanese)
6. Shinomiya K, Mutoh N, Furuya K (1992) Study of experimental cervical spondylotic myelopathy. Spine 17:S383–S387
7. Tarlov IM, Klinger H, Vitale S (1953) Spinal cord compression studies. I. Experimental techniques to produce acute and gradual compression. AMA Arch Neurol Psychiatry 70:813–819
8. Lonstein JE, Winter RB, Moe JH et al (1980) Neurological deficits secondary to spinal deformity. A review of the literature and a report of 43 cases. Spine 5:331–355
9. Craig JB, Govender S (1992) Neurofibromatosis of the cervical spine. J Bone Joint Surg Br 74: 575–578
10. Curtis BH, Fisher RL, Butterfield WL et al (1969) Neurofibromatosis with Paraplegia. Report of eight cases. J Bone Joint Surg Am 51:843–861
11. Kumano K, Okai K, Tsuyama N et al (1975) A characteristic and the natural history of scoliosis in Recklinghausen's disease. Seikeigeka 26:829–836 (in Japanese)
12. Winter RB, Moe JH, Wang JF (1973) Congenital Kyphosis. Its natural history and treatment as observed in a study of one hundred and thirty patients. J Bone Joint Surg Am 55:223–256
13. James JIP (1973) Congenital kyphoscoliosis. Israel J Med Sci 9:728–731
14. Winter RB, Lonstein JE, Anderson M (1988) Neurofibromatosis hyperkyphosis: a review of 33 patients with kyphosis of 80 degrees or greater. J Spinal Disord 1:39–49
15. Yato Y, Fujimura Y, Nakamura M et al (1997) Decreased choline acetyltransferase activity in the murine spinal cord motoneurons under chronic mechanical compression. Spinal Cord 35:729–734
16. Hirai M (1953) Study about vascularization mechanism of birds spinal cord. The first-edition about vascularization mechanism of house cocks spinal cord. Igakukenkyu 23:127–140 (in Japanese)
17. Turnbull I, Breig A, Hassler O (1966) Effects of mechanical stresses on the spinal cord in cervical spondylosis. A study on fresh cadaver material. J Neurosurg 25:45–56
18. Turnbull IM (1971) Microvasculature of the human spinal cord. J Neurosurg 35:141–147
19. Dommisse GF (1974) The blood supply of the spinal cord. J Bone Joint Surg Br 56:225–235

Part III
Neuroprotection

Chapter 13
Granulocyte Colony-Stimulating Factor-Mediated Neuroprotective Therapy for Spinal Cord Injury

Masao Koda, Takeo Furuya, Taigo Ianada, Koshiro Kamiya, Mitsutoshi Ota, Satoshi Maki, Akihiko Okawa, Kazuhisa Takahashi, and Masashi Yamazaki

Abstract To prove the efficacy of granulocyte colony-stimulating factor (G-CSF) for spinal cord injury (SCI), we performed several animal experiments in rodent SCI models. Through those experiments, we showed G-CSF's mechanisms of action for SCI.

G-CSF showed efficacy for SCI through mobilization of bone marrow-derived cells. G-CSF attenuated neuronal cell death in vitro and in vivo, resulting in promotion of functional recovery after SCI. Expression of IL-1β and TNF-α was significantly suppressed by G-CSF in the acute phase of SCI. G-CSF promoted upregulation of anti-apoptotic protein Bcl-Xl on oligodendrocytes and suppressed apoptosis of oligodendrocytes after SCI. G-CSF exerted neuroprotective effects via promotion of angiogenesis after SCI.

G-CSF's current use in the clinic for hematopoietic stimulation and its ongoing clinical trial for brain infarction make it an appealing molecule that could be rapidly placed into trials for acute SCI patients. G-CSF is one of the hopeful candidates for clinical application.

Keywords G-CSF • Neuroprotection • Secondary injury

13.1 Introduction

The pathologies following acute spinal cord injury (SCI) are divided into two sequential events: the primary injury and the secondary injury [1]. Direct mechanical trauma induces the primary injury, which includes the spinal cord tissue damage.

M. Koda (✉) • T. Furuya • T. Ianada • K. Kamiya • M. Ota • S. Maki • A. Okawa • K. Takahashi
Department of Orthopaedic Surgery, Chiba University Graduate School of Medicine, Chiba, Japan
e-mail: masaokod@gmail.com

M. Yamazaki
Department of Orthopaedic Surgery, University of Tsukuba, Tsukuba, Japan

K. Uchida et al. (eds.), *Neuroprotection and Regeneration of the Spinal Cord*,
DOI 10.1007/978-4-431-54502-6_13,

This initial insult then triggers a progressive wave of secondary injury, which exacerbates the injury to the spinal cord via the activation of pathophysiological mechanisms.

Known pathophysiological mechanisms of the secondary injury after SCI include ischemia, posttraumatic inflammatory response mediated by resident microglia and blood-derived inflammatory cells, release of excitatory amino acids, generation of reactive oxygen species, influx of Ca^{2+}, and so on [1]. Those multiple mechanisms instigate neuronal and glial cell death, resulting in exaggeration of tissue damage after SCI.

Secondary injury is the main therapeutic target for various kinds of drug therapies. Thus a huge effort has been expended by clinicians, basic scientists, and industry to discover effective neuroprotective agents which can act against mechanisms of the secondary injury following SCI [1].

Currently, high-dose methylprednisolone sodium succinate (MPSS) is the only clinically available treatment for acute SCI to reduce the secondary injury. In recent years, however, the use of high-dose MPSS in acute SCI has become controversial, largely based on the risk of serious adverse effects versus what is perceived to be a modest neurological benefit [2]. Therefore, development of new SCI drug therapies that could replace high-dose MPSS is an area of intense study.

Granulocyte colony-stimulating factor (G-CSF) is a 19.6 kDa glycoprotein that was identified initially as a serum component that induced differentiation of the murine myelomonocytic leukemic cell line and is capable of inducing the survival, proliferation, and differentiation of cells of neutrophil lineage [3, 4]. In addition to its effects as a hematopoietic cytokine, it was recently reported that G-CSF has the potential to promote the survival of other types of cells, including in ischemic myocardium [5]. In the central nervous system, G-CSF has direct neuroprotective effects against glutamate-induced neuronal death and stroke [6, 7]. Most recently, clinical trials have reported on the safety and feasibility of G-CSF administration following stroke, supporting the hypothesis that G-CSF may also be an effective therapeutic for SCI [8].

To prove the efficacy of G-CSF for SCI, we performed several animal experiments in rodent SCI models. Here we show the results of those experiments, indicating G-CSF's mechanism of action for SCI.

13.1.1 G-CSF Receptor Expression

To assess the expression of G-CSF receptor (G-CSFR), we performed immunofluorescence double staining on histological sections of spinal cords. The data revealed that G-CSFR was expressed on neurons, astrocytes, and oligodendrocytes in normal spinal cord (Fig. 13.1). According to the expression pattern of G-CSFR, we speculated that G-CSF can act on neuron, astrocyte, and oligodendrocyte.

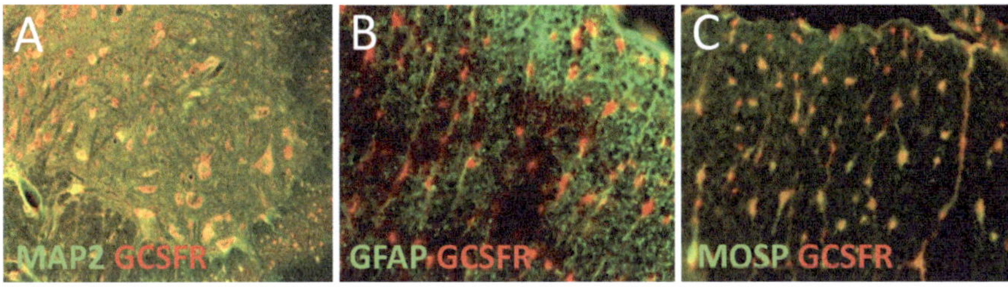

Fig. 13.1 Expression of granulocyte colony-stimulating factor receptor (G-CSFR) in normal spinal cord. Immunohistochemistry for G-CSFR and cell type markers was performed. G-CSFR was expressed by MAP2+ neurons (**a**), GFAP+ astrocytes (**b**), and MOSP+ oligodendrocytes (**c**)

13.1.2 G-CSF Promotes Migration of Bone Marrow-Derived Stem Cells into Injured Spinal Cord

To elucidate the effects of G-CSF-mediated mobilization of bone marrow-derived stem cells on the injured spinal cord, we constructed bone marrow chimera mice. Bone marrow cells of green fluorescent protein (GFP) transgenic mice were transplanted into lethally irradiated C57BL/6 mice. Four weeks after bone marrow transplantation, a large part of the bone marrow cells of those chimera mice was GFP-positive, enabling the tracking of bone marrow-derived cells by green fluorescence. SCI was produced by a static load (20 g, 5 min) at T8 level on those chimera mice. G-CSF (200 μg/kg/d) was injected subcutaneously for 5 days. Immunohistochemistry for GFP and cell lineage markers was performed to evaluate G-CSF-mediated mobilization of bone marrow-derived cells into injured spinal cord. Hind limb locomotor recovery was assessed for 6 weeks.

Immunohistochemistry revealed that G-CSF increased the number of GFP-positive cells in injured spinal cord, indicating that G-CSF promoted mobilization of bone marrow-derived cells and enhanced migration of those cells into injured spinal cord. The numbers of double-positive cells for GFP and glial markers were larger in the G-CSF-treated mice than in the control mice. G-CSF-treated mice showed significant recovery of hind limb function compared to that of the control mice. G-CSF showed efficacy for SCI treatment through mobilization of bone marrow-derived cells [9].

13.1.3 G-CSF Suppresses Apoptosis of Neurons After SCI

To elucidate the direct neuroprotective effect of G-CSF, we performed in vitro experiments using cultured neurons and in vivo experiments using mouse compressive SCI model. We found that G-CSF is neuroprotective against glutamate-induced cell death of cerebellar granule neurons in vitro.

Next, we used a mouse model of compressive SCI to examine the neuroprotective potential of G-CSF in vivo. Histological assessment with cresyl violet staining revealed that the number of surviving neurons in the injured spinal cord was significantly increased in G-CSF-treated mice. Immunohistochemistry for neuronal apoptosis revealed that G-CSF suppressed neuronal apoptosis after SCI. Moreover, administration of G-CSF promoted hind limb functional recovery. G-CSF might promote functional recovery by inhibiting neuronal apoptosis after SCI [10].

13.1.4 G-CSF Suppresses Inflammatory Cytokine Expression After SCI

To elucidate the potential therapeutic effect of G-CSF for SCI in rats, rat contusive SCI was introduced using the infinite horizon impactor (magnitude, 200 kilodyne). Recombinant human G-CSF (15.0 μg/kg) was administered by tail vein injection for 5 days. To detect the anti-inflammatory effects of G-CSF in the SCI model, we performed real-time PCR for inflammatory cytokines on the spinal cord sample of G-CSF and control rats. Twelve hours after surgery, expression of IL-1β and TNF-α mRNAs was significantly suppressed in the G-CSF group compared to the vehicle control group. The results of real-time PCR for the other factors showed no significant difference between the vehicle and G-CSF-treated groups. According to these results, G-CSF suppresses inflammatory cytokine expression after SCI [11].

13.1.5 G-CSF Suppresses Apoptosis of Oligodendrocytes and Protects Myelin After SCI

To elucidate anti-apoptotic effect of G-CSF on oligodendrocyte, in vivo experiments using rat contusive SCI introduced by the IH impactor (200 kilodyne) were performed. Recombinant human G-CSF (15.0 μg/kg) was administered by tail vein injection for 5 days. Histological assessment with luxol fast blue staining revealed that the area of white matter spared in the injured spinal cord was significantly larger in G-CSF-treated rats. Immunohistochemical analysis showed that G-CSF promoted upregulation of anti-apoptotic protein Bcl-Xl on oligodendrocytes and suppressed apoptosis of oligodendrocytes after SCI (Fig. 13.2). Moreover, administration of G-CSF promoted better functional recovery of hind limbs assessed by BBB locomotor scale [11].

13.1.6 G-CSF Promotes Angiogenesis After SCI

Because the degree of angiogenesis in the subacute phase after SCI correlates with regenerative responses, it is possible that G-CSF's neuroprotective effects after SCI are due to enhancement of angiogenesis. We utilized the contusive SCI rat model using IH impactor and randomly divided subjects between a G-CSF-treated group and a control group. In the G-CSF-treated rats, the total number of vessels was

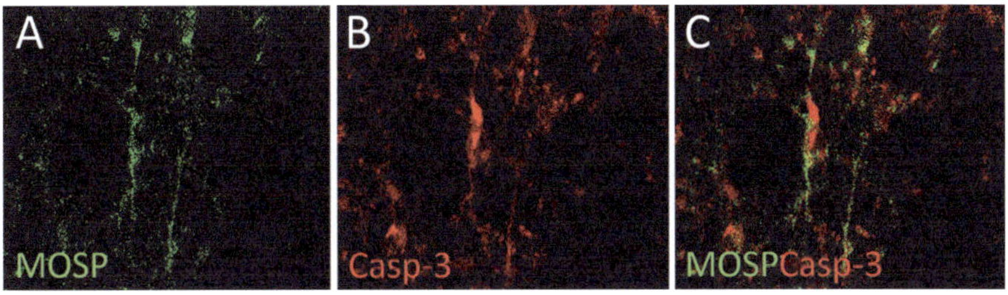

Fig. 13.2 Apoptosis of oligodendrocytes. Immunohistochemistry for oligodendrocyte marker MOSP (**a**) and apoptosis marker cleaved caspase-3 (Casp-3) (**b**) was performed. There were a lot of (**c**) MOSP- and Casp-3 double-positive apoptotic oligodendrocytes in injured spinal cord 1 week after SCI. In G-CSF-treated rats, the number of apoptotic oligodendrocytes decreased

significantly larger, and expression of angiogenic cytokines including bFGF, VEGF, and HGF was significantly higher than those in the control group. The G-CSF-treated group showed significant recovery of hind limb function compared to that of the control group. These results suggest that G-CSF exerts neuroprotective effects via promotion of angiogenesis after SCI [12].

13.2 Discussion

One of the major obstacles for conducting clinical trials for neuroprotective drugs is to first establish the safety and competency for use in human subjects. The complexity, size, and duration of clinical trials of novel drugs often make them quite costly to conduct and may impede the development of therapeutics that could have a significant impact in clinical practice. Therefore, although the efficacy of various drug therapies in models of SCI has been reported, few drugs have been practically carried into clinical trials. Thus, drugs with proven clinical exploitability have a significant advantage for clinical trials for novel therapeutic purposes. From this point of view, G-CSF's current use in the clinic for hematopoietic stimulation and its ongoing clinical trial for brain infarction make it an appealing molecule that could be rapidly placed into trials for acute SCI patients. Although many hurdles such as optimal dosage, therapeutic time window, and more precise mechanism of action still need to be resolved, the present results encourage us to make steps towards future clinical trials of G-CSF for acute SCI patients.

13.3 Conclusion

G-CSF exerts neuroprotective action for SCI via the abovementioned pleiotropic effects. Therefore G-CSF is one of the hopeful candidates for clinical application.

Acknowledgement Masao Koda declares that he has no conflict of interest.

References

1. Rabchevsky AG, Patel SP, Springer JE (2011) Pharmacological interventions for spinal cord injury: where do we stand? how might be we step forward? Pharmacol Ther 132:15–29
2. Matsumoto T, Tamaki T, Kawakami M et al (2001) Early complications of high-dose methylprednisolone sodium succinate treatment in the follow-up of acute cervical spinal cord injury. Spine 26:426–430
3. Nicola NA, Metcalf D, Matsumoto M et al (1983) Purification of a factor inducing differentiation in murine myelomonocytic leukemia cells. Identification as granulocyte colony-stimulating factor. J Biol Chem 258:9017–9023
4. Roberts AW (2005) G-CSF: a key regulator of neutrophil production, but that's not all! Growth Factors 23:33–41
5. Harada M, Qin Y, Takano H et al (2005) G-CSF prevents cardiac remodeling after myocardial infarction by activating the Jak-Stat pathway in cardiomyocytes. Nat Med 11:305–311
6. Schäbitz WR, Kollmar R, Schwaninger M et al (2003) Neuroprotective effect of granulocyte colony-stimulating factor after focal cerebral ischemia. Stroke 34:745–751
7. Schneider A, Kruger C, Steigleder T et al (2005) The hematopoietic factor G-CSF is a neuronal ligand that counteracts programmed cell death and drives neurogenesis. J Clin Invest 115:2083–2098
8. Shyu WC, Lin SZ, Lee CC et al (2006) Granulocyte colony-stimulating factor for acute ischemic stroke: a randomized controlled trial. CMAJ 174:927–933
9. Koda M, Nishio Y, Kamada T, Someya Y, Okawa A et al (2007) Granulocyte colony-stimulating factor (G-CSF) mobilizes bone marrow-derived cells into injured spinal cord and promotes functional recovery after compression-induced spinal cord injury in mice. Brain Res 1149:223–231
10. Nishio Y, Koda M, Kamada T, Someya Y, Kadota R et al (2007) Granulocyte colony-stimulating factor (G-CSF) attenuates neuronal death and promotes functional recovery after spinal cord injury in mice. J Neuropathol Exp Neurol 66:724–731
11. Kadota R, Koda M, Kawabe J et al (2012) Granulocyte colony-stimulating factor (G-CSF) protects oligodendrocyte and promotes hindlimb functional recovery after spinal cord injury in rats. PLoS One 7(11):e50391. doi:10.1371
12. Kawabe J, Koda M, Hashimoto M et al (2011) Neuroprotective effects of granulocyte colony-stimulating factor and relationship to promotion of angiogenesis after spinal cord injury in rats: laboratory investigation. J Neurosurg Spine 15:414–421

Chapter 14
Recombinant Human Hepatocyte Growth Factor Promotes Functional Recovery After Spinal Cord Injury

Kazuya Kitamura, Akio Iwanami, Kanehiro Fujiyoshi, Jun-ichi Yamane, Keigo Hikishima, Hiroshi Funakoshi, Toshikazu Nakamura, Masashi Aoki, Yoshiaki Toyama, Hideyuki Okano, and Masaya Nakamura

Abstract Hepatocyte growth factor (HGF), which is a potent mitogen for mature hepatocytes and a mediator of the inflammatory responses to tissue injury, was recently highlighted as a potent neurotrophic factor in the central nervous system. We revealed that introducing exogenous HGF into the injured rat spinal cord using

K. Kitamura
Department of Orthopedic Surgery, Keio University School of Medicine,
Tokyo, Shinjuku-ku 160-8582, Japan

Department of Orthopedic Surgery, Hiratsuka City Hospital,
Hiratsuka, Kanagawa 254-0065, Japan

A. Iwanami • K. Fujiyoshi • J.-i. Yamane • Y. Toyama • M. Nakamura (✉)
Department of Orthopedic Surgery, Keio University School of Medicine,
Tokyo, Shinjuku-ku 160-8582, Japan
e-mail: masa@a8.keio.jp

K. Hikishima
Department of Physiology, Keio University School of Medicine,
Tokyo, Shinjuku-ku 160-8582, Japan

Central Institute for Experimental Animals,
Tonomachi, Kawasaki, Kanagawa 210-0821, Japan

H. Funakoshi
Center for Advanced Research and Education, Asahikawa Medical University,
Midorigaoka, Asahikawa, Hokkaido 078-8510, Japan

T. Nakamura
Kringle Pharma Joint Research Division for Regenerative Drug Discovery, Center for Advanced Science and Innovation, Osaka University, Osaka 565-0871, Japan

M. Aoki
Department of Neurology, Tohoku University School of Medicine,
Sendai, Miyagi 980-8574, Japan

H. Okano
Department of Physiology, Keio University School of Medicine,
Tokyo, Shinjuku-ku 160-8582, Japan

K. Uchida et al. (eds.), *Neuroprotection and Regeneration of the Spinal Cord*,
DOI 10.1007/978-4-431-54502-6_14, © Springer Japan 2014

a herpes simplex virus-1 vector significantly reduces the area of damaged tissue and promotes functional recovery. However, this rat study did not examine the therapeutic effects of administering HGF after injury, which is the most critical issue for clinical application. To translate this strategy to human treatment, we induced a contusive cervical SCI in the common marmoset, a primate, and then administered recombinant human HGF (rhHGF) intrathecally. Motor function was assessed using an original open-field scoring system focusing on manual function, including reach-and-grasp performance and hand placement in walking. The intrathecal rhHGF preserved the corticospinal fibers and myelinated areas, thereby promoting functional recovery. This study demonstrates the therapeutic effects, safety, and clinical efficacy of intrathecal rhHGF treatment for SCI in adult nonhuman primates and the possibility that this novel therapy may be suitable for clinical application.

Keywords Clinical application • Hepatocyte growth factor • Nonhuman primate • Recombinant human hepatocyte growth factor • Spinal cord injury

14.1 Introduction

Spinal cord injury (SCI) is followed by secondary degeneration, which is characterized by progressive tissue necrosis. Many experimental interventions have focused on this posttraumatic inflammatory process, using neurotrophic factors to reduce the damaged area and to promote axonal regeneration through the lesion epicenter. Neurotrophins such as nerve growth factor (NGF) [1, 2], brain-derived neurotrophic factor (BDNF) [3], neurotrophin-3 (NT-3) [4, 5], and glial cell line-derived neurotrophic factor (GDNF) [6, 7] have been reported to enhance axonal growth in the injured spinal cord; some of these studies also showed that neurotrophins promoted behavioral recovery after SCI [3, 7]. Both neurotrophic support and angiogenesis are critical to the endogenous regenerative response to trauma after SCI [8, 9]. The initial damage to local blood vessels is decisive for the progression of destructive events during secondary degeneration [10], and strategic treatments to improve angiogenesis after SCI have shown a relationship between blood flow and functional recovery [11, 12].

Hepatocyte growth factor (HGF) was first identified as a potent mitogen for mature hepatocytes [13, 14] and a natural ligand for the c-Met proto-oncogene product [15]. Recent studies have revealed that HGF acts as a neurotrophic factor for a variety of neuron types [16–20] and that administering HGF enhances angiogenesis, improves microcirculation, inhibits destruction of the blood–brain barrier [21], and exerts a neuroprotective effect after cerebral ischemia [22, 23] and in the transgenic amyotrophic lateral sclerosis (ALS) rat model [24].

In this study, we first examined the changes in endogenous HGF and c-MET expression in rat spinal cord before and after SCI and then determined whether the administration of exogenous HGF into the injured spinal cord using herpes simplex virus-1 (HSV-1) vector had positive effects on histological changes and the motor function after SCI. Accordingly, we revealed that introducing exogenous HGF into the spinal cord significantly reduces the damaged area and promotes functional recovery in adult rats [25]. However, this strategy, which involved injecting a HSV-1 vector into the spinal cord prior to SCI, can never be applied to clinical treatment. Furthermore, rodent SCI models are limited in their ability to ensure the efficacy and safety of treatments for humans. It is critical to examine potential treatments in nonhuman primates before proceeding to clinical trials.

Then, we started another in vivo study, a total of 400 μg of recombinant human HGF (rhHGF) was infused intrathecally for 4 weeks immediately after C5-level contusive SCI in adult common marmosets, as a preclinical trial. Contusive injury is considered the most relevant to human SCI when evaluating therapies and predicting their translation to human treatment. However, to assess hand dexterity recovery, we needed an open-field rating scale for a primate cervical SCI model that would be comparable to the BBB scale in rodents [26]. Therefore, we established an original open-field rating scale to evaluate hand neurological performance after contusive cervical SCI. We found that intrathecal rhHGF infusion significantly reduced the areas of damaged tissue in the spinal cord and promoted functional recovery, consistent with our rat study.

Here we report how we established a novel strategy for SCI using HGF and present the efficacy of rhHGF for SCI.

14.2 Upregulation of Endogenous HGF is Delayed Compared to That of c-Met in Spinal Cord During the Acute Phase of Injury

To determine the dynamics of the HGF–c-Met system in adult rat spinal cord after SCI, the levels of HGF and c-Met mRNA expression in injured spinal cord were analyzed using real-time reverse-transcriptase polymerase chain reaction (RT-PCR) and the amounts of HGF protein in injured spinal cord and plasma were also analyzed using an enzyme-linked immunosorbent assay (ELISA) at multiple time points after SCI. While the level of c-Met mRNA expression in injured spinal cord drastically increased from 1 day after SCI (Fig. 14.1a), the level of HGF mRNA expression gradually increased and peaked at 2 weeks after SCI (Fig. 14.1b). Thus HGF and c-Met mRNA expression peaked at different time points after SCI. Consistent with the level of HGF mRNA expression, the amount of HGF protein in injured spinal cord gradually increased, peaking at around 4 weeks after SCI (Fig. 14.1c). In contrast, the amount of HGF protein in the plasma did not increase after SCI (Fig. 14.1d).

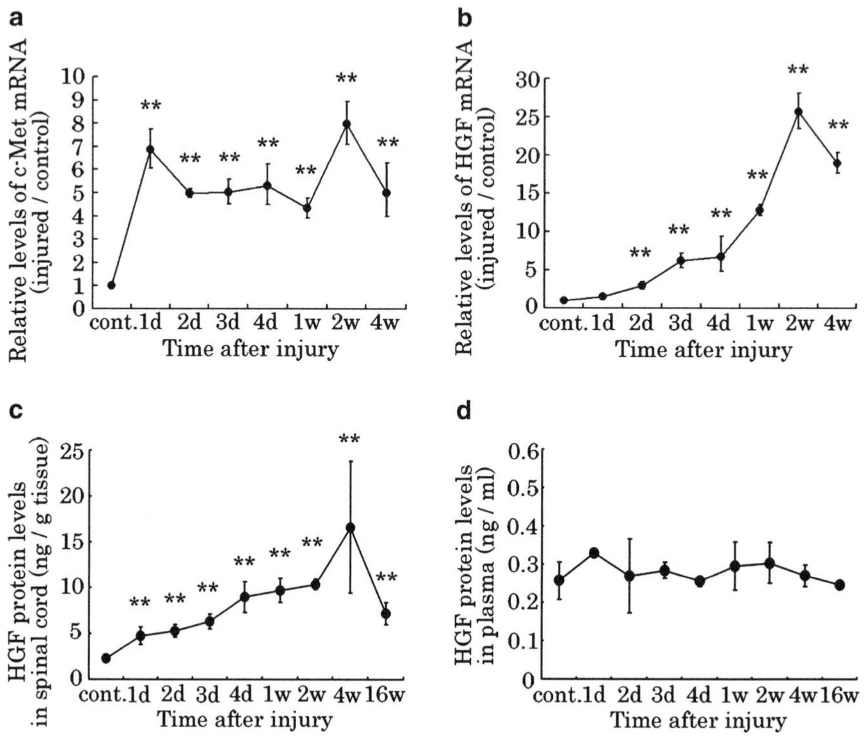

Fig. 14.1 Endogenous regulation of HGF and c-Met expression after SCI. The levels of c-Met mRNA and HGF mRNA expression after SCI in a 4-mm segment of spinal cord from the lesion epicenter were analyzed using real-time RT-PCR. In contrast to a drastic increase in c-Met mRNA expression during the acute phase of SCI (**a**), HGF mRNA expression showed a gradual increase only during the subacute phase (**b**). ELISA data shows that the amount of HGF protein in a 4-mm segment of spinal cord from the lesion epicenter gradually increased during the subacute phase of SCI (**c**), similar to the pattern of HGF mRNA expression, and the plasma HGF levels did not increase significantly after SCI (**d**). All data were reported as the mean ± SEM. $^{**}p<0.01$. $n>3$ each. Figure adapted from [25]

14.3 Exogenous HGF Promoted Endogenous Repair and Functional Recovery After Spinal Cord Injury in Rat

14.3.1 Introduction of Exogenous HGF into Spinal Cord Using HSV-1 Vector and Thoracic SCI Model

Replication-incompetent HSV-1 vector, HSV-HGF (HGF group) or HSV-LacZ (LacZ group), was injected into the spinal cord at thoracic (T)10 level after laminectomy in adult female Sprague–Dawley rats. To examine the distribution and amount of HGF protein in uninjured spinal cord after gene delivery, the spinal cord tissues were harvested and processed for an ELISA and HGF immunostaining at 3 days after the HSV-1 vectors injection. While HGF immunoreactivity (IR) showed a remarkable expansion putatively in the extracellular matrix in the HGF group at 3 days after injection, very little HGF-IR was observed in the LacZ group (data not shown). Injection of the HSV-1 vectors resulted in a significantly higher amount of HGF protein in the HGF group (11.5 ± 0.8 ng/g tissue), compared with that in the LacZ group (3.4 ± 0.1 ng/g tissue), at 3 days after injection (data not shown) [25].

Based on these findings, at 3 days after HSV-1 vectors injection, contusive SCI was induced at the injection site using the Infinite Horizon impactor (200 kdyn, Precision Systems, Lexington, KY) to investigate therapeutic effects of HGF on injured spinal cord.

14.3.2 HGF Promotes Survival of Neurons and Oligodendrocytes After SCI

To determine the effects of exogenous HGF on the injured spinal cord, we performed several quantitative histological analyses. First, the cavity area of the injured spinal cord at 6 weeks after SCI was significantly smaller in the HGF group than the LacZ group (Fig. 14.2a). Second, the HGF group obviously had more preserved myelinated areas than the LacZ group at 6 weeks after SCI. Of note, the HGF group exhibited a significantly spared rim of white matter, even at the lesion epicenter, whereas the LacZ group exhibited severely demyelinated white matter throughout the lesion epicenter (Fig. 14.2b). Next, to determine the effect of HGF on motoneurons, the numbers of ChAT-positive motoneurons in the ventral horns were quantified at 6 weeks after SCI. Although almost all the ChAT-positive motoneurons disappeared at the lesion epicenter in both groups, a significantly larger number of ChAT-positive motoneurons were observed at the site rostral to the epicenter in the HGF group, compared with that in the LacZ group (Fig. 14.2c). These findings suggested that HGF exerted protective effects on motoneurons and oligodendrocytes and contributed to tissue sparing after SCI [25].

Next, to determine whether HGF inhibited the activation of caspase-3 after SCI, immunoblotting analyses using anti-cleaved caspase-3 antibody were performed at 1, 3, and 7 days after SCI. Cleaved caspase-3 was strongly induced after SCI and was most detectable at 3 days after SCI in both the HGF and LacZ groups (data not shown). Quantitative analysis revealed that the induction of cleaved caspase-3 was significantly attenuated in the HGF group, compared with the LacZ group, at 3 days after SCI (data not shown). Furthermore, double immunostaining using anti-cleaved caspase-3 antibody and antibodies for neurons or oligodendrocytes showed that the numbers of NeuN and cleaved caspase-3 double-positive motoneurons in the ventral horns and GST-π and cleaved caspase-3 double-positive oligodendrocytes were obviously reduced in the HGF group, compared with the LacZ group (data not shown). These results suggested that HGF significantly reduced the levels of cleaved caspase-3 activation in neurons and oligodendrocytes after SCI, thereby promoting their survival [25].

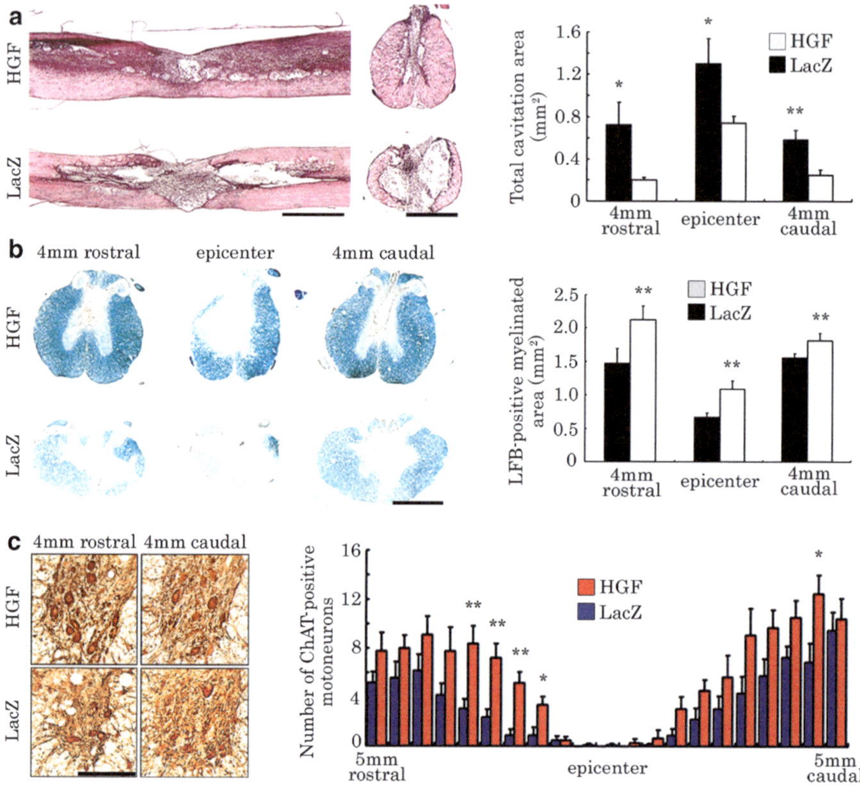

Fig. 14.2 A significant reduction in the size of damaged parenchyma in the HGF group. HE staining of midsagittal sections and the axial sections of lesion epicenter at 6 weeks after injury showed significantly smaller cavitation areas of damage in the HGF group, compared with the LacZ group. $n=5$ each (**a**). The axial sections of lesion epicenter stained with Luxol fast blue (LFB) at 6 weeks after injury showed a significant reduction in the area of demyelination in the HGF group, compared with the LacZ group. $n=5$ each (**b**). The number of ChAT-positive motoneurons in the ventral horns at the lesion epicenter and adjacent sections up to 5 mm rostral and caudal to the epicenter in 0.5-mm increments was quantified at 6 weeks after SCI. The pictures show magnified views of right ventral horns of axial sections at 4 mm rostral to the epicenter. Significant differences between the two groups were observed mainly in the sections rostral to the epicenter. $n=5$ each (**c**). $*p<0.05$, $**p<0.01$. Scale bars = 2 mm in (**a**) *left*; 1 mm in (**a**) *right* and (**b**); 150 μm in (**c**). Figure adapted from [25]

14.3.3 HGF Enhances Angiogenesis After SCI

To examine the effect of HGF on vascular endothelial cells after SCI, immunostaining with anti-RECA-1 antibody was performed. In intact thoracic spinal cord, the vessels had delicate walls composed of homogeneously stained endothelial cells. While most of the vessels disappeared at the epicenter at 1 week after SCI, several vessels were stained intensely and showed abnormally large lumina with thick wall, which were not observed in the intact spinal cord (data not shown). We found that significantly larger number of RECA-1-positive vessels with lumina larger than 20 μm, representing newly formed vessels [8], were observed in the HGF group compared with the LacZ group at the epicenter and at 4 mm rostral to the epicenter at 1 week after SCI (data not shown) [25].

14.3.4 HGF Promotes Regrowth of Serotonergic Fibers and Functional Recovery After SCI

To determine the effects of HGF on the axonal growth after SCI, axial sections of injured spinal cords were immunostained with anti-5HT antibody at 1 week and 6 weeks after SCI. 5HT-positive raphe-spinal serotonergic fibers were observed mainly in the gray matter in each group. Quantitative analyses revealed that while 5HT-positive fibers were almost undetectable in either group at 1 week after SCI, a significantly greater abundance of 5HT-positive fibers was detected, even in an area 4 mm caudal to the epicenter, in the HGF group as compared with that in the LacZ group at 6 weeks after SCI (data not shown). Furthermore, at 1 week after SCI, the 5HT-positive fibers also showed c-Met-IR, and at 6 weeks after SCI, they expressed GAP-43, which has been used as a marker of axonal regeneration [27–30], even in a region 4 mm caudal to the epicenter (data not shown).

The contusive SCI resulted in complete paralysis followed by gradual recovery, reaching a plateau (BBB score 6.6 ± 1.1) at 6 weeks after SCI in the LacZ group. Significant differences in the BBB scores were observed between the two groups from 7 days after SCI (data not shown). We believe that the difference between a BBB score of 8 (sweeping of hindlimbs) and BBB score of 9 (weight support on hindlimbs) is clinically substantial. From a clinical perspective, the recovery of the HGF group to weight-supported plantar steps (BBB score 10.1 ± 0.6) was noteworthy [25].

14.4 Recombinant Human HGF Promotes Hand Function in Nonhuman Primate After Spinal Cord Injury

14.4.1 Cervical Contusive SCI Model in Common Marmoset

What we did first in marmoset study was to investigate the distribution of motoneurons in intact spinal cord that innervate the hand muscles by injecting cholera toxin B subunit (CTB) into the forearm flexor and extensor muscles. Immunohistological analysis using anti-CTB antibody revealed that the wrist and finger extensor motoneurons were mainly located in lamina IX of the cervical (C)4–C7 segments and wrist flexor motoneurons were in lamina IX of the C6–T1 segments (data not shown) [31]. Based on this finding, we induced contusive SCI at C5 level and almost all of the wrist extensor and flexor motoneurons were located at a site caudal to the lesion epicenter. After a laminectomy at the C5 level, the dura mater was exposed and a 20-g weight was dropped from a height of 50 mm onto the dura using a modified NYU impactor as reported previously [32–34] in adult female common marmosets ($n=6$ for the rhHGF group; $n=5$ for the PBS group). Right after contusive SCI at the C5 level, a C7 laminectomy was carried out and an intrathecal catheter was inserted from the C7 level. An osmotic mini pump, filled with 400 μg rhHGF (HGF group) or PBS (control group), was connected to a catheter and placed in the subcutaneous space on the right side of the animal's back [31]. The pump was left in place to deliver the total 400 μg dose of rhHGF for 4 weeks; dosage was based on previous results from intrathecal rhHGF administration in ALS rats [24], which have about the same body weight as marmosets.

14.4.2 Motor Function Recovery over Time and Original Open-Field Rating Scale Development

All animals showed severe quadriplegia 1 day after injury; they lay on the floor in a prone position, with little limb movement, and could not roll over or move forward by themselves. After C5-level SCI, irrespective of therapeutic intervention, the animals showed progressive recovery of motor function. To access the recovery of motor function and evaluate the therapeutic effects of intrathecal rhHGF, we established an original open-field rating scale with three main categories: upper limbs, lower limbs, and trunk stability (Table 14.1). This study's injury model, cervical SCI, requires a detailed analysis of upper limb function to precisely evaluate motor function recovery. Thus, the upper limb category was divided into three subdivisions: weight bearing, reach-and-grasp performance, and somatosensory function (Table 14.1) [31].

Table 14.1 Original open-field rating scale (adapted from [31])

Upper limbs maximum 20 points		
1. Weight bearing		
Weight bearing in stance	Anterior chest on the floor, no weight support of upper limbs	+0
	Anterior chest lifted up from the floor with weight support of upper limbs	+1
Weight bearing in walking	Anterior chest on the floor, no weight support of upper limbs	+0
	Anterior chest lifted up from the floor with weight support of upper limbs	
	With forearm dragged	+1
	With hand dragged	+1
	Stepping with hand clearance from the floor	+1
	Coordinated steps with lower limbs	+1
Hand position in walking	Below shoulder	+0
	Between shoulder and head	+1
	Above head	+1

(continued)

Table 14.1 (continued)

Hand placement in walking	Dorsal placement (dropped wrist)	+0
	Ulnar placement, not pronated	+1
	Pronated, but no palmar placement	+1
	Pronated with palmar placement	+1
2. Reach-and-grasp performance		
	Elevation below head height	+0
	Cannot grasp a pen	+0
	Grasp a pen	+1
	Elevation up to head height	+1
	Cannot grasp a pen at head height	+0
	Grasp a pen perpendicular to the body plane	+1
	Grasp a pen parallel to the body plane	+1
	Elevation up to 3 cm above head height	+1
	Cannot grasp a pen at 3 cm above head height	+0
	Grasp a pen perpendicular to the body plane	+1
	Grasp a pen parallel to the body plane	+1
3. Somatosensory function		
Somatosensory	Drop upper limbs through gaps in the cage bars up to	
	Humerus	+0
	Elbow	+1
	Only hand	+1
	Never drop	+1
Trunk stability maximum 3 points		
	Cannot roll over from supine to prone position	+0
	Roll over from supine to prone position	+1
	Keep sitting position	+1
	Keep standing position	+1
Lower limbs maximum 7 points		
ROM and weight bearing	Slight movement of lower limbs	+0
	Extensive movement of lower limbs	+1
	Move forward with weight bearing of lower limbs	+1
	Jump	+1
	Jump successively	+1
Somatosensory	Drop lower limbs through gaps in the cage bars up to	
	Thigh	+0
	Knee	+1
	Only foot	+1
	Never drop	+1

Definitions

Dorsal placement: wrist joint is dropped and dorsal side of the hand is placed on the floor

Ulnar placement: pronation of forearm is insufficient and little finger of the hand (ulnar side of the hand) is placed on the floor

Pronated, but no palmar placement: forearm is pronated, wrist joint is extended, but no palmar placement due to limited fingers extension

Pronated with palmar placement: palmar placement with forearm pronated and wrist and fingers extended

Keep sitting or standing position: keep sitting or standing position more than 5 s in the cage

Slight movement of lower limbs: partial joint movement through less than half of the range of the three joints motion

Extensive movement of lower limbs: movement through more than half of the range of the three joints motion

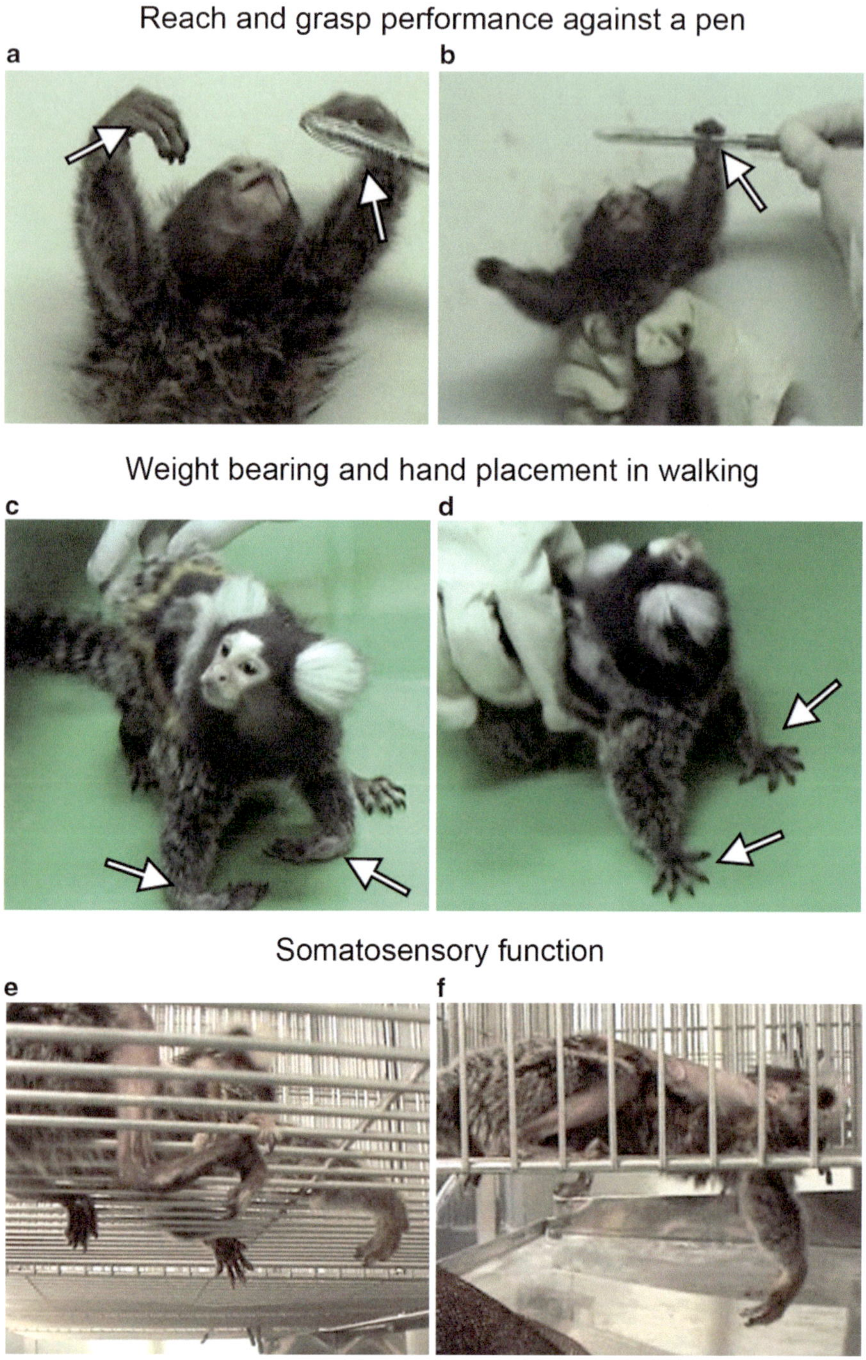
Reach and grasp performance against a pen
a
b
Weight bearing and hand placement in walking
c
d
Somatosensory function
e
f

The hand position (below shoulder, between shoulder and head, or above head) and placement in walking (dorsal placement, ulnar placement but not pronated, pronated but no palmar placement, or palmar placement) were highlighted in the subdivision of weight bearing (Table 14.1, Fig. 14.3c, d). The assessment of reach-and-grasp performance highlighted finger flexion and extension, wrist extension, forearm pronation, and shoulder flexion (Table 14.1, Fig. 14.3a, b). To access somatosensory function, we evaluated the distance the limb was dropped through gaps in the cage, as follows: lower limbs up to the thigh, knee, or foot only and upper limbs up to the humerus, elbow, or hand only (Table 14.1, Fig. 14.3e, f). Because there were various combinations of improvement in multiple subdivisions and attributes, we adopted a point-addition scoring system in this original open-field rating scale, unlike the system used in the BBB scale [26]. Details of motor function recovery over time and precise category definitions of the original open-field rating scale are described in [31].

14.4.3 *rhHGF Promoted Recovery of Hand Function After SCI*

The evaluation of motor function by the original open-field scale showed significant differences between the two groups (Fig. 14.4a–c). Animals in both groups gradually recovered, reaching a plateau around 8 weeks after SCI, and the original score of the upper limbs (pre-injury score = 20) recovered to 15.9 ± 0.8 and 7.8 ± 1.8 in the rhHGF and PBS groups, respectively, 12 weeks after SCI (Fig. 14.4a). Significant differences between the two groups were observed at most time points from 14 days onward after SCI in the open-field upper limb scores (Fig. 14.4a) [31].

Fig. 14.3 Representative images of marmosets after SCI at C5. An animal in the PBS group showed good elevation of upper limbs up to the head level 8 weeks after SCI. However, this animal could not grasp a pen parallel to the body plane because of insufficient forearm pronation and wrist and finger extension (**a**, *arrows*). An animal in the rhHGF group could reach for a pen at 3 cm above head height and could grasp a pen even when parallel to the body plane. Note that the forearm was well pronated, with the wrist joint fully extended (**b**, *arrows*). The same animal as in (**a**) walked with the anterior chest lifted up from the floor by bearing its weight on the upper limbs. However, the wrist joints dropped completely, and the dorsal surfaces of the hands were placed and dragged on the floor (**c**, *arrows*). On the other hand, the same animal as in (**b**) showed good palmar placement of the hands, with the wrist joints completely extended (**d**, *arrows*), and walked with its hands clear of the floor. One week after SCI, an animal in the PBS group dropped its limbs through gaps in the cage floor as far as the humerus or thigh and could not raise the dropped limb quickly (**f**). The animal gradually recovered and, at 6 weeks after SCI, rarely dropped its limbs to the humerus or thigh level, but still often dropped them as far as the elbow or knee (**e**). Figure adapted from [31]

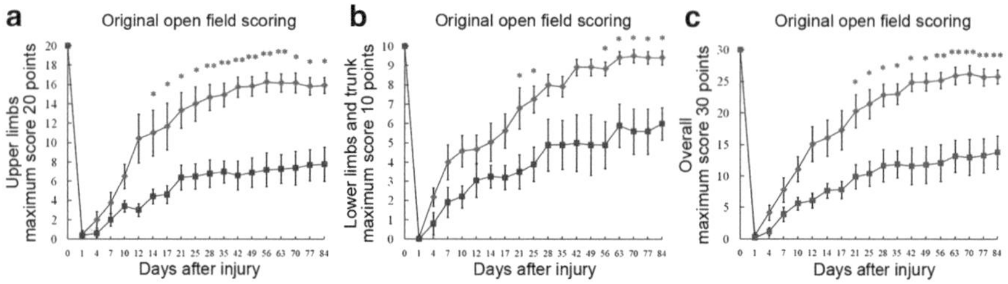

Fig. 14.4 Behavioral analyses were performed by the original open-field rating scale for the upper limbs (maximum, 20 points) (**a**), for the lower limbs and trunk (maximum, 10 points) (**b**), and combined (maximum 30 points) (**c**). All three methods showed significant recovery in the rhHGF group compared with the PBS group. *$p<0.05$, **$p<0.01$. ($n=6$ for the rhHGF group; $n=5$ for the PBS group). Figure adapted from [31]

14.4.4 rhHGF Significantly Preserved the Corticospinal Tract Pathway and LFB-Positive Myelinated Areas

Twelve weeks after injury, the ChAT-positive motoneurons around the lesion epicenter had almost disappeared, consistent with our rat study. However, we did not detect any significant differences in the number of surviving C2–T1 ChAT-positive motoneurons between the two groups (data not shown) [32]. We next investigated the pattern of the corticospinal tract (CST) pathway and its terminations in common marmosets. Axial sections of intact and injured spinal cords were immunostained with an anti-calmodulin-dependent kinaseIIα (CaMKIIα) antibody [35]. We previously found that CaMKIIα immunoreactivity (IR) labels the CST in the marmoset spinal cord [32, 34, 36], although its specificity remains to be demonstrated. In this study, we made the following observations. First, in the intact spinal cord, CaMKIIα-IR was detected in the lateral column of white matter, the dorsal horn, and the intermediate zone (IMZ) of the gray matter (Fig. 14.5a), suggesting that the CST in the common marmoset is located in lateral columns, unlike in rodents, in which the CST projects mainly to dorsal horn neurons and premotor spinal circuits [37]. Second, we did not detect CaMKIIα-IR in either the ventral white matter column or the ventral gray matter horn, suggesting that, as in rodents, the proportion of the ventral CST extending into the white matter is small and that the CST does not project directly to cervical motoneurons in the ventral horns [31].

Whereas CaMKIIα-IR in the lateral column was obviously reduced in segments caudal to the lesion site in the PBS group compared with the intact spinal cord control, the CaMKIIα-IR was well maintained, even caudal to the lesion site, in the rhHGF group (Fig. 14.5b arrowheads). Stereological quantification of the CaMKIIα-positive area in the lateral column showed significant differences between the two groups at the segments caudal to the lesion site (Fig. 14.5d). CaMKIIα-IR was detected in the IMZ (laminae VI–VII) cell bodies, which could include segmental interneurons (sINs) and propriospinal neurons (PNs). CaMKIIα-positive neurons in the IMZ at C5 had

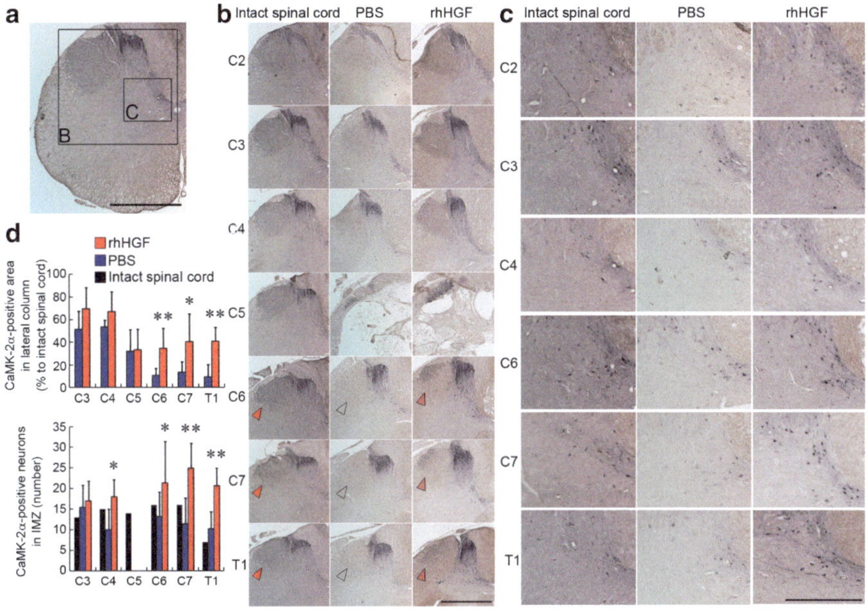

Fig. 14.5 CaMKIIα immunoreactivity (IR) in the lateral column of the white matter and in the intermediate zone (IMZ) of the gray matter in an intact spinal cord (**a**) and injured spinal cord 12 weeks after SCI (**b**, **c**). In the intact spinal cord, CaMKIIα-IR was detected in the lateral column, dorsal horn, and intermediate zone of the gray matter. No CaMKIIα-IR was detected in the ventral horn of the gray matter. Scale bar, 1 mm (**a**). CaMKIIα-IR in the lateral column, suggesting the corticospinal tract (CST) pathway, was significantly preserved even at sites caudal to the lesion epicenter (*arrowheads*) in the rhHGF group compared with the PBS group. Scale bar, 1 mm (**b**). CaMKIIα-IR was detected in cell bodies at the IMZ (laminae VI-VII), suggested to be segmental interneurons and propriospinal neurons. There were significantly more IMZ CaMKIIα-positive neurons at the C4 and C6–Th1 segments in the rhHGF group than in the PBS group. IMZ CaMKIIα-positive neurons were absent from the C5 segment in both groups. Scale bar, 500 μm (**c**). Quantitative analyses of the CaMKIIα-IR showed significant differences between the two groups (**d**). $*p<0.05$, $**p<0.01$. ($n=6$ for the rhHGF group; $n=5$ for the PBS group; $n=1$ for the intact spinal cord). Figure adapted from [31]

disappeared at 12 weeks after SCI in both groups (Fig. 14.5b, c). The rhHGF group had obviously greater numbers of these neurons around the lesion epicenter, as compared with the PBS group (Fig. 14.5c). Quantitative analysis of these neurons showed significant differences between the two groups at the C4 and C6–Th1 segments (Fig. 14.5d). Note that in some segments, the number of neurons was greater in the rhHGF and PBS groups than in the intact spinal cord (Fig. 14.5d) [31].

To examine rhHGF's tissue-sparing effects, we stained axial sections with Luxol fast blue (LFB) at 12 weeks after SCI. There was a significant rim of spared myelinated white matter even at the lesion epicenter in the rhHGF group, consistent with our rat study (data not shown). Stereological quantitative analysis of the LFB-positive myelinated areas revealed significant differences around the lesion epicenter between the two groups (data not shown) [31].

14.5 Discussions

Previous studies have shown that the HGF–c-Met system is involved in the mediation of inflammatory responses to tissue injury. In animal models in which the liver [38–40], lung [41], or kidney [40, 42] tissues were experimentally damaged, the HGF mRNA expression and HGF activity were found to increase markedly in the damaged organs, peaking within 24 h after the insult. Consistent with these increased expressions, the plasma HGF level also increased within 24 h after the damage, suggesting that HGF could be delivered to these injured organs from other organs through the blood supply via an endocrine mechanism, in addition to being produced endogenously in these organs [40]. In the CNS, on the other hand, it was reported that HGF mRNA was upregulated exclusively in the peri-infarct region at 14 days after cerebral ischemia [43]. In this study, we demonstrated that the HGF mRNA expression level gradually increased, peaking at 2 weeks after SCI, while the c-Met mRNA expression level increased markedly within a day of SCI. In addition, no increase in the plasma HGF levels was found after SCI. These findings suggest that the injured spinal cord cannot produce a sufficient amount of HGF by itself, as compared with the remarkable increase in c-Met expression after SCI, nor can HGF be supplied through an endocrine mechanism, in contrast to the case following damage to other organs, as mentioned above. These results prompted us to perform in vivo studies to determine whether the application of exogenous HGF into the injured spinal cord during the acute phase of SCI might exert a beneficial effect and promote functional recovery.

We showed that the application of exogenous HGF into spinal cord during the acute phase of SCI in rat exerted significant neuroprotective and anti-apoptotic effects to promote the survival of neurons and oligodendrocytes and also enhanced angiogenesis around the lesion epicenter after SCI. These effects significantly reduced the area of damage and provided a better scaffold for axonal regeneration. Furthermore, HGF directly acted on the 5HT-positive fibers to promote their regrowth, which likely contributed to the significantly better recovery of the motor functions during the chronic phase of SCI [25].

To begin to translate this HGF strategy to the treatment of human SCI, we performed intrathecal rhHGF infusion during the acute phase of cervical SCI in marmosets. A major advantage of using nonhuman primates in translational research is the ability to assess fine motor control recovery in the forelimbs. Another advantage of using marmosets is the similarity of their neuroanatomy to that of human beings.

Some features of motor projections have undergone pronounced changes from rodents to primates. The CST is a major pathway for voluntary movement control. It is a phylogenetically new system that appeared first in mammals and developed predominantly in primates [44, 45]. Over the course of the evolution of human and nonhuman primates, the CST has changed its location from the dorsal to lateral columns of the spinal cord [46] and changed its terminations. Whereas in rodents the CST axons project mainly to dorsal horn neurons and premotor spinal circuits, in primates, a significant proportion of the CST axons project to the ventral horn, and some synapse directly onto motoneurons innervating hand and forearm muscles, as direct cortico-motoneuronal (CM) connections [47]. Direct CM connections predominantly developed in higher primates such as macaque monkeys, apes, and humans [48–50]. Moreover, previous studies have suggested a strong correlation between the number of direct CM connections and the level of manual dexterity of nonhuman primate species [47, 48, 51, 52]; the appearance of direct CM connections is correlated with the emergence of precision grip between the thumb and the index finger, which is observed in macaque monkeys but not in marmosets. Thus, macaque monkeys have been used in many experiments because they have more advanced finger dexterity than marmosets or squirrels. In previous experiments in macaque monkeys, a unilateral transection of the spinal cord was made to interrupt the CST, including direct CM connections, at the designated cervical segment, and the recovery of precision grip was assessed after SCI [53–56]. However, to evaluate and predict the therapeutic effects of interventions as human treatments, contusive injury is considered most relevant to human SCI. Furthermore, for precise assessments, the monkeys used in a translational study should be of the same age, sex, and body weight, which is problematic in experiments using macaque monkeys but feasible in marmosets [57].

In this study, as shown in Fig. 14.5, the CaMKIIα-positive putative CST axons in marmosets were located in the lateral column, unlike in rodents, but projected mainly to the dorsal horn and IMZ without a visible CM connection, as in rodents, indicating the possibility that the marmoset CST is intermediate in the course of evolution from rodents to macaque monkeys and humans. Marmosets cannot perform a precise finger–thumb grip, but can be evaluated by reach-and-grasp prehensile tasks with a pen and by hand placement while walking. However, we could not evaluate these precise tasks using the previously reported bar grip test, cage-climbing test, or monitoring of spontaneous motor activity [33, 34]. Therefore, we established an original open-field rating scale, which enabled us to evaluate the neurological hand performance after cervical SCI in marmosets. As mentioned above, almost all of the wrist extensor and flexor motoneurons were located at a site caudal to the lesion epicenter at C5, suggesting the usefulness of evaluating wrist and finger extension and forearm pronation, which are important for performing reach-and-grasp prehensile tasks with a pen and for hand placement while walking. However, the number of surviving ChAT-positive motoneurons, which innervate forearm muscles, showed no significant differences between the HGF-treated and control groups, in contrast with our rat study. Based on this finding, it was necessary to reexamine the direct and indirect CM pathways after cervical SCI.

Compared with the direct CM pathway, the role of indirect pathways from the cerebral cortex to motoneurons, via subcortical or spinal interneuronal systems, has received much less attention, even though such pathways contribute the majority of motoneuron input [58]. In primates, many neuroanatomical studies have shown that the majority of corticospinal fiber terminations are not distributed in lamina IX, but in the IMZ of the spinal gray matter where various types of interneurons are located [59, 60], and PNs located in the C3–C4 segments can mediate the disynaptic excitation to motoneurons [61, 62]. Furthermore, an evaluation of finger dexterity (precision grip with the tips of the index finger and thumb) suggests that the C3–C4 PNs play a significant role in recovering precision grip after a CST lesion at the border between C4 and C5, in which direct CM connections to forelimb motoneurons are interrupted, while a major portion of the C3–C4 PN descending axons (indirect CM connections) remain intact [53]. In contrast, precision grip does not recover after a CST lesion at C1/C2, which interrupts corticospinal input to the C3–C4 PNs [63]. These findings suggest that after a CST lesion at C4/C5, indirect CM connections can be used to control the reach-and-grasp hand movements requiring a precision grip in macaque monkeys.

In this study, we induced a C5-level contusive injury, that is, caudal to the C3–C4 PNs and rostral to almost all forelimb motoneurons. This interrupted almost all the direct CM connections to forelimb motoneurons, whereas the majority of corticospinal input to the C3–C4 PNs remained intact. Therefore, this cervical SCI model is appropriate for investigating the involvement and role of C3–C4 PNs in the recovery of hand dexterity. Significantly greater numbers of CaMKIIα-positive interneurons in the IMZ at C4 and C6–Th1 segments were observed in the rhHGF group than the PBS group, suggesting that C3–C4 PNs played a major role in the recovery of hand movement after SCI in marmosets, as also described in macaques [53, 55, 56]. In spite of severe spinal cord damage around the lesion epicenter in the rhHGF group, motor function in the four extremities was recovered to a considerable extent, presumably by the endogenous plasticity of motor pathways, including indirect CM connections.

Intrathecal rhHGF infusion significantly reduced the damaged areas and promoted functional recovery after SCI, consistent with our rat study [25]. Although HGF's anti-apoptotic, neurotrophic, and angiogenic effects were not investigated during the acute phase of SCI [25] due to the small number of animals involved in this study, the LFB-positive myelinated areas and CaMKIIα-positive fibers were significantly preserved in the rhHGF group. These effects resulted in significantly better neurological hand performance, which was successfully assessed by our original open-field rating scale.

We believe that intrathecal administration would also be the most effective administration route in the clinical application of rhHGF for SCI patients, because the blood–brain barrier significantly limits the translocation of rhHGF from blood to the spinal cord. We observed that the subcutaneous injection of rhHGF was ineffective in ALS rats (Funakoshi et al. unpublished result), while the intrathecal administration of rhHGF showed significant therapeutic effects in these animals [24]. In this study, we administered 400 μg of rhHGF intrathecally over 4 weeks in marmosets, which corresponds to 0.05 μg/kg/day. Although we could not determine the HGF concentrations in the CSF of marmosets, we revealed that the HGF levels in the spinal cord was elevated around threefold compared to the control level in rat thoracic SCI model, when therapeutic effects of exogenous HGF were observed [25]. Therefore, we assume that the enhancement of HGF concentration in the spinal cord to no more than threefold above the control level would be sufficient to show therapeutic effects and the dosage to be used in clinical applications of HGF by intrathecal administration needs to be carefully assessed. We also revealed that not only 200 μg of intrathecal rhHGF over 2 weeks from right after SCI but also delayed administration of 200, 40, or 8 μg of intrathecal rhHGF over 2 weeks even from

4 days after SCI significantly promoted functional recovery respectively in rat thoracic SCI model (Kitamura et al. unpublished result). These findings support the concept that there is probably no need to increase the HGF concentration to an extremely high level and suggest the clinical efficacy of delayed intrathecal administration of rhHGF. Regarding the safety of intrathecal catheter insertion, infusion from the lumbar level has a great advantage over that from the cervical or thoracic level. Moreover, catheter insertion at the lumbar level might be useful for nonoperated people with SCI. This information needs to be assessed further to establish a therapeutic dose range and the optimal administration site for use in future clinical studies in SCI patients.

14.6 Conclusions

We revealed that injured spinal cord cannot produce a sufficient amount of HGF by itself during the acute phase of SCI and introduction of exogenous HGF into injured spinal cord exerts multiple therapeutic effects. We developed this strategy from an experimental one using HSV-1 vector in rat to a preclinical one using rhHGF in marmoset. This study demonstrates the therapeutic effects, safety, and clinical efficacy of intrathecal rhHGF treatment for SCI in adult nonhuman primates and the possibility that this novel therapy may be suitable for clinical application. Phase 1 clinical trial of intrathecal rhHGF in ALS patients has been started in Tohoku University, and we are proceeding to the final step to start a clinical trial in people with SCI in the very near future.

Acknowledgements This work was supported by grants from Grants-in-Aid for Scientific Research from JSPS and the Ministry of Education, Culture, Sports, Science and Technology of Japan (MEXT), the Project for Realization of Regenerative Medicine and Support for the Core Institutes for iPS Cell Research from MEXT, and by a grant-in-aid for the Global COE program from MEXT to Keio University. Research on Measures for Intractable Diseases from the Japanese Ministry of Health Labor and Welfare of Japan, and by "Super Special Consortia" for Supporting the Development of Cutting-edge Medical Care. The funders had no role in study design, data collection and analysis, decision to publish, or preparation of the manuscript.

Conflict of Interest Dr. Toshikazu Nakamura had reported that he was employed by Osaka University as a professor of Kringle Pharma Joint Research Division for Regenerative Drug Discovery in Osaka University, which is sponsored by Kringle Pharma, Inc. (KP), Osaka, Japan. rhHGF protein used in this study was kindly provided by KP. Dr. Funakoshi has served as a scientific advisor of KP. The other authors have declared that no competing interests exist.

References

1. Tuszynski MH, Peterson DA, Ray J, Baird A, Nakahara Y, Gage FH (1994) Fibroblasts genetically modified to produce nerve growth factor induce robust neuritic ingrowth after grafting to the spinal cord. Exp Neurol 126(1):1–14. doi:S0014488684710375 [pii]
2. Tuszynski MH, Gabriel K, Gage FH, Suhr S, Meyer S, Rosetti A (1996) Nerve growth factor delivery by gene transfer induces differential outgrowth of sensory, motor, and noradrenergic

neurites after adult spinal cord injury. Exp Neurol 137(1):157–173. doi:S0014-4886(96)90016-3 [pii] 10.1006/exnr.1996.0016
3. Jakeman LB, Wei P, Guan Z, Stokes BT (1998) Brain-derived neurotrophic factor stimulates hindlimb stepping and sprouting of cholinergic fibers after spinal cord injury. Exp Neurol 154(1):170–184. doi:S0014-4886(98)96924-2 [pii] 10.1006/exnr.1998.6924
4. McTigue DM, Horner PJ, Stokes BT, Gage FH (1998) Neurotrophin-3 and brain-derived neurotrophic factor induce oligodendrocyte proliferation and myelination of regenerating axons in the contused adult rat spinal cord. J Neurosci 18(14):5354–5365
5. Grill R, Murai K, Blesch A, Gage FH, Tuszynski MH (1997) Cellular delivery of neurotrophin-3 promotes corticospinal axonal growth and partial functional recovery after spinal cord injury. J Neurosci 17(14):5560–5572
6. Blesch A, Tuszynski MH (2001) GDNF gene delivery to injured adult CNS motor neurons promotes axonal growth, expression of the trophic neuropeptide CGRP, and cellular protection. J Comp Neurol 436(4):399–410
7. Liu LJ, Zhu JK, Xiao JD (1999) Rescue of motoneuron from brachial plexus nerve root avulsion induced cell death by Schwann cell derived neurotrophic factor. Zhongguo Xiu Fu Chong Jian Wai Ke Za Zhi 13(5):295–298
8. Casella GT, Marcillo A, Bunge MB, Wood PM (2002) New vascular tissue rapidly replaces neural parenchyma and vessels destroyed by a contusion injury to the rat spinal cord. Exp Neurol 173(1):63–76
9. Loy DN, Crawford CH, Darnall JB, Burke DA, Onifer SM, Whittemore SR (2002) Temporal progression of angiogenesis and basal lamina deposition after contusive spinal cord injury in the adult rat. J Comp Neurol 445(4):308–324. doi:10.1002/cne.10168 [pii]
10. Mautes AE, Weinzierl MR, Donovan F, Noble LJ (2000) Vascular events after spinal cord injury: contribution to secondary pathogenesis. Phys Ther 80(7):673–687
11. Guizar-Sahagun G, Ibarra A, Espitia A, Martinez A, Madrazo I, Franco-Bourland RE (2005) Glutathione monoethyl ester improves functional recovery, enhances neuron survival, and stabilizes spinal cord blood flow after spinal cord injury in rats. Neuroscience 130(3):639–649. doi:S0306-4522(04)00918-2 [pii] 10.1016/j.neuroscience.2004.09.056
12. Glaser J, Gonzalez R, Perreau VM, Cotman CW, Keirstead HS (2004) Neutralization of the chemokine CXCL10 enhances tissue sparing and angiogenesis following spinal cord injury. J Neurosci Res 77(5):701–708. doi:10.1002/jnr.20204
13. Nakamura T, Nawa K, Ichihara A (1984) Partial purification and characterization of hepatocyte growth factor from serum of hepatectomized rats. Biochem Biophys Res Commun 122(3):1450–1459. doi:0006-291X(84)91253-1 [pii]
14. Nakamura T, Nishizawa T, Hagiya M, Seki T, Shimonishi M, Sugimura A, Tashiro K, Shimizu S (1989) Molecular cloning and expression of human hepatocyte growth factor. Nature 342(6248):440–443. doi:10.1038/342440a0
15. Bottaro DP, Rubin JS, Falctto DL, Chan AM, Kmiccik TE, Vandc Woudc GF, Aaronson SA (1991) Identification of the hepatocyte growth factor receptor as the c-met proto-oncogene product. Science 251(4995):802–804
16. Caton A, Hacker A, Naeem A, Livet J, Maina F, Bladt F, Klein R, Birchmeier C, Guthrie S (2000) The branchial arches and HGF are growth-promoting and chemoattractant for cranial motor axons. Development 127(8):1751–1766
17. Maina F, Klein R (1999) Hepatocyte growth factor, a versatile signal for developing neurons. Nat Neurosci 2(3):213–217. doi:10.1038/6310
18. Hamanoue M, Takemoto N, Matsumoto K, Nakamura T, Nakajima K, Kohsaka S (1996) Neurotrophic effect of hepatocyte growth factor on central nervous system neurons in vitro. J Neurosci Res 43(5):554–564. doi:10.1002/(SICI)1097-4547(19960301)43:5<554::AID-JNR5>3.0.CO;2-H [pii] 10.1002/(SICI)1097-4547(19960301)43:5<554::AID-JNR5>3.0.CO;2-H
19. Honda S, Kagoshima M, Wanaka A, Tohyama M, Matsumoto K, Nakamura T (1995) Localization and functional coupling of HGF and c-Met/HGF receptor in rat brain: implication as neurotrophic factor. Brain Res 32(2):197–210

20. Funakoshi HNT (2011) Hepatocyte growth factor (HGF): neurotrophic functions and therapeutic implications for neuronal injury/diseases. Curr Trans Sig Ther 6(2):156–167
21. Date I, Takagi N, Takagi K, Kago T, Matsumoto K, Nakamura T, Takeo S (2004) Hepatocyte growth factor improved learning and memory dysfunction of microsphere-embolized rats. J Neurosci Res 78(3):442–453. doi:10.1002/jnr.20263
22. Miyazawa T, Matsumoto K, Ohmichi H, Katoh H, Yamashima T, Nakamura T (1998) Protection of hippocampal neurons from ischemia-induced delayed neuronal death by hepatocyte growth factor: a novel neurotrophic factor. J Cereb Blood Flow Metab 18(4):345–348. doi:10.1097/00004647-199804000-00001
23. Shimamura M, Sato N, Waguri S, Uchiyama Y, Hayashi T, Iida H, Nakamura T, Ogihara T, Kaneda Y, Morishita R (2006) Gene transfer of hepatocyte growth factor gene improves learning and memory in the chronic stage of cerebral infarction. Hypertension 47(4):742–751. doi:01.HYP.0000208598.57687.3e [pii] 10.1161/01.HYP.0000208598.57687.3e
24. Ishigaki A, Aoki M, Nagai M, Warita H, Kato S, Kato M, Nakamura T, Funakoshi H, Itoyama Y (2007) Intrathecal delivery of hepatocyte growth factor from amyotrophic lateral sclerosis onset suppresses disease progression in rat amyotrophic lateral sclerosis model. J Neuropathol Exp Neurol 66(11):1037–1044
25. Kitamura K, Iwanami A, Nakamura M, Yamane J, Watanabe K, Suzuki Y, Miyazawa D, Shibata S, Funakoshi H, Miyatake S, Coffin RS, Nakamura T, Toyama Y, Okano H (2007) Hepatocyte growth factor promotes endogenous repair and functional recovery after spinal cord injury. J Neurosci Res 85(11):2332–2342. doi:10.1002/jnr.21372
26. Basso DM, Beattie MS, Bresnahan JC (1995) A sensitive and reliable locomotor rating scale for open field testing in rats. J Neurotrauma 12(1):1–21
27. Kaneko S, Iwanami A, Nakamura M, Kishino A, Kikuchi K, Shibata S, Okano HJ, Ikegami T, Moriya A, Konishi O, Nakayama C, Kumagai K, Kimura T, Sato Y, Goshima Y, Taniguchi M, Ito M, He Z, Toyama Y, Okano H (2007) A selective Sema3A inhibitor enhances regenerative responses and functional recovery of the injured spinal cord. Nat Med 12(12):1380–1389
28. Kobayashi NR, Fan DP, Giehl KM, Bedard AM, Wiegand SJ, Tetzlaff W (1997) BDNF and NT-4/5 prevent atrophy of rat rubrospinal neurons after cervical axotomy, stimulate GAP-43 and Talpha1-tubulin mRNA expression, and promote axonal regeneration. J Neurosci 17(24):9583–9595
29. Ikegami T, Nakamura M, Yamane J, Katoh H, Okada S, Iwanami A, Watanabe K, Ishii K, Kato F, Fujita H, Takahashi T, Okano HJ, Toyama Y, Okano H (2005) Chondroitinase ABC combined with neural stem/progenitor cell transplantation enhances graft cell migration and outgrowth of growth-associated protein-43-positive fibers after rat spinal cord injury. Eur J Neurosci 22(12):3036–3046
30. Ramon-Cueto A, Plant GW, Avila J, Bunge MB (1998) Long-distance axonal regeneration in the transected adult rat spinal cord is promoted by olfactory ensheathing glia transplants. J Neurosci 18(10):3803–3815
31. Kitamura K, Fujiyoshi K, Yamane J, Toyota F, Hikishima K, Nomura T, Funakoshi H, Nakamura T, Aoki M, Toyama Y, Okano H, Nakamura M (2011) Human hepatocyte growth factor promotes functional recovery in primates after spinal cord injury. PLoS One 6(11):e27706. doi:10.1371/journal.pone.0027706 PONE-D-11-12341 [pii]
32. Iwanami A, Yamane J, Katoh H, Nakamura M, Momoshima S, Ishii H, Tanioka Y, Tamaoki N, Nomura T, Toyama Y, Okano H (2005) Establishment of graded spinal cord injury model in a nonhuman primate: the common marmoset. J Neurosci Res 80(2):172–181. doi:10.1002/jnr.20435
33. Iwanami A, Kaneko S, Nakamura M, Kanemura Y, Mori H, Kobayashi S, Yamasaki M, Momoshima S, Ishii H, Ando K, Tanioka Y, Tamaoki N, Nomura T, Toyama Y, Okano H (2005) Transplantation of human neural stem cells for spinal cord injury in primates. J Neurosci Res 80(2):182–190. doi:10.1002/jnr.20436
34. Yamane J, Nakamura M, Iwanami A, Sakaguchi M, Katoh H, Yamada M, Momoshima S, Miyao S, Ishii K, Tamaoki N, Nomura T, Okano HJ, Kanemura Y, Toyama Y, Okano H (2010) Transplantation of galectin-1-expressing human neural stem cells into the injured spinal cord of adult common marmosets. J Neurosci Res 88(7):1394–1405. doi:10.1002/jnr.22322

35. Terashima T, Ochiishi T, Yamauchi T (1994) Immunohistochemical detection of calcium/calmodulin-dependent protein kinase II in the spinal cord of the rat and monkey with special reference to the corticospinal tract. J Comp Neurol 340(4):469–479. doi:10.1002/cne.903400403
36. Fujiyoshi K, Yamada M, Nakamura M, Yamane J, Katoh H, Kitamura K, Kawai K, Okada S, Momoshima S, Toyama Y, Okano H (2007) In vivo tracing of neural tracts in the intact and injured spinal cord of marmosets by diffusion tensor tractography. J Neurosci 27(44):11991–11998. doi:27/44/11991 [pii] 10.1523/JNEUROSCI.3354-07.2007
37. Courtine G, Bunge MB, Fawcett JW, Grossman RG, Kaas JH, Lemon R, Maier I, Martin J, Nudo RJ, Ramon-Cueto A, Rouiller EM, Schnell L, Wannier T, Schwab ME, Edgerton VR (2007) Can experiments in nonhuman primates expedite the translation of treatments for spinal cord injury in humans? Nat Med 13(5):561–566. doi:nm1595 [pii] 10.1038/nm1595
38. Matsumoto K, Nakamura T (1997) Hepatocyte growth factor (HGF) as a tissue organizer for organogenesis and regeneration. Biochem Biophys Res Commun 239(3):639–644
39. Noji S, Tashiro K, Koyama E, Nohno T, Ohyama K, Taniguchi S, Nakamura T (1990) Expression of hepatocyte growth factor gene in endothelial and Kupffer cells of damaged rat livers, as revealed by in situ hybridization. Biochem Biophys Res Commun 173(1):42–47
40. Kono S, Nagaike M, Matsumoto K, Nakamura T (1992) Marked induction of hepatocyte growth factor mRNA in intact kidney and spleen in response to injury of distant organs. Biochem Biophys Res Commun 186(2):991–998
41. Yanagita K, Matsumoto K, Sekiguchi K, Ishibashi H, Niho Y, Nakamura T (1993) Hepatocyte growth factor may act as a pulmotrophic factor on lung regeneration after acute lung injury. J Biol Chem 268(28):21212–21217
42. Igawa T, Matsumoto K, Kanda S, Saito Y, Nakamura T (1993) Hepatocyte growth factor may function as a renotropic factor for regeneration in rats with acute renal injury. Am J Physiol 265(1 Pt 2):F61–F69
43. Nagayama T, Nagayama M, Kohara S, Kamiguchi H, Shibuya M, Katoh Y, Itoh J, Shinohara Y (2004) Post-ischemic delayed expression of hepatocyte growth factor and c-Met in mouse brain following focal cerebral ischemia. Brain Res 999(2):155–166
44. Phillips CG, Porter R (1977) Corticospinal neurones. Their role in movement. Monogr Physiol Soc 34(v–xii):1–450
45. Shapovalov AI (1975) Neuronal organization and synaptic mechanisms of supraspinal motor control in vertebrates. Rev Physiol Biochem Pharmacol 72:1–54
46. Rouiller EM, Moret V, Tanne J, Boussaoud D (1996) Evidence for direct connections between the hand region of the supplementary motor area and cervical motoneurons in the macaque monkey. Eur J Neurosci 8(5):1055–1059
47. Lemon RN, Kirkwood PA, Maier MA, Nakajima K, Nathan P (2004) Direct and indirect pathways for corticospinal control of upper limb motoneurons in the primate. Prog Brain Res 143:263–279. doi:S0079-6123(03)43026-4 [pii] 10.1016/S0079-6123(03)43026-4
48. Heffner R, Masterton B (1975) Variation in form of the pyramidal tract and its relationship to digital dexterity. Brain Behav Evol 12(3):161–200
49. Heffner RS, Masterton RB (1983) The role of the corticospinal tract in the evolution of human digital dexterity. Brain Behav Evol 23(3–4):165–183
50. Palmer E, Ashby P (1992) Evidence that a long latency stretch reflex in humans is transcortical. J Physiol 449:429–440
51. Bernhard CG, Bohm E, Petersen I (1953) New investigations on the pyramidal system in *Macaca mulatta*. Experientia 9(3):111–112
52. Lemon RN (2008) Descending pathways in motor control. Ann Rev Neurosci 31:195–218
53. Sasaki S, Isa T, Pettersson LG, Alstermark B, Naito K, Yoshimura K, Seki K, Ohki Y (2004) Dexterous finger movements in primate without monosynaptic corticomotoneuronal excitation. J Neurophysiol 92(5):3142–3147. doi:10.1152/jn.00342.2004 00342.2004 [pii]
54. Freund P, Schmidlin E, Wannier T, Bloch J, Mir A, Schwab ME, Rouiller EM (2006) Nogo-A-specific antibody treatment enhances sprouting and functional recovery after cervical lesion in adult primates. Nat Med 12(7):790–792. doi:nm1436 [pii] 10.1038/nm1436

55. Nishimura Y, Onoe H, Morichika Y, Perfiliev S, Tsukada H, Isa T (2007) Time-dependent central compensatory mechanisms of finger dexterity after spinal cord injury. Science 318(5853):1150–1155. doi:318/5853/1150 [pii] 10.1126/science.1147243
56. Nishimura Y, Morichika Y, Isa T (2009) A subcortical oscillatory network contributes to recovery of hand dexterity after spinal cord injury. Brain 132(Pt 3):709–721
57. Mansfield K, Tardif S, Eichler E (2004) White paper for complete sequencing of the common marmoset (*Callithrix jacchus*) genome. http://www.genome.gov/Pages/Research/Sequencing/SeqProposals/MarmosetSeq.pdf
58. Gelfan S (1964) Neuronal interdependence. Prog Brain Res 11:238–260
59. Bortoff GA, Strick PL (1993) Corticospinal terminations in two new-world primates: further evidence that corticomotoneuronal connections provide part of the neural substrate for manual dexterity. J Neurosci 13(12):5105–5118
60. Ralston DD, Ralston HJ 3rd (1985) The terminations of corticospinal tract axons in the macaque monkey. J Comp Neurol 242(3):325–337. doi:10.1002/cne.902420303
61. Alstermark B, Isa T, Ohki Y, Saito Y (1999) Disynaptic pyramidal excitation in forelimb motoneurons mediated via C(3)-C(4) propriospinal neurons in the *Macaca fuscata*. J Neurophysiol 82(6):3580–3585
62. Isa T, Ohki Y, Seki K, Alstermark B (2006) Properties of propriospinal neurons in the C3-C4 segments mediating disynaptic pyramidal excitation to forelimb motoneurons in the macaque monkey. J Neurophysiol 95(6):3674–3685. doi:00103.2005 [pii] 10.1152/jn.00103.2005
63. Isa T, Ohki Y, Alstermark B, Pettersson LG, Sasaki S (2007) Direct and indirect cortico-motoneuronal pathways and control of hand/arm movements. Physiology (Bethesda) 22:145–152. doi:22/2/145 [pii] 10.1152/physiol.00045.2006

Chapter 15
The Proteoglycan-Degrading Enzymes Promote Functional Recovery After Spinal Cord Injury: Keratan Sulfate and Chondroitin Sulfate

Shiro Imagama, Zenya Ito, Kei Ando, Yukihiro Matsuyama, Yoshihiro Nishida, and Naoki Ishiguro

Abstract Failure of axonal regrowth is a major obstacle to the treatment of injuries of the adult central nervous system (CNS), and proteoglycans are strong inhibitory cues. Chondroitin sulfate (CS) proteoglycans are strong inhibitors of neuronal injuries of the adult CNS. Besides CS chains, keratan sulfate (KS) chains are also covalently attached to some proteoglycans. However, the biological significance of KS remains to be not well understood. Here we investigated the role of KS in functional recovery and neural plasticity after spinal cord injury (SCI), using KS knockout mice and KS-degrading enzyme, keratanase II (K-II). Motor function recovery with enhanced axonal regeneration/sprouting was promoted in the KS-deficient mice and KS-degrading rats after the thoracic SCI. In vitro assays also demonstrated that KS proteoglycans were required for the proteoglycan-mediated inhibition of neurite outgrowth after SCI. Unexpectedly, K-II and the CS-degrading enzyme chondroitinase ABC (C-ABC) showed comparable effects in vivo and in vitro, but these two enzymes worked neither additively nor synergistically. These data and further in vitro studies suggested that all the three components of the proteoglycan moiety, i.e., the core protein, CS chains, and KS chains, were required for the inhibitory activity of proteoglycans. Our data indicate that KS is essential for and has a comparable impact as CS on post-injury plasticity. Our study also demonstrated that KS and CS are independently required for the proteoglycan-mediated inhibition of axonal regeneration/sprouting, and KS is a candidate target for the treatment of neuronal injuries.

Keywords Chondroitin sulfate • Keratan sulfate • Neural plasticity • Proteoglycan • Spinal cord injury

S. Imagama (✉) • Z. Ito • K. Ando • Y. Nishida • N. Ishiguro
Departments of Orthopedic Surgery, Nagoya University Graduate School of Medicine, 65 Tsurumai-cho, Showa-ku, Nagoya 466-8550, Japan
e-mail: imagama@med.nagoya-u.ac.jp

Y. Matsuyama
Department of Orthopedic Surgery, Hamamatsu University School of Medicine, 1-20-1 Handayama, 431-3192 Hamamatsu, Japan

K. Uchida et al. (eds.), *Neuroprotection and Regeneration of the Spinal Cord*,
DOI 10.1007/978-4-431-54502-6_15, © Springer Japan 2014

15.1 Introduction

Neuronal axons of the adult mammalian central nervous system (CNS) hardly regenerate after injuries, and many factors contribute to this lack of repair. The CNS extracellular matrix (ECM) may maintain the neuronal network by inhibiting axonal growth and suppress the formation of additional inadequate synapses. The disorganized production of proteoglycans in the ECM leads to the inhibition of structural rearrangement of the neuronal network after neuronal injury. Among proteoglycans, chondroitin sulfate proteoglycans (CSPGs) have been well focused [1–4], and CSPGs inhibit neurite outgrowth in vitro. The chondroitin sulfate (CS)-degrading enzyme chondroitinase ABC (C-ABC) promotes axonal regeneration after nigrostriatal tract transaction [5] and functional recovery after spinal cord injury (SCI) [6]. Therefore, the CS chains are recognized as principal for the inhibition of axonal regrowth and functional recovery.

Proteoglycans consist of a core protein and covalently attached long sugar chains of repeating disaccharide units with sulfation, i.e., glycosaminoglycans. Four sulfated glycosaminoglycans, CS, dermatan sulfate, heparan sulfate, and keratan sulfate (KS) are known. In in vitro study, digestion of KS restores neurite outgrowth on proteoglycan-coated substratum, which KS has been suggested in the regulation of axon guidance and/or axonal regeneration/sprouting [7, 8]. However, KS has been poorly studied. KS is composed of repeating disaccharide units of galactose and *N*-acetylglucosamine (GlcNAc), where the C6 position of GlcNAc is always sulfated. As GlcNAc sulfation at the C6 position is necessary for KS chain elongation [9], deficiency of human *N*-acetylglucosamine 6-*O*-sulfotransferase-5 (GlcNAc6ST-5) leads to loss of KS synthesis [10]. Then the lack of mouse GlcNAc6ST-1 causes loss of reactivity to the anti-KS antibody 5D4 in the brain and shows better axonal growth than wild-type mice after a cortical stab wound [11].

In this chapter, to evaluate whether KS is target of treatment for SCI, we introduce the study that we applied a contusion SCI model to *N*-acetylglucosamine 6-*O*-sulfotransferase-1-deficient mice (KS knockout mice) and found that these mice showed better functional recovery than their wild-type counterparts [12]. However, as these knockout mice lose *N*-acetylglucosamine 6-*O*-sulfotransferase-1 in every cell in the body, critical questions remain to be answered, e.g., whether KS specifically works in the spinal cord and how much impact KS has on functional disturbance. Then, we used keratanase II (K-II), which specifically degrades KS, and investigated the role of KS in post-injury plasticity [13]. We found that KS and CS have a comparable impact on this form of plasticity. We also examined whether KS collaborates with CS, or works independently, and determined the structural basis of proteoglycan-mediated inhibition of neural plasticity.

15.2 KS Knockout Mice (*N*-Acetylglucosamine 6-*O*-sulfotransferase-1-Deficient Mice) Show Better Functional Recovery After Spinal Cord Injury

15.2.1 Induction of KS Expression After Spinal Cord Injury in Wild-Type Mice

We made a contusion injury of the spinal cord at the tenth thoracic level with 100 kdyn using an infinite horizon (IH) impactor. 5D4, an anti-KS monoclonal antibody, was used to evaluate the expression and localization of KS. 5D4-reactive KS expressed around the lesion epicenter and reached a maximum level around 5–7 days after injury in wild-type mice (Fig. 15.1a). On the other hand, KS was not detected at all in GlcNAc6ST-1–/– mice (Fig. 15.1b–d). In injured wild-type mice, GlcNAc6ST-1 expression was also detected (Fig. 15.1e). As for CS expression, there was no significant difference between GlcNAc6ST-1–/– mice and wild-type mice (Fig. 15.1f).

15.2.2 Motor Functional Tests and Motor-Evoked Potential

To evaluate motor functional recovery after SCI, we performed the footfall test and footprint test. For the footfall test, mice were placed on a lattice of thin metal wires. The wire grid was positioned flat and was 7 × 11 in with grid squares of 0.35 × 0.35 in. This test can evaluate accurate limb placement and precise motor control. Intact animals cross the grid without making footfalls, whereas a paralytic foot tends to fall from the lattice during movement. The numbers of footfalls were almost the same between wild-type and GlcNAc6ST-1–/– mice 3 days after injury (Fig. 15.2a). At 4–6 weeks after injury, GlcNAc6ST-1–/– mice showed the functional recovery comparable to that of sham-operated mice and a significantly better recovery than wild-type mice (Fig. 15.2a). The stride length examination also demonstrated a significantly better functional recovery in GlcNAc6ST-1–/– mice (Fig. 15.2b). The Basso mouse scale (BMS) score [14] for 8 weeks also showed a significantly better recovery in the GlcNAc6ST-1–/– mice than in the wild-type mice (Fig. 15.2c).

Then we measured the latency of motor-evoked potential (MEP) to further objectively evaluate motor function. Mice received electrical stimuli at the occipito-cervical area, and MEP was recorded at both hind limbs. The onset latency of MEP was measured from the onset of the stimulus to the first response of each wave. At 6 weeks after injury, the latency of GlcNAc6ST-1–/– mice became comparable to that of the sham-operated controls and significantly shorter than wild-type mice (Fig. 15.2d, e). From these data, the functional recovery was significantly better in GlcNAc6ST-1–/– mice.

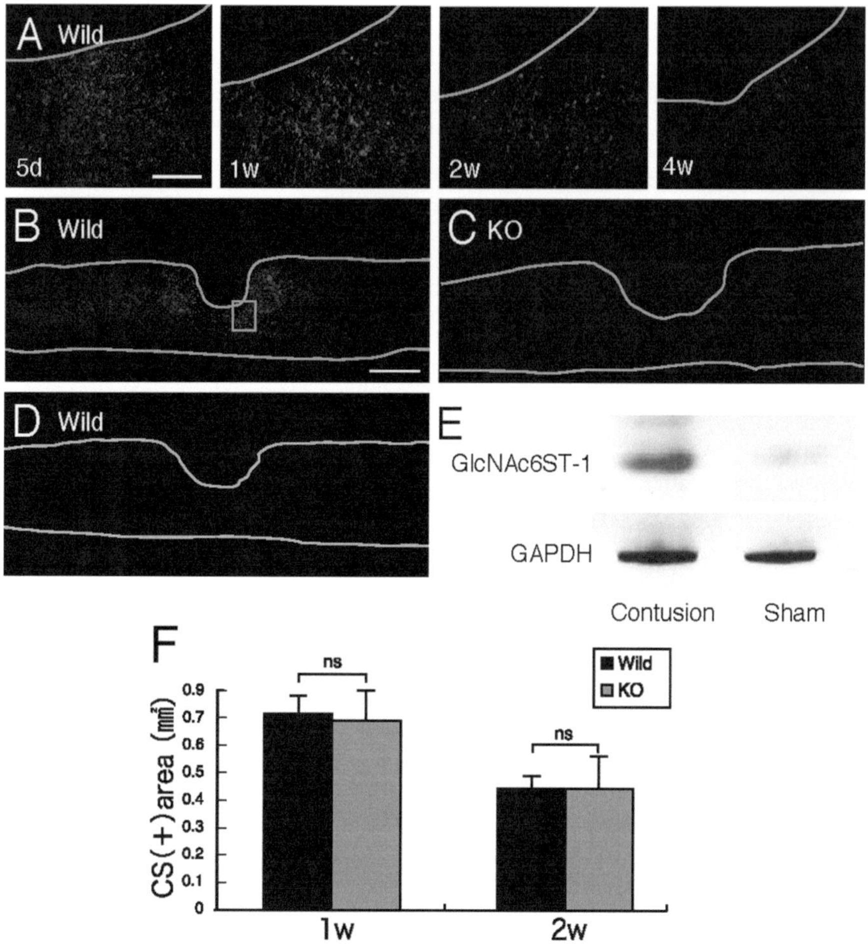

Fig. 15.1 KS and CS expression after spinal cord injury. (**a**) Expression profile of 5D4-reactive KS in wild-type mice after spinal cord injury. Scale bar, 100 μm. (**b–d**) KS was expressed around the lesion center 7 days after injury in wild-type mice (**b**) but was not detected in GlcNAc6ST-1–/– mice (**c**) or isotype-matched IgG controls (**d**). (**e**) RT-PCR for GlcNAc6ST-1 and GAPDH was performed for samples from the wild-type mouse spinal cord 7 days after injury or sham operation. (**f**) Quantification of CS expression. Quantification data are the means ± SEM. ns, not significant (Student's *t*-test). The sections shown are midline sagittal sections of the injured spinal cord. The *drawn lines* indicate the margins of the lesion core (**a**) and the outline of the spinal cord (**b**, **c**)

15.2.3 Glial Scar Formation

We next examined collagen IV, which expresses in the late stages of glial scarring [15]. Collagen IV expression at 1 week after injury was apparent, but the margin was unclear in both wild-type and GlcNAc6ST-1–/– mice. There was no difference

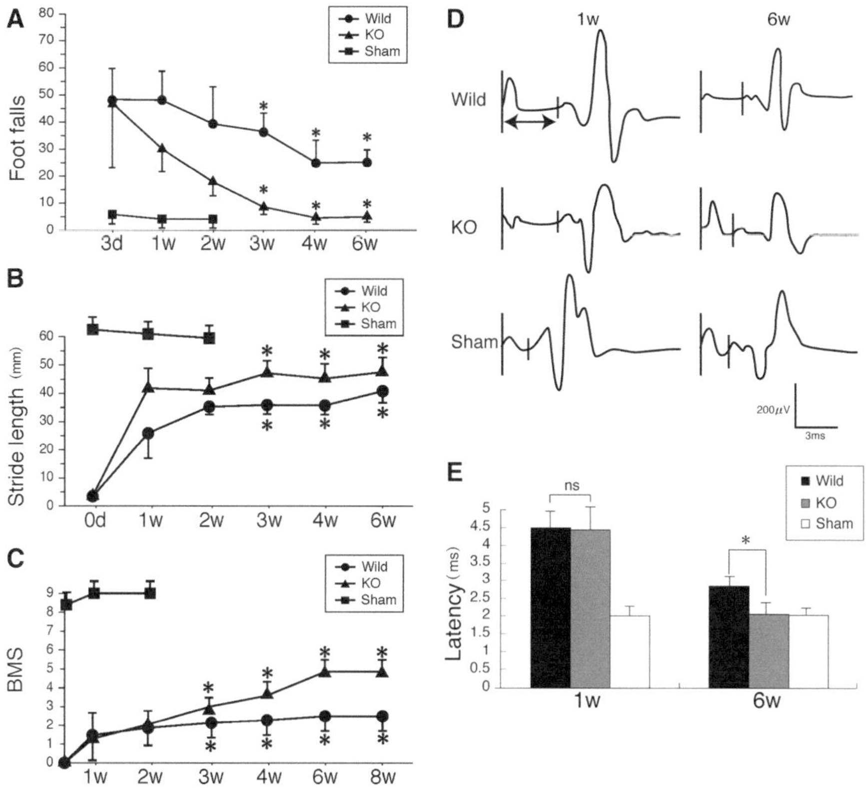

Fig. 15.2 Footfall, footprint tests, and BMS scoring. (**a**) Footfall test. The graph shows data for each genotype at each time point. *$p<0.05$ (wild-type vs. GlcNAc6ST-1−/− mice). (**b**) Data of the footprint test taken 4 weeks after injury are quantified. *$p<0.05$ (wild-type vs. GlcNAc6ST-1−/− mice). Quantification data are the means ± SEM (repeated measures ANOVA and the Mann–Whitney *U*-test). (**c**) BMS scoring. *$p<0.05$ (wild-type vs. GlcNAc6ST-1−/− mice). (**d**, **e**) Motor-evoked potential. (**d**) Representative profiles of motor-evoked potential are shown. (**e**) Latency times were quantified. *$p<0.05$. Quantification data are the means ± SEM (one-way ANOVA)

in the collagen IV-positive area at 1 week between these mice. The margin of the scar area became clear at 4 weeks after injury, and the scar area was significantly reduced in GlcNAc6ST-1−/− mice (Fig. 15.3a, b).

15.2.4 Neuronal Axon Growth

We stained tissues 5 mm distal to the lesion for 5-hydroxytryptamine (5HT) as the serotonergic descending raphespinal tract. 5HT-positive fibers were significantly more in the ventral horn of the gray matter in GlcNAc6ST-1−/− mice than in wild-type mice (5HT-positive area: wild-type, 972 ± 1,080 vs. GlcNAc6ST-1−/−,

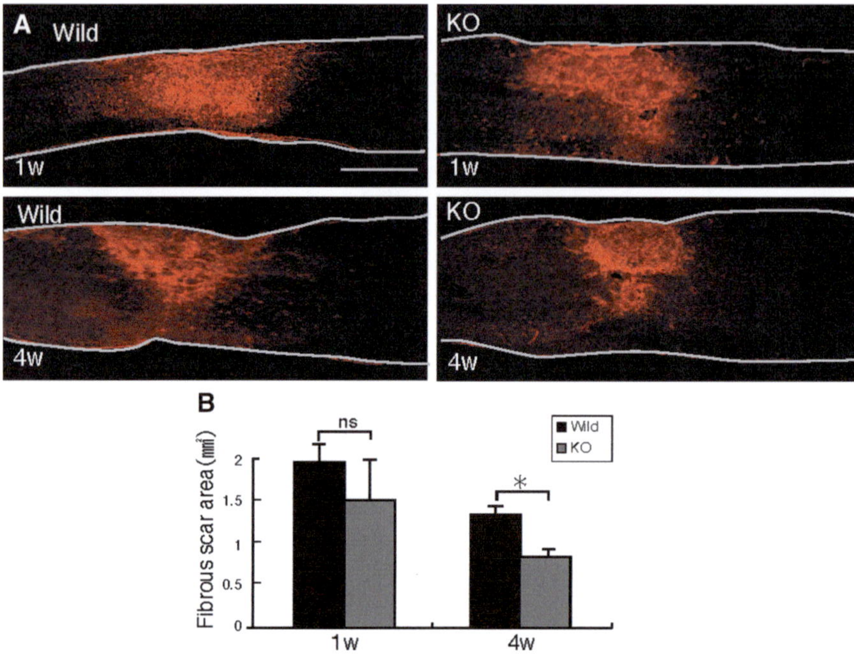

Fig. 15.3 Glial scar assessment by collagen IV deposition. (**a**) Representative photos for collagen IV expression are shown. Scale bar, 500 μm. The *drawn lines* indicate the outline of the spinal cord. (**b**) The collagen IV-positive areas are summarized in the graph. $*p<0.05$. Quantification data are the means ± SEM (Student's *t*-test). The sections shown are midline sagittal sections of the injured spinal cord

7,120 ± 1,168 μm²; $p<0.005$) (Fig. 15.4a–c). GAP43-positive axons which reflect axon regeneration and sprouting were also more in GlcNAc6ST-1−/− mice than in wild-type mice at 4 weeks after injury (GAP43-positive fiber counts/150,000 μm²: wild-type, 1,962 ± 1,522 vs. GlcNAc6ST-1−/−, 6,631 ± 1,090; $p<0.005$) (Fig. 15.4d–f). In tracer-fiber counts for the corticospinal tract (CST), the number of biotin-dextran amine (BDA)-positive fibers was increased in the region caudal to the epicenter in GlcNAc6ST-1−/− mice, particularly in the gray matter (Fig. 15.4g–i). The quantification of the number of labeled BDA fibers was performed in the gray matter 5 mm caudal to the lesion and divided by the number of labeled corticospinal axons 10 mm rostral to the lesion for each animal. There was a significant difference between wild-type and GlcNAc6ST-1−/− mice (BDA-positive fibers in caudal region/rostral region: wild-type, 1.9 ± 1.1% vs. GlcNAc6ST-1−/−, 6.9 ± 1.0 %; $p<0.005$).

15.2.5 Spot Assay

We used the spot assay to examine the activity of mouse brain proteoglycans. We confirmed both KS and CS in the mouse brain proteoglycans (Fig. 15.5a). We then spotted these proteoglycans with rhodamine B, which appeared red (Fig. 15.5b).

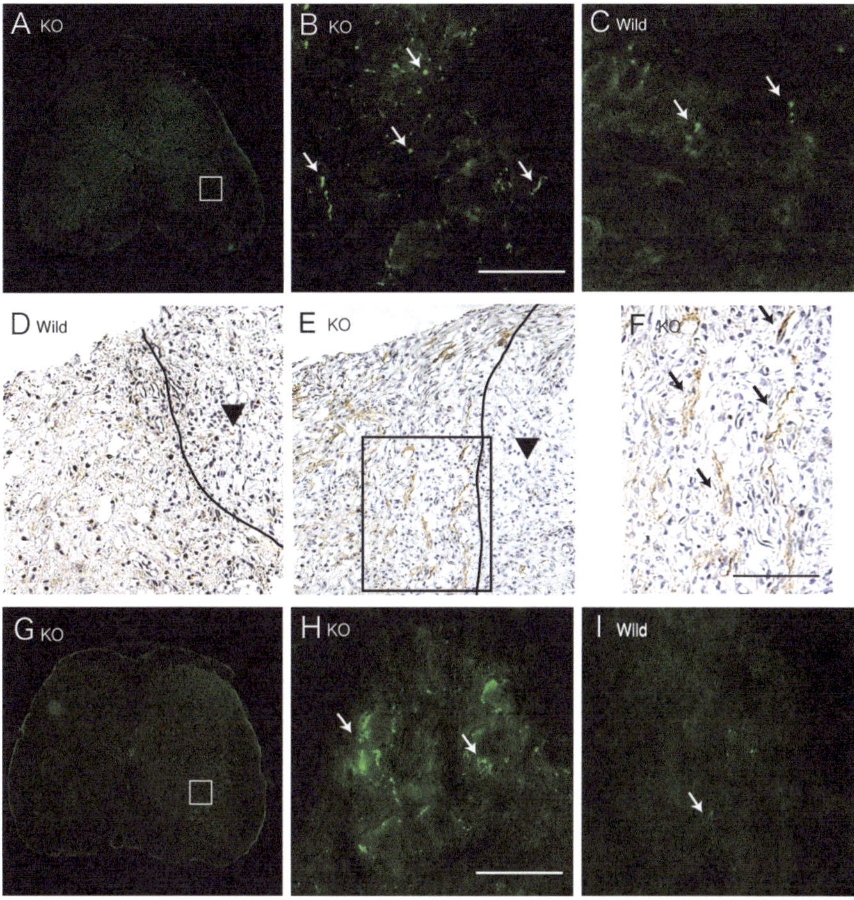

Fig. 15.4 Axonal growth. 5HT staining of the ventral horn (**a**–**c**; 5 mm distal to the lesion), GAP43 staining (**d**–**f**), and tracer-fiber counts of the corticospinal tract (BDA-positive fibers) (**g**–**i**; 5 mm caudal to the lesion) are shown for GlcNAc6ST-1–/– (**a**, **b**, **e**, **f**, **g**, **h**) and wild-type (**c**, **d**, **i**) mice. Scale bar, 50 μm. Higher magnification figures of the *boxed areas* in **a**, **e**, and **g** are shown in **b**, **f**, and **h**, respectively. The *arrows* in **b**, **c**, **f**, and **h**, **i** indicate 5HT-positive, GAP43-positive, and BDA-positive fibers, respectively. The *arrowheads* in **d** and **e** indicate the contusion area. The *drawn lines* indicate the margins of the lesion core. Five mice were used for each genotype at 4 weeks after injury. The sections in **a**, **b**, **c**, **g**, **h**, and **i** are the axial sections of the injured spinal cord. The sections in **d**, **e**, and **f** are the midline sagittal sections of the injured spinal cord

While neurites of the primary neurons frequently crossed into the spots in the control (rhodamine B alone, the upper panel of Fig. 15.5b), neurites of neurons in the surrounding area did not cross into the spots of the mouse brain proteoglycans (the middle panel of Fig. 15.5b). On the other hand, neurites of neurons in the surrounding area could enter the spots of the proteoglycans which were treated with keratanase (the bottom panel of Fig. 15.5b). This finding was clearer when the

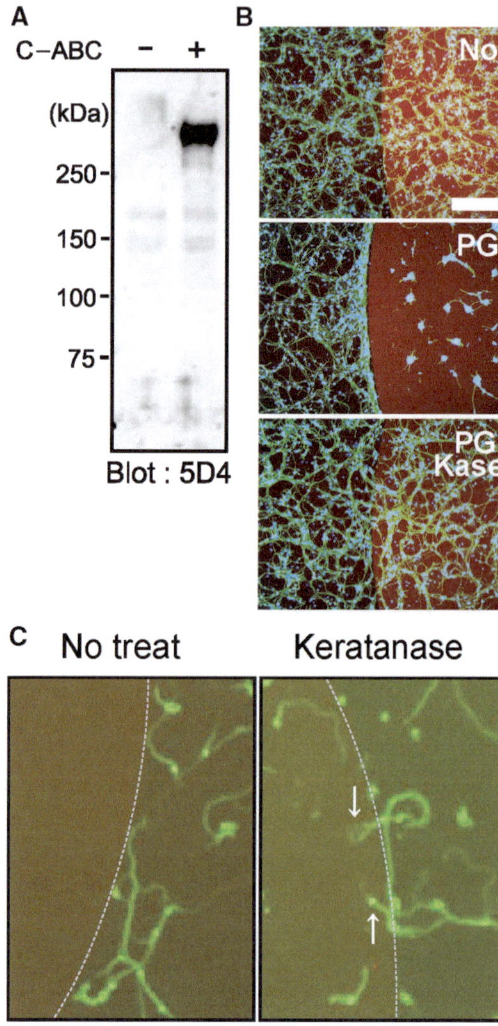

Fig. 15.5 Spot assay. (**a**) Proteoglycans from mouse brain were subjected to Western blot analysis. Note that C-ABC treatment revealed KS epitopes. (**b**, **c**) Spot assay. Mouse brain proteoglycans at 3 μg/mL were spotted, and primary granular neurons from the rat cerebellum were seeded. Proteoglycans inhibited neurite entry into the spot, whereas keratanase treatment allowed entry. Different cell numbers were used for (**b**) and (**c**) (1.0×10^6 or 1.0×10^5/well, respectively). Scale bar, 100 μm

seeded cell number was decreased (Fig. 15.5c). Therefore, this in vitro assay employing brain proteoglycans mimicked the in vivo failure of axonal regrowth into the lesions of SCI and the reversal of this failure in KS-deficient mice.

From these results, KS knockout mice (*N*-acetylglucosamine 6-*O*-sulfotransferase-1-deficient mice) show better functional recovery after SCI with axon regeneration/sprouting. Next study was conducted to evaluate whether KS-degrading enzyme promotes axonal regrowth and functional recovery after SCI in rats.

15.3 Keratan Sulfate-Degrading Enzyme (Keratanase II) Promotes Axonal Regeneration and Functional Recovery After Spinal Cord Injury

15.3.1 Degradation of KS by K-II In Vitro and In Vivo

We purified K-II from *Bacillus circulans* which showed keratanase activity only [16]. This enzyme is thermostable and keeps its enzymatic activity for at least 120 h at 37 °C (100 ± 1.606 % at 0 h vs. 91.9 ± 4.014 % at 120 h). We made contusion injuries using a force of 200 kdyn with IH impactor in the rat spinal cord at the ninth thoracic vertebral level. This contusion model completely destroyed the dorsal columns and dorsal CST in the spinal cord.

Di-sulfated KS and CS-C contents increased after injury, peaking around 7 days (Fig. 15.6a, b). K-II or C-ABC was administered to the injured site for 2 weeks after contusion injuries using an osmotic pump with K-II (0.05 units/200 μL), C-ABC (0.05 units/200 μL) (Seikagaku, Tokyo, Japan), or saline (as a vehicle control) (200 μL solution, 0.5 μL/h, 14-day delivery; Alzet pump model 2002 [Durect Co., Cupertino, CA]).

K-II degraded di-sulfated KS contents to the noninjury level (Fig. 15.6a). Western blot and immunohistochemistry revealed that the reactivity to KS antibody 5D4 (Seikagaku, Tokyo, Japan) was lost in rats treated with K-II for 7 days after injury, but not in C-ABC-treated rats (Fig. 15.6c, d). The smear appearance in Western blot is the nature of proteoglycans, which is due to the long sugar chains. The granular staining profile of microglia represented the main source of KS expression. (Fig. 15.6e). From these data, K-II worked in vivo although not completely abolished KS. The in vivo degradation of CS by C-ABC, but not that by K-II, was also confirmed (Fig. 15.6b, c).

Furthermore, we also performed immunohistochemistry of collagen IV for glial scar evaluation at 2 weeks after SCI. The area of collagen IV-positive scarring was significantly decreased in K-II- and C-ABC-treated rats (Fig.15.6f).

15.3.2 Motor Function Recovery by K-II Administration

Motor function recovery was evaluated with the Basso, Beattie, and Bresnahan (BBB) scores [17] and %grip test. In %grip test, paw placement for each limb on the grid bar was assessed as the animal walked on a plastic-coated wire mesh grid (50-cm length × 33-cm width × 20-cm height, with 2.5 × 2.5-cm openings) for 3 min. Steps in which the paw gripped the grid bar and supported the animal's weight were counted as correct. The percentage of correct paw placements was calculated for each hind limb and averaged. K-II led to a striking recovery of motor function; the effect was similar to that of C-ABC (Fig. 15.7a, b). To determine an appropriate

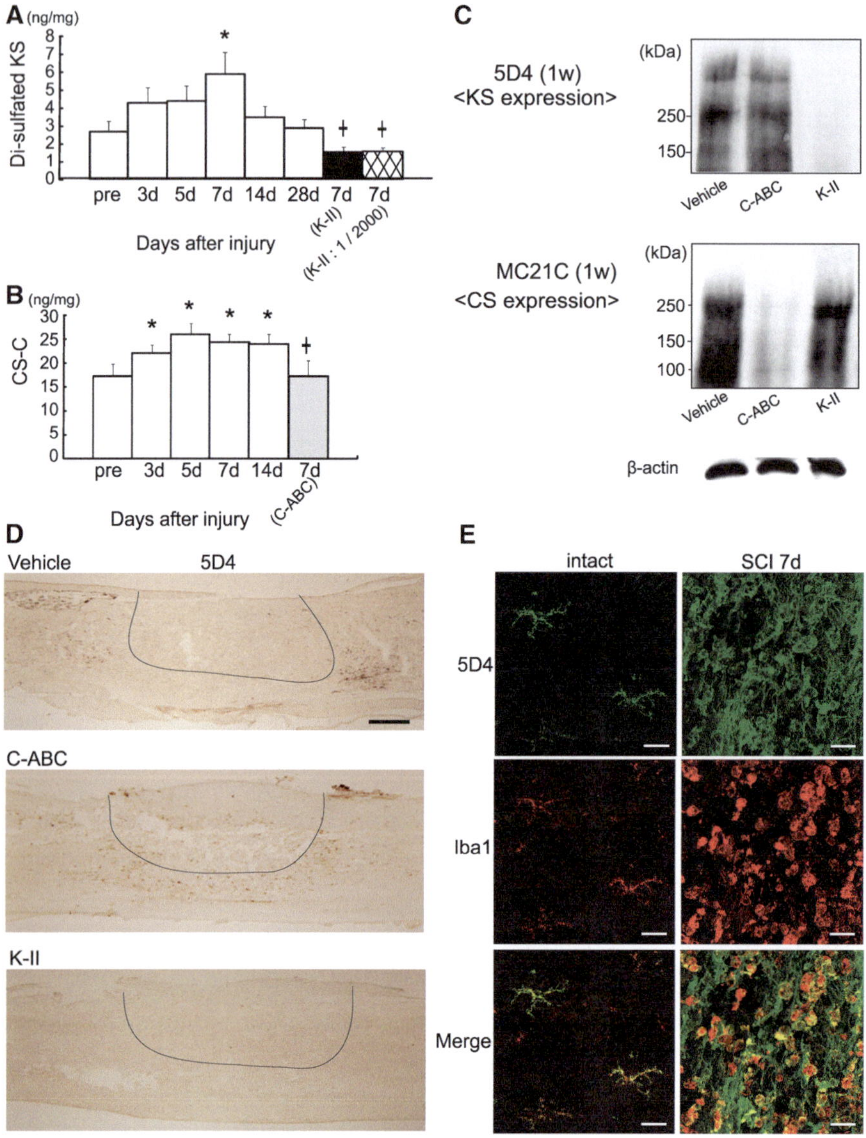

Fig. 15.6 Specific degradation of KS by K-II. (**a**) Amounts of di-sulfated KS after SCI. A 10-mm fragment of the injured spinal cord was subjected to the analysis. Data represent the means ± SEM. *$p<0.05$ vs. the preinjured specimen (pre). +, $p<0.05$ vs. 7 days. $n=5$ in each group. K-II, 0.05 units of K-II were administered to the spinal cord; K-II 1/2000, 0.0000025 units of K-II were administered to the spinal cord. (**b**) Amounts of CS-C after SCI. *$p<0.05$ vs. pre. +, $p<0.05$ vs. 7 days. $n=6$ in each group. C-ABC, 0.05 units of C-ABC were administered to the spinal cord. (**c**) Rats were treated with K-II or C-ABC for 1 week after spinal cord injury. A 10-mm specimen of the injured spinal cord was subjected to Western blot analysis for 5D4-reactive KS, MC21C-reactive CS, and β-actin. (**d**) 5D4-reactive KS was visible in the penumbra region in vehicle-treated and C-ABC-treated rats, but not in K-II-treated rats. These rats were treated with the

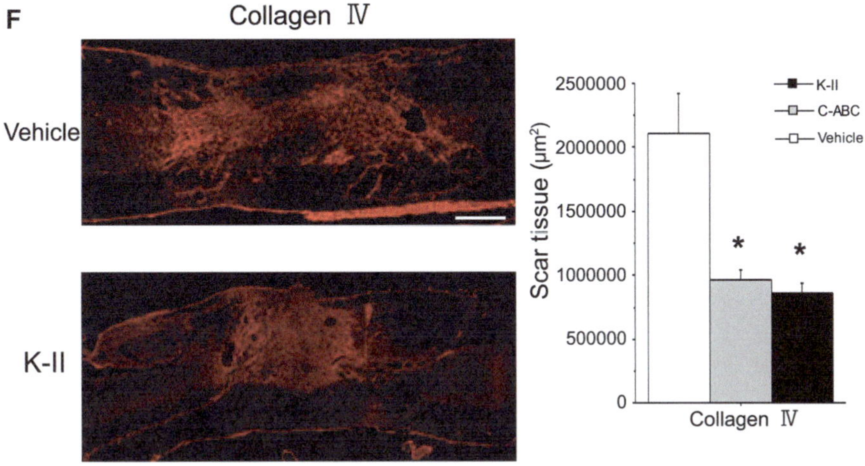

Fig. 15.6 (continued) indicated enzyme for 1 week after spinal cord injury. Scale bars, 500 μm. All photos are of sagittal sections with the left side rostral. (**e**) Double staining for KS (5D4) and microglia (Iba1). The *left panels* show the intact spinal cord, and the *right panels* show the spinal cord 1 week after injury. Most 5D4-reactive cells overlapped Iba1-positive cells, which indicated that KS was mainly expressed by microglia. The *left images* showed ramified microglia expressing 5D4-KSPG. The *right images* show that 5D4-KSPG expression is seen on characteristic cellular profiles with short processes and a less ramified morphology after SCI. Scale bars, 20 μm. (**f**) Immunohistochemistry of collagen IV at 2 weeks after SCI. The area of collagen IV-positive scarring was significantly decreased in K-II- and C-ABC-treated rats. Scale bar, 500 μm. *Right side*, quantitative analysis of the expression of collagen IV was performed at 2 weeks after SCI. 2,900 × 2,200 μm counting frames around a lesion were analyzed. Data represent the means ± SEM. *$p<0.01$ vs. the vehicle control ($n=5$ vehicle; $n=5$ C-ABC; $n=5$ K-II)

dose of C-ABC, we examined several doses and found that at the doses of 0.05, 0.1, and 1.0 units/200 μL, C-ABC showed a comparable effect on motor function recovery, while the dose of 0.025 units/200 μL showed a less potent effect (Fig. 15.7c). Therefore, we used 0.05 units/200 μL of C-ABC in this study. We also determined the dose of 0.05 units/200 μL of K-II (Fig.15.7d). The MEP was also performed as the observed motor function recovery, in which an electric stimulus is given at the thoracic level (Th7) and a response is taken at the gastrocnemius muscles (Fig. 15.7e). This functional recovery was due to the enzymatic activity of K-II, as heat-inactivated K-II did not promote motor function recovery at all (Fig. 15.7f). Interestingly, the combination of K-II and C-ABC showed neither additive nor synergistic effects (Fig. 15.7e, g).

15.3.3 Sensory Function Recovery by K-II Administration

Thermal hyperalgesia and mechanical allodynia were revealed after SCI (Fig. 15.8a, b). The tail-immersion test was used to determine the somatic thermo-threshold of rats preoperatively and then weekly after the operation. Briefly, rats were gently lifted

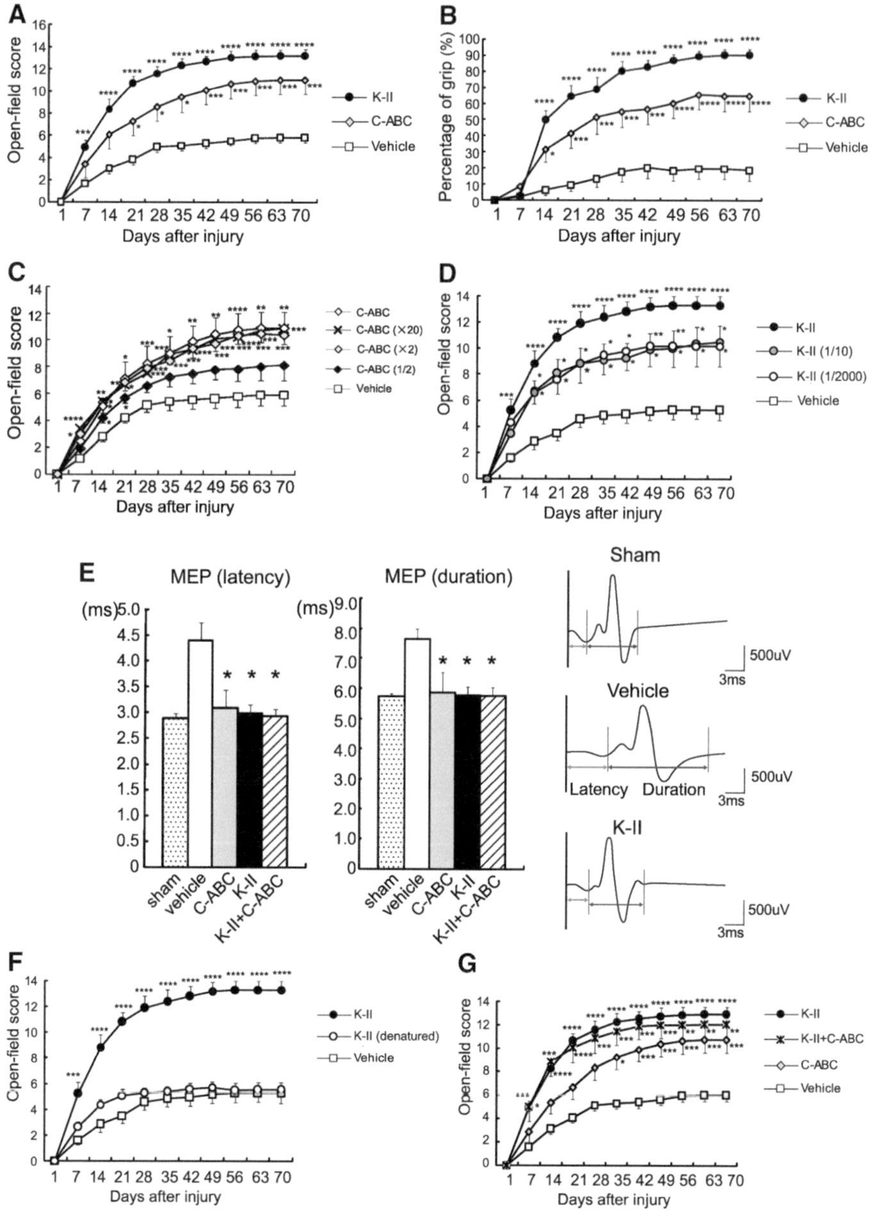

Fig. 15.7 Motor function recovery by K-II after SCI. (**a**, **b**) The BBB score and %grip test data after SCI. Recovery was significantly better in the K-II and C-ABC treatment groups than in the vehicle-administered control. Data represent the means ± SEM. $*p<0.05$; $***p<0.005$; $****p<0.001$ vs. the vehicle control ($n=10$ K-II (0.05 units); $n=7$ C-ABC (0.05 units); $n=10$ vehicle). (**c**) Motor function recovery after SCI in rats treated with C-ABC at various doses. C-ABC promoted functional recovery at the doses of 0.05 units, 0.1 units (×2), and 1.0 units (×20) better than 0.025 units (1/2). Data represent the means ± SEM. $*p<0.05$; $**p<0.01$; $***p<0.005$; $****p<0.001$ vs. the vehicle control ($n=5$ in each group). (**d**) Motor function recovery after SCI in rats treated with K-II at various doses. K-II promoted functional recovery at a concentration of

from their home cages and taken to the test room, where the withdrawal latency of the tail to a temperature stimulus was measured by immersing the tail in a 55 ± 0.5 °C water bath. Graded von Frey hair (vFH) monofilaments were applied to the plantar surface of the foot with the up–down method as a touch test [18]. From these data, thermal hyperalgesia and mechanical allodynia were recovered by K-II or C-ABC treatment, reaching an almost normal level 10 weeks after injury (Fig. 15.8a, b). Sp-SCEP, in which an epidural electric stimulus was given at the Th11 level and a response was taken at the Th7 level, showed that the sensory function was recovered by K-II or C-ABC treatment at 8 weeks after injury (Fig. 15.8c). The reinjury of K-II-treated rats lost the recovered response of sp-SCEP (Fig. 15.8c). The combination of K-II and C-ABC showed neither additive nor synergistic effects on sensory function recovery, as well as motor function recovery (Fig. 15.8c, d).

15.3.4 Histological Analysis After SCI

The GAP43 (Chemicon International, Temecula, CA) and 5HT (Immunostar, Hudson, WI) immunohistochemistry were assessed as a percentage along the longitudinal axis of the spinal cord (Fig. 15.9a, b). These fibers were significantly enhanced in both the rostral and caudal regions in K-II- or C-ABC-treated rats as compared with vehicle control rats (Fig. 15.9b). Representative photos of GAP43 and 5HT staining around the lesion were consistent with the fact that K-II or C-ABC significantly promoted axonal regrowth after SCI (Fig. 15.9c). Furthermore, we performed anterograde labeling of CST to evaluate axonal growth and sprouting. Eight weeks after injury, descending CST fibers were labeled with biotin-dextran amine (BDA: 10 % in saline, 3.5 μl per cortex, molecular weight 10,000; Invitrogen, Carlsbad, CA) injected under anesthesia into the left and right motor cortices (coordinates: 2 mm posterior and 2 mm lateral to the bregma, 1.5 mm depth). For each injection, 0.25 μl of BDA was delivered for a period of 30 s via a 15–20-μm inner diameter glass capillary attached to a microliter syringe (ITO Corporation, Shizuoka, Japan). In these tracer-fiber counts at 2 weeks after BDA injection, many fibers were

Fig. 15.7 (continued) 0.05 units and even restored motor function at concentrations of 0.005 units (1/10) and 0.0000025 units (1/2000). Data represent the means ± SEM. $*p<0.05$; $**p<0.01$; $***p<0.005$; $****p<0.001$ vs. the vehicle control ($n=7$ K-II; $n=5$ K-II (1/10); $n=6$ K-II (1/2000); $n=7$ vehicle). (**e**) Electrophysiologic tests using motor-evoked potential (MEP) also showed functional recovery in the treatment groups at 8 weeks after SCI. Data represent the means ± SEM. $*p<0.05$ vs. the vehicle control ($n=8$ sham; $n=9$ vehicle; $n=5$ C-ABC (0.05 units); $n=7$ K-II (0.05 units); $n=7$ K-II+C-ABC (0.05 units each)). (**f**) Heat-denatured K-II failed to promote motor function recovery after spinal cord injury. Data represent the means ± SEM. $***p<0.005$, $****p<0.001$ vs. the vehicle control ($n=7$ K-II (0.05 units); $n=5$ heat-denatured K-II; $n=7$ vehicle). (**g**) The combination of K-II and C-ABC did not show additive or synergistic effects on motor function (BBB score). Data represent the means ± SEM. $*p<0.05$; $**p<0.01$; $***p<0.005$; $****p<0.001$ vs. the vehicle control [$n=9$ vehicle; $n=7$ C-ABC (0.05 units); $n=11$ K-II (0.05 units); $n=7$ K-II+C-ABC (0.05 units each)]

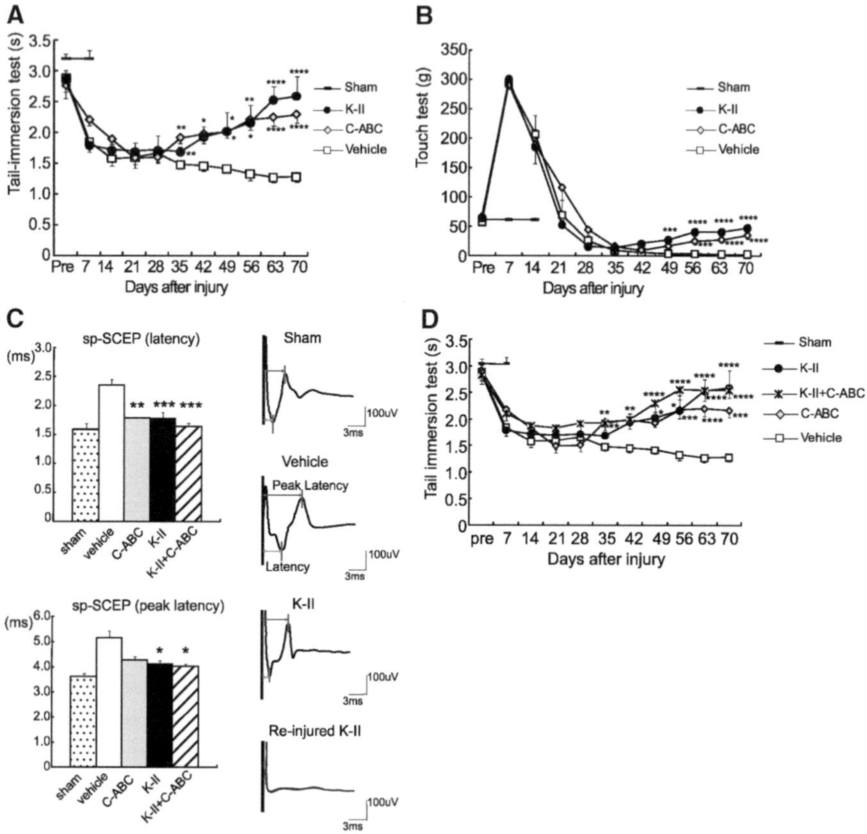

Fig. 15.8 Sensory function recovery by K-II after SCI. (**a**) The tail-immersion test indicated that there was little allodynia in the K-II- and C-ABC-treated rats. Data represent the means ± SEM. *$p<0.05$, **$p<0.01$, ****$p<0.001$ vs. the vehicle control ($n=7$ sham; $n=5$ K-II; $n=7$ C-ABC; $n=9$ vehicle). (**b**) The touch test also indicated that there was little allodynia in the K-II- and C-ABC-treated rats. Data represent the means ± SEM. *$p<0.05$, ***$p<0.005$ vs. the vehicle control ($n=7$ sham; $n=5$ K-II; $n=7$ C-ABC; $n=9$ vehicle). (**c**) Electrophysiologic tests using sp-SCEP showed not only motor functional recovery but also sensory recovery in the treatment groups at 8 weeks after SCI. The reinjury of K-II-treated rats lost the recovered response of sp-SCEP. Data represent the means ± SEM. *$p<0.05$, **$p<0.01$, ***$p<0.005$ vs. the vehicle control ($n=8$ sham; $n=7$ vehicle; $n=5$ C-ABC; $n=6$ K-II; $n=5$ K-II+C-ABC). (**d**) The combination of K-II and C-ABC did not show additive or synergistic effects on sensory function (tail-immersion test). Data represent the means ± SEM. *$p<0.05$; **$p<0.01$; ***$p<0.005$; ****$p<0.001$ vs. the vehicle control ($n=8$ sham; $n=9$ vehicle; $n=7$ C-ABC; $n=11$ K-II; $n=7$ K-II+C-ABC)

detected in the region rostral to the epicenter, and there was no difference among the three groups in the rostral region (Fig. 15.9d). In the vehicle group, BDA-positive fibers were barely expressed in the caudal region (Fig. 15.9d, e). In contrast, in K-II- and C-ABC-treated rats, the number of BDA-positive fibers was significantly increased in the region caudal to the epicenter, particularly in the gray matter (Fig. 15.9d, e).

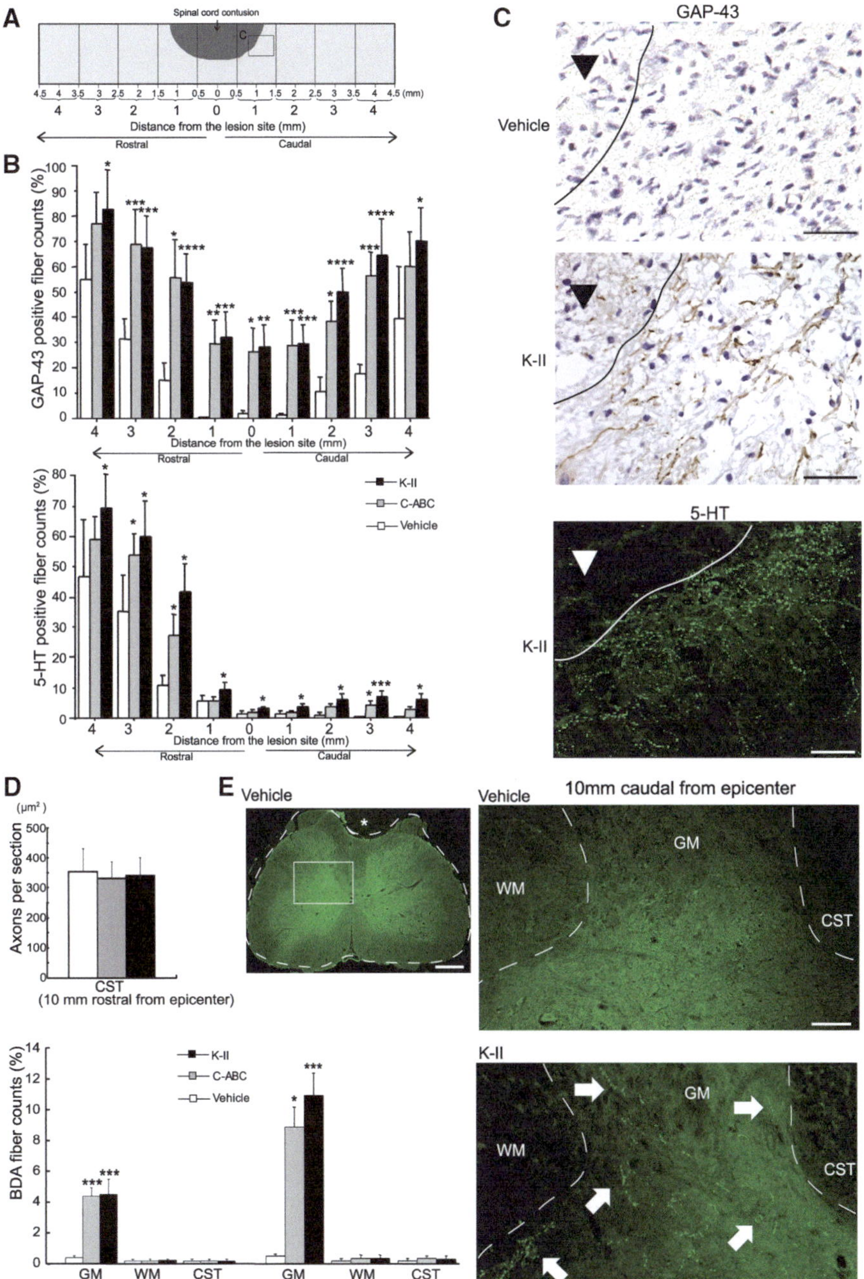

Fig. 15.9 Histological analysis. (**a**) The scheme of the methods to reconstruct serial sagittal sections. On each section, the number of GAP43- and 5HT-positive fibers was counted from 4 mm rostral to 4 mm caudal the lesion site. The number was calculated as a percentage of the fibers seen in the sham-operated spinal cord. All serial sections were evaluated at 10 weeks after SCI.

These BDA-positive fibers in the gray matter may reflect growth or sprouting of proximal or spared axons.

15.3.5 Restoration of Neurite Outgrowth by K-II

We used proteoglycans that purified from the brains of chicks contain both KS and CS. The proteoglycans strongly inhibited neurite outgrowth (Fig. 15.10a, b), which was blocked by K-II and C-ABC to same amount. The combination of K-II and C-ABC showed neither synergistic nor additive effects (Fig. 15.10b), which was consistent to motor function recovery. The heat-denatured proteoglycans as well as reduced/alkylated proteoglycans also lost their inhibitory effect (Fig. 15.10c), suggesting that the conformation of the core protein structure is also essential to this inhibition, since proteins rather than sugar chains are labile to heat or reduction/alkylation.

K-II digests KS into oligosaccharides consisting of two to four saccharides. KS-derived oligosaccharides (Fig. 15.10d) showed no impact on neurite growth (Fig. 15.10e). These results suggest that K-II directly blocks the inhibition of neurite outgrowth by proteoglycans, not induced from the K-II-induced degradation products of KS.

15.3.6 Neurite Growth Inhibition by KS/CSPG

From these in vivo and in vitro results, we investigated whether K-II and C-ABC work on the same axis. Aggrecan, which is a representative proteoglycan in the CNS and harbors both KS and CS chains, strikingly inhibited axonal outgrowth

Fig. 15.9 (continued) (**b**) Reconstruction of serial parasagittal section of the number of GAP43- and 5HT-positive fibers, represented as a percentage of the fibers seen in the sham-operated spinal cord. Data represent the means ± SEM. *$p<0.05$; **$p<0.01$; ***$p<0.005$; ****$p<0.001$ vs. the vehicle control ($n=5$ vehicle; $n=5$ C-ABC; $n=6$ K-II). (**c**) Immunohistochemical analysis of GAP43 and 5HT (serotonin) expression in the injured spinal cord of the boxed area in scheme (**a**) at 10 weeks after SCI. Scale bars, 50 μm for the panels of GAP43; 100 μm for the panel of 5HT. All images are of sagittal section with the left side rostral. *Arrowheads* indicate the contusion area. (**d**) BDA labeling of CST. The *upper graph* represents the number of labeled corticospinal axons 10 mm rostral to the lesioned site. No significant difference was observed between treatment groups. The *lower graph* represents the ratio of labeled corticospinal axons 4 mm and 10 mm caudal vs. 10 mm rostral to the lesioned site. K-II-treated rats had significantly more BDA-positive fibers at 4 mm and 10 mm caudal to the lesioned site than vehicle-treated rats. Data represent the means ± SEM. *$p<0.05$; ** $p<0.005$ vs. the vehicle control ($n=7$ vehicle; $n=6$ C-ABC; $n=5$ K-II). CST, corticospinal tract. (**e**) Representative axial sections of the spinal cord taken from 10 mm caudal from the lesion site at 10 weeks after SCI. The *boxed areas* are magnified on the *right side* of the panel. BDA-positive fibers were clearly seen in the section of K-II-treated rat (*arrows*). Scale bars, 500 μm for the *left panel*; 100 μm for the *right panels*. The thin silicone tube of an osmotic mini pump (*) remained at a point 10 mm caudal from the epicenter. *WM* white matter, *GM* gray matter

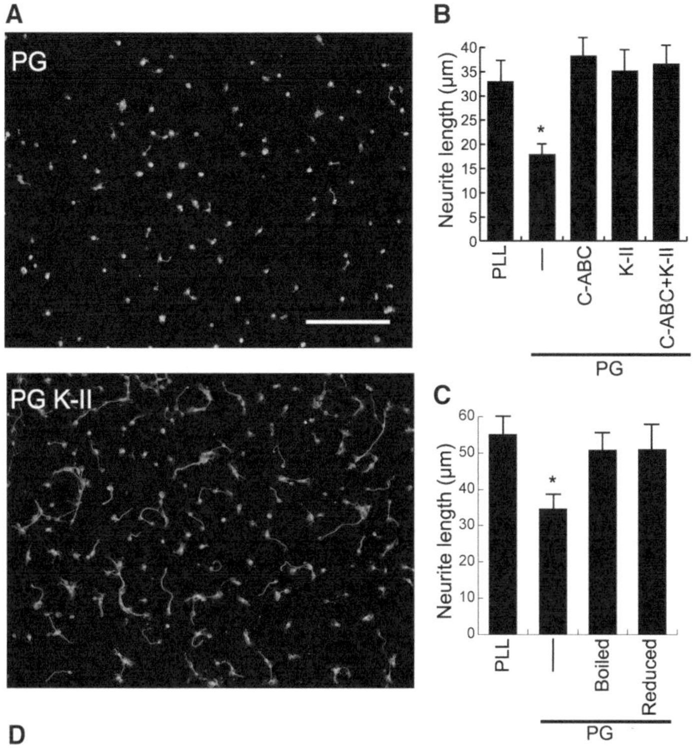

D

OS-1	GlcNAc6S
OS-2	Galβ1 →4GlcNAc
OS-3	Gal6Sβ1 →4GlcNAc6S
OS-4	GlcNAc6Sβ1 →3Gal6S
OS-5	Galβ1 →4GlcNAcβ1 →3Galβ1 →4GlcNAc6S
OS-6	Galβ1 →4GlcNAc6Sβ1 →3Galβ1 →4GlcNAc6S
OS-7	Galβ1 →4GlcNAc6Sβ1 →3Gal6Sβ1 →4GlcNAc6S
OS-8	Gal6Sβ1 →4GlcNAc6Sβ1 →3Gal6Sβ1 →4GlcNAc6S
OS-9	Neu5Ac α2 →3Galβ1 →4GlcNAc6Sβ1 →3Gal6Sβ1 →4GlcNAc6S

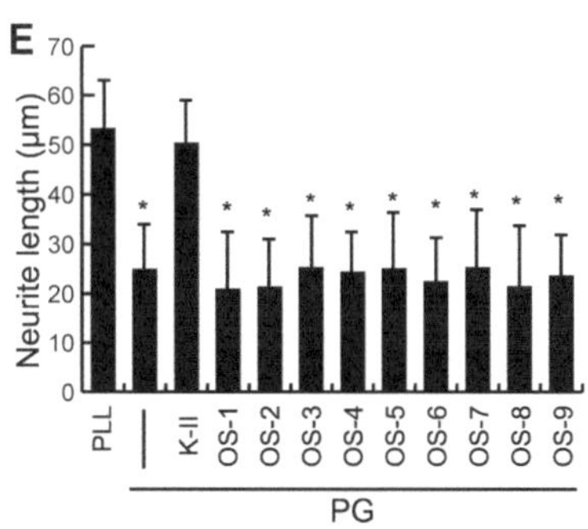

Fig. 15.10 Restoration of neurite outgrowth by K-II. (**a**) P8 rat cerebellar granular neurons were cultured on proteoglycan (PG) extracted from chick brains. K-II treatment restored neurite outgrowth (PG K-II). Scale bar, 100 μm. (**b**) The quantification of (**a**). $*p<0.05$ vs. PLL. PG (300 ng/mL), C-ABC (200 mU/mL), and K-II (5 mU/mL) were used. Data represent the average neurite length ± SD. (**c**), Heat-denatured proteoglycan lost its neurite outgrowth-inhibitory activity. Data represent the average neurite length ± SD. $*p<0.05$ vs. PLL. (**d**) Structures of the oligosaccharides used in this experiment. (**e**) P8 rat cerebellar granular neurons were cultured on chick brain PG substrate in the absence or presence of oligosaccharides (1 μg/mL). Data represent the average neurite lengths ± SD. $*p<0.05$ vs. PLL

(Fig. 15.11a–c), consistent with previous studies [19, 20]. The inhibitory effect of aggrecan was as strong as that by a mixture of proteoglycans (Fig. 15.11c). Interestingly, this inhibition was reversed by K-II as well as C-ABC, and the combination of these enzymes did not demonstrate additive or synergistic effects (Fig. 15.11c).

Keratanase digested mono-sulfated KS only, but K-II digested both mono-sulfated and di-sulfated KS. Keratanase and endo-β-galactosidase, which digests KS and polylactosamine, also reversed aggrecan-mediated inhibition of neurite outgrowth (Fig. 15.11b, c). From these results, KS of aggrecan is required for the aggrecan-mediated inhibition of neurite outgrowth.

Furthermore, we investigated the efficacy among the three components of KS/CSPG (core protein, CS chains, and KS chains) for the inhibitory activity. We generated an artificial proteoglycan consisting of bovine serum albumin (BSA), KS, and CS. However, KS/CS-BSA, KS-BSA, and CS-BSA never inhibited neurite outgrowth (Fig. 15.11d), which revealed the necessity of core protein for neurite inhibition as well as CS and KS chains.

15.3.6.1 Statistical Analysis

We performed statistical analysis with an unpaired two-tailed Student's *t*-test for single comparisons and one-way ANOVA for multiple comparisons. For the BBB score, %grip test, touch test, and tail-immersion test, we used repeated measures ANOVA and Tukey's test. In all statistical analyses, significance was accepted at $p<0.05$.

15.4 Discussion

15.4.1 KS-Degrading Enzyme is a Good Candidate Target for the Treatment of SCI

The relation between KS and the nervous system has not been extensively studied. KS is expressed in the roof plate and has been induced after SCI and axotomy of the nigrostriatal tract, suggesting that it may play a role in the inhibition of axonal growth [21–23]. In the first study of this chapter, GlcNAc6ST-1−/− mice exhibited better motor function recovery and enhanced regeneration of the serotonergic descending raphespinal tract axons and CST axons after SCI, as compared with wild-type mice. This study is the first to demonstrate a link between KS and neurological function and indicates that GlcNAc6ST-1−/− mice are a good model for investigating the roles of KS in the CNS. However, as these knockout mice lose *N*-acetylglucosamine 6-*O*-sulfotransferase-1 in the body, we next performed the experiments with the KS-degrading enzyme K-II as the second study in this chapter. K-II strongly degraded KS both in vivo and in vitro, promoted axonal regrowth, and

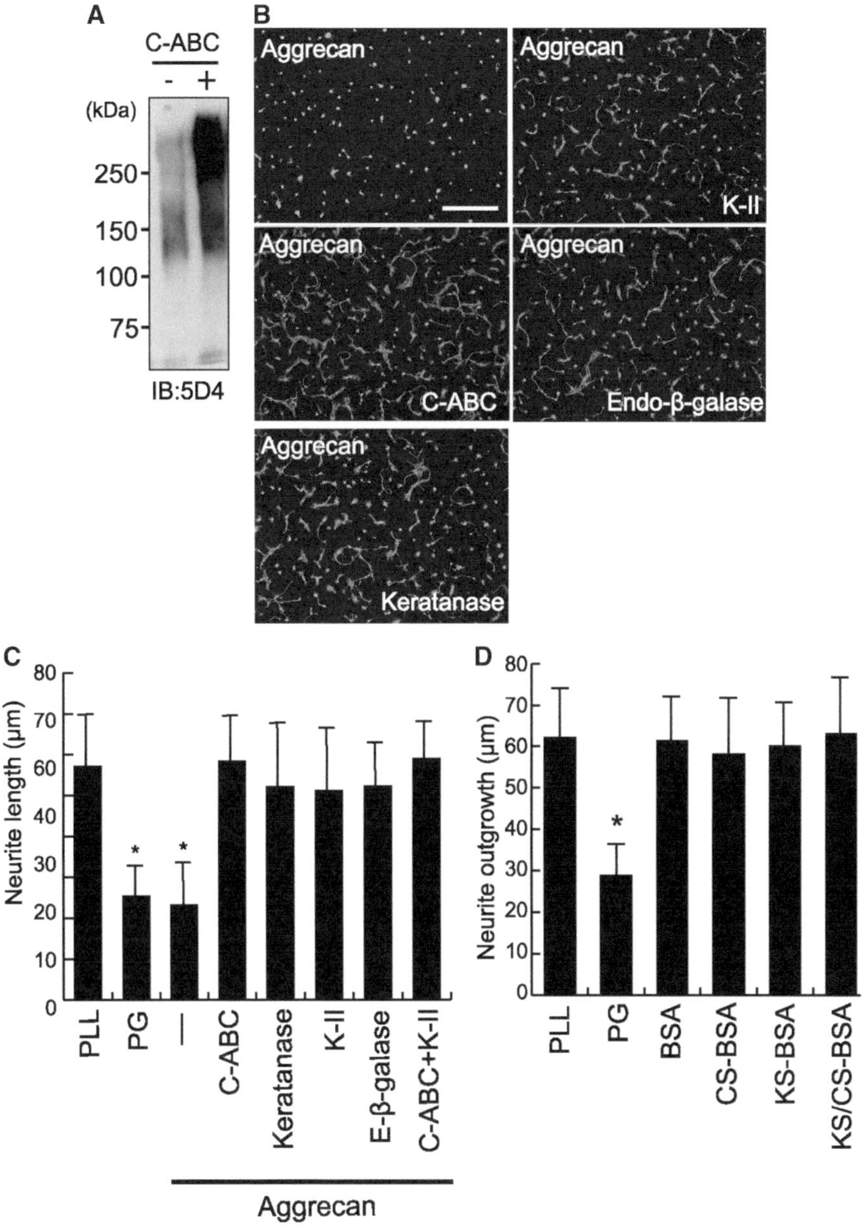

Fig. 15.11 Effects of KS/CSPGs on neurite outgrowth. (**a**) Bovine aggrecan was digested with C-ABC (500 mU/mL) and subjected to SDS-PAGE using 5D4. Note that C-ABC treatment exposed KS epitopes. (**b**) P8 rat cerebellar granule neurons were cultured on aggrecan (5 μg/mL). Degradation of CS or KS restored neurite outgrowth. Scale bar, 100 μm. (**c**) The quantification of (**b**) Data represent the average neurite length ± SD. $*p<0.05$ vs. PLL. (**d**) There was no inhibition of neurite outgrowth by CS-BSA, KS-BSA, or KS/CS-BSA (300 ng/mL each). Data represent the average neurite length ± SD. $*p<0.05$ vs. PLL

led to sensory and motor functional recovery after SCI. Our data strongly suggest that the KS plays a critical role in functional disturbance after SCI and is a good candidate target for therapy of SCI. It is also important to consider that KS degradation may cause maladaptive plasticity. However, as shown in Fig. 15.8, K-II administration promoted recovery from thermal hyperalgesia and mechanical allodynia. In this context, KS degradation never induced unwanted adverse effect on sensory function. As another advantage of KS degradation, there is a much smaller amount of KS than CS in the CNS (Fig. 15.6a–c). The family of keratan sulfate proteoglycans (KSPGs) is also smaller than that of CSPGs [24–26]. From this aspect, KS degradation can minimize the adverse effects of therapy. Surprisingly, K-II shows comparable activity to C-ABC in promoting axonal regrowth and both sensory and motor function recovery after SCI in vivo and in vitro. For these reasons, KS-degrading enzyme, K-II, is one of the attractive targets for the treatment of SCI.

15.4.2 Structure and Function Relationship Between CS and KS in the Proteoglycan-Mediated Inhibition of Neurite Growth

KSPGs have been studied independently from CSPGs, but our study has integrated KS and CS into a common axis. We found that the effects of K-II and C-ABC on in vivo and in vitro were comparable to each other, whereas the combination of these two enzymes showed neither additive nor synergistic effects. Considering each glycosaminoglycan exists as an independent sugar chain, our study has demonstrated that KS and CS are independently required for the inhibition of post-injury neural plasticity and neurite outgrowth. Furthermore, we suggested the necessity of core protein for proteoglycan-mediated inhibition, as well as CS and KS chains. Our data demonstrated that neurite outgrowth was never inhibited by heat-denatured proteoglycans, reduced/alkylated proteoglycans, nor an artificial KS/CSPG (KS/CS-BSA), whereas the natural KS/CSPG aggrecan inhibited neurite outgrowth. From these data, we insist that the three components (KS, CS, and core protein) of the proteoglycan are independently required for proteoglycan-mediated inhibition after neuronal injuries (Fig. 15.12a). Recently PTPσ is reported as a receptor for CS and mediates the inhibitory activity of CSPGs on axonal regeneration [27]. Then, we speculate the KS-specific receptors may also exist so that KS and CS are independently required for the inhibition of neurite outgrowth (summarized in Fig. 15.12b).

15.5 Conclusion

Our study integrated KS and CS into a common axis. Since KS expression was closely associated with functional disturbance after SCI, KS digestion promoted the remarkable motor and sensory function recovery after SCI in rats with enhanced axonal regeneration/sprouting. K-II and C- ABC exerted comparable effects in vivo

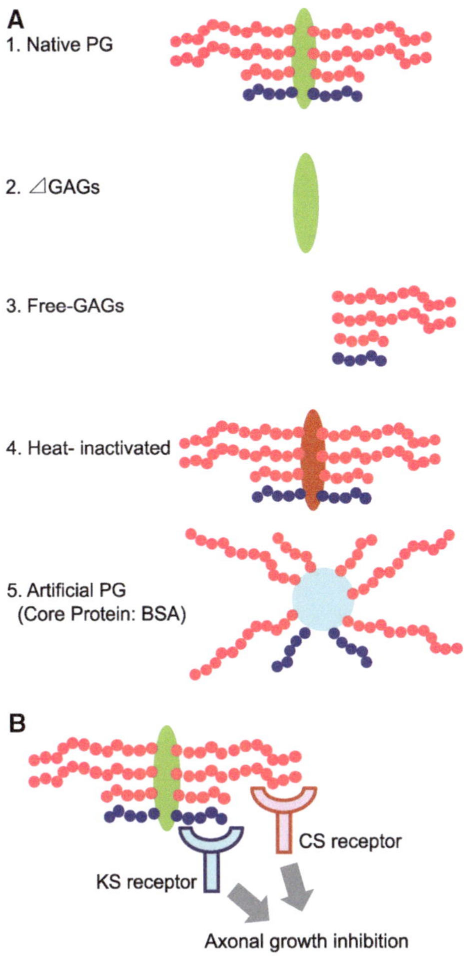

Fig. 15.12 Structure and function relationship in the proteoglycan-mediated inhibition of neurite growth. (**a**) The present study has revealed that KS and CS have a comparable impact on proteoglycans-mediated inhibition of neurite growth. Considering our previous results that neither KS nor CS is sufficient for neurite growth inhibition [12], our data suggest that all three components of the proteoglycans moiety (core protein, CS, and KS) are required for this inhibition activity. (**b**) This scheme shows a speculated mechanism underlying the proteoglycan-mediated inhibition of axonal growth

and in vitro, but these two enzymes worked neither additively nor synergistically. All the three components of the proteoglycan moiety, i.e., the core protein, CS chains, and KS chains, were independently required for the inhibitory activity of proteoglycans. Therefore, KS is essential for the inhibitory effect of proteoglycans and is a good candidate target for therapy of neuronal injuries.

Acknowledgments We wish to thank K. Kadomatsu (Nagoya University), K. Sakamoto (Nagoya University), and T. Yamashita (Osaka University) for their advising us throughout these studies, K. Suzuki, Y. Kurahashi, and A. Tanaka (Sekagaku Corporation) for performing the stability test of K-II and the HPLC analysis of sugar, M. Sawada (Nagoya University) for guidance with the primary culture of neurons, and N. Ozaki (Nagoya University) for guidance with the sensory tests. We also thank T. Natori (Yamanashi-Gakuin University), M. Iida, Y. Naito, S. Nakashima, N. Misawa, and Y. Miwa (Nagoya University) for their excellent technical assistance.

Conflict of Interest All authors declare that they have no conflict of interest.

References

1. Davies SJ, Goucher DR, Doller C, Silver J (1999) Robust regeneration of adult sensory axons in degenerating white matter of the adult rat spinal cord. J Neurosci 19(14):5810–5822
2. Grimpe B, Silver J (2004) A novel DNA enzyme reduces glycosaminoglycan chains in the glial scar and allows microtransplanted dorsal root ganglia axons to regenerate beyond lesions in the spinal cord. J Neurosci 24(6):1393–1397. doi:10.1523/JNEUROSCI.4986-03.200424/6/1393 [pii]
3. Silver J, Miller JH (2004) Regeneration beyond the glial scar. Nat Rev Neurosci 5(2):146–156. doi:10.1038/nrn1326nrn1326 [pii]
4. Tom VJ, Steinmetz MP, Miller JH, Doller CM, Silver J (2004) Studies on the development and behavior of the dystrophic growth cone, the hallmark of regeneration failure, in an in vitro model of the glial scar and after spinal cord injury. J Neurosci 24(29):6531–6539. doi:10.1523/JNEUROSCI.0994-04.200424/29/6531 [pii]
5. Moon LD, Asher RA, Rhodes KE, Fawcett JW (2001) Regeneration of CNS axons back to their target following treatment of adult rat brain with chondroitinase ABC. Nat Neurosci 4(5):465–466. doi:10.1038/8741587415 [pii]
6. Bradbury EJ, Moon LD, Popat RJ, King VR, Bennett GS, Patel PN, Fawcett JW, McMahon SB (2002) Chondroitinase ABC promotes functional recovery after spinal cord injury. Nature 416(6881):636–640. doi:10.1038/416636a416636a [pii]
7. Powell EM, Fawcett JW, Geller HM (1997) Proteoglycans provide neurite guidance at an astrocyte boundary. Mol Cell Neurosci 10(1–2):27–42. doi:S1044-7431(97)90629-1 [pii]10.1006/mcne.1997.0629
8. Snow DM, Steindler DA, Silver J (1990) Molecular and cellular characterization of the glial roof plate of the spinal cord and optic tectum: a possible role for a proteoglycan in the development of an axon barrier. Dev Biol 138(2):359–376. doi:0012-1606(90)90203-U [pii]
9. Kitayama K, Hayashida Y, Nishida K, Akama TO (2007) Enzymes responsible for synthesis of corneal keratan sulfate glycosaminoglycans. J Biol Chem 282(41):30085–30096. doi:10.1074/jbc.M703695200
10. Akama TO, Nishida K, Nakayama J, Watanabe H, Ozaki K, Nakamura T, Dota A, Kawasaki S, Inoue Y, Maeda N, Yamamoto S, Fujiwara T, Thonar EJ, Shimomura Y, Kinoshita S, Tanigami A, Fukuda MN (2000) Macular corneal dystrophy type I and type II are caused by distinct mutations in a new sulphotransferase gene. Nat Genet 26(2):237–241. doi:10.1038/79987
11. Zhang H, Muramatsu T, Murase A, Yuasa S, Uchimura K, Kadomatsu K (2006) *N*-Acetylglucosamine 6-*O*-sulfotransferase-1 is required for brain keratan sulfate biosynthesis and glial scar formation after brain injury. Glycobiology 16(8):702–710. doi:cwj115 [pii]10.1093/glycob/cwj115
12. Ito Z, Sakamoto K, Imagama S, Matsuyama Y, Zhang H, Hirano K, Ando K, Yamashita T, Ishiguro N, Kadomatsu K (2010) *N*-acetylglucosamine 6-*O*-sulfotransferase-1-deficient mice show better functional recovery after spinal cord injury. J Neurosci 30(17):5937–5947. doi:30/17/5937 [pii]10.1523/JNEUROSCI.2570-09.2010

13. Imagama S, Sakamoto K, Tauchi R, Shinjo R, Ohgomori T, Ito Z, Zhang H, Nishida Y, Asami N, Takeshita S, Sugiura N, Watanabe H, Yamashita T, Ishiguro N, Matsuyama Y, Kadomatsu K (2011) Keratan sulfate restricts neural plasticity after spinal cord injury. J Neurosci 31(47):17091–17102. doi:10.1523/JNEUROSCI.5120-10.2011
14. Basso DM, Fisher LC, Anderson AJ, Jakeman LB, McTigue DM, Popovich PG (2006) Basso mouse scale for locomotion detects differences in recovery after spinal cord injury in five common mouse strains. J Neurotrauma 23(5):635–659. doi:10.1089/neu.2006.23.635
15. Liesi P, Kauppila T (2002) Induction of type IV collagen and other basement-membrane-associated proteins after spinal cord injury of the adult rat may participate in formation of the glial scar. Exp Neurol 173(1):31–45. doi:10.1006/exnr.2001.7800
16. Yamagishi K, Suzuki K, Imai K, Mochizuki H, Morikawa K, Kyogashima M, Kimata K, Watanabe H (2003) Purification, characterization, and molecular cloning of a novel keratan sulfate hydrolase, endo-beta-*N*-acetylglucosaminidase, from *Bacillus circulans*. J Biol Chem 278(28):25766–25772. doi:10.1074/jbc.M212183200M212183200 [pii]
17. Basso DM, Beattie MS, Bresnahan JC (1995) A sensitive and reliable locomotor rating scale for open field testing in rats. J Neurotrauma 12(1):1–21
18. Hutchinson KJ, Gomez-Pinilla F, Crowe MJ, Ying Z, Basso DM (2004) Three exercise paradigms differentially improve sensory recovery after spinal cord contusion in rats. Brain 127(Pt 6):1403–1414. doi:10.1093/brain/awh160awh160 [pii]
19. Asher RA, Scheibe RJ, Keiser HD, Bignami A (1995) On the existence of a cartilage-like proteoglycan and link proteins in the central nervous system. Glia 13(4):294–308. doi:10.1002/glia.440130406
20. Johnson WE, Caterson B, Eisenstein SM, Hynds DL, Snow DM, Roberts S (2002) Human intervertebral disc aggrecan inhibits nerve growth in vitro. Arthritis Rheum 46(10):2658–2664. doi:10.1002/art.10585
21. Cole GJ, McCabe CF (1991) Identification of a developmentally regulated keratan sulfate proteoglycan that inhibits cell adhesion and neurite outgrowth. Neuron 7(6):1007–1018. doi:0896-6273(91)90345-Z [pii]
22. Jones LL, Tuszynski MH (2002) Spinal cord injury elicits expression of keratan sulfate proteoglycans by macrophages, reactive microglia, and oligodendrocyte progenitors. J Neurosci 22(11):4611–4624. doi:2002646422/11/4611 [pii]
23. Moon LD, Asher RA, Rhodes KE, Fawcett JW (2002) Relationship between sprouting axons, proteoglycans and glial cells following unilateral nigrostriatal axotomy in the adult rat. Neuroscience 109(1):101–117. doi:S0306452201004572 [pii]
24. Funderburgh JL (2000) Keratan sulfate: structure, biosynthesis, and function. Glycobiology 10(10):951–958
25. Funderburgh JL (2002) Keratan sulfate biosynthesis. IUBMB Life 54(4):187–194. doi:10.1080/15216540214932
26. Margolis RK, Margolis RU (1993) Nervous tissue proteoglycans. Experientia 49(5):429–446
27. Shen Y, Tenney AP, Busch SA, Horn KP, Cuascut FX, Liu K, He Z, Silver J, Flanagan JG (2009) PTPsigma is a receptor for chondroitin sulfate proteoglycan, an inhibitor of neural regeneration. Science 326(5952):592–596. doi:1178310 [pii]10.1126/science.1178310

Chapter 16
Targeted Retrograde Gene Delivery into the Injured Spinal Cord Using Recombinant Adenovirus Vector Carrying Neurotrophic Factor Gene

Hideaki Nakajima, Kenzo Uchida, Takafumi Yayama, Kazuya Honjoh, Takumi Sakamoto, and Hisatoshi Baba

Abstract We investigated the efficacy of retrograde gene delivery via the sternomastoid muscle of recombinant adenovirus vector (AdV) carrying brain-derived neurotrophic factor (BDNF) gene for the rescue of injured rat spinal cord. AdV-BDNF gene or AdV-β-galactosidase (AdV-LacZ) gene was injected into the sternomastoid muscle immediately after traumatic C4 spinal cord injury. Localization of β-galactosidase expression produced by LacZ gene or AdV-BDNF gene transfection was examined by immunofluorescence staining and double staining of cell markers (NeuN, RIP, GFAP, OX-42, and NG2) in the injured spinal cord. TUNEL-positive cells were counted, and immunoreactivity to active caspase-3 and NG2 was examined after gene injection. Retrograde delivery of LacZ marker gene was identified in cervical spinal cord neurons and glial cells including oligodendrocytes in the white matter. AdV-BDNF transfection resulted in a significant decrease in the number of TUNEL-positive apoptotic cells by downregulating the caspase apoptotic pathway, with significant promotion of NG2 expression in injured spinal cord, compared with AdV-LacZ injection. Our results suggest that targeted retrograde BDNF gene delivery suppresses apoptosis of neurons and oligodendrocytes in the injured rat spinal cord.

Keywords Adenoviral vector (AdV) • Apoptosis • Brain-derived neurotrophic factor (BDNF) • Retrograde gene transfer • Spinal cord injury

---

H. Nakajima (✉) • K. Uchida • T. Yayama • K. Honjoh • T. Sakamoto • H. Baba
Faculty of Medical Sciences, Department of Orthopaedics and Rehabilitation Medicine, University of Fukui, Matsuoka Shimoaizuki 23-3, Eiheiji, Fukui 910-1193, Japan
e-mail: nhideaki@u-fukui.ac.jp

K. Uchida et al. (eds.), *Neuroprotection and Regeneration of the Spinal Cord*,
DOI 10.1007/978-4-431-54502-6_16,

16.1 Introduction

Traumatic spinal cord injury can cause neural tissue damage and reduce neuronal cell survival activity including protein synthesis, necrosis, and apoptosis. Several studies have demonstrated the rapid appearance of apoptotic neurons and glial cells in the injured cord segments and adjacent areas following spinal cord insult [1–4]. In addition to neuronal apoptosis, programmed cell death of oligodendrocytes was also observed along the longitudinal axis of the spinal cord, which could be involved in delayed and prolonged process of demyelination and deterioration of sensorimotor function of the cord [3, 5]. Because prevention of apoptosis that occurs after spinal cord injury could potentially lead to spinal cord tissue restoration and motor function improvement, it has become a target for drug therapy. A number of clinical trials have reported success in suppressing apoptotic cell death after spinal cord injury [6, 7].

Neurotrophic factors are required for neuronal survival and influence axonal elongation during normal development [8–10]. Deficiency of endogenous neurotrophic factors is a serious problem for neuronal cell survival [8, 11]; therefore, exogenous administration of neurotrophic factors has been proposed as one potential treatment for spinal cord injury [12–14]. Effective neurotrophin delivery promotes neuronal cell survival, prevents neuronal cell atrophy, and potentially facilitates axonal regeneration. In this context, targeted neurotrophin gene delivery through peripheral nerves or target muscle transmitted by adenoviral vectors (AdV) is less invasive with the potential of repeated administration [15, 16], compared with direct administration of gene transduction to the nervous system by intrathecal, intracerebroventricular, or intraparenchymal infusion [17]. Our group has also reported the feasibility of retrograde delivery of adenovirus genome to the cervical and lumbar segments through injection of an adenovirus vector into the target muscles using AdV carrying β-galactosidase (AdV-LacZ) gene [18–20] (Fig. 16.1). In the spinal hyperostotic mouse (*twy/twy*), our group has confirmed that AdV-mediated brain-derived neurotrophic factor (BDNF) gene via retrograde axonoplasmic transport could be transfected into cervical spinal cord neurons and some glial cells [21].

However, it is not clear whether the AdV-BDNF suppresses neuronal and glial cell apoptosis in the acute spinal cord injury model, and there is no report that describes cell death, particularly apoptosis, following retrograde neurotrophin gene transfection. The present study was designed to investigate the effects of retrograde AdV-BDNF gene delivery on apoptosis of neurons and glial cells (oligodendrocytes) after traumatic spinal cord injury.

16.1.1 Animal Model of Spinal Cord Injury and Targeted AdV-BDNF Gene Delivery

AdV-mediated BDNF was prepared using the instruction provided with the Adenovirus Expression Vector Kit (Takara Biomedical, Otsu, Japan). As a control marker gene, a recombinant adenovirus vector coding for bacterial β-galactosidase

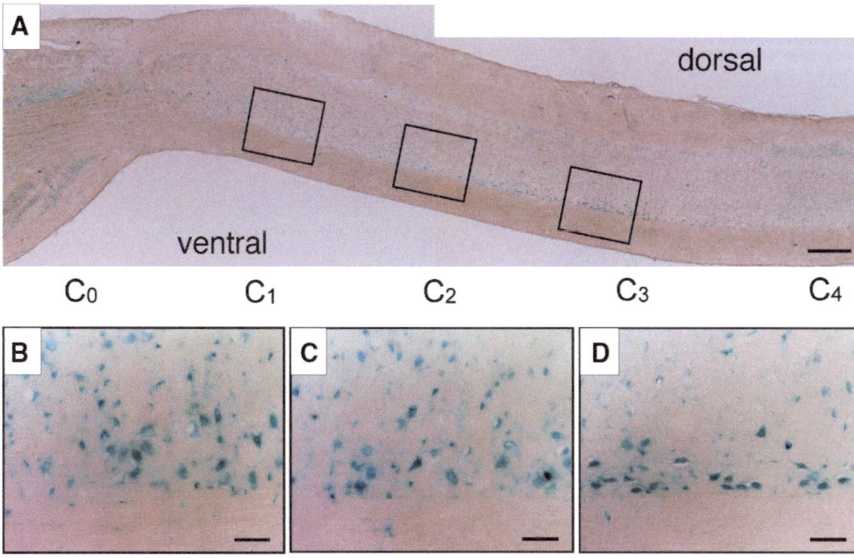

Fig. 16.1 Targeted retrograde gene delivery of recombinant adenovirus vector-mediated LacZ gene through the sternomastoid muscle innervated by spinal accessory nerves. (**a**) Lower magnification, (**b–d**) high-power photomicrograph of the box area

cDNA was isolated using the same procedure (AdV-LacZ). The final titers of the adenovirus vector contained 5.0×10^8 plaque forming units/mL.

Experiments were conducted in adult male Sprague–Dawley rats (Clea, Tokyo), aged 8–10 weeks. At the C4 vertebral level (C5 cord segment), the dorsal dural surface of the spinal cord was compressed extradurally using a 50 g static load (custom-made rod, 2×3 mm in diameter) for 5 min, as we described previously [19]. Immediately after the injury, the sternomastoid muscles were exposed on both sides while the rat was positioned in supine position using a stereotaxic surgical frame, taking utmost care in preserving branches of the spinal accessory nerves that innervate the muscles. Using a microsyringe (Hamilton, Reno, NV), each 100 μL of AdV encoding LacZ (5.0×10^8 PFU) or BDNF (5.0×10^8 PFU) was injected carefully and slowly into the middle belly of the superficial layer of the bilateral sternomastoid muscles simultaneously. AdV-LacZ injection without spinal cord injury (only operation for laminectomy) was used as normal groups (i.e., positive controls).

16.1.2 Distribution of β-Galactosidase Expression in the Spinal Cord by Retrograde Gene Delivery

To assess the distribution of β-galactosidase following retrograde gene delivery into the normal (Fig. 16.2a) and injured (Fig. 16.2e) spinal cord, immunofluorescence staining was performed. β-Galactosidase-positive cells were observed mainly in the

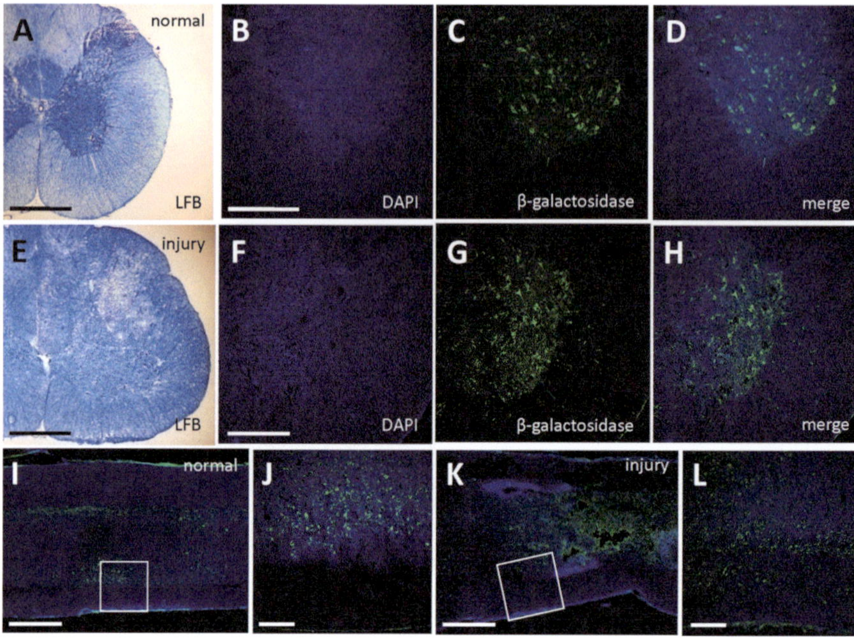

Fig. 16.2 Photomicrographs showing immunofluorescence for β-galactosidase in axial and sagittal sections of normal (**a**–**d**) and (**i**, **j**) and injured (**e**–**h**) and (**k**, **l**) spinal cord at 1 week after AdV-LacZ gene injection. (**a**, **e**) Luxol fast blue (LFB) staining. (**b**, **f**) DAPI. (**c**, **g**) β-galactosidase. (**d**, **h**–**l**) merged. Scale bar = 500 μm (**a**, **b**, **e**, and **f**), 1 mm (**i**, **k**), 100 μm (**j**, **l**) (Reprinted, with permission, from [20])

gray matter including motoneurons and interneurons in the normal spinal cord on axial (Fig. 16.2b–d) and sagittal sections (Fig. 16.2i, j) of positive controls, while they were observed in all (gray matter and white matter) of the injured spinal cord on axial (Fig. 16.2f–h) and sagittal (Fig. 16.2k, l) sections.

16.1.3 Apoptosis of Neurons and Oligodendrocytes

Histological evaluation and immunoblot analysis were applied to assess the effects of retrograde BDNF gene delivery on apoptotic cell death in the injured spinal cord. A number of TUNEL-positive cells were found in both gray and white matters of the cord after AdV-LacZ gene transfection. In comparison, TUNEL-positive cells were markedly decreased in the injured cord after treatment with AdV-BDNF gene transfection. The number of TUNEL-positive cells per cross section significantly decreased in the AdV-BDNF-injected group compared to the AdV-LacZ-injected group at 3 days, 1 and 2 weeks after injury in the rostral and caudal adjacent site (Fig. 16.3a, c), and at 1 week after the injury in the epicenter (Fig. 16.4b).

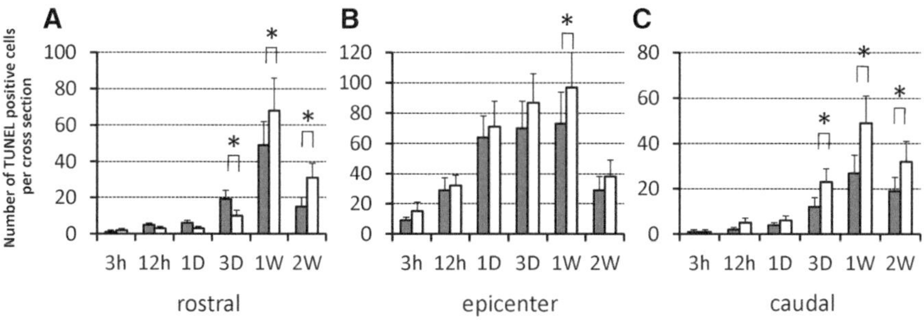

Fig. 16.3 Bar graphs show results of quantitative analysis of TUNEL-positive cells per cross section following AdV-LacZ or AdV-BDNF transfection at rostral (**a**), epicenter (**b**), and caudal (**c**) sites of the injured cervical cord. Data are mean ± SD. *$p<0.05$ (Reprinted, in part, with permission, from [20])

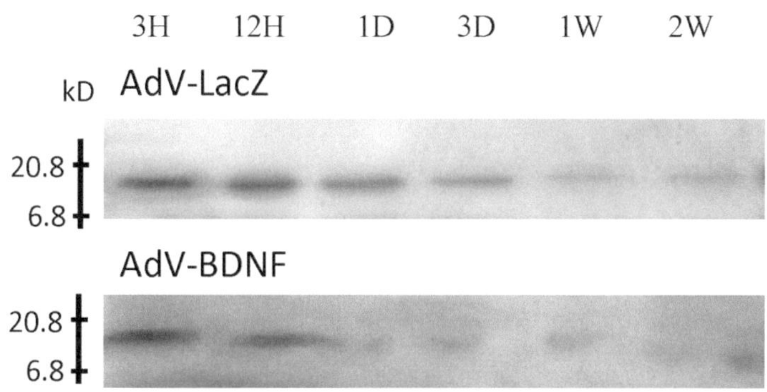

Fig. 16.4 Immunoblot analysis for the expression of active caspase-3 following AdV-LacZ or AdV-BDNF gene transfection into the injured cervical cord (Reprinted, in part, with permission, from [20])

Figure 16.4 shows the results of immunoblot analysis and double immunofluorescence staining carried out to investigate the effect of retrograde gene transfection on the expression of active caspase-3. A band of active caspase-3 was evident from 3 h to 1 week after spinal cord injury in AdV-LacZ-treated rats, while the band appeared 3–12 h later in AdV-BDNF gene-injected animals.

16.1.4 Effects of Retrograde AdV-BDNF Gene Delivery on Endogenous Oligodendrocyte Progenitor Cells

Expression of NG2 (precursor of oligodendrocyte lineage) in the white matter of the cord was investigated at 4 weeks after retrograde injection of AdV-BDNF. Abundant NG2-positive cells were noted in the white matter of AdV-BDNF- than

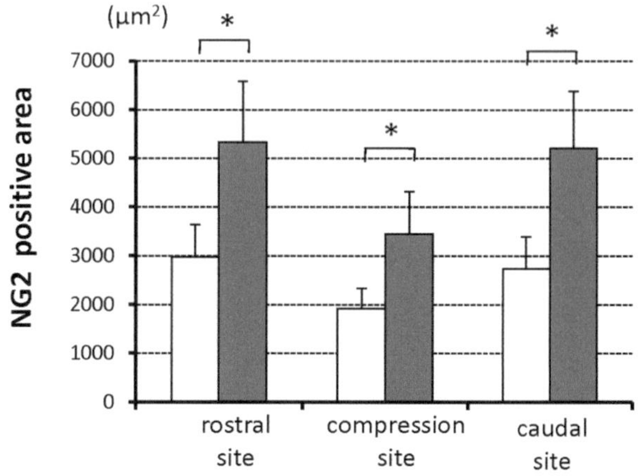

Fig. 16.5 Quantitative analysis of the NG2-positive area in the axial sections showed a significant increase of NG2 expression after AdV-BDNF gene injection. Data are mean ± SD. $*p<0.05$ (Reprinted, in part, with permission, from [20])

AdV-LacZ-injected rats in transaxial (Fig. 16.5a, b) sections. Quantitative analysis of NG2-positive area in AdV-BDNF-treated rats showed significant increase in all three anatomic sites (Fig. 16.5c).

16.2 Discussion

The delivery of neuroprotective genes such as neurotrophic factors can be potentially beneficial for restoration of neural tissue function after spinal cord injury [9, 10, 13, 16]. Development of virus vector for gene delivery is a practically feasible tool for transduction of neurotrophic peptides [22]. However, effective administration of neuroprotective genes into the injured site of the cord remains a major challenge. Direct routes for administration of neuroprotective genes have been used for gene delivery. However, there are difficulties and serious concerns regarding the possible spread of traumatic neural injury and worsening of neural insult, including necrosis, and apoptosis as well as cell death [23]. In contrast, targeted retrograde gene delivery through the peripheral nervous system or by muscle injection of adenovirus vectors seems a less invasive method that can be conducted repeatedly [16].

In a series of experiments, our group evaluated the feasibility and efficacy of retrograde gene delivery into the injured cervical spinal cord using recombinant adenovirus vector through the sternomastoid muscle, which is innervated by the spinal accessory nerve [18–21], applying modified wheat germ agglutinin-horseradish peroxidase labeling method of cervical motoneurons pool [9]. β-Galactosidase (AdV-LacZ) gene expression was found in the cervical spinal cord from 4 to 6 weeks after injection of adenovirus vector, reaching peak expression level at 1–2 weeks and exhibiting transduction efficacy (survival rate of cervical spinal cord motoneurons: 87.5–98.9 % within 3 days after injection) [18, 19]. Transduction of interneurons and glial cells (microglia, reactive astrocytes, and oligodendrocytes) induced by primary or secondary wave of injury could be verified with X-gal staining at early time after the trauma. The efficiency of retrograde delivery of neuropeptide genes could be influenced by various factors [24], but our group has confirmed that AdV-LacZ is transported via retrograde axonoplasmic flow rather than through systemic circulation because no gene expression was observed in various peripheral organs [20]. Accordingly, targeted retrograde AdV-LacZ gene and hopefully AdV-BDNF gene delivery is considered feasible from a methodological point of view.

Exogenous administration of BDNF promotes neural cell survival, alleviates neuronal atrophy [13], facilitates axonal regeneration, prevents apoptosis, enhances differentiation of neuronal stem cells to neurons followed by improvement of motor function [14], and induces glial cell proliferation, axonal outgrowth, and myelination. Our group has reported that retrograde AdV-BDNF gene transduction in the injured cervical cord plays a positive role in maintaining surviving neurons following trauma [25], but there was no evidence of whether the same treatment suppressed neuronal and glial cell apoptosis. Apoptosis of neurons and oligodendrocytes involves the activation of casepase-3. Activation of casepase-3 and upregulation of these caspase mRNA levels occur immediately after spinal cord trauma. Under-expression of these neuropeptides suggests suppression of neural cell apoptosis. The retrograde delivery of AdV-BDNF to the epicenter and around injured site resulted in a significant decrease in the number of TUNEL-positive cells at early stage following traumatic cord insult, suggesting anti-apoptotic effect of the treatment. Our observation also suggests that AdV-BDNF transduction immediately after the injury is attributable to downregulation of caspase-3-mediated pathway, particularly neurons and oligodendrocytes in animals with injured cervical spinal cord.

Oligodendrocytes that survive even under demyelinating insult to the cord were believed to be uncorrelated to remyelination [26]. Instead, the presence of NG2-labeled endogenous oligodendrocyte progenitor cells in the lesion indicates the proliferation of cycling cells [27] and considered to contribute to myelin repair [28]. After spinal cord injury, expression and localization of NG2 were identified in the residual white matter, and in the present study, they were also found in the traumatized and adjacent sites. In the present study, we found increased NG2 immunoreactivity after AdV-BDNF gene injection and potential anti-apoptotic effect of BDNF that is conveyed to the neural cells via axonoplasmic transport. BDNF is reported to induce proliferation of oligodendrocytes and myelination of regenerating axons after spinal cord injury [29]. Accordingly, it is conceivable that increased NG2 immunoreactivity following AdV-BDNF gene transfection represents anti-apoptotic effect on neural cells including oligodendrocytes.

16.3 Conclusion

We have described the potential roles of targeted retrograde AdV-BDNF gene transfection to the traumatically injured cervical spinal cord in terms of significant reduction in the number of TUNEL-positive neurons and oligodendroglia. This action seems to be mediated by downregulation of caspase-3-mediated apoptotic cascade. Retrograde BDNF gene delivery is a potentially feasible method to promote the survival of neurons and oligodendroglia after traumatic spinal cord injury.

Acknowledgment This work was supported in part by Grants-in-Aid for General Scientific Research of the Ministry of Education, Science and Culture of Japan (grants numbers C15591571, B16390435, B18390411, and B19791023).

Conflict of Interest All authors declare that they have no conflict of interest.

References

1. Katoh K, Ikata T, Katoh S et al (1996) Induction and its spread of apoptosis in rat spinal cord after mechanical trauma. Neurosci Lett 216:9–12
2. Li GL, Brodin G, Farooque M et al (1996) Apoptosis and expression of bcl-2 after compression trauma to rat spinal cord. J Neuropathol Exp Neurol 55:280–289
3. Crowe MJ, Bresnahan JC, Shuman SL et al (1997) Apoptosis and delayed degeneration after spinal cord injury in rats and monkeys. Nat Med 3:73–76
4. Nakahara S, Yone K, Sakou T et al (1999) Induction of apoptosis signal regulating kinase 1 (ASK1) after spinal cord injury in rats: possible involvement of ASK1-JNK and p38 pathways in neuronal apoptosis. J Neuropathol Exp Neurol 58:442–450
5. Abe Y, Yamamoto T, Sugiyama Y et al (1999) Apoptotic cells associated with Wallerian degeneration after experimental spinal cord injury: a possible mechanism of oligodendroglial death. J Neurotrauma 16:946–952
6. Ray SK, Wilford GG, Matzelle DC et al (1999) Calpetin and methylprednisolone inhibit apoptosis in rat spinal cord injury. Ann N Y Acad Sci 860:261–269
7. Wada S, Yone K, Ishidou Y et al (1999) Apoptosis following spinal cord injury in rats and preventive effect of *N*-methyl-D-aspartate receptor antagonist. J Neurosurg 91:98–104
8. Bregman BS (2000) Transplants and neurotrophins modify the response of developing and mature CNS neurons to spinal cord injury. Axonal regeneration and recovery of function. In: Kalb RG, Strittmatter SM (eds) Neurobiology of spinal cord injury. Humana, Totowa, pp 169–194
9. Uchida K, Baba H, Maezawa Y et al (1998) Histological investigation of spinal cord lesions in the spinal hyperostotic mouse (*twy/twy*): morphological changes in anterior horn cells and immunoreactivity to neurotrophic factors. J Neurol 245:781–793
10. Uchida K, Nakajima H, Inukai T et al (2008) Adenovirus-mediated transfer of neurotrophin-3 gene enhances survival of anterior horn neurons of twy/twy mice with chronic mechanical compression of the spinal cord. J Neurosci Res 86:1789–1800
11. Nakamura M, Bregman BS (2001) Differences in neurotrophic factor gene expression profiles between neonate and adult rat spinal cord after injury. Exp Neurol 169:407–415
12. Kobayashi NR, Fan DP, Giehl KM et al (1997) BDNF and NT-4/5 prevent atrophy of rat rubrospinal neurons after cervical axonotomy, stimulate GAP-43 and T alpha 1-tubulin mRNA expression, and promote axonal regeneration. J Neurosci 17:9583–9595
13. Novikova LN, Novikov LN, Kellerth JO (2000) Survival effects of BDNF and NT-3 on axonotomized rubrospinal neurons depends on the temporal pattern of neurotrophin administration. Eur J Neurosci 12:776–780
14. Blits B, Boer GJ, Verhaagen J (2002) Pharmacological, cell, and gene therapy strategies to promote spinal cord regeneration. Cell Transplant 11:593–613
15. Ruitenberg MJ, Eggers R, Boer GJ et al (2002) Adeno-associated viral vectors as agents for gene delivery: application in disorders and trauma of the central nervous system. Methods 28:182–194

16. Hendriks WT, Ruitenberg MJ, Blits B et al (2004) Viral vector-mediated gene transfer of neurotrophins to promote regeneration of the injured spinal cord. Prog Brain Res 146:451–476
17. Mannes AJ, Caudle RM, O'Connell BC et al (1998) Adenoviral gene transfer to spinal-cord neurons: intrathecal vs. intraparenchymal administration. Brain Res 793:1–6
18. Nakajima H, Uchida K, Kobayashi S et al (2005) Targeted retrograde gene delivery into the injured cervical spinal cord using recombinant adenovirus vector. Neurosci Lett 385:30–35
19. Nakajima H, Uchida K, Kobayashi S et al (2008) Target muscles for retrograde gene delivery to specific spinal cord segments. Neurosci Lett 435:1–6
20. Nakajima H, Uchida K, Yayama T et al (2010) Targeted retrograde gene delivery of brain-derived neurotrophic factor suppresses apoptosis of neurons and oligodendroglia after spinal cord injury in rats. Spine 35:497–504
21. Xu K, Uchida K, Nakajima H et al (2006) Targeted retrograde transfection of adenovirus vector carrying brain-derived neurotrophic factor gene prevents loss of mouse (*twy/twy*) anterior horn neurons in vivo sustaining mechanical compression. Spine 31:1867–1874
22. Hermens WT, Verhaagen J (1998) Viral vectors, tools for gene transfer in the nervous system. Prog Neurobiol 55:399–432
23. Boulis NM, Turner DE, Imperiale MJ et al (2002) Neuronal survival following remote adenovirus gene delivery. J Neurosurg Spine 96:212–219
24. Haase G, Pettmann B, Vigne E et al (1998) Adenovirus-mediated transfer of the neurotrophin-3 gene into skeletal muscle of *pmn* mice: therapeutic effects and mechanisms of action. J Neurol Sci 160:S97–S105
25. Nakajima H, Uchida K, Kobayashi S et al (2007) Rescue of rat anterior horn neurons after spinal cord injury by retrograde transfection of adenovirus vector carrying brain-derived neurotrophic factor gene. J Neurotrauma 24:703–712
26. Keirstead HS, Levine JM, Blakemore WF (1998) Response of the oligodendrocyte progenitor cell population (defined by NG2 labeling) to demyelination of the adult spinal cord. Glia 22: 161–170
27. Polite A, Reynolds R (2005) NG2-expressing cells as oligodendrocyte progenitors expressing in the normal and demyelinated adult central nervous system. J Anat 207:707–716
28. Levine JM, Reynolds R (1999) Activation and proliferation of endogenous oligodendrocyte precursor cells during ethidium bromide-induced demyelination. Exp Neurol 160:333–347
29. McTiger DM, Horner PJ, Strokes BT et al (1998) Neurotrophin-3 and brain-derived neurotrophic factor induce oligodendrocyte proliferation and myelination of regenerating axons in the contused adult rat spinal cord. J Neurosci 18:5354–5365

Chapter 17
Blockade of Interleukin-6 Effects on Cytokine Profiles and Macrophage Activation After Spinal Cord Injury in Mice

Alexander Rodriguez Guerrero, Kenzo Uchida, Hideaki Nakajima, Shuji Watanabe, Masaya Nakamura, Seiji Okada, William E.B. Johnson, and Hisatoshi Baba

Abstract The objective of this study was to clarify the effects of a temporal blockade of IL-6/IL-6 receptor (IL-6R) engagement, using an anti-mouse IL-6R monoclonal antibody (MR16-1), on macrophage activation and the inflammatory response in the acute phase after spinal cord injury (SCI) in mice. MR16-1 antibodies versus isotype control antibodies or saline alone was administered immediately after thoracic SCI in mice. MR16-1-treated group samples showed increased neuronal regeneration and locomotor recovery compared with controls. Immunoblot analysis of the MR16-1-treated samples identified downregulation of Th1 and upregulation of Th2 cytokines. MR16-1 treatment promoted arginase-1-positive, CD206-positive

A.R. Guerrero
Department of Orthopaedics and Rehabilitation Medicine, Faculty of Medical Sciences, University of Fukui, Fukui, Japan

Service of Neurosurgery, Hospital Nacional Rosales, University of El Salvador, San Salvador, El Salvador

K. Uchida (✉) • H. Nakajima • S. Watanabe • H. Baba
Department of Orthopaedics and Rehabilitation Medicine, Faculty of Medical Sciences, University of Fukui, Matsuoka Shimoaizuki 23-3, Eiheiji, Fukui 910-1193, Japan
e-mail: kuchida@u-fukui.ac.jp

M. Nakamura
Department of Orthopaedic Surgery, School of Medicine, Keio University, Tokyo 160-8582, Japan

S. Okada
Department of Advance Medical Initiatives, Orthopedics, Graduate School of Medical Sciences, Kyushu University, Fukuoka, Japan

W.E.B. Johnson
Life and Health Sciences, Aston University, Aston Triangle, Birmingham B4 7ET, UK

K. Uchida et al. (eds.), *Neuroprotection and Regeneration of the Spinal Cord*,
DOI 10.1007/978-4-431-54502-6_17,

M2 macrophages, with preferential localization of these cells at the injury site and enhanced positivity for Mac-2 and Mac-3, suggestive of increased phagocytic behavior. The results suggest that temporal blockade of IL-6 signaling after SCI abrogates damaging inflammatory activity and promotes functional recovery by promoting the formation of alternatively activated M2 macrophages.

Keywords Alternatively activated macrophage • Interleukin (IL)-6/IL-6 receptor (R) • Spinal cord injury • T helper (Th) cytokine

17.1 Introduction

Spinal cord injury (SCI) is followed by disruption of the blood–brain barrier and influx of inflammatory cells producing various pro-inflammatory cytokines, inducing a reactive process of secondary cell death in the tissue surrounding the original site of injury [1]. Evidence suggests that such inflammation may be beneficial; for example, macrophages phagocytose the myelin debris present in the injured spinal cord, which is known to inhibit axonal regeneration [2], promoting neuronal regeneration and tissue repair [3]. However, macrophages can also produce excessive inflammation, axonal retraction, and axonal dieback [4, 5]. Such variation could be the result of macrophages undergoing different activation pathways, generating subpopulations with divergent abilities [6].

This divergence is referred to as macrophage polarization. Two subtypes of macrophages have attracted great interest in the field of SC regeneration: classically activated (M1 phenotype) and alternatively activated (M2 phenotype) macrophages [7, 8]. Classically activated macrophages are the product of exposure to T helper (Th)1 cytokines, such as interferon (IFN)-γ and tumor necrosis factor (TNF)-α; alternatively activated macrophages are activated via Th2 cytokines, such as interleukin (IL)-4, IL-10, and IL-13, which lead to an M2 phenotype that has enhanced phagocytic behavior, anti-inflammatory roles, as well as neuroprotective effects [9].

IL-6 is an early and key factor that triggers the inflammatory response after SCI [10, 11]. Complete blockade of IL-6 has detrimental effects on recovery from SCI [12]; however, a temporal blockade of IL-6 has been shown to downregulate the expression of pro-inflammatory cytokines in the acute phase of SCI, while preserving the beneficial effects of inflammation in the later stages of recovery [13, 14]. Interestingly, IL-6 blockade increases the number of microglia recruited to the injured SC [15]. Microglia are the major source of the Th2 cytokines IL-4 [16] and IL-13 [17] in the normal central nervous system, although neutrophils and macrophages also act as a source of IL-4 [18, 19].

We investigated the effects of temporal blockade of IL-6/IL-6 receptor (IL-6R) engagement during this response, using a rat anti-mouse IL-6R monoclonal antibody (MR16-1) [20, 21], focusing particularly on the different pathways of macrophage activation.

17.1.1 Anti-Interleukin (IL)-6 Receptor (MR16-1) Treatment Promoted Neuroregeneration and Locomotor Recovery After SCI

The area of spared myelin in the MR16-1-treated group was significantly greater than that in the rat IgG control group at 42 days (Fig. 17.1a, b), also showing significantly larger GAP-43-positive area (Fig. 17.1c–f) and NF-H-positive area (Fig. 17.1g–j).

The contusive SCI resulted in immediate complete paralysis. At 7 days post-injury, the MR16-1-treated group showed a significant improvement in Basso Mouse Scale (BMS) locomotor score; this difference continued up to 6 weeks post-injury (Fig. 17.1k). At that point, the BMS score of the MR16-1-treated group was 5.0 ± 0.3, whereas that of the control group was 2.8 ± 0.3 points.

17.1.2 MR16-1 Treatment Reduced Th1 Cytokine and Increased Th2 Cytokine Levels at Injury Site After SCI

Using immunoblot analysis (Fig. 17.2), we evidenced that IFN-γ levels (28 kDa band) (Fig. 17.2a) and TNF-α levels (19 kDa band) were markedly reduced in the MR16-1-treated group from 1 to 14 days after injury (Fig. 17.2b), with increased protein levels of IL-4 (18 kDa band) reaching a peak at 7 days post-injury (Fig. 17.2c) as well as IL-13 levels (13 kDa band) (Fig. 17.2d).

17.1.3 MR16-1 Treatment Promoted M1 Macrophages Decrease and M2 Macrophages Increase at Lesion Site After SCI

Rat IgG control group showed larger lesion sites with cells extending from the epicenter (in posttraumatic hematoma) in contrast to MR16-1-treated group (Fig. 17.3a–d). Greater numbers of iNOS-positive cells at 3 days post-injury were found in the rat IgG control group (Fig. 17.3e–h). By contrast, arginase-1-positive cells at 3 days post-injury populated the lesion site in the MR16-1-treated group (Fig. 17.3k, l) in higher numbers than in the control group (Fig. 17.3i, j). The patterns of immunopositivity for iNOS and arginase matched the distribution of CD11b-positive cells (activated macrophages).

At the lesion epicenter, the MR16-1-treated group showed decreased numbers of iNOS- or CD16/32-expressing macrophages with increased populations of arginase-1- or CD206-expressing macrophages, up to 14 days post-injury.

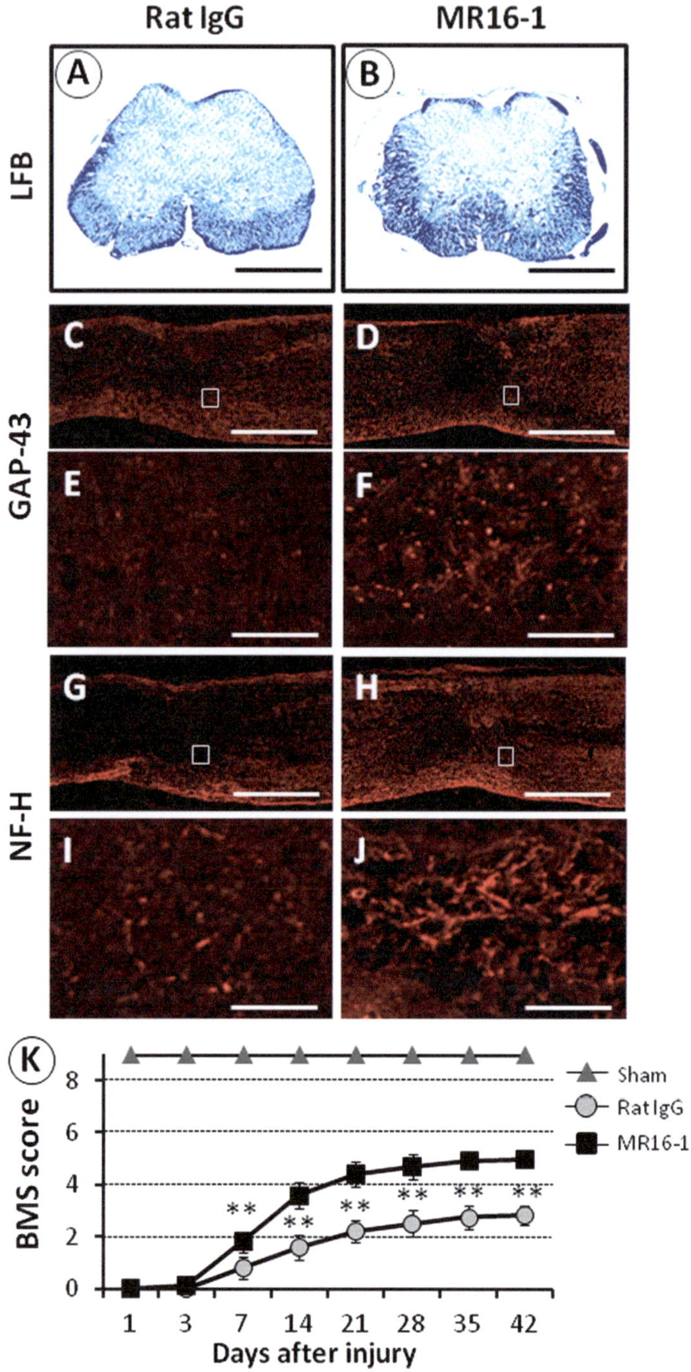

Fig. 17.1 Histological and behavioral evaluation after anti-interleukin (IL)-6 receptor (MR16-1) treatment. Luxol fast blue (LFB) stained axial sections at the injury epicenter (42 days post-injury) showed remarkable reduction in the area of demyelination in the MR16-1-treated group (**a**, **b**), greater abundance of growth-associated protein (**c**–**f**), and neurofilament heavy 200 kDa-positive nerve fibers (**g**–**j**) compared with rat IgG control group. (**k**) Basso Mouse Scale (BMS) score showed significant hind limb motor function improvement in the MR16-1-treated group. Scale bar (**a**, **b**) 200 μm, (**c**, **d**, **g**, **h**) 500 μm, (**e**, **f**, **i**, **j**) 50 μm. (**c**–**f**) GAP-43 conjugated to Alexa Fluor 568 (*red*); (**g**–**j**) NF-H conjugated to Alexa Fluor 568 (*red*) (Reprinted, in part, with permission, from [21])

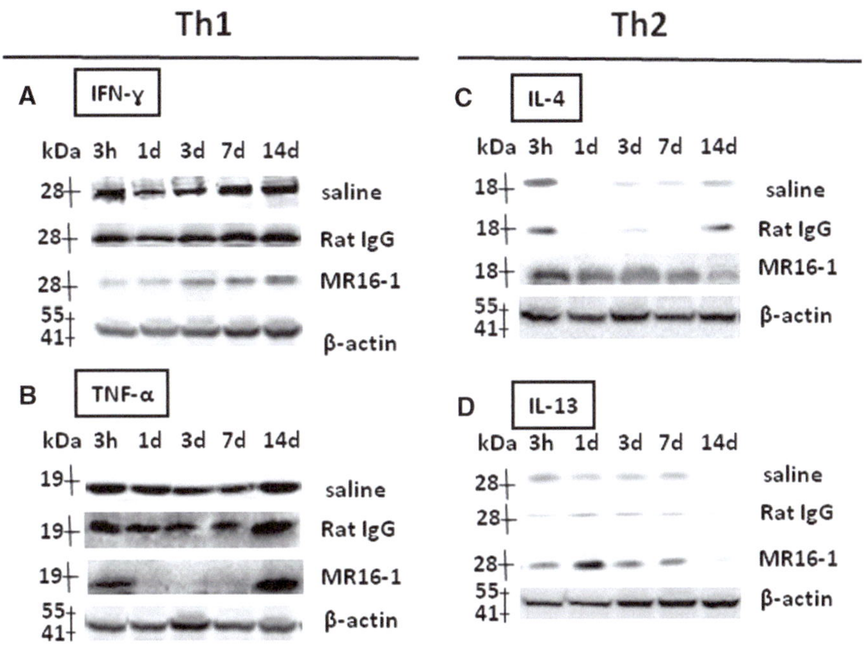

Fig. 17.2 Immunoblot analysis of T helper (Th)1 and Th 2 cytokines after MR16-1 treatment. Compared with control groups, MR16-1-treated group samples showed decreased levels of interferon (IFN)-γ (**a**) and tumor necrosis factor (TNF)-α (**b**), with increased expression of interleukin (IL)-4 (**c**) and IL-13 (**d**). Band intensity normalized to that of β-actin (Reprinted, in part, with permission, from [21])

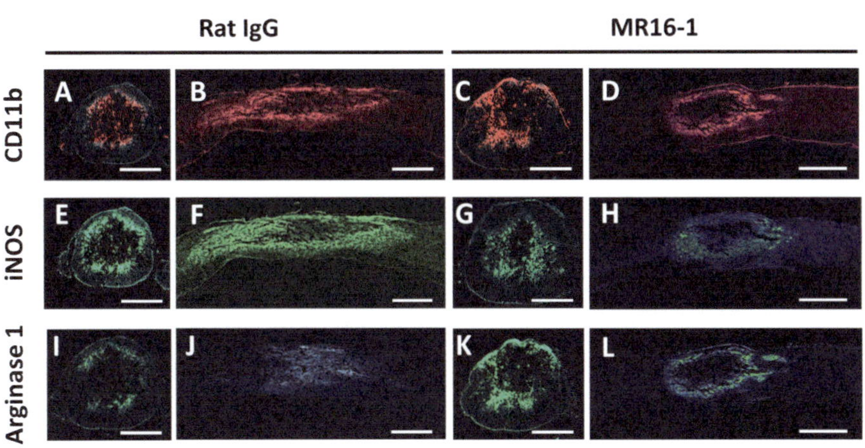

Fig. 17.3 Distribution of classically activated (M1) and alternatively activated (M2) phenotype macrophages in the injured spinal cord at 3 days after MR16-1 treatment. MR16-1-treated group samples showed smaller injury sites with centralized presence of CD11b-positive cells (**a**–**d**). Inducible nitric oxide synthase (iNOS)-positive cells were predominant and distributed over the same CD11b-positive area in the rat IgG control group, (**e**–**h**), whereas MR16-1-treated group showed larger numbers of arginase-1-positive cells, localized more specifically to the injury site (**i**–**l**). (**a**–**d**) CD11b conjugated to Alexa Fluor 568 (*red*); (**e**–**h**) iNOS conjugated to Alexa Fluor 488 (*green*); (**i**–**l**) arginase-1 conjugated to Alexa Fluor 488 (*green*); (**a**–**l**) DAPI used for nuclear counterstaining (*blue*). Scale bar: (**a**, **c**, **e**, **g**, **i**, **k**) 200 μm, (**b**, **d**, **f**, **h**, **j**, **l**) 500 μm (Reprinted, with permission, from [21])

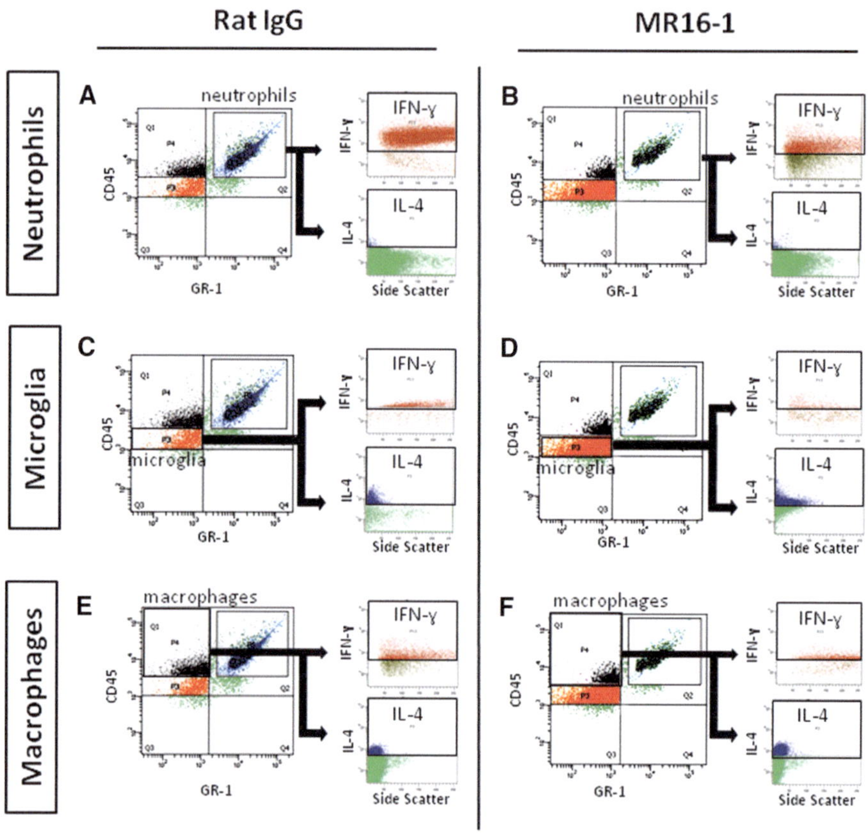

Fig. 17.4 Semiquantitative flow cytometry analysis of interferon (IFN)-γ and interleukin (IL)-4 levels in neutrophils, microglia, and macrophages after MR16-1 treatment. Flow cytometry plots at 1 day post-injury showed reduction of neutrophils positive for intracellular IFN-γ in MR16-1-treated group (**a**, **b**). At 3 days post-injury, MR16-1-treated group samples had larger numbers of IL-4-positive microglia (**c**, **d**) and reduced total number of macrophages with increased IL-4 expression and decreased IFN-γ expression (**e**, **f**) (Reprinted, in part, with permission, from [21])

17.1.4 MR16-1 Treatment Inhibited Interferon (IFN)-γ Production by Neutrophils and Increased Interleukin (IL)-4 Expression in Microglia and Macrophages

Flow cytometry analysis showed significantly lower numbers of IFN-γ-positive neutrophils infiltrating the injured SC from 1 to 7 days after injury in the MR16-1-treated group (Fig. 17.4a, b).

Significantly larger numbers of IL-4-positive microglia were present in the MR16-1-treated group at 3 days after injury (Fig. 17.4c, d). The number of macrophages infiltrating the SC after injury was reduced in the MR16-1-treated group

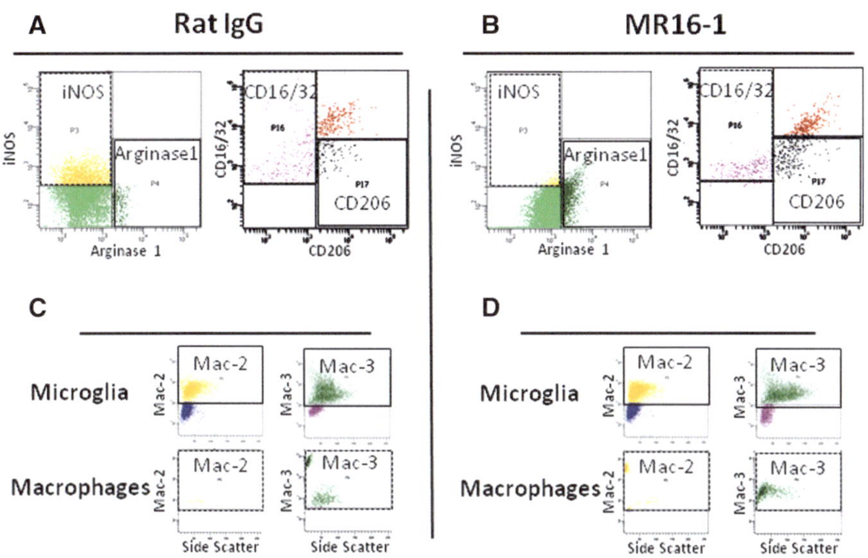

Fig. 17.5 Semiquantitative flow cytometry analysis of phagocytic and digestive activities of alternatively activated macrophages after MR16-1 treatment. (**a**, **b**) Three days post-injury: MR16-1-treated group showed lower numbers of iNOS-positive and CD16/32-positive macrophages with an increased arginase-1-positive and CD206-positive macrophage population. (**c**, **d**) Microglia of both groups showed no difference in Mac-2 and Mac-3 expression; however, the number of Mac-2- and Mac-3-positive cells within the population of arginase-1-positive macrophages was significantly larger in the MR16-1-treated group than in the rat IgG control group (Reprinted, in part, with permission, from [21])

compared with the rat IgG control group (Fig. 17.4e, f); such macrophage population showed increased intracellular IL-4 levels at days 1 and 3 after injury, with decreased intracellular IFN-γ levels at 3 days after injury.

17.1.5 MR16-1 Treatment Changed the Predominant Phenotype of Macrophages and Their Abilities After SCI

Flow cytometry analysis showed that MR16-1 treatment was associated with a marked shift from an iNOS-positive to arginase-1-positive macrophage population, from 1 to 7 days post injury, and from CD16/32-positive to CD206-positive macrophage population, from 3 up to 14 days after injury (Fig. 17.5a, b), matching the results of immunostaining.

Arginase-1-positive macrophages of the MR16-1-treated group had enhanced positivity for Mac-2 and Mac-3 compared with the rat IgG control group, and these differences were significant from 1 up to 7 days post-injury (Fig. 17.5c, d).

17.2 Discussion

IL-6 is a multifunction cytokine crucial for T-/B-cell differentiation and proliferation, immunoglobulin secretion, acute phase protein production, and macrophage/monocyte function [22]. In the pathophysiology of SCI, IL-6 is considered to be a pro-inflammatory cytokine that triggers secondary injury [10]. Once IL-6 is released, it binds to the membrane-bound IL-6R in an IL-6/IL-6R complex that associates with gp130 to exert a signal into cells [13]. MR16-1 is a rat anti-mouse IL-6R antibody that competitively inhibits the binding of IL-6 to IL-6R dose dependently, has a half-life of about 3 days in mice, and exhibits anti-inflammatory properties in rheumatoid arthritis [23] and SCI [13, 14]. In the present study of SCI, the MR16-1-treated group had smaller injury sites with less connective tissue formation secondary to the blockade of reactive astrogliosis reported previously [14]. Increased myelin sparring and an enhanced SC repair process, as shown by an increased prevalence of NF-H-positive and GAP-43-positive fibers at 42 days post-injury, were probably the consequence of increased neuronal survival in response to a diminished inflammatory cascade [24]. In addition, MR16-1 treatment improved locomotor BMS score from 7 days after SCI compared with the control groups, suggesting anatomical improvement, as reported by previous researchers [14, 15, 24]. We also found that MR16-1 treatment reduced the levels of the Th1 cytokines IFN-γ and TNF-α, with a parallel increase in levels of the Th2 cytokines IL-4 and IL-13 at the site of the spinal lesion in the acute phase after SCI. Hence, we hypothesized that a temporal blockade of IL-6 signaling by MR16-1 treatment changed the profile of cytokines present in the injured SC into an alternative macrophage-activating environment. In agreement with previous research, significant increases in IL-4 and IL-13 levels [7, 9, 25] and simultaneous reduction in IFN-γ and TNF-α levels would promote the formation of alternatively activated macrophages and inhibit that of the classically activated macrophages [26].

Based on the results of this study, we considered that administration after SCI of the IL-6 blocking antibody MR16-1 promotes changes in the microenvironment of the injury site, reducing TNF-α expression and its effects, restraining the entry of neutrophils into the injured spinal cord, reducing the levels of IFN-γ (as a result of low production of recruiting cytokines), and augmenting IL-4-expressing and IL-13-expressing microglia [10, 27]. The high levels of these Th2 cytokines (IL-4, IL-13) will activate hematogenous macrophages and resident macrophages through the IL-4Rα/JAK/STAT signaling pathway into alternatively activated M2 macrophages, whereas the low levels the of Th1 cytokines (TNF-α, IFN-γ) will prevent the macrophages shifting back into an M1 phenotype associated with classic activation [6, 7]. Such alternatively activated macrophages have increased phagocytic abilities because of the presence of endosomes/lysosomes and pinocytic structures with digestive enzymes [9, 28], efficiently removing scar tissue and growth inhibitors present in myelin debris and allowing axonal regeneration with subsequent locomotor recovery [29].

The use of MR16-1 antibody in vivo seems promising, as it produced lasting effects not limited to the half-life of the drug itself, exerting anti-inflammatory properties after a single dose. MR16-1 treatment could be a feasible option for translational research of therapeutic approaches for SCI in humans in the near future, since a humanized version is already available for the treatment of rheumatoid arthritis and approved by the US FDA and the European Union (as Actemra® and RoActemra®, respectively, Hoffman-La Roche, Nutley, NJ, USA).

17.3 Conclusion

A temporal blockade of IL-6 signaling by MR16-1 antibody could promote the generation of alternatively activated macrophages (M2 phenotype) and thus modify the inflammatory response after SCI to promote SC regeneration with functional recovery.

Acknowledgment This work was supported in part by Grants-in-Aid to HN, KU, and HB for General Scientific Research of the Ministry of Education, Science and Culture of Japan (grants numbers B19791023, C21591895, C21791389, B22390287, and B23791631).

Conflict of Interest All authors declare that they have no conflict of interest.

References

1. Pineau I, Lacroix S et al (2007) Proinflammatory cytokine synthesis in the injured mouse spinal cord: multiphasic expression pattern and identification of the cell types involved. J Comp Neurol 500:267–285
2. Giger RJ, Hollis ER, Tuszynski MH et al (2010) Guidance molecules in axon regeneration. Cold Spring Harb Perspect Biol 2:a001867
3. David S, Bouchard C, Tsatas O et al (1990) Macrophages can modify the nonpermissive nature of the adult mammalian central nervous system. Neuron 5:463–469
4. Busch SA, Horn KP, Silver DJ et al (2009) Overcoming macrophage-mediated axonal dieback following CNS injury. J Neurosci 29:9967–9976
5. Gensel JC, Nakamura S, Guan Z et al (2009) Macrophages promote axon regeneration with concurrent neurotoxicity. J Neurosci 29:3956–3968
6. Mosser DM, Edwards JP (2008) Exploring the full spectrum of macrophage activation. Nat Rev Immunol 8:958–969
7. Gordon S (2003) Alternative activation of macrophages. Nat Rev Immunol 3:23–35
8. David S, Kroner A (2011) Repertoire of microglial and macrophage responses after spinal cord injury. Nat Rev Neurosci 12:388–399
9. Kigerl KA, Gensel JC, Ankeny DP et al (2009) Identification of two distinct macrophage subsets with divergent effects causing either neurotoxicity or regeneration in the injured mouse spinal cord. J Neurosci 29:13435–13444
10. Gruol DL, Nelson TE (1997) Physiological and pathological roles of interleukin-6 in the central nervous system. Mol Neurobiol 15:307–339
11. Van Wagoner NJ, Benveniste EN (1999) Interleukin-6 expression and regulation in astrocytes. J Neuroimmunol 100:124–139
12. Cafferty WB, Gardiner NJ, Das P et al (2004) Conditioning injury-induced spinal axon regeneration fails in interleukin-6 knock-out mice. J Neurosci 24:4432–4443

13. Okazaki M, Yamada Y, Nishimoto N et al (2002) Characterization of anti-mouse interleukin-6 receptor antibody. Immunol Lett 84:231–240
14. Okada S, Nakamura M, Mikami Y et al (2004) Blockade of interleukin-6 receptor suppresses reactive astrogliosis and ameliorates functional recovery in experimental spinal cord injury. J Neurosci Res 76:265–276
15. Mukaino M, Nakamura M, Yamada O et al (2010) Anti-IL-6-receptor antibody promotes repair of spinal cord injury by inducing microglia-dominant inflammation. Exp Neurol 224:403–414
16. Ponomarev ED, Maresz K, Tan Y et al (2007) CNS-derived interleukin-4 is essential for the regulation of autoimmune inflammation and induces a state of alternative activation in microglial cells. J Neurosci 27:10714–10721
17. Shin WH, Lee DY, Park KW et al (2004) Microglia expressing interleukin-13 undergo cell death and contribute to neuronal survival in vivo. Glia 46:142–152
18. Brandt E, Woerly G, Younes AB et al (2000) IL-4 production by human polymorphonuclear neutrophils. J Leukoc Biol 68:125–130
19. Pouliot P, Turmel V, Gelinas E et al (2005) Interleukin-4 production by human alveolar macrophages. Clin Exp Allergy 35:804–810
20. Tamura T, Udagawa N, Takahashi N et al (1993) Soluble interleukin-6 receptor triggers osteoclast formation by interleukin 6. Proc Natl Acad Sci U S A 90:11924–11928
21. Rodriguez Guerrero A, Uchida K, Nakajima H et al (2012) Blockade of interleukin-6 signaling inhibits the classic pathway and promotes an alternative pathway of macrophage activation after spinal cord injury in mice. J Neuroinflammation 9:40
22. Kishimoto T, Akira S, Narazaki M et al (1995) Interleukin-6 family of cytokines and gp130. Blood 86:1243–1254
23. Choy EH, Isenberg DA, Garrood T et al (2002) Therapeutic benefit of blocking interleukin-6 activity with an anti-interleukin-6 receptor monoclonal antibody in rheumatoid arthritis: a randomized, double-blind, placebo-controlled, dose-escalation trial. Arthritis Rheum 46:3143–3150
24. Okano H, Okada S, Nakamura M et al (2005) Neural stem cells and regeneration of injured spinal cord. Kidney Int 68:1927–1931
25. Ma J, Chen T, Mandelin J et al (2003) Regulation of macrophage activation. Cell Mol Life Sci 60:2334–2346
26. Stout RD, Jiang C, Matta B et al (2005) Macrophages sequentially change their functional phenotype in response to changes in microenvironmental influences. J Immunol 175:342–349
27. Ethuin F, Gerard B, Benna JE et al (2004) Human neutrophils produce interferon gamma upon stimulation by interleukin-12. Lab Invest 84:1363–1371
28. Schwartz M (2010) "Tissue-repairing" blood-derived macrophages are essential for healing of the injured spinal cord: from skin-activated macrophages to infiltrating blood-derived cells? Brain Behav Immun 24(7):1054–1057
29. Bomstein Y, Marder JB, Vitner K et al (2003) Features of skin-coincubated macrophages that promote recovery from spinal cord injury. J Neuroimmunol 142:10–16

Chapter 18
Oxidative Stress as Secondary Injury Mechanism After Mechanical Trauma in the Spinal Cord

Shinsuke Katoh, Yoshitaka Hamada, and Takashi Chikawa

Abstract The secondary pathological changes following mechanical trauma to the spinal cord cause deterioration of its function, and oxidative stress is known to contribute to the process. The roles of intercellular adhesion molecule-1 (ICAM-l) and nitric oxide in the process were investigated using rat incomplete spinal cord injury model.

ICAM-1mRNA expression reached its maximum at 6 h after SCI. By the intravenous injection of ICAM-1 monoclonal antibody (ICAM-l mAb) after SCI, post-traumatic polynuclear cell infiltration seemed to decrease and motor recovery was enhanced. Nitric oxide (NO) increased in the injured spinal cord. The expression of mRNA of constitutive NOS (c-NOS) did not change, whereas that of inducible NOS (i-NOS) increased after injury. Inhibiting the activity of c-NOS made motor function worse and that of i-NOS enhanced motor recovery.

Lecithinized superoxide dismutase (PC-SOD) was developed to increase half-life and permeability in vivo, and PC-SOD was used in this model to lessen oxidative stress. Intravenous injection of PC-SOD after injury suppressed the expression of IL-1β, ICAM-1, and i-NOS mRNAs, enhanced the expression of mRNA of neurotrophin-3, and caused motor recovery better than methylprednisolone injection.

These results indicated that oxidative stress enhances neuronal damage after mechanical trauma and suggested that it is important to suppress the oxidative stress.

Keywords Intercellular adhesion molecule-1 • Lecithinized superoxide dismutase • Nitric oxide • Oxidative stress • Secondary injury

---

S. Katoh (✉) • Y. Hamada • T. Chikawa
Departments of Rehabilitation and Orthopedics, Tokushima University Hospital, 2-50-1 Kuramoto, Tokushima 770-8503, Japan
e-mail: skatoh@tokushima-u.ac.jp

K. Uchida et al. (eds.), *Neuroprotection and Regeneration of the Spinal Cord*,
DOI 10.1007/978-4-431-54502-6_18, © Springer Japan 2014

18.1 Introduction

It is not uncommon that neurological deterioration occurs several days after traumatic spinal cord injury (SCI) if neurological conditions are properly evaluated. In patients with cervical SCI, neurological deterioration occurs in about 15 % of patients with complete cervical injury on an average of 2.4 days after injury if minor deterioration included [1]. Secondary self-destructive processes after mechanical trauma in the spinal cord enhance the structural and functional losses of the spinal cord [2]. The diminishing of these processes may lead to reduction of neurological deterioration and enhancement of neurological recovery. The processes are time-dependent and the oxidative stress plays one of the pivotal roles [3]. There are many sources of oxidative stresses including free radical production through activation of arachidonic acid, conversion of xanthine dehydrogenase to xanthine oxidase, and activation of neutrophils [4, 5]. As lipid peroxidation and arachidonate metabolites were demonstrated experimentally to reach peak values immediately after SCI, they seem to be unsuitable as targets for pharmacological treatment of SCI in clinical practice. Neutrophilic leukocytes (NLs) appear in the walls of and adjacent to veins and venules within 4 h of injury, and large numbers of NLs are observed in the injured tissue from 8 to 24 h after SCI [6]. Xu and his co-workers also demonstrated that an increase of myeloperoxidase (MPO), an indicator of the extent of posttraumatic polymorphonuclear leukocyte (PMN) infiltration, reached its maximum level 4 h after SCI in rats [7]. Therefore, some of the processes of the oxidative stresses can be the target for the treatment.

Steroid was used in clinical practice to enhance neurological recovery. It has two different effects, one against the inflammation and the other against the oxidative stress. The first National Acute Spinal Cord Injury Study (NASCIS 1) had employed the dosage of methylprednisolone sodium succinate (MP) against the inflammation, which had not demonstrated any positive clinical effects [8]. The dosage of MP as the bolus injection in the second (NASCIS 2) and the third (NASCIS 3) studies was 5.6-fold as compared with that in the first study, which had been targeting on the oxidative stress, not on inflammation. NASCIS 2 and 3 trials showed statistically significant clinical outcome; however, they caused controversies for a decade [9, 10]. Several clinical studies showed significant increase of the complications and insignificant neurological improvement, and the usage of MP in the treatment of acute SCI has no longer been standard care [11, 12]. However, suppressing the secondary injury processes occurred in the injured spinal cord is still important to lessen the extent of spinal cord damage, and precise mechanisms have to be elucidated.

In this chapter, we will introduce experimental studies to elucidate the mechanisms and to lessen the processes. SCI model used in this series is as follows: young adult male Wistar rats were used, laminectomy was performed at Th10, compression injury was induced by placing a weight, and severity of injury was changed by the choice of the weight and duration of the placement [4].

18.2 Intercellular Adhesion Molecule-1 [13]

Intercellular adhesion molecule-1 (ICAM-l; CD54) is a ligand for CD11a/CD18 and CD11b/CD18, and these interactions are important determinants of leukocyte–endothelial cell adhesion (Springer, 1990). In the central nervous system, ICAM-1 expresses on vascular endothelial cells, parenchymal cells, and microglial cells [14, 15]. Neutrophils and vascular endothelial cells activated by the cell adhesion molecule may produce reactive oxygen species (ROS) and may exacerbate damage to reperfused tissue by physically obstructing capillaries [16, 17]. The amount expression of ICAM-1 mRNA after moderate and severe SCI was measured by semiquantitative reverse transcription polymerase chain reaction (RT-PCR) in rats. The roles of ICAM-1 was investigated by evaluating the effect of ICAM-l mAb on MPO, spinal cord edema, spinal cord blood flow (SCBF) in the injured tissues, and motor function.

18.2.1 Expression of ICAM-1 mRNA After SCI and the Effect of Intravenous Injection of ICAM-1 Monoclonal Antibody

In the normal spinal cord, ICAM-l mRNA was not detected and was observed 3 h after injury; it reached its maximum value after 6 h and decreased after 12 h, and its expression correlated with the severity of injury (Fig. 18.1).

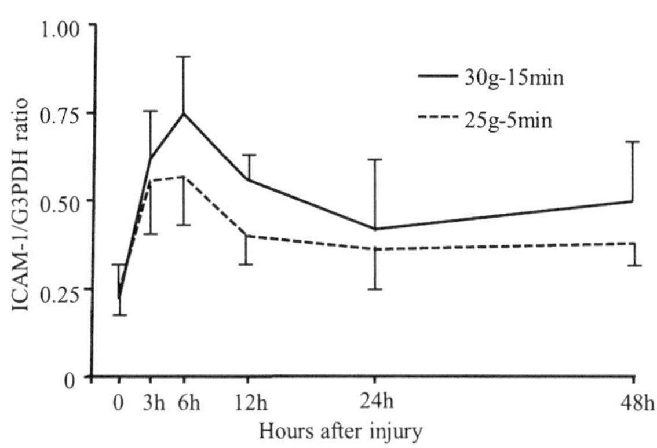

Fig. 18.1 Change with time in the ICAM-1 mRNA/G3PDH mRNA ratio after compression injury. The relative amount of ICAM-1 mRNA was quantified by densitometry and expressed as the ICAM-1/G3PDH ratio. *Points* and *bars* show the mean ± SD of values obtained in three rats at each determination point. The ratio increased after injury, and the amount of increase was bigger in severe injury [13]

MPO increased after SCI by 688.9 % at 4 h and 476.7 % at 24 h. In the mild incomplete injury model (25-g weight for 5 mm), intravenous administration of ICAM-1 mAb (1 mg/kg; ICAM-l-mAb-treated group) 30 mm after significantly inhibited the increase of MPO at 4 and 24 h after injury by 43.0 % and 26.6 %, respectively. The injury caused spinal cord edema and water content of the cord increased by 2.7 %, and 1CAM-1 mAb treatment significantly reduced this edema by 1.1 %. After SCI, SCBF measured by H_2 clearance method decreased from 45.2 ± 3.5 before injury to 31.0 ± 3.5 mL/min/100 g at 1 h, 30.5 ± 5.1 mL/min/100 g at 2 h, and 29.4 ± 5.6 mL/min/100 g at 4 h. The decrease of SCBF was partially prevented by ICAM-l mAb injection; it was 39.9 ± 6.0 mL/min/l00 g at 1 h ($p < 0.05$), but not at 2 h (32.3 ± 3.4 mL/min/l00 g) or 4 h (30.8 ± 3.4 mL/min/l00 g) after SCI.

Motor function was evaluated using several parameters. In the control group injected saline, motor dysfunction increased in the first 24 h after SCI as assessed by Tarlov's motor scale and the inclined plane test, the deterioration of motor function was not observed in the ICAM-1-mAb-treated group. The ICAM-l-mAb-treated group showed significantly better recovery than the control group throughout 3 weeks after injury (Fig. 18.2a, b). The footprint analysis before and 3 weeks after SCI showed that the distance between the central pads of the hindfeet increased significantly by 73.4 %, and the stride lengths of the right hind limb decreased significantly by 34.6 % after SCI in the control group, but did not change significantly in the ICAM-l-mAb-treated group (Fig. 18.3). Joint angles during swing (swing) and at the beginning of stance (beginning stance) decreased 34.3 % and 12.0 %, respectively, in the control rats, but not in ICAM-l-mAb-treated rats.

18.3 Nitric Oxide [18]

Nitric oxide (NO) was found to be an endothelium-derived relaxing factor [19]. In the central nervous system, NO may be neurotoxic by causing overstimulation of the *N*-methyl-*n*-aspartate receptor or cause hypotension and hyperalgesia and may be neuroprotective through anti-inflammatory or antioxidant effects [20–22]. We measured the expression of NO and NO synthase (NOS) after mechanical trauma in the spinal cord. Its roles in the secondary injury processes were investigated by evaluating the effects of an NOS inhibitor at different time point of mechanical trauma.

18.3.1 Expression of NO and Its Correlation with Oxidative Stress

Because of its short life in vivo and a small amount of expression, it could detect the expression of NO in the injured spinal cord only when we used highly sensitive procedure for quantitative measurement of NO by a modified spin-trapping method [23]. To confirm the signal was that of NO, we investigated the effect of an NOS inhibitor, NG-nitro-L-arginine methyl ester (L-NAME), a strong selective inhibitor

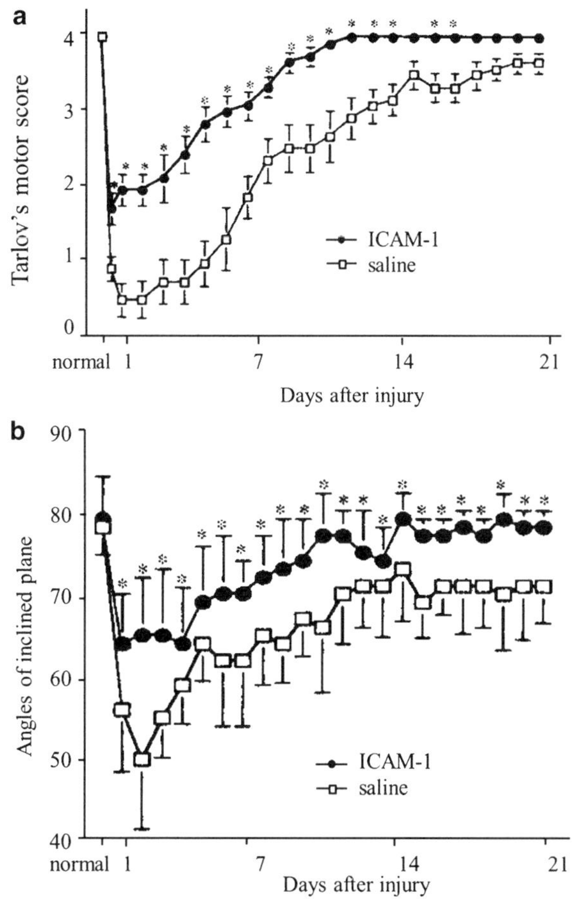

Fig. 18.2 Effect of ICAM-1 mAb treatment on the hind limb motor function after compression of the spinal cord for 5 min with a 25-g weight. ICAM-1 mAb (1 mg/kg) was injected via the tail vein 30 min after injury. Data are mean ± SEM values of Tarlov's motor scale and mean ± SD values of the other analysis for 12 rats. The degree of motor function was assessed every day for 21 days after injury according to Tarlov's criteria (**a**) and the inclined plane test (**b**). Tarlov's motor scale is as follows: 0, no voluntary movement; 1, perceptible movement of joints; 2, good movement of joints but inability to stand; 3, ability to stand and walk; 4, complete recovery. In the inclined plane test, the maximum inclination of the plane, at which rats could maintain themselves for 5 s. *Values for the ICAM-1-mAb-treated group were significantly different from those for controls (Mann–Whitney *U*-test in Tarlov's criteria and Student's unpaired *t*-test in the inclined plane test) [13]

of brain and endothelial cell NO synthesis, on the NO spectrum. The spectrum was not seen after intravenous injection of L-NAME (30 mg/kg) 15 min before SCI. After spinal cord compression, the NO level was increased 3.3-fold in the injured region and 4.9-fold in the adjacent central region.

The value of the thiobarbituric acid reactive substances (TBARS) representing the amount of lipid peroxide was 33.1 ± 6.1 nmol/g wet weight in the normal spinal cord, and the value increased after 30 min to 2.2-fold (66.9 ± 5.9) in the injured

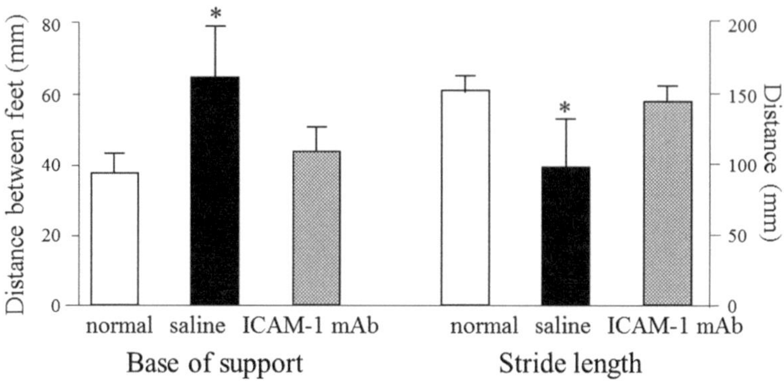

Fig. 18.3 Footprint analysis 3 weeks after injury. The base of support was determined by measuring the distance between the central pads of the hind paws. The stride lengths of the right and left hind paws were measured in two consecutive prints. A significant increase in the base of support and a significant decrease in the right stride length were observed in the saline-treated group, but not in the ICAM-1-mAb-treated group. *Significantly different from normal and ICAM-1-mAb-treated rats (Student's unpaired *t*-test) [13]

region and to 1.8-fold (58.5 ± 9.9) in the adjacent central region. Intravenous infusion of L-NAME (30 mg/kg) for 15 min before injury increased the TBARS value in the injured spinal cord to 2.6-fold (86.3 ± 8.1) at 30 min after injury. These results showed the close correlation of NO production and the oxidative stress after mechanical trauma to the spinal cord.

18.3.2 Expression of Constitutive and Inducible NOS in the Spinal Cord

There are several forms of NOS, and we measured the expression of mRNAs of constitutive NOS (c-NOS) and inducible NOS (i-NOS) since c-NOS has been reported to be short-acting and to play protective roles, whereas i-NOS to be long-acting and cytotoxic in the central nervous system. We measured c-NOS mRNA expression before and in the subacute phase after SCI and found that the level of the c-NOS signal did not change after SCI. No appreciable i-NOS signal was detected in RNA from the control spinal cord; it was observed in RNA from 3 h after injury (30-g weight, 15 min compression) and reached maximum after 24 h (Fig. 18.4).

18.3.3 Effect of NOS Inhibitor on Lipid Peroxidation and Motor Disturbance After Mechanical Trauma

We investigated the effects of L-NAME on the level of TBARS, MPO activity, and motor function in order to determine the correlation between the level of NO and oxidative injury after injury.

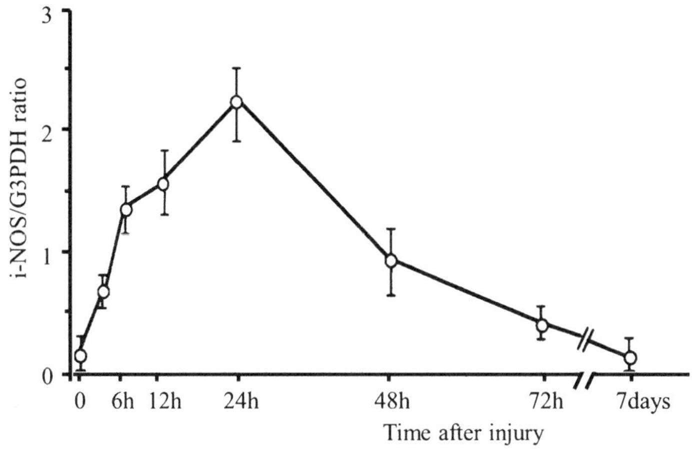

Fig. 18.4 Change with time in i-NOS mRNA/G3PDH mRNA ratio after compression injury with a 30-g weight for 15 min. The relative amount of i-NOS mRNA was quantified by densitometry and expressed as i-NOS/G3PDH ratio. *Points* and *bars* show the mean ± SD of values obtained in three rats at each determination point [18]

We injected a single dose of L-NAME at 30 mg/kg 15 min before injury intravenously to decrease the activity of c-NOS which is present in the spinal cord at the time of injury. The MPO activity was 27.3 ± 6.6 unit/g net weight in the normal spinal cord and increased to 205.8 ± 18.2 in the injured region 4 h after SCI. Pretreatment with L-NAME increased the MPO activity to 497.2 ± 85.2 in the injured spinal cord 4 h after SCI, and the recovery of motor function was poorer.

Low-dose L-NAME injections (0.1 mg/kg, 4 injections) after injury were used to elucidate the roles of i-NOS induced after injury. Low-dose intravenous injection of L-NAME at this dose 5 min and 3, 6, and 24 h after injury significantly reduced motor disturbance except half a day after injury. Injection of the same dose of L-NAME 6, 24, 48, and 72 h after SCI also significantly reduced motor disturbance (Fig. 18.5).

18.4 Preventive Effects of Lecithinized Superoxide Dismutase (PC-SOD) Against Oxidative Stress [24, 25]

Superoxide dismutase (SOD), an enzyme that scavenges superoxide anions [26], was effective on experimental ischemic SCI [27]. However, its short half-life in vivo and low cell membrane or tissue affinity prevented further development. Lecithinization of SOD (PC-SOD) may increase its half-life and its affinity, which made its applicability higher (Fig. 18.6) [28]. We compared the effects with MP which has been shown to be effective to improve spinal cord function after injury in the experimental models.

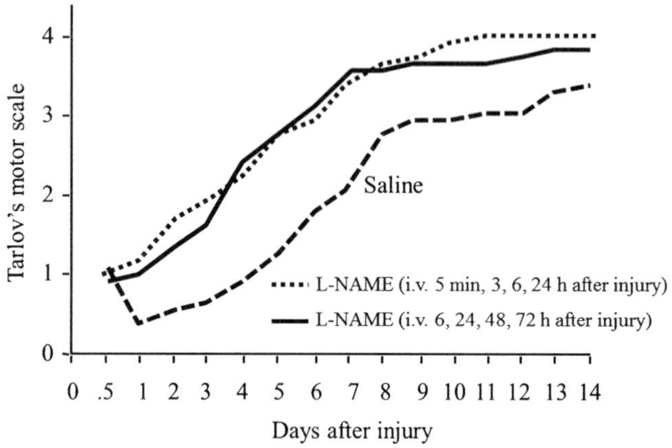

Fig. 18.5 Effect of L-NAME treatment on the hind limb motor function after injury to the spinal cord for 5 min with a 30-g weight. The hind limb motor function was assessed every day until 14 days after SCI by Tarlov's criteria. L-NAME (0.1 mg/kg) was injected into a tail vein 5 min and 3, 6, and 24 h (*dot line*) or 6, 24, 48, and 72 h (*line*) after injury. Values are means for ten rats. Values for L-NAME-treated groups are significantly different from those for the control group by the Mann–Whitney *U*-test at all times except 0.5 day after injury [18]

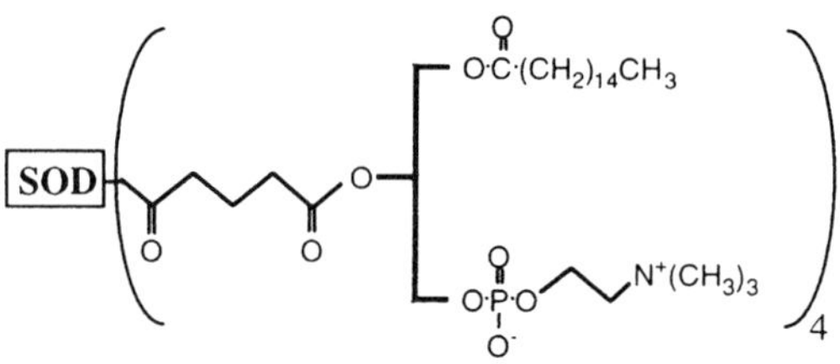

Fig. 18.6 Structure of PC-SOD [24]

18.4.1 Effect of PC-SOD Injection on Lipid Peroxidation in theSpinal Cord Injury

SOD activity in spinal cord tissue increased by 32.4 % ($p<0.01$) 4 h after SCI. Intravenous injection of unmodified SOD 30 min after injury did not alter SOD level, but that of PC-SOD significantly increased it by 58.7 % ($p<0.01$). These changes were not observed in the plasma [24].

We also examined their effects on lipid peroxidation. The value of TBARS increased from 66.2 ± 12.8 nmol MDA/g tissue in the normal spinal cord to 192.2 ± 16.8 nmol MDA/tissue 1 h after SCI in the injured region. Intravenous bolus infusion of 30 min after SCI reduced the increase in the TBARS value in the injured spinal cord to 142.9 ± 8.2 in the PC-SOD (40,000 units/kg) group, 143.2 ± 5.70 in the MP (30 mg/kg) group, and 83.2 ± 10.6 in the PC-SOD+MP group. PC-SOD and MP had additive effects on the TBARS level [25].

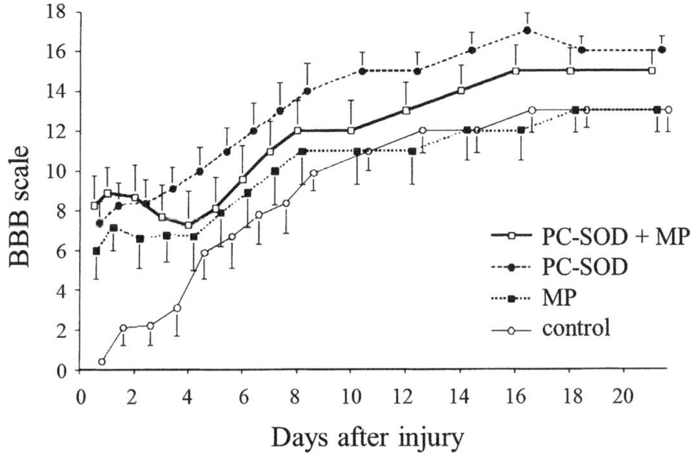

Fig. 18.7 BBB open field locomotor scale after injury by placing weight of 30 g for 5 min. PC-SOD group showed significantly higher scale at all times after injury, whereas, the scales of MP group were not different except for the first 3 days. The scales of PC-SOD group were significantly higher than those in the MP group [25]

18.4.2 Comparison of the Effect of PC-SOD on Motor Function [25]

Recovery of hind limb motor function after moderate incomplete injury was compared among rats treated with intravenous injection of PC-SOD (40,000 units/kg), that with MP and that with both PC-SOD and MP. The BBB open field locomotor scores of three groups were significantly higher than that of the control group in the first 3 days ($p<0.05$). The score of the PC-SOD group increased, whereas that of the MP group showed a temporary decrease from day 3 to 5 and then it gradually recovered. The scores in all groups reached a plateau about 18 days after SCI. The PC-SOD+MP group showed similar tendency to that of the MP group (Fig. 18.7). The angle of rotation in footprint analysis 6 weeks after injury showed significantly better function in PC-SOD group and PC-POD+MP group than MP group (Fig. 18.8).

18.4.3 Comparison of the Effect of PC-SOD on Inflammatory and Neurotrophic Genes [25]

In order to elucidate the discrepancy between the effect on lipid peroxidation and the effect on motor function, we measured the expression of inflammatory and neurotrophic genes in the spinal cord after injury.

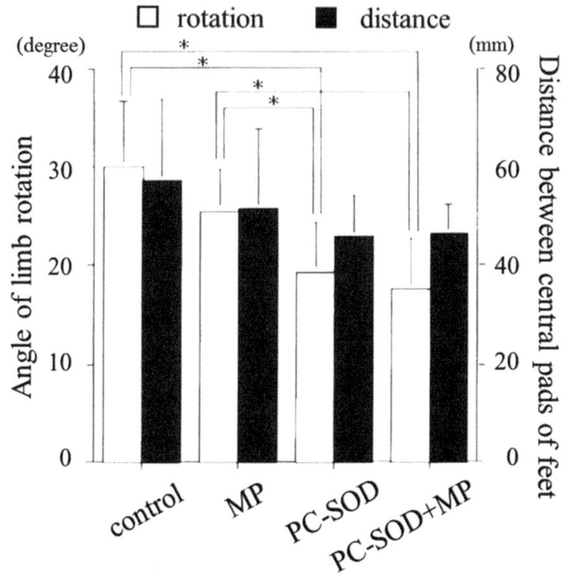

Fig. 18.8 Footprint analyses of hind limb motor function 6 weeks after injury by placing weight of 30 g for 5 min. The *black axis* shows the distance between the central pads of the feet, and the *white axis* shows the angle of limb rotation. *Significant difference among four groups by one-way ANOVA and Fisher's PLSD test [25]

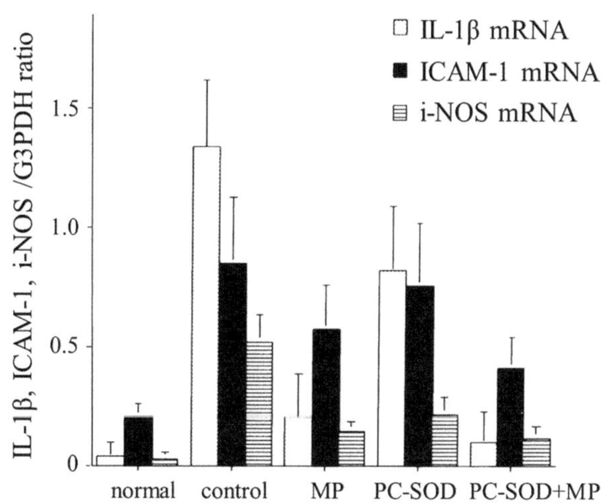

Fig. 18.9 Expression of mRNAs of IL-1β, ICAM-1, and i-NOS in control rats and those treated with MP, PC-SOD, and both. IL-1β was measured at 3 h, ICAM-1 at 6 h, and i-NOS 24 h after injury. The relative amount of mRNAs of the substances was quantified by densitometry and expressed as the ratio to G3PDH mRNA. *Columns* and *bars* show the mean ± SD of values [25]

The levels of inflammatory genes, interleukin (IL)-1β mRNA measured at 3 h after injury, ICAM-l at 6 h, and i-NOS mRNA at 24 h, were reduced by all three treatments. The relative mRNA levels of IL-1β, ICAM-l, and i-NOS were 14.9 %, 67.1 %, and 27.8 % as compared to the control in the MP-treated group, 61.3 %, 88.2 %, and 40.9 % in the PC-SOD-treated group, and 7.3 %, 48.2 %, and 22.0 % in the PC-SOD + MP-treated group, respectively. The suppression of expression of all three mRNAs was greater by MP than by PC-SOD, the effect being greatest on IL-1β mRNA, and ICAM-l mRNA was not significantly affected by PC-SOD alone. PC-SOD + MP treatment showed biggest suppression effects on all three mRNAs (Fig. 18.9).

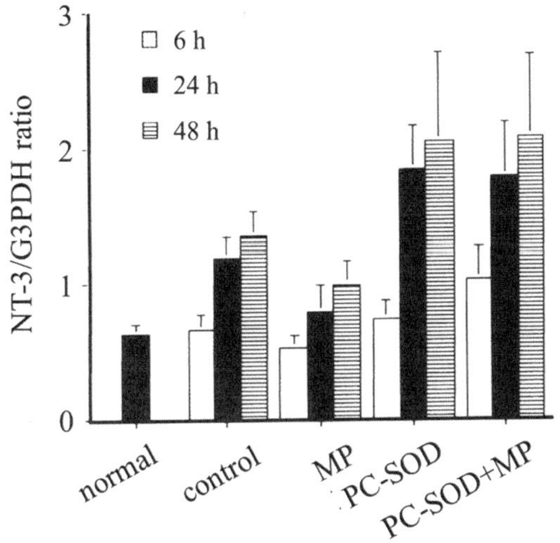

Fig. 18.10 Expression of mRNA of NT-3 at 6, 24, and 48 h after injury in control rats and those treated with MP, PC-SOD, and both. *Columns* and *bars* show the mean ± SD of values [25]

We measured the expression of neurotorphin-3 (NT-3) mRNA as a representative of neurotrophic genes. The levels of NT-3 mRNA suppressed in MP-treated group (−21.5 % at 6 h, −33.9 % at 24 h, and −27.4 % at 48 h of sham-treated group). The expression of NT-3 mRNA was enhanced by PC-SOD treatment (+12.3 % at 6 h, +55.9 % at 24 h, and +51.3 % at 48 h of sham control). The enhancement was not augmented significantly by combination with MP (+39.7 % at 6 h, −3.3 % at 24 h, and +1.2 % at 48 h of PC-SOD) (Fig. 18.10).

18.5 Discussion

The secondary injuries after mechanical trauma are time-dependent and the time course should be into consideration to plan the tactics to lessen the injuries (Table 18.1). As shown by the results from ICAM-1 study, passive immunization of ICAM-1 resulted in decrease of oxidative stress, which led spinal cord edema decreased and motor recovery enhanced. Blocking of infiltration of activated PMN to the spinal cord through the damaged vascular wall seems to be one of the important targets, since it occurs several hours after injury. There are many substances and mechanisms that are involved in the infiltration, and other clinically applicable tactics could be found to lessen the infiltration. In the management of SCI, it is well known that preventing the complications is important not only for earlier rehabilitation but also for neurological recovery [29, 30]. These clinical facts are supported by the experimental studies.

NO has been regarded to have double-edged roles in the central nervous system [31]. The results presented here also showed that NO produced by c-NOS seemed to be neuroprotective and that by i-NOS to be neurotoxic. Because of relatively prolonged expression of i-NOS mRNA shown in the experimental studies,

Table 18.1 Secondary injury after mechanical trauma

Seconds	Hemorrhage, ischemia, hypoxia, ⇩ATP
Minutes	⇧stress genes, ⇧mical microglia, ⇧pro-inflammatory cytokines Inflammation, ⇩ cytoskeleton, ⇧glutamate exitotoxicity
Hours	⇧free radicals, ⇧edema, neutrophil infiltration, lipid peroxidation, ⇧nitric oxide, ⇧ICAM-1, ⇧protease
Days	⇧TGF-β, necrosis, neural apoptosis, astrogliosis, axon demyelination
Week	Severe axon degeneration, cyst formation, permanent loss of spinal cord function

monitoring or control of i-NOS expression should be considered when planning tactics against secondary injury.

SOD had been regarded as a possible candidate to reduce secondary injury, but it had been failed even in the experimental studies because of its biological characteristics. PC-SOD was developed to overcome them, and it was shown to be a clinically applicable drug. The experimental study showed that antioxidant effect was not better than MP, and the suppression of pro-inflammatory substances was smaller than MP. Its effect on motor function, however, was better in some way of evaluation of hind limb function. Enhancing the expression of NT-3 can play some role, but further study is necessary to elucidate the mechanism of beneficial effect of PC-SOD.

18.6 Conclusion

Oxidative stress plays one of the pivotal roles in the secondary pathological changes after mechanical trauma. There are many sources of oxidative stresses, and some of them occur in clinically treatable time window after mechanical trauma. Further studies are necessary to elucidate the mechanisms and to lessen the neuronal damages.

Conflict of Interest All authors declare that they have no conflict of interest.

References

1. Katoh S, el Masry WS (1994) Neurological recovery after conservative treatment of cervical cord injuries. J Bone Joint Surg Br 76(2):225–228
2. Janssen L, Hansebout R (1989) Pathogenesis of spinal cord injury and newer treatments. A review. Spine 14
3. Demopoulos H, Flamm E, Pietronigro D, Sligman M (1980) The free radical pathology and the microcirculation in the major central nervous disorders. Acta Physiol Scand Suppl 492:91–119
4. Iwasa K, Ikata T, Fukuzawa K (1989) Protective effect of vitamin E on spinal cord injury by compression and concurrent lipid peroxidation. Free Radic Biol Med 6:599–606

5. Mitsuhashi T, Ikata T, Morimoto K, Tonai T, Katoh S (1994) Increased production of eicosanoids, TXA2, PGI2 and LTC4 in experimental spinal cord injuries. Paraplegia 32(8):524–530
6. Means ED, Anderson DK (1983) Neuronophagia by leukocytes in experimental spinal cord injury. J Neuropathol Exp Neurol 42(6):707–719
7. Xu JA, Hsu CY, Liu TH, Hogan EL, Perot PL Jr, Tai HH (1990) Leukotriene B4 release and polymorphonuclear cell infiltration in spinal cord injury. J Neurochem 55(3):907–912
8. Bracken MB, Shepard MJ, Hellenbrand KG, Collins WF, Leo LS, Freeman DF, Wagner FC, Flamm ES, Eisenberg HM, Goodman JH et al (1985) Methylprednisolone and neurological function 1 year after spinal cord injury. Results of the national acute spinal cord injury study. J Neurosurg 63(5):704–713
9. Bracken M, Shepard M, Collins W, Holford T, Young W, Baskin D, Eisenberg H, Flamm E, Leo-Summers L, Maroon J, Marshall L, Perot PJ, Piepmeier J, Sonntag V, Wagner F, Wilberger J, Winn H (1990) A randomized, controlled trial of methylprednisolone or naloxone in the treatment of acute spinal-cord injury. Results of second national acute spinal cord injury study. N Engl J Med 322:1405–1411
10. Bracken MB, Shepard MJ, Holford TR, Leo-Summers L, Aldrich EF, Fazl M, Fehlings MG, Herr DL, Hitchon PW, Marshall LF, Nockels RP, Pascale V, Perot PL Jr, Piepmeier J, Sonntag VK, Wagner F, Wilberger JE, Winn HR, Young W (1998) Methylprednisolone or tirilazad mesylate administration after acute spinal cord injury: 1-year follow up. Results of the third national acute spinal cord injury randomized controlled trial. J Neurosurg 89(5):699–706
11. Ito Y, Sugimoto Y, Tomioka M, Kai N, Tanaka M (2009) Does high dose methylprednisolone sodium succinate really improve neurological status in patient with acute cervical cord injury?: a prospective study about neurological recovery and early complications. Spine (Phila Pa 1976) 34(20):2121–2124. doi:10.1097/BRS.0b013e3181b613c7
12. Matsumoto T, Tamaki T, Kawakami M, Yoshida M, Ando M, Yamada H (2001) Early complications of high-dose methylprednisolone sodium succinate treatment in the follow-up of acute cervical spinal cord injury. Spine 26(4):426–430
13. Hamada Y, Ikata T, Katoh S, Nakauchi K, Niwa M, Kawai Y, Fukuzawa K (1996) Involvement of an intercellular adhesion molecule 1-dependent pathway in the pathogenesis of secondary changes after spinal cord injury in rats. J Neurochem 66(4):1525–1531
14. Clark WM, Madden KP, Rothlein R, Zivin JA (1991) Reduction of central nervous system ischemic injury by monoclonal antibody to intercellular adhesion molecule. J Neurosurg 75(4):623–627. doi:10.3171/jns.1991.75.4.0623
15. Zielasek J, Archelos JJ, Toyka KV, Hartung HP (1993) Expression of intercellular adhesion molecule-1 on rat microglial cells. Neurosci Lett 153(2):136–139
16. Fujita H, Morita I, Murota S (1994) A possible mechanism for vascular endothelial cell injury elicited by activated leukocytes: a significant involvement of adhesion molecules, CD11/CD18, and ICAM-1. Arch Biochem Biophys 309(1):62–69. doi:S000398618471085X [pii]
17. Hallenbeck JM, Dutka AJ, Tanishima T, Kochanek PM, Kumaroo KK, Thompson CB, Obrenovitch TP, Contreras TJ (1986) Polymorphonuclear leukocyte accumulation in brain regions with low blood flow during the early postischemic period. Stroke 17(2):246–253
18. Hamada Y, Ikata T, Katoh S, Tsuchiya K, Niwa M, Tsutsumishita Y, Fukuzawa K (1996) Roles of nitric oxide in compression injury of rat spinal cord. Free Radic Biol Med 20(1):1–9
19. Furchgott RF, Zawadzki JV (1980) The obligatory role of endothelial cells in the relaxation of arterial smooth muscle by acetylcholine. Nature 288(5789):373–376
20. Li P, Tong C, Eisenach JC, Figueroa JP (1994) NMDA causes release of nitric oxide from rat spinal cord in vitro. Brain Res 637(1–2):287–291. doi:0006-8993(94)91246-7 [pii]
21. Wink DA, Hanbauer I, Laval F, Cook JA, Krishna MC, Mitchell JB (1994) Nitric oxide protects against the cytotoxic effects of reactive oxygen species. Ann N Y Acad Sci 738:265–278
22. Kubes P, Suzuki M, Granger DN (1991) Nitric oxide: an endogenous modulator of leukocyte adhesion. Proc Natl Acad Sci U S A 88(11):4651–4655
23. Tominaga T, Sato S, Ohnishi T, Ohnishi ST (1993) Potentiation of nitric oxide formation following bilateral carotid occlusion and focal cerebral ischemia in the rat: in vivo detection of the nitric oxide radical by electron paramagnetic resonance spin trapping. Brain Res 614(1–2):342–346

24. Nakauchi K, Ikata T, Katoh S, Hamada Y, Tsuchiya K, Fukuzawa K (1996) Effects of lecithinized superoxide dismutase on rat spinal cord injury. J Neurotrauma 13(10):573–582
25. Chikawa T, Ikata T, Katoh S, Hamada Y, Kogure K, Fukuzawa K (2001) Preventive effects of lecithinized superoxide dismutase and methylprednisolone on spinal cord injury in rats: transcriptional regulation of inflammatory and neurotrophic genes. J Neurotrauma 18(1):93–103
26. McCord JM, Fridovich I (1969) Superoxide dismutase. An enzymic function for erythrocuprein (hemocuprein). J Biol Chem 244(22):6049–6055
27. Cuevas P, Carceller-Benito F, Reimers D (1989) Administration of bovine superoxide dismutase prevents sequelae of spinal cord ischemia in the rabbit. Anat Embryol (Berl) 179(3):251–255
28. Igarashi R, Hoshino J, Ochiai A, Morizawa Y, Mizushima Y (1994) Lecithinized superoxide dismutase enhances its pharmacologic potency by increasing its cell membrane affinity. J Pharmacol Exp Ther 271:1672–1677
29. el Masry WS (1993) Physiological instability of the spinal cord following injury. Paraplegia 31(5):273–275
30. Katoh S, Ikata T, Tsubo M, Hamada Y, el Masry WS (1997) Possible implication of leukocytes in secondary pathological changes after spinal cord injury. Injury 28(3):215–217
31. Lipton SA, Choi YB, Pan ZH, Lei SZ, Chen HS, Sucher NJ, Loscalzo J, Singel DJ, Stamler JS (1993) A redox-based mechanism for the neuroprotective and neurodestructive effects of nitric oxide and related nitroso-compounds. Nature 364(6438):626–632. doi:10.1038/364626a0

Part IV
Transplantation

Chapter 19
Regenerative Medicine for Spinal Cord Injury Utilizing iPS Cells

Osahiko Tsuji, Satoshi Nori, Yoshiomi Kobayashi, Kanehiro Fujiyoshi, Hideyuki Okano, Yoshiaki Toyama, and Masaya Nakamura

Abstract Reports of functional recovery from spinal cord injury (SCI) after the transplantation of rat-fetus-derived neural stem/precursor cells (NS/PCs) and murine embryonic stem cells (ES cells) have raised great expectations for the successful clinical trial of stem cell transplantation therapy. However, the ethical issues concerning about destroying human embryos or fertilized oocytes to obtain such stem cells have been a major impediment to developing clinically useful stem cell sources and to use them in clinical applications. Recently, induced pluripotent stem

O. Tsuji
Department of Orthopaedic Surgery, School of Medicine, Keio University, 35 Shinanomachi, Tokyo, Shinjuku 160-8582, Japan

Department of Orthopaedic Surgery, Saitama Social Insurance Hospital, 4-9-3 Kitaurawa, Urawa, Saitama, Saitama 330-0074, Japan

S. Nori
Department of Orthopaedic Surgery, School of Medicine, Keio University, 35 Shinanomachi, Tokyo, Shinjuku 160-8582, Japan

Department of Orthopaedic Surgery, Tokyo Dental College Ichikawa General Hospital, 5-11-13 Sugano, Ichikawa, Chiba 272-8513, Japan

Y. Kobayashi • Y. Toyama • M. Nakamura (✉)
Department of Orthopaedic Surgery, School of Medicine, Keio University, 35 Shinanomachi, Tokyo, Shinjuku 160-8582, Japan
e-mail: masa@a8.keio.jp

K. Fujiyoshi
Department of Orthopaedic Surgery, School of Medicine, Keio University, 35 Shinanomachi, Tokyo, Shinjuku 160-8582, Japan

Department of Orthopedic Surgery, National Hospital Organization, Murayama Medical Center, 2-37-1 Gakuen, Musashimurayama, Tokyo 208-0011, Japan

H. Okano
Department of Physiology, School of Medicine, Keio University, 35 Shinanomachi, Tokyo, Shinjuku 160-8582, Japan

K. Uchida et al. (eds.), *Neuroprotection and Regeneration of the Spinal Cord*, DOI 10.1007/978-4-431-54502-6_19, © Springer Japan 2014

cells (iPS cells), which can serve as a source of autologous cell transplantation, have been attracting a lot of attention as a clinically practical alternative to stem cells obtained directly from tissues. In this chapter, we outline the neural induction of murine and human iPS cells, their therapeutic efficacy in mouse and primate SCI models, and their safety in vivo.

Keywords Cell transplantation • Induced pluripotent stem cells • Neural differentiation • Safety • Spinal cord injury

19.1 Introduction

At the start of the twentieth century, Spanish neuroanatomist Santiago Ramón y Cajal wrote, "Once the development was ended, the fonts of growth and regeneration…dried up irrevocably," neatly articulating the long-unchallenged dogma that neurogenesis does not occur in adult mammals and that, once injured, the adult mammalian central nervous system, especially the spinal cord, can never regenerate. In 1992, however, cells with the potential to generate new neurons, neural stem cells, were identified by Reynolds and Weiss et al. [1]. Subsequently, methods were established to culture mammalian neural progenitor cells, including stem cells, from animals and humans [2–4].

When the molecular biological properties of neural stem cells in the developing and adult central nervous system were elucidated [5–9], attempts were made to take advantage of their pluripotency to regenerate nervous system cells and tissues that had been lost as a result of neurodegenerative disease or injury. While being maintained in an undifferentiated state, neural stem cells divide and proliferate. These cells possess the potential for self-renewal, i.e., for giving rise to cells that are identical to themselves, and for pluripotency, i.e., giving rise to neurons, astrocytes, and oligodendrocytes, the three cell types that comprise the nervous system. Moreover, they can be cultured in vitro by a variety of methods, including as spherical bodies by the neurosphere method. Therefore, as many neural stem cells as needed can be generated in culture, and these cells show promise for transplantation cell therapy, particularly in spinal cord injury (SCI) research, since the transplantation of fetal spinal cord tissue leads to functional recovery from SCI in the rat [10].

Following this report, studies were conducted in our laboratories to establish the safety and efficacy of transplanting in vitro-expanded stem cells to treat SCI. We tested the efficacy of transplanting (a) rat fetal spinal cord-derived NS/PCs to treat rat SCI during the subacute stage after injury [11], (b) mouse fetal striatum-derived NS/PCs to treat SCI in mice (an experiment that used luciferase luminescence to bioimage the transplanted cells) [12], and (c), as part of a preclinical trial, human fetal brain-derived NS/PCs to treat SCI in a nonhuman primate, the common marmoset (*Callithrix jacchus*) [13]. We found and reported good functional recovery in all three cases. These results led to strong expectations that human neural stem cells that had been cultured and expanded in vitro would be applied to nerve regeneration in humans. However, the fact that these cells always had to be collected from the brains of aborted fetuses of both mice and human has been a major factor in precluding the clinical use of human neural stem cells, and even now there are still no prospects for their clinical application in Japan.

In recent years, mouse and human induced pluripotent stem (iPS) cells that possess embryonic stem (ES) cell-like pluripotency and proliferative capacity have been produced by transducing several different genes into somatic cells [14–16]. If it were possible to perform custom cell transplantation therapy by generating iPS cells from patients themselves and transplanting them into SCI sites after the iPS cells had been induced to differentiate into neural stem/progenitor cells, it would also be possible to avoid both the ethical problem of using human fetal tissue and the possibility of immunological rejection. In this chapter we will outline the in vitro culture methods of inducing ES-cell- and iPS-cell-derived NS/PCs, discuss their safety upon transplantation, and describe current research on their transplantation into mouse and primate SCI models in vivo.

19.2 ES-Cell-Derived Neural Stem Cells

19.2.1 In Vitro Models of Neural Development and Mouse ES-Cell-Derived Neural Stem Cells

As stated above, neural stem cells are defined as having self-renewal potential and pluripotency. However, their ability to differentiate and proliferate is strictly governed by their time and place of birth, and not all neural stem cells have the exact same properties. Neural stem cells are already present around embryonic day 5 (E5.5) and can be cultured in the presence of leukemia inhibitory factor (LIF) [17]. Soon thereafter and still at a relatively early stage of embryonic development (E8.5–12.5), the neural stem cells can be cultured in vitro in the presence of fibroblast growth factor-2 (FGF-2). From this stage until the late stage of embryonic development, the radial glia located around the cerebral ventricle possess the properties of neural stem cells, self-renewing by symmetric cell division and producing neurons by asymmetric cell division [18, 19]. In the late stage of embryonic development, neural stem cells proliferate in vitro in response to epidermal growth factor (EGF) as well as FGF-2. However, the neural stem cells that emerge from this stage onward are no longer able to produce early-born projection neurons, such as forebrain-type cholinergic neurons, dopaminergic neurons, or motor neurons, which are born only in the early stage of development. Finally, from the late stage of embryonic development through the neonatal period and into adulthood, neural stem cells in the brain are mainly present around the cerebral ventricles and produce glial cells (astrocytes and oligodendrocytes) as well as neurons [20]. Thus, the differentiation and proliferation capacity of neural stem cells is strictly controlled by the spatial and temporal specificities that the cells are endowed with at the time and place where they are born.

In a report from our group, Okada et al. [21] used mouse ES cells derived from the inner cell mass to induce neural stem cells with high plasticity that are present in a relatively early stage of development. That is, they succeeded in constructing a neural development model culture system in vitro that mimics neural development and reflects its temporal and spatial specificity. This culture system eliminates the requirement for LIF to maintain the ES cells in their undifferentiated state, and by using floating cultures it allows the formation of embryoid bodies (EBs), which contain cells derived from the three germ layers. EBs contain relatively early-stage neural stem cells, and by growing EBs in floating cultures containing serum-free neural stem cell culture medium supplemented with FGF-2, it is possible to selectively culture neural stem cells in the form of neurospheres. Moreover, inhibiting bone morphogenetic protein (BMP) during EB formation promotes differentiation into neuroepithelium, and adding a low concentration of Noggin, which plays an important role in the formation of the forebrain, or retinoic acid (RA), which is important in neural induction and the development of the hindbrain and anterior spinal cord, increases the proportion of neural stem cells in the EBs and the efficiency of neurosphere formation.

Primary neurospheres (PNSs) formed in this way can be subcultured as secondary (SNSs) and tertiary neurospheres. Intriguingly, although PNSs produce neurons almost exclusively, SNSs and tertiary neurospheres produce glial cells, including astrocytes and oligodendrocytes, as well as neurons. The ability of neurospheres to be subcultured repeatedly and to produce all three cell lineages of the nervous system demonstrates that mouse ES-cell-derived neurospheres contain neural stem cells, as defined by their potential for self-renewal and their pluripotency. Moreover, the changes in differentiation potential associated with subculturing closely reflect the temporal changes seen in the development of the nervous system in vivo, where only neurons are born in the initial stage of development and glial cells first begin to be born in the middle stage of development. Furthermore, by adding Noggin or changing the concentration of RA during EB formation, neural stem cells with anterior-posterior axis region-specific properties can be induced. Similarly, dorsal-ventral region-specific control has been achieved by adding the ventralization factor Sonic Hedgehog (SHH) or the dorsalization factor BMP4 or Wnt3a to the culture during the formation of PNSs [21]. Based on these findings, adding the right factor at the right time during culture appears to permit the region-specific control of neural stem cell properties.

19.2.2 Transplantation of Mouse ES-Cell-Derived Neural Stem Cells into Injured Spinal Cords

The self-renewal potential, pluripotency, and genetic adaptability of ES cells make them an attractive cell source for therapeutic transplantation. Methods of inducing mouse ES cells to form neurons have already been widely investigated [22], and ES-cell-derived NS/PCs seem ideal as a source of cells for transplantation. Furthermore, the differentiation stage of the transplanted cells can be specified, from undifferentiated ES cells to EBs to differentiated neurons. However, as the degree of differentiation decreases, the rate of teratoma formation by the transplanted cells increases [23].

In terms of the efficacy of ES cell transplantation for treating SCI, in 1999, McDonald et al. formed EBs from mouse ES cells and reported good functional recovery when they were transplanted into rats with an SCI [24]. However, their study did not rule out the risk of tumorigenicity over a longer observation period or as a result of transplanting less-differentiated EBs. Keirstead et al. [25] established a method for efficiently inducing human ES cells to form very pure populations of oligodendrocyte progenitor cells by using a liquid culture medium that contained a factor, such as insulin or thyroid hormone, that promotes oligodendrocyte differentiation. They reported the remyelination of demyelinated axons and hind limb function recovery when they transplanted these cells into the injured spinal cords of rats. Later, Yamada et al. [26] formed EBs from ES cells and transplanted them into injured spinal cords, after applying an electrical stimulus to the EBs that caused the selective induction of neuronal differentiation. These authors found that a higher proportion of the electrically induced EBs differentiated into neurons than did control EBs. They also showed that the proliferative ability of the EBs that had been exposed to the electrical stimulus was lower than that of EBs that were not exposed to the electrical stimulus. They therefore concluded that electrical stimulation was an effective method for safely inducing neuronal differentiation; however, it did not lead to the recovery of hind limb function after SCI. The stage at which neural progenitor cells induced from ES cells are most suitable for transplantation therapy in the subacute stage after injury was not clear from any of these studies.

In another report from our group, Kumagai et al. [27] used Okada's culture system, described above (Sect. 18.2.1), to induce the formation of PNSs from mouse ES cells via EBs and then of SNSs, by subculturing the PNSs. They transplanted PNSs and SNSs into a mouse spinal cord contusive injury model in the subacute stage, on day 9 after the injury, and conducted a study of their treatment efficacy. As stated above, differentiation from the PNS cells was almost entirely into neurons, whereas the SNS cells tended to differentiate into all three cell lineages, i.e., astrocytes and oligodendrocytes as well as neurons [21]. However, post-transplantation luciferase bioimaging of the PNSs and SNSs showed that approximately 20 % of the cells had survived. Furthermore, the cells from the transplanted PNSs and SNSs tended to differentiate into all three nervous system cell lineages in vivo.

In addition, the atrophy and demyelination that followed the contusive injury were significantly mitigated in the SNS-transplant group compared with the PNS-transplant group, and more extensive angiogenesis within the injured spinal cord was observed in the SNS-transplant group. The evaluation of hind limb function on the Basso Mouse Scale showed that only the SNS-transplant group had good functional recovery, which was statistically significant compared with the control group (which received vehicle only).

Besides the reduction in atrophy and demyelination, and the increased angiogenesis, the functional recovery was apparently attributable to axon regrowth promoted by the transplanted cells and to remyelination by transplanted cells that differentiated into oligodendrocytes. These findings suggested that when applying ES cells to the treatment of SCI, it is preferable to transplant ES-derived cells that have formed neural stem/progenitor cells able to give rise to both glial cells and neurons, rather than neural stem/progenitor cells that generate almost only neurons. Thus, these findings are extremely important for future attempts to implement ES cell and iPS cell transplantation therapy.

However, even though aborted fetuses were not used to obtain these cells, which were established from excess embryos from infertility treatments, the ethical issues remain. The same is true of fetus-derived neural stem cells, but their use is even more problematic, because these cells would generally be used as allografts, which could trigger immunological rejection.

19.3 iPS-Cell-Derived Neural Stem Cells

19.3.1 Assessment of the Safety of Using Mouse iPS-Cell-Derived Neural Stem Cells

A breakthrough in regard to resolving the problems associated with using stem cells described thus far was provided by Nobel laureate Professor Shinya Yamanaka and colleagues at Kyoto University, who established iPS cells from mouse and human fibroblasts in 2006 and 2007, respectively [14, 15]. iPS cells are somatic cells that have been reprogrammed by transducing such genes as *Oct3/4*, *Sox2*, *Klf4*, and *c-Myc* into mouse or human fibroblasts. They are pluripotent stem cells that have the same proliferative ability and differentiation potential as ES cells. It appears possible to generate iPS cells from the somatic cells of individual patients, a technology that is expected to resolve the ethical and immunological problems that hinder the use of ES cells. Nonetheless, some concerns regarding the use of iPS remain (1) the potential introduction of transgenes (e.g., as a result of using viral vectors) and (2) a possibly greater risk of tumor formation than with even ES cells, if the fibroblasts are not completely reprogrammed.

We recently demonstrated great differences in the tumorigenicity and responsiveness to neural induction signals of iPS cells derived from various somatic tissues [28]. We generated 36 independent mouse iPS cell clones from various tissues and induced them to differentiate into neurospheres. We then evaluated their differentiation capacity and post-transplantation safety in vivo by transplanting them into the corpus striatum of the brains of NOD/SCID mice. Almost all of the iPS cell clones could differentiate into neurospheres. However, detailed analyses of the cells by flow cytometry revealed that the percentages of undifferentiated Nanog-EGFP-positive cells present in the neurospheres after differentiation induction varied greatly with the source of the somatic cells that were reprogrammed into iPS cells.

For example, iPS cell clones derived from mouse embryo fibroblasts (MEFs) showed equal responsiveness to neural differentiation-inducing signals as ES cells, and hardly any undifferentiated cells remained in the neurospheres. Post-transplantation teratoma formation in mice with transplants of MEF-iPS-cell-clone-derived neurospheres was both as infrequent and as minor as in the group transplanted with ES-cell-derived neurospheres. Moreover, no teratoma formation was observed during a 16-week observation period of mice with transplants of two iPS cell clones derived from adult gastric epithelial cells (Stm) [29].

By contrast, iPS cell clones derived from adult tail-tip fibroblasts (TTFs) displayed statistically significant resistance to differentiation, and many undifferentiated cells remained in the neurospheres after the induction of differentiation. Furthermore, the TTF-iPS-derived neurospheres formed significantly larger teratomas when transplanted into NOD/SCID mice, many of which soon became debilitated or died. Neurospheres derived from iPS cell clones from adult liver, (Hep)-derived iPS cells, were intermediate between the MEF-iPS cell clones and TTF-iPS cell clones for both responsiveness to neural differentiation signals and tumorigenesis.

Interestingly, neither the transduction of *c-Myc* nor screening of the reprogrammed cells with a reporter molecule was associated with the responsiveness of the iPS cells to the induction of differentiation or with their safety after transplantation. It appears that the above-described persistence of gene expression patterns of the original somatic cells from which the iPS cells were derived may explain the variations in their differentiation capacity, but an urgent need remains for a detailed analysis of the properties of iPS cells derived from different tissues.

19.3.2 Transplantation of "Safe" Mouse iPS-Cell-Clone-Derived Neural Stem Cells to Treat Spinal Cord Injury

In light of the above studies in relation to safety, we first assessed the safety of each clone by transplanting neurospheres into the brain of the NOD/SCID mice, as described above. Next, we used a mouse iPS cell clone whose safety had been confirmed (38C2 clone), to study the effectiveness of treating SCI by transplanting neurospheres derived from it into the lesion site in a mouse model [30]. Neurosphere transplantation was performed in the subacute stage on day 9 after the injury. As described above for the experiments with ES cells, the results of luciferase bioimaging showed that approximately 20 % of the transplanted neurospheres survived within the injured spinal cord and that they differentiated into neurons, astrocytes, and oligodendrocytes. Severe atrophic change and demyelination had occurred in the injured spinal cord after the contusive injury, but the changes were significantly mitigated in the group treated with the iPS-cell-derived neurospheres. Evaluation of the motor function of the hind limbs on the Basso Mouse Scale showed significantly better recovery of function in the group treated with iPS-cell-derived neurospheres than in the control groups (PBS-treated group and fibroblast-transplanted group). This functional recovery was apparently attributable to effects such as the

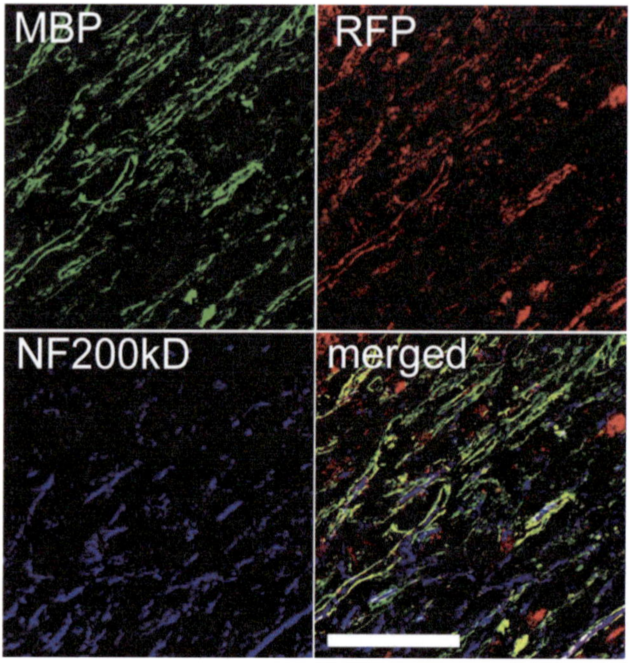

Fig. 19.1 Immunohistochemistry of 38C2-MEF-iPS-SNS-derived mature oligodendrocytes (MBP+). Grafted cells (RFP+) were integrated into the myelin sheath and differentiated into myelinating oligodendrocytes and myelinating the neurofilaments of host. Scale bar: 20 μm [30]

promotion of axonal regrowth in the raphespinal tract and remyelination by the transplanted cells (Fig. 19.1), in addition to the mitigation of the atrophic change and demyelination mentioned above.

19.3.3 Adult-Tissue-Derived "Safe" iPS Cell Clones and "Unsafe" iPS Cell Clones

Next, we conducted a similar transplantation experiment using adult-tissue (TTF)-derived iPS cells as a model that was closer to actual clinical application. There were six TTF-derived clones among the 36 mouse iPS cell clones used in our joint safety study with Miura et al. [28], but only one of them, clone 335D1, was confirmed to be safe in our teratoma assay. We used clone 335D1 along with two "unsafe" clones (256H13, 256H18) in a transplantation experiment, in which we induced the clones to form neurospheres and transplanted them into the mouse SCI model, as described for clone 38C2.

We found that, although functional recovery was achieved after transplantation of the neurospheres from all of the clones (335D1, 256H13, 256H18) into the injured spinal cord, the improvement was suddenly lost, 6 weeks after the injury, in the mice with transplants of the "unsafe"-clone-derived neurospheres. Most of these mice then died suddenly.

A histological analysis revealed huge teratomas within the spinal cords of the animals that had been treated with neurospheres derived from the "unsafe" clones. Moreover, these grafted "unsafe" cells exhibited Nanog and Oct3/4 immunoreactivity, suggesting that the grafted and surviving "unsafe"-clone-derived cells were in the undifferentiated state. By contrast, when the "safe" 335D1 clone was used, no tumor formation was observed in any of the mice, as expected, and their functional recovery was statistically significant in comparison with the control group and equivalent to that obtained with ES-cell-derived neurospheres.

These findings showed that adult-tissue-derived iPS cell clones were not as safe as clones derived from embryonic tissue, and while there was extremely wide variation among the clones in relation to their safety after transplantation, if their safety is rigorously assessed in advance, they may be a useful source of cells for the treatment of SCI [30].

19.3.4 Transplantation of "Safe" Human-iPS-Cell-Clone-Derived Neural Stem Cells into the Injured Spinal Cord of NOD/SCID Mouse

Based on the successful results of mouse-iPS-cell-derived neural stem cell transplantation into the injured spinal cord of mice, we progressed to the next step utilizing human-iPS-cell-derived neural stem/precursor cells [31]. For the transplanting of human-iPS-cell-derived NS/PCs, to avoid the immune rejection concerning with xenograft, we first made contusive thoracic SCI on NOD/SCID mice. We used a clone from human iPS cells (hiPSCs) that we established from adult human dermal fibroblasts (hDFs) by the retroviral transduction of four reprogramming factors; for the clone used in this study, 201B7, the factors were Oct3/4, Sox2, Klf4, and c-Myc [15]. Using this 201B7 clone, we harvested and induced NS/PCs through embryoid body formation according to the protocols reported as previously [21]. These grafted hiPSC-NS/PCs, pre-labeled with Venus (fluorescent protein) lentivirally, survived, migrated, and differentiated into the three neural lineages in the injured spinal cord on 56 post-injury days. Immunohistochemical analyses revealed that engrafted hiPSC-NS/PCs differentiated into neuronal nuclei (NeuN)-positive and β-tubulin isotype III (βIII tubulin)-positive neurons, glial fibrillary acidic protein (GFAP)-positive astrocytes, and adenomatous polyposis coli CC-1 (APC)-positive oligodendrocytes. The βIII tubulin$^+$/Venus$^+$ neurons comprised 49.1 ± 2.0 % of the Venus$^+$ cells, and the mature NeuN$^+$/Venus$^+$ neurons comprised 22.9 ± 1.0 %. Thus, 56 days after SCI, about 50 % of the grafted hiPSC-NSs had differentiated into neurons, about half of which were mature neurons. GFAP$^+$/Venus$^+$ astrocytes comprised 17.0 ± 1.2 %, but APC$^+$/Venus$^+$ oligodendrocytes were rare (3.0 ± 0.4 %). Nestin$^+$/Venus$^+$ NS/PCs made up 10.7 ± 2.2 % of the total. Since 22.9 % of the hiPSC-NSs

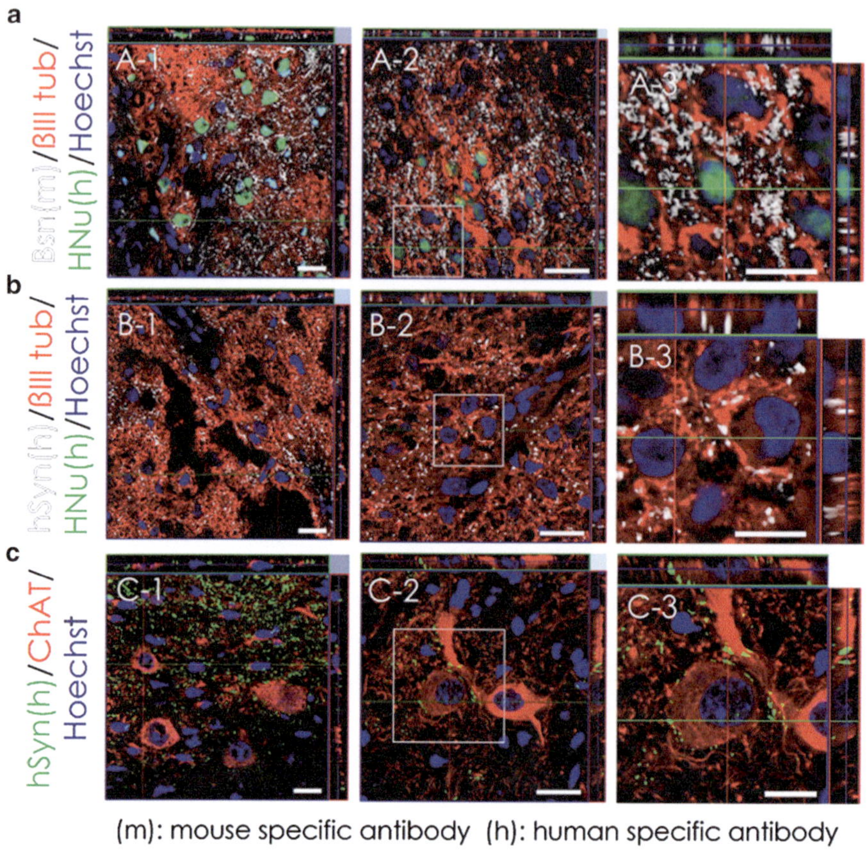

Fig. 19.2 Evidence for synapse formation between hiPSC-derived neurons and host mouse spinal cord neurons. (**a**) Sections were triple stained with HNu (*green*), βIII tubulin (*red*), and the presynaptic marker Bassoon (Bsn, *white*). The Bsn antibody used here recognized the rat and mouse, but not human, protein. (**b**) Sections triple stained for HNu (*green*), βIII tubulin (*red*), and the human-specific presynaptic marker hSyn (*white*). (**c**) Confocal images showing a large number of somatic and dendritic terminals from graft-derived nerve cells on host motor neurons at the ventral horns (scale bars, 20 μm in *A-1*, *A-2*, *B-1*, *B-2*, *C-1*, and *C-2*; 10 μm in *A-3*, *B-3*, and *C-3*) [31]

differentiated into NeuN-positive mature neurons, we next examined their neurotransmitter phenotype using neurotransmitter-specific markers. Of the Venus$^+$ cells, 15.8 ± 2 % were glutamic acid decarboxylase 67 (GAD67)-positive, indicating that 69 % (15.8 %/22.9 % = 69.0 %) of the hiPSC-NS-derived mature neurons were GABAergic. We also found small numbers of Venus$^+$ tyrosine hydroxylase (TH)-positive neurons and choline acetyltransferase (ChAT)-positive cholinergic neurons. These hiPSC-derived neurons integrated with the host neural circuitry and also possessed synaptic activity, proved by histological and immune electron microscopy analyses (Fig. 19.2) [31].

These grafted hiPSC-NSs promoted angiogenesis and axonal regrowth and preserved myelination, and some formed synapses with host mouse neurons as mentioned above. These positive effects promoted functional recovery that persisted for up to 112 days after SCI, without tumor formation [31]. We evaluated the motor functional recovery by BMS score, Rotarod test, and the DigiGait system. The BMS score showed significantly better functional recovery in the hiPSC-NS than the control group 21 days after SCI and thereafter. In the Rotarod test, the hiPSC-NS group showed a significantly longer running time than the control group 56 days post-SCI. The DigiGait system measures the treadmill gait, as an objective evaluation of motor function. While all the hiPSC-NS-grafted mice could walk on the treadmill at 8 cm/s, a subset of the control mice could not maintain this speed. The profile of stride length at 8 cm/s clearly demonstrated a significantly better recovery of motor function in the hiPSC-NS-grafted mice compared to the control mice that could walk at this speed.

Motor-evoked potential (MEP) was used to measure the functional recovery in all the mice electrophysiologically. The latency of the MEP was also measured, from the onset of stimulus to the first response of each wave. At 112 days after SCI, waves were detected in most of the hiPSC-NS group, but none were detected in the control group (0 of 15 mice). The average signal-to-response latency in the hiPSC-NS group was 4.6 ± 0.1 ms.

The transplantation of hiPSC-NS/PCs could result in a wide range of positive effects, including angiogenesis, axonal regeneration, and local-circuitry reconstruction, which have been reported in previous studies using rodent ES or iPS cells for SCI treatment [30, 32]. All these mechanisms could contribute to motor functional recovery after hiPSC-NS transplantation for SCI.

These findings indicated that NS/PCs derived from hiPSCs are a potential cell source for transplantation therapy for SCI.

19.3.5 Pre-evaluated "Safe" Human-iPS-Cell-Derived Neural Stem Cells Promote Functional Recovery After Spinal Cord Injury in Common Marmoset Without Tumorigenicity

As mentioned above, murine and human iPSC-NS/PCs promote functional recovery following transplantation into the injured spinal cord in rodents (NOD/SCID mice). For future clinical applicability, it is critical to obtain the proof of the concept on the efficacy of grafted human iPSC-NS/PCs (hiPSC-NS/PCs) for the repair of SCI in a nonhuman primate model, considering the differences in the anatomy and functions of the spinal cord between rodents and primates. Our next study employed a pre-evaluated "safe" hiPSC-NS/PC clone, 201B7, and an adult common marmoset (*C. jacchus*) model of contusive SCI. SCI was induced at the fifth cervical level (C5), followed by transplantation of hiPSC-NS/PCs at 9 days after injury [33]. All animals received daily ampicillin for 1 week after cell transplantation and subcutaneous cyclosporine injections until they were sacrificed for analysis at 12 weeks after cell engraftment.

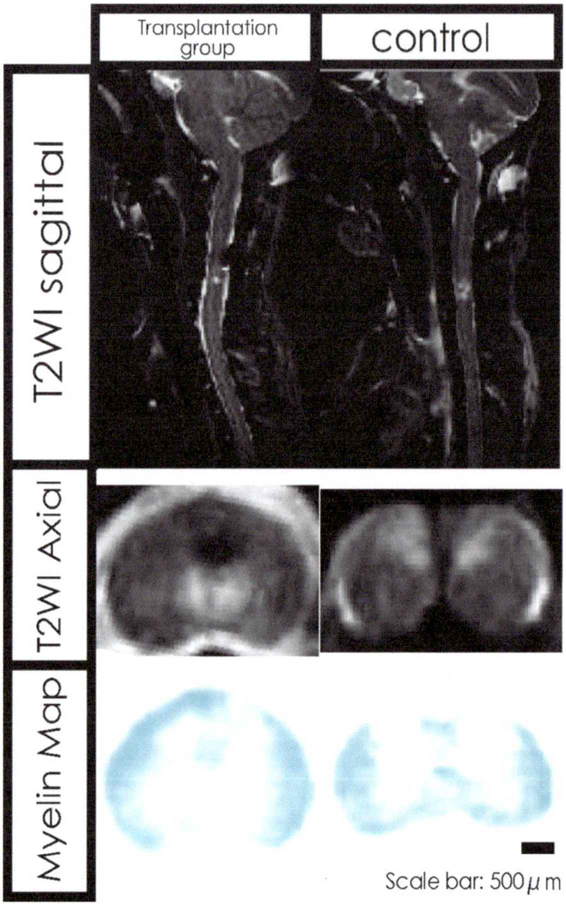

Fig. 19.3 Conventional MRI and myelin map of the spinal cord was carried out at 12 weeks after hiPSC-NS/PCs engraftment [33]

Grafted hiPSC-NS/PCs survived and differentiated into all three neural lineages, NeuN-positive mature neurons, GFAP-positive astrocytes, and Olig1-positive oligodendrocytes. Furthermore, transplantation of hiPSC-NS/PCs enhanced the axonal sparing/regrowth and angiogenesis and prevented the demyelination after SCI compared with the vehicle control animals. Notably, no tumor formation occurred for at least 12 weeks after transplantation through histological analyses. Quantitative RT-PCR showed that mRNA expression levels of human neurotrophic factors were significantly higher in cultured hiPSC-NS/PCs than in hDFs.

On MRI analyses in vivo, T2-weighted images (T2WIs) showed that an intramedullary high signal intensity area at the lesion site was prominent in the vehicle control group, which was significantly larger than the comparable area in the transplantation group. Furthermore, the myelin map showed that the overall myelin-positive area at the lesion epicenter was significantly larger in the transplantation group than in the control group (Fig. 19.3). In consistent with these MRI data, Luxol fast blue (LFB) and Eriochrome cyanine (EC) staining showed that an area of spared myelination was prominent in the transplantation group than in control. Quantification of the myelinated areas in the lesion sites revealed significant differences between the transplantation and control groups at 12 weeks after cell engraftment.

Several behavioral tests (the open field test, bar grip test, and cage climbing test), which are our originally established, showed that hiPSC-NS/PCs promoted functional recovery after SCI in the common marmoset [33].

Taken together, these results indicate that pre-evaluated safe hiPSC-NS/PCs are a potential source of cells for the treatment of SCI in the clinic.

19.4 Discussion

As indicated above, iPS cells may have great potential as a source of cells for autologous transplantation. In recent years, it has become possible to generate human iPS cells from a single drop of blood [34], and iPS cell research is advancing rapidly. However, retroviruses and lentiviruses are used to transduce reprogramming factors during iPS cell establishment, and because these viruses are often integrated in the vicinity of gene promoters, there is a risk of altering the pattern of expression of nearby endogenous genes and causing tumor formation. Actual examples of leukemia developing in two of ten patients with X-linked severe combined immunodeficiency (X-SCID) who underwent gene therapy with a retrovirus vector have been reported [35]. Fortunately, in recent years, iPS cells have been successfully produced without using retroviruses or lentiviruses by means of transient gene expression [34, 36–38] and protein transduction [39, 40] and by replacing some of the previously transduced genes with drug treatment [41, 42]. The use of iPS cells produced without inserting exogenous genes appears to be preferable for cell transplantation therapy. However, detailed comparisons of the properties of iPS clones generated by these various methods will be necessary to determine whether their pluripotency and in vitro differentiation capacity are comparable to those of iPS cells produced with retroviruses.

The greatest potential drawback of hiPSC-based therapies is their potential for tumorigenicity. Therefore, we observed the treated animals for an extended period [31, 33]. Within the observation period, no tumor occurred at all. However, strictly, we cannot exclude the risk of tumorigenesis derived from undifferentiated Nestin-positive neural progenitor cells after several months of post-transplantation. Thus, considering the fail safe system of future clinical trial, we should establish the selective ablation of the grafted cell using such as the herpes simplex thymidine kinase (HSV-TK) and "suicide" gene system [43, 44], if tumor formation occurred after human iPS-NS/PC transplantation.

At the beginning of 2009, although the United States Food and Drug Administration (FDA) approved a clinical trial (Phase 1) in the United States of Geron Corporation's ES-cell-derived oligodendrocyte progenitor cells to treat acute stage SCI, which has attracted a great deal of attention worldwide. However, unfortunately this attractive trial fizzled out at 2011 for lack of fund. Anyway, the use of human ES cells is problematic among people with certain ethical and religious viewpoints. iPS cells have attracted a great deal of attention as a technology that can resolve these problems, but the difficulties that currently prevent the use of these cells in the clinic, and the needed investigations, including developing new methods of inducing the cells and establishing their tumorigenicity, must first be resolved. In particular, hiPSCs established by delivering the reprogramming factors using a different method, such as an integration-free virus system [45] or a virus-free [46] or transgene-free system [39, 47, 48], or by using (HLA)-homozygous-donor-derived cells [49] should be evaluated. Further study using integration-free hiPSC [36, 37, 39–42, 47, 50–52]-derived NS/PCs is required to validate the safety of such cells for stem cell interventions following SCI.

19.5 Conclusion

Pre-evaluated safe mouse- and human-iPSC-clone-derived NS/PCs survived and differentiated into three neural lineage cells within the injured spinal cord of mice and adult common marmosets, with no evidence of tumor formation within our observation periods (several months). The hiPSC-NS/PCs also contributed to significant functional recovery in this nonhuman primate model of SCI. Although hiPSCs hold great promise as a cell source for the study and treatment of human diseases and disorders, it is critical to carefully assess safety concerns prior to their use in the clinic [53].

Acknowledgements The original investigation on iPS cells was performed in collaboration with Prof. Shinya Yamanaka (Center for iPS Cell Research and Application, Kyoto University, Japan). This work was supported by grants from Grants-in-Aid for Scientific Research from JSPS and the Ministry of Education, Culture, Sports, Science and Technology of Japan (MEXT); the Project for Realization of Regenerative Medicine and support for the core institutes for iPS cell research from MEXT; Research Fellowships for Young Scientists from the Japan Society for the Promotion of Science; Keio Gijuku Academic Development Funds; and by a Grant-in-Aid for the Global COE program from MEXT to Keio University.

References

1. Reynolds BA, Weiss S (1992) Generation of neurons and astrocytes from isolated cells of the adult mammalian central nervous system. Science 255:1707–1710
2. Kilpatrick TJ, Bartlett PF (1993) Cloning and growth of multipotential neural precursors: requirements for proliferation and differentiation. Neuron 10:255–265
3. Davis AA, Temple S (1994) A self-renewing multipotential stem cell in embryonic rat cerebral cortex. Nature 372:263–266
4. Palmer TD, Ray J, Gage FH (1995) FGF-2-responsive neuronal progenitors reside in proliferative and quiescent regions of the adult rodent brain. Mol Cell Neurosci 6:474–486
5. Doetsch F, Caille I, Lim DA, Garcia-Verdugo JM, Alvarez-Buylla A (1999) Subventricular zone astrocytes are neural stem cells in the adult mammalian brain. Cell 97:703–716

6. Alvarez-Buylla A, Garcia-Verdugo JM, Tramontin AD (2001) A unified hypothesis on the lineage of neural stem cells. Nat Rev Neurosci 2:287–293
7. Seri B, Garcia-Verdugo JM, McEwen BS, Alvarez-Buylla A (2001) Astrocytes give rise to new neurons in the adult mammalian hippocampus. J Neurosci 21:7153–7160
8. van Praag H, Schinder AF, Christie BR, Toni N, Palmer TD, Gage FH (2002) Functional neurogenesis in the adult hippocampus. Nature 415:1030–1034
9. Eriksson PS, Perfilieva E, Bjork-Eriksson T, Alborn AM, Nordborg C, Peterson DA, Gage FH (1998) Neurogenesis in the adult human hippocampus. Nat Med 4:1313–1317
10. Bregman BS, Kunkel-Bagden E, Reier PJ, Dai HN, McAtee M, Gao D (1993) Recovery of function after spinal cord injury: mechanisms underlying transplant-mediated recovery of function differ after spinal cord injury in newborn and adult rats. Exp Neurol 123:3–16
11. Ogawa Y, Sawamoto K, Miyata T, Miyao S, Watanabe M, Nakamura M, Bregman BS, Koike M, Uchiyama Y, Toyama Y, Okano H (2002) Transplantation of in vitro-expanded fetal neural progenitor cells results in neurogenesis and functional recovery after spinal cord contusion injury in adult rats. J Neurosci Res 69:925–933
12. Okada S, Ishii K, Yamane J, Iwanami A, Ikegami T, Katoh H, Iwamoto Y, Nakamura M, Miyoshi H, Okano HJ, Contag CH, Toyama Y, Okano H (2005) In vivo imaging of engrafted neural stem cells: its application in evaluating the optimal timing of transplantation for spinal cord injury. FASEB J 19:1839–1841
13. Iwanami A, Kaneko S, Nakamura M, Kanemura Y, Mori H, Kobayashi S, Yamasaki M, Momoshima S, Ishii H, Ando K, Tanioka Y, Tamaoki N, Nomura T, Toyama Y, Okano H (2005) Transplantation of human neural stem cells for spinal cord injury in primates. J Neurosci Res 80:182–190
14. Takahashi K, Yamanaka S (2006) Induction of pluripotent stem cells from mouse embryonic and adult fibroblast cultures by defined factors. Cell 126:663–676
15. Takahashi K, Tanabe K, Ohnuki M, Narita M, Ichisaka T, Tomoda K, Yamanaka S (2007) Induction of pluripotent stem cells from adult human fibroblasts by defined factors. Cell 131:861–872
16. Yu J, Vodyanik MA, Smuga-Otto K, Antosiewicz-Bourget J, Frane JL, Tian S, Nie J, Jonsdottir GA, Ruotti V, Stewart R, Slukvin II, Thomson JA (2007) Induced pluripotent stem cell lines derived from human somatic cells. Science 318:1917–1920
17. Hitoshi S, Seaberg RM, Koscik C, Alexson T, Kusunoki S, Kanazawa I, Tsuji S, van der Kooy D (2004) Primitive neural stem cells from the mammalian epiblast differentiate to definitive neural stem cells under the control of Notch signaling. Genes Dev 18:1806–1811
18. Miyata T, Kawaguchi A, Okano H, Ogawa M (2001) Asymmetric inheritance of radial glial fibers by cortical neurons. Neuron 31:727–741
19. Noctor SC, Flint AC, Weissman TA, Dammerman RS, Kriegstein AR (2001) Neurons derived from radial glial cells establish radial units in neocortex. Nature 409:714–720
20. Temple S (2001) The development of neural stem cells. Nature 414:112–117
21. Okada Y, Matsumoto A, Shimazaki T, Enoki R, Koizumi A, Ishii S, Itoyama Y, Sobue G, Okano H (2008) Spatiotemporal recapitulation of central nervous system development by murine embryonic stem cell-derived neural stem/progenitor cells. Stem Cells 26:3086–3098
22. Bibel M, Richter J, Schrenk K, Tucker KL, Staiger V, Korte M, Goetz M, Barde YA (2004) Differentiation of mouse embryonic stem cells into a defined neuronal lineage. Nat Neurosci 7:1003–1009
23. Brederlau A, Correia AS, Anisimov SV, Elmi M, Paul G, Roybon L, Morizane A, Bergquist F, Riebe I, Nannmark U, Carta M, Hanse E, Takahashi J, Sasai Y, Funa K, Brundin P, Eriksson PS, Li JY (2006) Transplantation of human embryonic stem cell-derived cells to a rat model of Parkinson's disease: effect of in vitro differentiation on graft survival and teratoma formation. Stem Cells 24:1433–1440
24. McDonald JW, Liu XZ, Qu Y, Liu S, Mickey SK, Turetsky D, Gottlieb DI, Choi DW (1999) Transplanted embryonic stem cells survive, differentiate and promote recovery in injured rat spinal cord. Nat Med 5:1410–1412

25. Keirstead HS, Nistor G, Bernal G, Totoiu M, Cloutier F, Sharp K, Steward O (2005) Human embryonic stem cell-derived oligodendrocyte progenitor cell transplants remyelinate and restore locomotion after spinal cord injury. J Neurosci 25:4694–4705
26. Yamada M, Tanemura K, Okada S, Iwanami A, Nakamura M, Mizuno H, Ozawa M, Ohyama-Goto R, Kitamura N, Kawano M, Tan-Takeuchi K, Ohtsuka C, Miyawaki A, Takashima A, Ogawa M, Toyama Y, Okano H, Kondo T (2007) Electrical stimulation modulates fate determination of differentiating embryonic stem cells. Stem Cells 25:562–570
27. Kumagai G, Okada Y, Yamane J, Nagoshi N, Kitamura K, Mukaino M, Tsuji O, Fujiyoshi K, Katoh H, Okada S, Shibata S, Matsuzaki Y, Toh S, Toyama Y, Nakamura M, Okano H (2009) Roles of ES cell-derived gliogenic neural stem/progenitor cells in functional recovery after spinal cord injury. PLoS One 4:e7706
28. Miura K, Okada Y, Aoi T, Okada A, Takahashi K, Okita K, Nakagawa M, Koyanagi M, Tanabe K, Ohnuki M, Ogawa D, Ikeda E, Okano H, Yamanaka S (2009) Variation in the safety of induced pluripotent stem cell lines. Nat Biotechnol 27:743–745
29. Aoi T, Yae K, Nakagawa M, Ichisaka T, Okita K, Takahashi K, Chiba T, Yamanaka S (2008) Generation of pluripotent stem cells from adult mouse liver and stomach cells. Science 321:699–702
30. Tsuji O, Miura K, Okada Y, Fujiyoshi K, Mukaino M, Nagoshi N, Kitamura K, Kumagai G, Nishino M, Tomisato S, Higashi H, Nagai T, Katoh H, Kohda K, Matsuzaki Y, Yuzaki M, Ikeda E, Toyama Y, Nakamura M, Yamanaka S, Okano H (2010) Therapeutic potential of appropriately evaluated safe-induced pluripotent stem cells for spinal cord injury. Proc Natl Acad Sci U S A 107(28):12704–12709
31. Nori S, Okada Y, Yasuda A, Tsuji O, Takahashi Y, Kobayashi Y, Fujiyoshi K, Koike M, Uchiyama Y, Ikeda E, Toyama Y, Yamanaka S, Nakamura M, Okano H (2011) Grafted human-induced pluripotent stem-cell–derived neurospheres promote motor functional recovery after spinal cord injury in mice. Proc Natl Acad Sci U S A 108(40):16825–16830
32. Gage FH (2000) Mammalian neural stem cells. Science 287:1433–1438
33. Kobayashi Y, Okada Y, Itakura G, Iwai H, Nishimura S, Yasuda A, Nori S, Hikishima K, Konomi T, Fujiyoshi K, Tsuji O, Toyama Y, Yamanaka S, Nakamura M, Okano H (2012) Pre-evaluated safe human iPSC-derived neural stem cells promote functional recovery after spinal cord injury in common marmoset without tumorigenicity. PLoS One 7:e52787
34. Seki T, Yuasa S, Oda M, Egashira T, Yae K, Kusumoto D, Nakata H, Tohyama S, Hashimoto H, Kodaira M, Okada Y, Seimiya H, Fusaki N, Hasegawa M, Fukuda K (2010) Generation of induced pluripotent stem cells from human terminally differentiated circulating T cells. Cell Stem Cell 7:11–14
35. Hacein-Bey-Abina S, Von Kalle C, Schmidt M, McCormack MP, Wulffraat N, Leboulch P, Lim A, Osborne CS, Pawliuk R, Morillon E, Sorensen R, Forster A, Fraser P, Cohen JI, de Saint Basile G, Alexander I, Wintergerst U, Frebourg T, Aurias A, Stoppa-Lyonnet D, Romana S, Radford-Weiss I, Gross F, Valensi F, Delabesse E, Macintyre E, Sigaux F, Soulier J, Leiva LE, Wissler M, Prinz C, Rabbitts TH, Le Deist F, Fischer A, Cavazzana-Calvo M (2003) LMO2-associated clonal T cell proliferation in two patients after gene therapy for SCID-X1. Science 302:415–419
36. Yu J, Hu K, Smuga-Otto K, Tian S, Stewart R, Slukvin II, Thomson JA (2009) Human induced pluripotent stem cells free of vector and transgene sequences. Science 324:797–801
37. Kaji K, Norrby K, Paca A, Mileikovsky M, Mohseni P, Woltjen K (2009) Virus-free induction of pluripotency and subsequent excision of reprogramming factors. Nature 458:771–775
38. Woltjen K, Michael IP, Mohseni P, Desai R, Mileikovsky M, Hamalainen R, Cowling R, Wang W, Liu P, Gertsenstein M, Kaji K, Sung HK, Nagy A (2009) piggyBac transposition reprograms fibroblasts to induced pluripotent stem cells. Nature 458:766–770
39. Zhou H, Wu S, Joo JY, Zhu S, Han DW, Lin T, Trauger S, Bien G, Yao S, Zhu Y, Siuzdak G, Scholer HR, Duan L, Ding S (2009) Generation of induced pluripotent stem cells using recombinant proteins. Cell Stem Cell 4:381–384
40. Kim D, Kim CH, Moon JI, Chung YG, Chang MY, Han BS, Ko S, Yang E, Cha KY, Lanza R, Kim KS (2009) Generation of human induced pluripotent stem cells by direct delivery of reprogramming proteins. Cell Stem Cell 4:472–476

41. Shi Y, Do JT, Desponts C, Hahm HS, Scholer HR, Ding S (2008) A combined chemical and genetic approach for the generation of induced pluripotent stem cells. Cell Stem Cell 2:525–528
42. Maherali N, Hochedlinger K (2009) Tgfbeta signal inhibition cooperates in the induction of iPSCs and replaces Sox2 and cMyc. Curr Biol 19:1718–1723
43. Eiges R, Schuldiner M, Drukker M, Yanuka O, Itskovitz-Eldor J, Benvenisty N (2001) Establishment of human embryonic stem cell-transfected clones carrying a marker for undifferentiated cells. Curr Biol 11:514–518
44. Schuldiner M, Itskovitz-Eldor J, Benvenisty N (2003) Selective ablation of human embryonic stem cells expressing a "suicide" gene. Stem Cells 21:257–265
45. Fusaki N, Ban H, Nishiyama A, Saeki K, Hasegawa M (2009) Efficient induction of transgene-free human pluripotent stem cells using a vector based on Sendai virus, an RNA virus that does not integrate into the host genome. Proc Jpn Acad Ser B Phys Biol Sci 85:348–362
46. Okita K, Nakagawa M, Hyenjong H, Ichisaka T, Yamanaka S (2008) Generation of mouse induced pluripotent stem cells without viral vectors. Science 322:949–953
47. Rhee YH, Ko JY, Chang MY, Yi SH, Kim D, Kim CH, Shim JW, Jo AY, Kim BW, Lee H, Lee SH, Suh W, Park CH, Koh HC, Lee YS, Lanza R, Kim KS, Lee SH (2011) Protein-based human iPS cells efficiently generate functional dopamine neurons and can treat a rat model of Parkinson disease. J Clin Invest 121:2326–2335
48. Warren L, Manos PD, Ahfeldt T, Loh YH, Li H, Lau F, Ebina W, Mandal PK, Smith ZD, Meissner A, Daley GQ, Brack AS, Collins JJ, Cowan C, Schlaeger TM, Rossi DJ (2010) Highly efficient reprogramming to pluripotency and directed differentiation of human cells with synthetic modified mRNA. Cell Stem Cell 7:618–630
49. Okita K, Matsumura Y, Sato Y, Okada A, Morizane A, Okamoto S, Hong H, Nakagawa M, Tanabe K, Tezuka K, Shibata T, Kunisada T, Takahashi M, Takahashi J, Saji H, Yamanaka S (2011) A more efficient method to generate integration-free human iPS cells. Nat Methods 8:409–412
50. Hu K, Yu J, Suknuntha K, Tian S, Montgomery K, Choi KD, Stewart R, Thomson JA, Slukvin II (2011) Efficient generation of transgene-free induced pluripotent stem cells from normal and neoplastic bone marrow and cord blood mononuclear cells. Blood 117:e109–e119
51. Jia F, Wilson KD, Sun N, Gupta DM, Huang M, Li Z, Panetta NJ, Chen ZY, Robbins RC, Kay MA, Longaker MT, Wu JC (2010) A nonviral minicircle vector for deriving human iPS cells. Nat Methods 7:197–199
52. Yusa K, Rad R, Takeda J, Bradley A (2009) Generation of transgene-free induced pluripotent mouse stem cells by the piggyBac transposon. Nat Methods 6:363–369
53. Okano H, Nakamura M, Yoshida K, Okada Y, Tsuji O, Nori S, Ikeda E, Yamanaka S, Miura K (2013) Steps toward safe cell therapy using induced pluripotent stem cells. Circ Res 112: 523–533

Chapter 20
Transplantation of Neural Stem Cells with Valproate for Spinal Cord Injury

Masahiko Abematsu and Kinichi Nakashima

Abstract The regenerative capacity of an injured spinal cord is limited, and once paralysis occurs, it is difficult to improve the situation. We have developed a treatment method called the HINT method (*H*DAC *I*nhibitor and *N*eural stem cell *T*ransplantation) that improves hind limb motor functionality in mice with severe spinal cord injuries by using a combination of antiepileptic drugs and neural stem cells. This chapter will introduce you to the new neural damage reconstruction mechanism employed in the HINT method.

Keywords Epigenetics • Neural stem cell • Regeneration • Spinal cord injury • Valproate

20.1 Introduction

"Once the central nervous system has sustained an injury, such as in the brain or the spinal cord, this damage cannot be restored." This concept was the common dogma in the medical community for many years, and in 1906, Nobel Prize was awarded to Dr. Santiago Ramón y Cajal who advocated it [1]. At present, once the paralysis of a patient with spinal cord injury is fixed, it is resistant to a variety of treatments, and improvement in symptoms is rarely observed.

M. Abematsu (✉)
Department of Orthopedic Surgery, Kagoshima Graduate School of Medical and Dental Science, Kagoshima, Japan

The Near-Future Locomotor Organ Medicine Creation Course (Kusunoki Kai), Kagoshima Graduate School of Medical and Dental Science, Kagoshima, Japan
e-mail: masa@m3.kufm.kagoshima-u.ac.jp

K. Nakashima
Stem Cell Biology and Medicine, Graduate School of Medical Sciences, Kyushu University, Fukuoka, Japan

K. Uchida et al. (eds.), *Neuroprotection and Regeneration of the Spinal Cord*,
DOI 10.1007/978-4-431-54502-6_20,

Over the past decades, many researchers have been conducting regenerative therapy studies using animal models of stroke and spinal cord injuries to solve this problem. To date, many treatment methods have been tested, including inflammation suppression of lesions that impede nerve regeneration [2], promotion of regrowth of damaged axons [3, 4], remyelination of demyelinated axons using transplanted cells [5], improvement of blood flow to the lesion area [6], and several other methods [7, 8]. Thus far, when therapeutic effects were observed, only a small number of those studies have discussed in detail the mechanisms involving such therapeutic effect. However, this is not sufficient for clinical applications, which rely on clear evidences.

It has been suggested from the research results to date that three steps are required to regenerate adult central nervous system circuitry [9]:

1. Axons must reach the appropriate destination neuron by re-elongation of axons that have been severed.
2. Remyelination of newly elongated axons.
3. Synapse formation between the newly elongated axon and the destination neuron.

Recently, neural stem cells have attracted attention as a tool for spinal cord regeneration therapy. It has been reported that a certain degree of therapeutic effects can be obtained by transplanting cells into the damaged spinal cord [5, 7, 8, 10, 11]. These cells are pluripotent, have the ability to self-regenerate, and can differentiate into the major cell types of the nervous system: neurons and glial cells (oligodendrocytes and astrocytes). In recent years, it has become possible to prepare and differentiate embryonic stem cells (ES) as well as induced pluripotent stem (iPS) cells with relative ease. In several reports [5], it was demonstrated that demyelinated axons within the damaged spinal cord were re-myelinated by transplanted cells derived from oligodendrocytes. It is suggested that hind limb motor function can be recovered using this procedure. There are also [7] suggesting that neurons derived from transplanted cells may contribute to the recovery of motor function; however, the exact mechanism is not known.

Previous studies have shown the occurrence of significant inflammatory responses within the damaged spinal cord and the formation of a glial scar in the lesion because of the inflamed cytokines. There have been attempts to transplant neural stem cells into the damaged region. However, most cells differentiate into astrocytes, and few reports have demonstrated dramatic therapeutic effects.

The promotion of neuronal differentiation was reported in two studies that used neural stem cells expressing neurogenin 2 from the neuronal differentiation promotion transcription factor in transplanted cells, and motor function recovery was observed when compared to nontreatment groups [11, 12]. Hofstetter et al. concluded that therapeutic effects were achieved in remyelination using transplanted cells derived from oligodendrocytes. A study by Perrin et al. concluded that the number of host-derived serotoninergic neurons increased, which is related to the recovery of motor function.

20.2 Title of Study

Recently, we reported that the antiepileptic drug valproate affects neuronal differentiation and promotion of neural stem cells via its inhibitory activity on histone deacetylase as well as on glial cell differentiation [13]. In this study, to resolve the problems described above, we exploited this effect. In addition to transplanting neural stem cells, we promoted neuronal differentiation and suppressed glial cell differentiation in transplanted neural stem cells using valproate. We have begun developing a therapy (termed the HINT method) based on the novel idea of rebuilding the damaged neural network [14]. We observed significant recovery of motor function (Fig. 20.1a) when we used the HINT method to treat mice with spinal cord injuries.

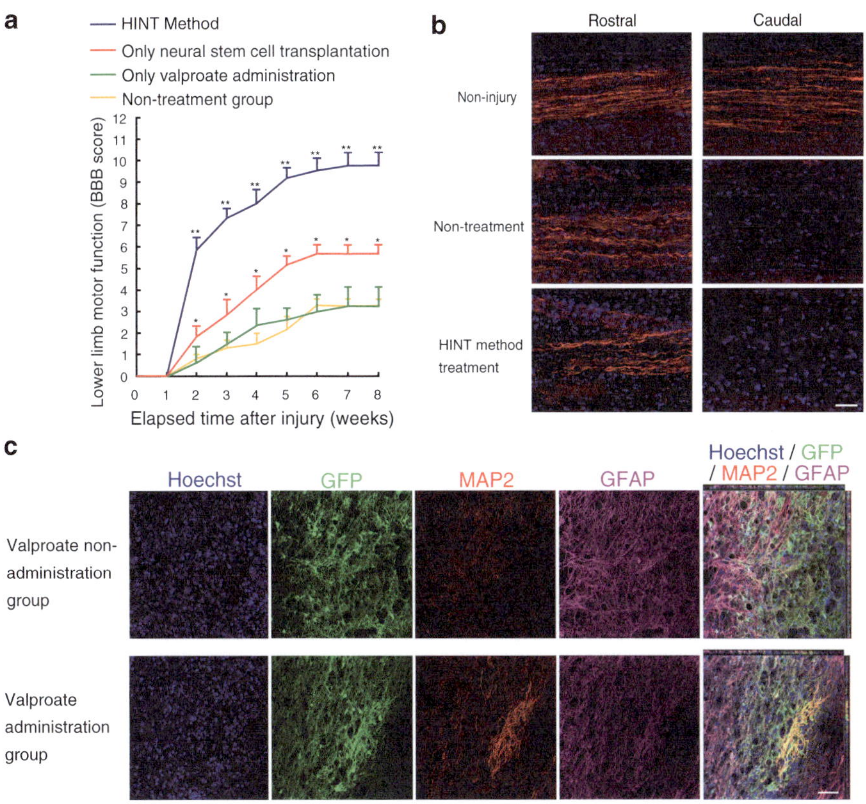

Fig. 20.1 (**a**) Temporal changes in the lower limb motor function in model mice with spinal cord injury. Significant improvement of lower limb motor function was observed by using the HINT treatment method. (**b**) Tracer experiment results of pyramidal tract primary neurons with biotinylated dextran amine. Re-elongation of severed axons was not observed despite the significant lower limb motor function improvement by the HINT treatment method. (**c**) With the administration of valproate, the differentiation of transplanted GFP-positive neural stem cells into MAP2-positive neurons was promoted, whereas differentiation into GFAP-positive astrocytes was inhibited

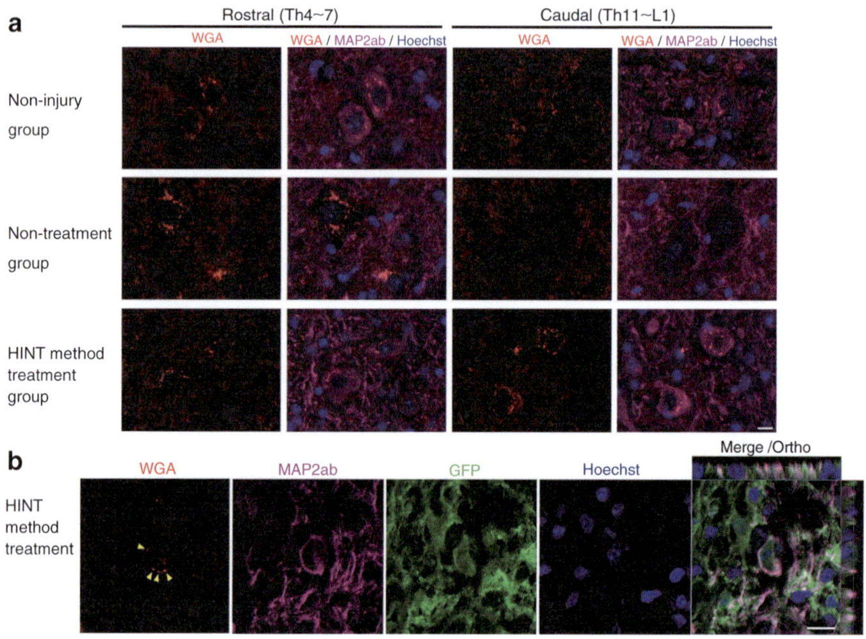

Fig. 20.2 (**a**) Evaluation of transsynaptic neural network regeneration using WGA. In the nontreatment group, WGA-positive neurons were almost nonexistent on the caudal side of the central injury location; however, in the HINT treatment method group, WGA-positive neurons were observed on the caudal side. (**b**) WGA-positive cells were observed in the neurons derived from transplanted cells in the vicinity of the central injury location

However, when we examined axonal regeneration of the primary neurons extending from the cortical motor cortex that had sustained damage, regeneration was not observed in the treatment group using this method (Fig. 20.1b).

Because the transplanted neural stem cells are involved in improving motor function, we first examined the differentiation trends. On the basis of immunohistochemistry analyses, we observed that with the HINT method, neuronal differentiation of transplanted cells was greatly enhanced in the treatment group (Fig. 20.1c). Many of the neuronal projections derived from transplanted cells extended to the cranial side and the caudal dorsal funiculus (pyramidal tract area) as well as to cells near the anterior cornu of the spinal cord. Furthermore, using electron microscopy, we observed neurons derived from transplanted cells had received axons from the host neurons, then projected to cells on the anterior cornu of the spinal cord, and finally formed synapses.

Next to examine the route the damaged neuron takes, we used adenoviral injection to forcibly express wheat germ agglutinin (WGA) tracer that is passed from the primary to the tertiary neuron through the synapse into the motor cortex area. Surprisingly, in the HINT treatment group, the WGA had travelled from the cerebral cortex to the primary motor neurons and transported to transplanted cell-derived neurons. We also observed that WGA had travelled from the lesion to the peripheral side of cells on the anterior cornu of the spinal cord (Fig. 20.2a, b).

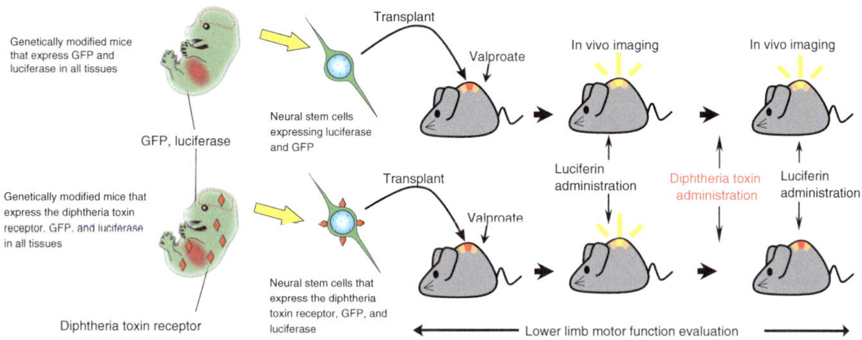

Fig. 20.3 Specific removal of the transplanted cells and observation of transplanted cell survival using in vivo imaging system. By the evaluation of specific removal of luciferase containing transplanted cells and observation of transplanted cell survival using in vivo imaging systems, it is possible to evaluate the amount of transplanted cells surviving in the same host. At the same time it is possible to specifically remove transplanted cells using the diphtheria toxin from a live host through the expression of the diphtheria toxin receptor on stem cells. Transplanted cells were evaluated by analyzing lower limb motor function whether or not they were directly involved in lower limb motor function improvement

Because host neurons were largely unobserved in the region around the lesion, it was strongly suggested that neurons derived from transplanted cells regenerate the damaged neural network in a relay fashion [14]. Moreover, to specifically remove the transplanted cells after treatment, we transplanted neural stem cells expressing the diphtheria toxin receptor. Once a treatment effect was observed, we administered diphtheria toxin to the mice (Fig. 20.3). We used an in vivo imaging system to verify that only transplanted cells were removed. By following the survival of transplanted cells over time, we observed that lower limb motor function again deteriorated to the same extent as in the nontreatment group. These data indicate that transplanted cells that undergo directed differentiation with valproate are directly involved in the improvement of lower limb motor function [14].

20.3 Discussion

Recently, we have begun to understand the importance of molecular epigenetic mechanisms in the maintenance of cell differentiation and differentiation traits, including cell reprogramming. In this study, through in vivo differentiation of transplanted neurons, we have succeeded in regenerating the neural network of the host that was damaged. We directed in vivo differentiation of transplanted stem cells to neuronal lineage by changing the chromatin structure to facilitate histone acetylation.

Following our results, Bonner et al. also succeeded in regeneration by forcing relay connections using fetal neural progenitor cell-derived neurons of the sensory neural network, which were destroyed by spinal cord injury [15]. The use of neurotrophic factors in axon guidance is very interesting. In addition to regenerating the damaged circuits by neurons derived from transplanted neural progenitor cells rather than host-derived cells, the development of complex therapies such as this will continue in future. Lu et al. transplanted a fibrin matrix containing neurotrophic factors and rat fetal-derived neural stem cells to the damaged portion of the rat spinal cord and dramatically improved lower limb function [16]. Similar to our results, transplanted cells derived from neurons extended many long projections and formed synapses with the neurons of the host. Taken together, these data showed that the proposed neural network reconstruction mechanism of the relay connection by neurons derived from transplanted cells, in fact, exists.

20.4 Conclusion

To achieve more efficient regeneration of damaged spinal cords, it is necessary for human clinical applications to change the required treatment according to the type and extent of damage rather than apply a standard treatment. For example, in demyelination, it was hypothesized that a therapy to replenish oligodendrocytes is necessary for the primary clinical condition. However, it is now thought that replenishing neurons of the damaged neural network is more appropriate. Several questions remain to be answered: for neuronal replacement, what kind of neuronal subtype is most necessary? Will the necessary cell types and subtypes be different according to the damaged anatomical area? Will it be necessary to regenerate the neuronal circuits step-by-step? These and many other aspects are still unknown and, thus, require further research.

Conflict of Interest The authors declare that they have no conflict of interest.

References

1. Llinás RR (2003) The contribution of Santiago Ramón y Cajal to functional neuroscience. Nat Rev Neurosci 4:77–80
2. Oudega M, Vargas CG, Weber AB et al (1999) Long-term effects of methylprednisolone following transection of adult rat spinal cord. Eur J Neurosci 11:2453–2464
3. Schnell L, Schwab ME (1990) Axonal regeneration in the rat spinal cord produced by an antibody against myelin-associated neurite growth inhibitors. Nature 343:269–272
4. Bregman BS, Kunkel-Bagden E, Schnell L et al (1995) Recovery from spinal cord injury mediated by antibodies to neurite growth inhibitors. Nature 378:498–501
5. Cummings BJ, Uchida N, Tamaki SJ et al (2005) Human neural stem cells differentiate and promote locomotor recovery in spinal cord-injured mice. Proc Natl Acad Sci U S A 102:14069–14074
6. Leist M, Ghezzi P, Grasso G et al (2004) Derivatives of erythropoietin that are tissue protective but not erythropoietic. Science 305:239–242
7. Setoguchi T, Nakashima K, Takizawa T et al (2004) Treatment of spinal cord injury by transplantation of fetal neural precursor cells engineered to express BMP inhibitor. Exp Neurol 189:33–44

8. Ogawa Y, Sawamoto K, Miyata T et al (2002) Transplantation of in vitro-expanded fetal neural progenitor cells results in neurogenesis and functional recovery after spinal cord contusion injury in adult rats. J Neurosci Res 69:925–933
9. Horner PJ, Gage FH (2000) Regenerating the damaged central nervous system. Nature 407:963–970
10. Okada S, Ishii K, Yamane J et al (2005) In vivo imaging of engrafted neural stem cells: its application in evaluating the optimal timing of transplantation for spinal cord injury. FASEB J 19:1839–1841
11. Hofstetter CP, Holmström NA, Lilja JA et al (2005) Allodynia limits the usefulness of intraspinal neural stem cell grafts; directed differentiation improves outcome. Nat Neurosci 8:346–353
12. Perrin FE, Boniface G, Serguera C et al (2010) Grafted human embryonic progenitors expressing neurogenin-2 stimulate axonal sprouting and improve motor recovery after severe spinal cord injury. PLoS One 5:e15914
13. Hsieh J, Nakashima K, Kuwabara T et al (2004) Histone deacetylase inhibition-mediated neuronal differentiation of multipotent adult neural progenitor cells. Proc Natl Acad Sci U S A 101:16659–16664
14. Abematsu M, Tsujimura K, Yamano M et al (2010) Neurons derived from transplanted neural stem cells restore disrupted neuronal circuitry in a mouse model of spinal cord injury. J Clin Invest 120:3255–3266
15. Bonner JF, Connors TM, Silverman WF et al (2011) Grafted neural progenitors integrate and restore synaptic connectivity across the injured spinal cord. J Neurosci 31:4675–4686
16. Lu P, Wang Y, Graham L et al (2012) Long-distance growth and connectivity of neural stem cells after severe spinal cord injury. Cell 150(6):1264–1273

Chapter 21
The Effects of Mesenchymal Stem Cell-Transduced Multineurotrophin to Improve Function Following Spinal Cord Injury

Gentaro Kumagai and W. Dalton Dietrich

Abstract Neurotrophins and the transplantation of bone marrow-derived stromal cells (MSCs) are both candidate therapies targeting experimental and clinical spinal cord injury (SCI). While some studies have suggested the ability of MSCs to transdifferentiate into neural cells, other SCI studies have proposed anti-inflammatory and other mechanisms underlying established beneficial effects. We grafted rat MSCs genetically modified to express MNTS1, a multineurotrophin that binds TrkA, TrkB and TrkC, and p75NTR receptors or MSC-MNTS1p75^{-} that binds mainly to the Trk receptors. Seven days after contusive SCI, PBS-only, GFP-MSC, MSC-MNTS1/GFP, or MSC-MNTS1/p75^{-}/GFP was delivered into the injury epicenter. All transplanted groups showed reduced inflammation and cystic cavity size compared to control SCI rats. Interestingly, transplantation of the MSC-MNTS1 and MSC-MNTS1/p75^{-}, but not the naïve MSCs, enhanced axonal growth and significantly prevented cutaneous hypersensitivity after SCI. Moreover, transplantation of MSC-MNTS1/p75^{-} promoted angiogenesis and modified glial scar formation. These findings suggest that MSCs transduced with a multineurotrophin are effective in promoting cell growth and improving sensory function after SCI. These novel data also provide insight into the neurotrophin-receptor-dependent mechanisms through which cellular transplantation leads to functional improvement after experimental SCI.

Keywords Axonal regeneration • Multineurotrophin • Rat bone marrow stromal cells • Spinal cord injury • Transplantation

---

G. Kumagai (✉)
Department of Orthopedic Surgery, Hirosaki University Graduate School of Medicine,
Hirosaki 036-8076, Japan
e-mail: gengen722@hotmail.com

W.D. Dietrich
Department of Neurological Surgery, The Miami Project to Cure Paralysis,
University of Miami Miller School of Medicine, Miami, FL 33136-1060, USA

K. Uchida et al. (eds.), *Neuroprotection and Regeneration of the Spinal Cord*,
DOI 10.1007/978-4-431-54502-6_21, © Springer Japan 2014

21.1 Introduction

Cellular transplantation strategies may protect and promote regeneration after spinal cord injury (SCI) [1–6]. Embryonic and induced pluripotent stem cells are reported to differentiate into neurons, astrocytes, and oligodendrocytes and improve motor function after SCI [7–9]. This chapter shows the review of marrow-derived stromal cells (MSCs) transplantation and our previous study. We grafted MSCs genetically modified to express MTNS1 or MNTS1/p75$^-$ following SCI [10]. Although transplanted groups attenuated acute inflammation and reduced cystic cavity, the transplantation of the MSC-MNTS1 and MSC-MNTS1/p75$^-$, but not MSCs, promoted axonal growth and prevented cutaneous hypersensitivity after SCI. Moreover, transplantation of MSC-MNTS1/p75$^-$ promoted angiogenesis and modified glial scar formation. These findings indicate that MSC-MNTS1 are beneficial for improving sensory function and support a novel cellular transplantation strategy that targets a clinically relevant quality of life issue.

21.2 Review of MSCs Transplantation for SCI

21.2.1 Transplantation of MSCs

Bone MSCs are tissue-specific stem cells that are capable of self-renewal and can differentiate into mature lineages of blood cells, stromal and skeletal tissue [11]. MSCs are a population of heterogeneous mesenchymal cells in the bone marrow [12] that consist of pluripotent mesenchymal stem cells, macrophages, and endothelial cells [13]. MSCs can readily be harvested and expanded and have the potential for either autologous transplantation or transplantation after genetic manipulation [14]. From both in vitro and in vivo studies, MSCs are reported to be able to differentiate into neural cells [15]. Therefore, MSCs are good candidates for use in cell transplantation therapies in SCI. The findings from several laboratories have also indicated that BMSC may play a guiding role in fostering host axons to grow in the grafted spinal cord [16–18]. Moreover, it has been indicated that the transplantation of MSCs promotes overall functional recovery after SCI [17, 19–22] and did not induce allodynia in response to mechanical or thermal stimulation [23]. Although some studies have suggested that MSCs can also differentiate into cells with neural phenotypes in demyelinated spinal cord [21, 24] or injured spinal cord [17], the ability of MSC to transdifferentiate into neural cells remains controversial [15, 25]. Given the door variability in the secretion profile of MSC to provide repair, genetic manipulation may be necessary for clinical application.

21.2.2 Transplantation of Neurotrophin-Transduced MSCs

Neurotrophins affect essentially all biological aspects of vertebrate neurons, including the survival, differentiation, growth, and apoptosis of neurons, by using a two-receptor system, which consists of Trk tyrosine kinases and the p75 neurotrophin receptor [26]. Three types of Trk receptors, namely, TrkA, TrkB, and TrkC, mediate the biological activity of neurotrophins. Trk receptor tyrosine kinases undergo rapid transphosphorylation following ligand binding, leading to a cascade of protein phosphorylation in the cell. The distinctive neuronal deficiencies in mice with null mutations in the trkA, trkB, and trkC genes are similar to those observed in mice with null mutations in the nerve growth factor (NGF), brain-derived neurotrophic factor (BDNF), and NGF genes, respectively. Therefore, the Trk seem to mediate the survival-promoting action of neurotrophins on developing neurons. Another receptor system for neurotrophins, specifically p75, belongs to a large family of receptors that includes tumor necrosis factor (TNF) receptors, Fas (Apo-1/CD95), RANK, CD40, and approximately 25 other members. One of the most prominent biological functions of p75 is that it induces cell death because it contains a death-domain sequence distantly related to the intracellular domains of Fas and TNF receptors. Neurotrophin binding to p75 induces apoptosis in vivo [26]. Neurotrophin binding to the p75 receptor has diverse effects, ranging from cell death to regulation of axon elongation [27]. Currently, a very promising experimental strategy for promoting neuronal survival and endogenous regeneration in injured spinal cord is local delivery of neurotrophic factors. Several neurotrophic factors, like BDNF, glial cell-derived neurotrophic factor (GDNF), neurotrophin (NT)3, and NGF, can stimulate neurogenesis in vitro and in vivo [28], and their importance for the development of the nervous system for axonal pathfinding and neuronal survival has made them promising targets to augment regeneration in the injured brain and spinal cord [15, 29]. Several approaches have been reported to deliver genetically modified MSC transplants into injured spinal cord [18, 30–32]. Bifunctional neurotrophin known as D15A which is capable of mimicking the downstream effects of BDNF and NT-3 through binding to both TrkB and TrkC receptors, respectively [33]. D15A has been applied to regeneration studies by using cell transplantation after SCI. Transplantation of NT3/D15A-expressing glial-restricted precursor cells in the subacute phase of SCI led to an increasement of myelin formation and the recovery of hindlimb locomotion [34]. Transplantation of NT3/D15A-expressing Schwann cells in the subacute phase of SCI also promoted the survival of transplants and increase of axon growth and myelination [35].

21.3 Transplantation of Multineurotrophin/p75^{-}-Transduced MSCs for SCI

21.3.1 Multineurotrophin (MNTS1)/p75^{-}

Neurotrophins exert most of their positive effects, neuronal survival and axonal growth, through the Ras/MAPK- and PI3K/Akt-signaling pathways by activating the Trk receptors [36]. Furthermore, neurotrophins also bind the p75NTR, a member of the tumor necrosis factor receptor (TNFR) superfamily [37, 38]. The pro-neurotrophin forms can activate p75NTR and trigger apoptosis during development

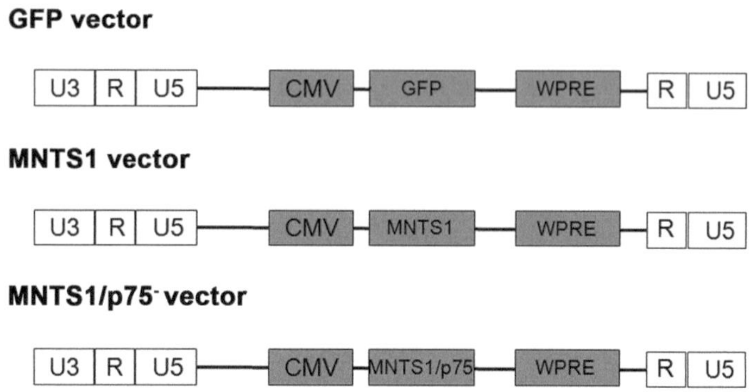

Fig. 21.1 Diagram of the GFP, MNTS1, and MNTS1/p75⁻ lentivirus vectors

or after injury [38]. In addition, this receptor can serve as a co-receptor for various ligands with different biological activities [38]. For example, p75NTR interacts with NgR and Lingo-1 [39] and has been reported to exhibit growth-inhibitory effects by modulating Rho GTPases [40–42]. Therefore, it is imperative to use neurotrophins that interact mainly with the Trk receptors to eliminate the possibility of these molecules to interact with p75NTR. For this purpose, we have made use of a multineurotrophin that can bind to all of the Trk receptors and therefore be able to target diverse neuronal populations that might respond to neurotrophins and created mutations to residues R113 and K114 to reduce the binding to p75NTR [10, 33].

21.3.2 The Effects of MSCs-Transduced MSC-MNTS1 or -MNTS1/p75⁻ [10]

The MNTS1 and MNTS1/p75⁻ cDNAs were produced synthetically by GeneArt and subcloned into the lentiviral vector pRRLsin.PPT.Th.CMV.MCS.Wpre described earlier (Fig. 21.1) [43]. MSCs were collected from femurs and tibias of adult GFP-expressing transgenic male Fischer rats. Before transplantation, MSCs were thawed and grown for 2 days before infecting with the lentivirus. LV/GFP/MNTS1- and LV/GFP/MNTS1/p75-infected MSCs exhibited robust transduction efficiency with GFP expression in greater than 70 % of the cells when we use an MOI of 50. All animal procedures and care were approved by the University of Miami Animal Care and Use Committee, in accordance with NIH and the Guide for the Care and Use of Animals. Adult female Fischer rats (180–200 g) ($n=48$) were used for the spinal cord injury model. The moderate contusion was created by the Infinite Horizon impactor (200 kdyn; Precision Systems, Lexington, KY) onto the exposed cord of T8 level. Animals were randomly divided into four implant groups: PBS-only, GFP-MSCs (MSCs), MNTS1/GFP-containing LV vector-transduced MSC (MSC-MNTS1), and MNTS1/p75⁻/GFP-containing LV vector-transduced MSC (MSC-MNTS1/p75⁻). We grafted PBS (control), MSCs, MSC-MNTS1, and

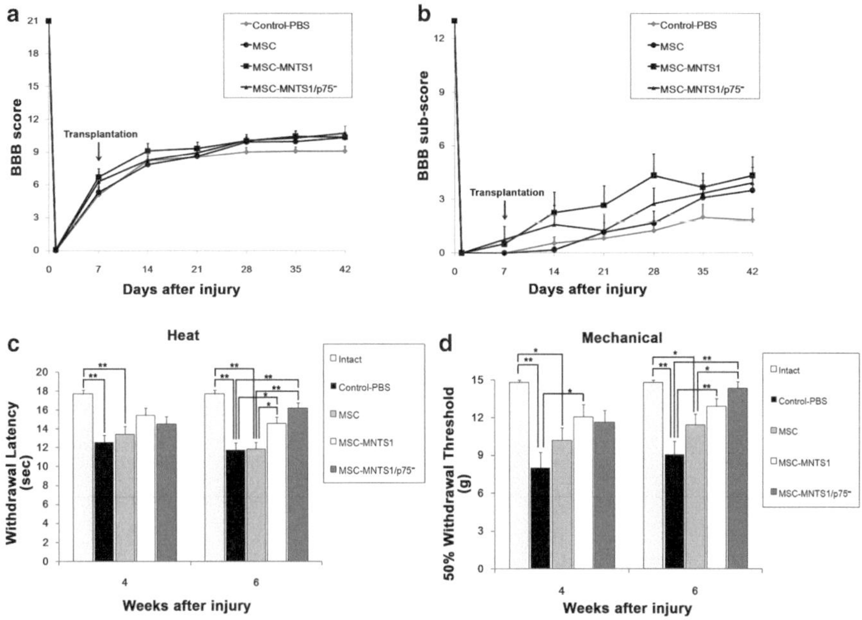

Fig. 21.2 Transplanted MSC-MNTS1 and MSC-MNTS1/p75⁻, but not MSCs, reduce the sensitivity of cutaneous hypersensitivity. (**a** and **b**) Open-field walking as determined by the BBB scores and BBB sub-score. *Downward arrow* indicates time of transplantation. Hindlimb function was assigned scores from 0 to 21 (flaccid paralysis to normal gait). Values are means ± SEM ($n=12$, each). (**c** and **d**) Rats were tested at 4 and 6 weeks following contusion and hind paw responses to noxious heat (heat) and innocuous mechanical (mechanical) stimuli were recorded. Values are means ± SEM ($n=12$, each). *: $P<0.05$. **: $P<0.01$

MSC-MNTS1/p75⁻ on 7 days after injury. One injection of 6 μl MSCs (4 × 105 cells) was performed over 3 min into the injury epicenter.

We monitored the locomotor functional recovery in all four groups: control, MSC, MSC-MNTS1, and MSC-MNTS1/p75⁻, respectively, using the BBB scoring scale and BBB sub-score [44, 45] (Fig. 21.2a, b). There was no significant difference in the BBB scores and BBB sub-score between the cell transplant and control groups. To evaluate the sensitivity of hindlimb cutaneous hypersensitivity, heat and mechanical stimuli were examined at 4 and 6 weeks after injury (Fig. 21.2c, d). Prior to contusion injury, the mean latency in second(s) to withdraw from a noxious heat stimulus was 17.7 ± 0.4 s (Intact group, $n=10$). Following contusion injury, withdrawal latencies to noxious heat in the control and MSC groups were significantly decreased at 4 or 6 weeks following injury (4 weeks; 12.5 ± 0.8 and 13.4 ± 0.9 s or 6 weeks; 11.7 ± 0.8 and 11.8 ± 0.7 s, respectively). On the other hand, the MSC-MNTS1 and MSC-MNTS1/p75⁻ group demonstrated significantly improved withdrawal thresholds compared to the control and MSC groups at 6 weeks after contusion, such that thresholds (6 weeks; 14.6 ± 0.7 and 16.2 ± 0.6 s, respectively) were no different from that of pre-contusion thresholds. Prior to contusion injury, the mean withdrawal threshold to innocuous mechanical stimuli was 14.8 ± 0.2

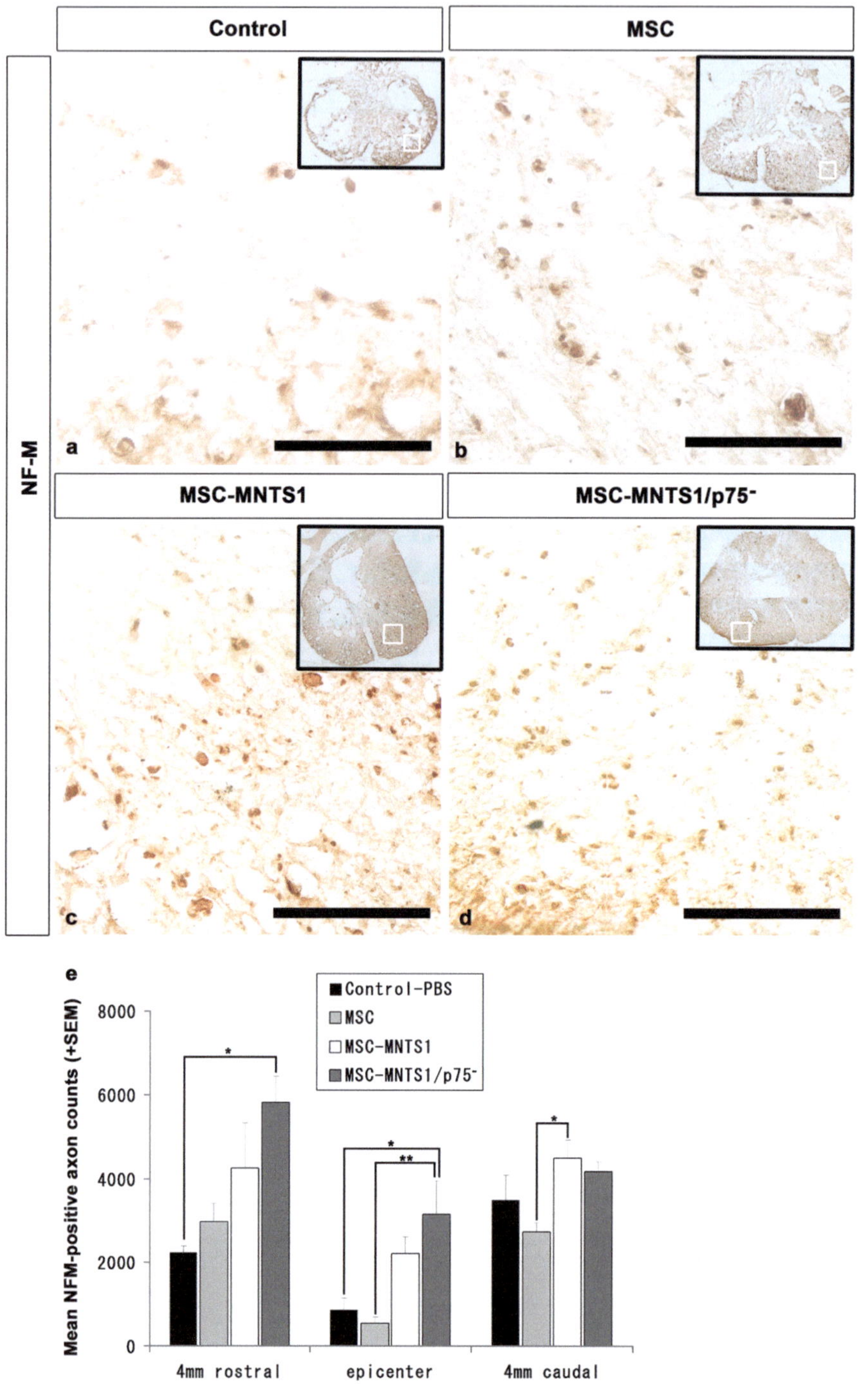

Fig. 21.3 Transplanted MSC-MNTS1 and -MNTS1/p75⁻, but not MSCs, promote axonal growth. (**a–d**) Representative images of axial sections stained for NF-M at the lesion epicenter in all four groups. Many more NF-M-positive axons were present in axial sections of the MSC-MNTS1

grams (Intact group, $n=10$). Following contusion injury, withdrawal latency to mechanical stimuli in the control and MSC groups was significantly decreased at 4 or 6 weeks following injury (4 weeks; 8.0 ± 1.2 and 10.2 ± 1.0 s or 6 weeks; 9.1 ± 1.0 and 11.4 ± 0.9 s, respectively). In contrast, the MSC-MNTS1 group demonstrated improved withdrawal thresholds compared to the control group at 4 or 6 weeks after contusion, such that thresholds (4 weeks; 12.1 ± 1.0 s, 6 weeks; 12.9 ± 0.6 s, respectively) were no different from that of pre-contusion thresholds. The MSC-MNTS1/p75⁻ group also demonstrated improved withdrawal thresholds compared to the control and MSC group at 6 weeks after contusion, such that thresholds (14.3 ± 0.5 s) were no different from that of pre-contusion thresholds.

Histopathological analysis of tissue by hematoxylin and eosin and luxol fast blue staining was based on area and volume values of contusion calculated by computer extrapolation using stereological methods from contour/analysis of single sections. Cavity, lesion, and preserved myelin volumes and area were obtained in the control and transplant groups. Cavity volume revealed significantly greater preservation in the MSC-MNTS1/p75⁻ group compared with the control group ($P=0.036$). Cavity area at 1,000 μm rostral to the epicenter revealed significantly greater preservation in MSC, MSC-MNTS1, and MSC-MNTS1/p75⁻ compared with the control group ($P=0.014$, $P=0.042$, and $P=0.011$, respectively). There was no significant difference in the lesion volume and area between the cell transplant and control groups. There was also no significant difference in preserved myelin volume and area between the cell transplant and control groups.

To assess the effect of increased neurotrophin on axonal growth by comparing the MSC, MSC-MNTS1, and MSC-MNTS1/p75⁻ groups, we examined neurofilament subunit (NF-M)-positive axons using stereology at the epicenter and at 4 mm rostral and caudal to the epicenter in axial sections (Fig. 21.3). While few NF-M-positive neuronal axons were observed at the rim of the lesion epicenter in both the control and MSC groups, there were significantly more NF-M-positive neuronal axonal counts in the MSC-MNTS1/p75⁻ group at the 4 mm site rostral to the lesion epicenter compared with the control group ($P=0.011$) and at the lesion epicenter compared with the control and MSC groups ($P=0.020$ and $P=0.009$, respectively). There were significantly more NF-M-positive axonal counts in the MSC-MNTS1 group at the 4 mm caudal to the lesion epicenter site compared with the MSC group ($P=0.043$).

To assess the effects of transplantation on the extent of angiogenesis after SCI, axial sections of the injured spinal cord were examined immunohistochemically

Fig. 21.3 (continued) (**c**) and MSC-MNTS1/p75⁻ (**d**) groups, when compared to control (**a**) or MSC (**b**) groups. Scale bar: 50 μm. (**e**) Quantitative analysis of the NF-M-positive axon counts at the epicenter and 4 mm rostral and caudal to the epicenter. While few NF-M-positive neuronal axons were observed at the rim of the lesion epicenter in the control group, there were significantly more NF-M-positive neuronal axon counts in the MSC-MNTS1/p75⁻ group at 4 mm rostral to the lesion epicenter site compared with the control group and at the lesion epicenter compared with the control and MSC groups. There were significantly more NF-M-positive neuronal axon counts in the MSC-MNTS1 group at 4 mm caudal to the lesion epicenter site compared with the MSC group. Values are means ± SEM ($n=4$, each). *: $P<0.05$, control versus MSC-MNTS1 or MSC-MNTS1/p75⁻. **: $P<0.01$, MSC versus MSC-MNTS1/p75⁻

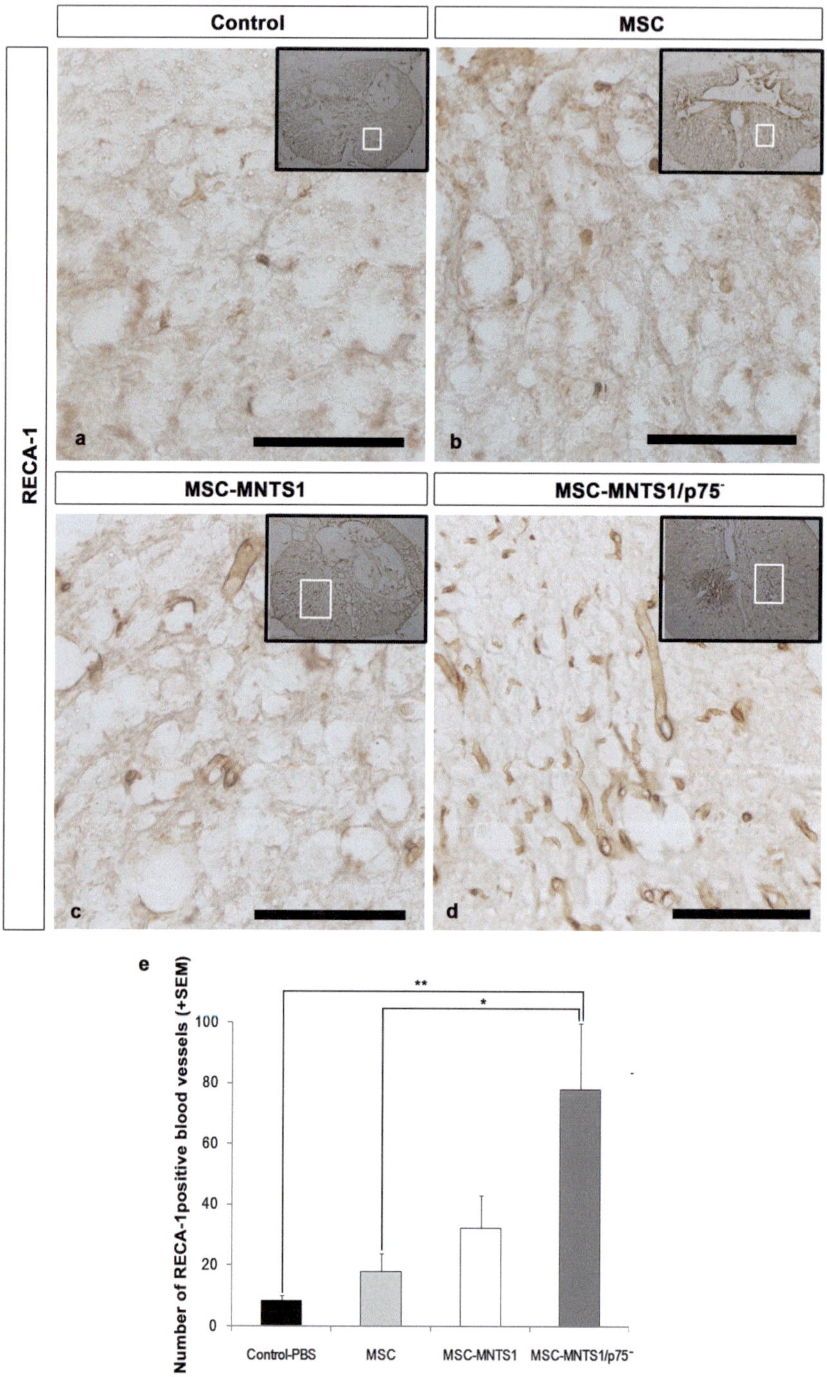

Fig. 21.4 Transplanted MSC-MNTS1, but not MSCs and MSC-MNTS1/p75⁻, promotes angiogenesis after SCI. (**a**–**d**) Representative images of axial sections stained for RECA-1 at the lesion epicenter in all groups. Many more RECA-1-positive blood vessels were present in axial sections

using stereology for RECA-1 (Fig. 21.4, a marker for endothelial cells). While a few RECA-1-positive blood vessels were observed at the lesion site in axial sections of the control and MSC groups, significantly more RECA-1-positive blood vessels were found in the MSC-MNTS1/p75$^-$ group compared with the control and MSC groups ($P<0.01$ and $P=0.024$, respectively).

Contusion injury to the spinal cord results in the chronic inflammatory events including activated microglia and macrophages. To assess the effects on the recruitment of these cells in the injury site, we examined ED-1 immuno-positive cells which are characterized as activated microglia/macrophages using stereology at the epicenter in axial sections. Quantitative analysis revealed that there were significantly more ED1-positive cells at the epicenter site compared with the MSC, -MNTS1, and -MNTS1/p75$^-$ groups ($P<0.01$, each). To assess the effects of transplantation on astrocyte reactivity after SCI, axial sections of the injured spinal cord were also examined immunohistochemically using stereology for GFAP. While GFAP immunoreactivities of the control and MSC groups were found in the white matter, those of the MSC-MNTS1 and -MNTS1/p75$^-$ groups were reduced in that area. There were also significantly more GFAP-positive cells in the control group at the epicenter site compared with the MSC-MNTS1/p75$^-$ groups ($P=0.037$).

To assess the cell survival of the MSC, -MNTS1, and -MNTS1/p75$^-$ grafted onto the injured spinal cord, coronal sections of the injured spinal cord were examined immunohistochemically for GFP. At three posttransplant periods, large numbers of transplanted cells were identified at 1 week after transplantation, followed by a gradual decrease around 4 weeks. In contrast, few grafted cells were found at 6 weeks after transplantation.

21.4 Discussion

Together our results indicate that cellular treatments after contusive SCI with MSC-MNTS1 or MSC-MNTS1/p75$^-$ reduce cutaneous hypersensitivity but do not improve recovery of motor function. Although our studies showed that in all transplanted groups the early survival of transplanted cells, attenuation of acute inflammation and a reduced cystic cavity volume, the transplantation of the MSC-MNTS1 and MNTS1/p75$^-$, but not the naïve MSCs, promoted axonal growth and prevented hypersensitivity after SCI. Moreover, transplantation of MSC-MNTS1/p75$^-$ promoted angiogenesis and modified glial scar formation. Finally, we provide for the first time evidence that treatment with transduced MSCs alleviated SCI-induced mechanical allodynia and thermal hyperalgesia of the hindlimb significantly better than documented with naïve MSCs.

Fig. 21.4 (continued) of the MSC-MNTS1/p75$^-$ groups (**d**), when compared to control (**a**), MSC (**b**), and MSC-MNTS1 (**c**) groups. Scale bar: 100 µm. (**e**) Quantitative analysis of blood vessels at the lesion epicenter. RECA-1 immunostaining revealed that significantly more RECA-1-positive vessels were observed at the lesion site in the MSC-MNTS1/p75$^-$ group compared with the control and MSC groups. Values are means ± SEM ($n=4$, each). *: $P<0.05$, control versus MSC-MNTS1/p75$^-$. **: $P<0.01$, MSC versus MSC-MNTS1/p75$^-$

Recently, transplantation of MSCs after SCI has been widely tested because they can be used as autografts, can be readily collected within a short time, and can be genetically modified to overexpress neurotrophic factors. Published studies indicate that the transplantation of MSCs promote overall functional recovery after SCI [17, 19–22] and do not induce allodynia in response to mechanical or thermal stimulation [23]. The mechanisms by which MSCs exert their effects on the injured spinal cord have also begun to be elucidated [6, 25, 46]. There is increasing evidence that MSCs may be immunosuppressive, synthesize a number of neurotrophic cytokines that stimulate nerve growth, including BDNF, NGF, and vascular endothelial growth factor (VEGF). These transplanted cells may also act as guides for regenerating axons across the lesion site of the injured spinal cord [25].

In contrast to reported positive findings, other studies indicate no significant improvements on BBB motor score after transplantation of MSCs into a contused or transected spinal cord [15, 47–49]. Here we report that naïve MSC also failed to promote functional recovery and reduce hypersensitivity after contusive SCI [10]. MSCs have been shown to attenuate chronic inflammation and injury-induced sensitivity to mechanical stimuli after experimental SCI [23]. Our results show that although there were significantly less ED1-positive cells in the naïve MSC-transplanted group compared with control, no significant prevention of hypersensitivity after SCI was observed with this cell treatment [10].

The generation of neuropathic pain after SCI is a major quality of life issue for many people living with SCI [50, 51]. Regarding the positive results of preventing hypersensitivity in the MSC-MNTS1 and -MNTS1/p75^{-} groups, several mechanisms may underlie the improvement of sensory function [52]. Neurotrophins affect essentially all biological aspects of neuronal function, including survival, differentiation, growth, and apoptosis by using a two-receptor system, consisting of Trk tyrosine kinases and the p75NTR neurotrophin receptor [26]. Three types of Trk receptors, namely, TrkA, TrkB, and TrkC, mediate the biological activity of neurotrophins. Trk receptor tyrosine kinases undergo rapid transphosphorylation following ligand binding, leading to a cascade of protein phosphorylation in the cell. The distinctive neuronal deficiencies reported in mice with null mutations of the TrkA, TrkB, and TrkC genes are similar to those observed in mice with null mutations in the NGF, BDNF, and NGF genes, respectively. Therefore, the Trk receptor appears to mediate the survival-promoting action of neurotrophins on developing neurons.

Multineurotrophin NT3/D15A is capable of mimicking the downstream effects of BDNF and NT-3 through binding to both TrkB and TrkC receptors, respectively [33]. Transplantation of NT3/D15A-expressing glial-restricted precursor cells in the subacute phase of SCI led to an increase of myelin formation and recovery of hindlimb locomotion [34]. Transplantation of NT3/D15A-expressing Schwann cells in the subacute phase of SCI also promoted the survival of transplants and increased myelination as well as 5-HT-, DβH-, and CGRP-positive fibers in the implants [35]. MNTS1, which contains only seven amino acid changes, binds all receptors of the Trk family. This molecule efficiently induces autophosphorylation of TrkA, TrkB, and TrkC and supports the survival of more sensory neurons from DRG and NG as well as sympathetic neurons than any of the neurotrophins individually [33].

One of the most prominent biological functions of p75NTR is that it induces cell death through the death-domain sequence which is distantly related to the intracellular domains of Fas and TNF receptors. This effect is mediated by the proneurotrophin form [26]. Neurotrophins and their receptors are essential growth factors in the formation of the heart and vascular system, and the complete ablation of the p75NTR causes severe developmental defects [53]. Also, p75NTR has been implicated in endothelial cell apoptosis [54]. Consistent with these findings, our study shows that animals receiving MSCs secreting the MNTS1/p75⁻ had more RECA-1-positive blood vessels within the injured spinal cord [10]. This result may be related to the Trk receptor activation which has been shown to promote angiogenesis. Although we observed reduced cavity volume and extensive axonal growth in the transplanted MSC-MNTS1 and -MNTS1/p75⁻ groups, this morphological finding did not result in improved locomotor functional recovery [10]. The failure to observe motor recovery is most likely due to the fact that the cell transplants may not have survived chronically in the present contusive SCI model. Thus, longer-term survival may be necessary for the cell transplants to influence the preservation of myelin and vital white matter tracts critical in the return of locomotor function after thoracic SCI. Also, additional studies are required to determine whether multiple MSC injections at possibly different pericontusional sites may be necessary to promote walking in this SCI model.

21.5 Conclusion

MSCs have a great potential as therapeutic agents against various human diseases including SCI. These cells can be readily obtained through established clinical procedures and are easy to isolate and expand for autotransplantation with limited risk of rejection. In this study, we have succeeded in preventing cutaneous hypersensitivity after SCI by the transplantation of MSCs secreting a multineurotrophin without p75 activity. Further studies are required to ensure the long-term safety and efficacy of manipulated MSCs to improve locomotor function and other quality-of-life issues after SCI.

Conflict of Interest The Authors declare that they have no conflict of interest.

References

1. Ogawa Y, Sawamoto K, Miyata T, Miyao S, Watanabe M, Nakamura M, Bregman BS, Koike M, Uchiyama Y, Toyama Y, Okano H (2002) Transplantation of in vitro-expanded fetal neural progenitor cells results in neurogenesis and functional recovery after spinal cord contusion injury in adult rats. J Neurosci Res 69(6):925–933
2. Cummings BJ, Uchida N, Tamaki SJ, Salazar DL, Hooshmand M, Summers R, Gage FH, Anderson AJ (2005) Human neural stem cells differentiate and promote locomotor recovery in spinal cord-injured mice. Proc Natl Acad Sci U S A 102(39):14069–14074

3. Hofstetter CP, Holmstrom NA, Lilja JA, Schweinhardt P, Hao J, Spenger C, Wiesenfeld-Hallin Z, Kurpad SN, Frisen J, Olson L (2005) Allodynia limits the usefulness of intraspinal neural stem cell grafts: directed differentiation improves outcome. Nat Neurosci 8(3):346–353
4. Iwanami A, Kaneko S, Nakamura M, Kanemura Y, Mori H, Kobayashi S, Yamasaki M, Momoshima S, Ishii H, Ando K, Tanioka Y, Tamaoki N, Nomura T, Toyama Y, Okano H (2005) Transplantation of human neural stem cells for spinal cord injury in primates. J Neurosci Res 80(2):182–190
5. Okada S, Ishii K, Yamane J, Iwanami A, Ikegami T, Katoh H, Iwamoto Y, Nakamura M, Miyoshi H, Okano HJ, Contag CH, Toyama Y, Okano H (2005) In vivo imaging of engrafted neural stem cells: its application in evaluating the optimal timing of transplantation for spinal cord injury. Faseb J 19(13):1839–1841
6. Rossi SL, Keirstead HS (2009) Stem cells and spinal cord regeneration. Curr Opin Biotechnol 20(5):552–562
7. Tsuji O, Miura K, Okada Y, Fujiyoshi K, Mukaino M, Nagoshi N, Kitamura K, Kumagai G, Nishino M, Tomisato S, Higashi H, Nagai T, Katoh H, Kohda K, Matsuzaki Y, Yuzaki M, Ikeda E, Toyama Y, Nakamura M, Yamanaka S, Okano H (2010) Therapeutic potential of appropriately evaluated safe-induced pluripotent stem cells for spinal cord injury. Proc Natl Acad Sci U S A 107(28):12704–12709
8. Keirstead HS, Nistor G, Bernal G, Totoiu M, Cloutier F, Sharp K, Steward O (2005) Human embryonic stem cell-derived oligodendrocyte progenitor cell transplants remyelinate and restore locomotion after spinal cord injury. J Neurosci 25(19):4694–4705
9. Kumagai G, Okada Y, Yamane J, Nagoshi N, Kitamura K, Mukaino M, Tsuji O, Fujiyoshi K, Katoh H, Okada S, Shibata S, Matsuzaki Y, Toh S, Toyama Y, Nakamura M, Okano H (2009) Roles of ES cell-derived gliogenic neural stem/progenitor cells in functional recovery after spinal cord injury. PLoS One 4(11):e7706
10. Kumagai G, Tsoulfas P, Toh S, McNiece I, Bramlett HM, Dietrich WD (2013) Genetically modified mesenchymal stem cells (MSCs) promote axonal regeneration and prevent hypersensitivity after spinal cord injury. Exp Neurol 248:369–380
11. Grove JE, Bruscia E, Krause DS (2004) Plasticity of bone marrow-derived stem cells. Stem Cells 22(4):487–500
12. Dexter TM (1982) Stromal cell associated haemopoiesis. J Cell Physiol Suppl 1:87–94
13. Van Damme A, Vanden Driessche T, Collen D, Chuah MK (2002) Bone marrow stromal cells as targets for gene therapy. Curr Gene Ther 2(2):195–209
14. Vaquero J, Zurita M (2009) Bone marrow stromal cells for spinal cord repair: a challenge for contemporary neurobiology. Histol Histopathol 24(1):107–116
15. Lu P, Tuszynski MH (2005) Can bone marrow-derived stem cells differentiate into functional neurons? Exp Neurol 193(2):273–278
16. Ankeny DP, McTigue DM, Jakeman LB (2004) Bone marrow transplants provide tissue protection and directional guidance for axons after contusive spinal cord injury in rats. Exp Neurol 190(1):17–31
17. Hofstetter CP, Schwarz EJ, Hess D, Widenfalk J, El Manira A, Prockop DJ, Olson L (2002) Marrow stromal cells form guiding strands in the injured spinal cord and promote recovery. Proc Natl Acad Sci U S A 99(4):2199–2204
18. Lu P, Jones LL, Tuszynski MH (2005) BDNF-expressing marrow stromal cells support extensive axonal growth at sites of spinal cord injury. Exp Neurol 191(2):344–360
19. Cizkova D, Rosocha J, Vanicky I, Jergova S, Cizek M (2006) Transplants of human mesenchymal stem cells improve functional recovery after spinal cord injury in the rat. Cell Mol Neurobiol 26(7–8):1167–1180
20. Himes BT, Neuhuber B, Coleman C, Kushner R, Swanger SA, Kopen GC, Wagner J, Shumsky JS, Fischer I (2006) Recovery of function following grafting of human bone marrow-derived stromal cells into the injured spinal cord. Neurorehabil Neural Repair 20(2):278–296
21. Chopp M, Zhang XH, Li Y, Wang L, Chen J, Lu D, Lu M, Rosenblum M (2000) Spinal cord injury in rat: treatment with bone marrow stromal cell transplantation. Neuroreport 11(13): 3001–3005

22. Wu S, Suzuki Y, Ejiri Y, Noda T, Bai H, Kitada M, Kataoka K, Ohta M, Chou H, Ide C (2003) Bone marrow stromal cells enhance differentiation of cocultured neurosphere cells and promote regeneration of injured spinal cord. J Neurosci Res 72(3):343–351
23. Abrams MB, Dominguez C, Pernold K, Reger R, Wiesenfeld-Hallin Z, Olson L, Prockop D (2009) Multipotent mesenchymal stromal cells attenuate chronic inflammation and injury-induced sensitivity to mechanical stimuli in experimental spinal cord injury. Restor Neurol Neurosci 27(4):307–321
24. Akiyama Y, Radtke C, Kocsis JD (2002) Remyelination of the rat spinal cord by transplantation of identified bone marrow stromal cells. J Neurosci 22(15):6623–6630
25. Wright KT, El Masri W, Osman A, Chowdhury J, Johnson WE (2011) Concise review: bone marrow for the treatment of spinal cord injury: mechanisms and clinical applications. Stem Cells 29(2):169–178
26. Kaplan DR, Miller FD (2000) Neurotrophin signal transduction in the nervous system. Curr Opin Neurobiol 10(3):381–391
27. Yamashita T, Fujitani M, Hata K, Mimura F, Yamagishi S (2005) Diverse functions of the p75 neurotrophin receptor. Anat Sci Int 80(1):37–41
28. Conte V, Royo N, Shimizu S, Saatman K, Watson D, Graham D, Stocchetti N, McIntosh T (2003) Neurotrophic factors. Eur J Trauma 29(6):335–355
29. Longhi L, Watson DJ, Saatman KE, Thompson HJ, Zhang C, Fujimoto S, Royo N, Castelbuono D, Raghupathi R, Trojanowski JQ, Lee VM, Wolfe JH, Stocchetti N, McIntosh TK (2004) Ex vivo gene therapy using targeted engraftment of NGF-expressing human NT2N neurons attenuates cognitive deficits following traumatic brain injury in mice. J Neurotrauma 21(12):1723–1736
30. Koda M, Kamada T, Hashimoto M, Murakami M, Shirasawa H, Sakao S, Ino H, Yoshinaga K, Koshizuka S, Moriya H, Yamazaki M (2007) Adenovirus vector-mediated ex vivo gene transfer of brain-derived neurotrophic factor to bone marrow stromal cells promotes axonal regeneration after transplantation in completely transected adult rat spinal cord. Eur Spine J 16(12):2206–2214
31. Zhang W, Yan Q, Zeng YS, Zhang XB, Xiong Y, Wang JM, Chen SJ, Li Y, Bruce IC, Wu W (2010) Implantation of adult bone marrow-derived mesenchymal stem cells transfected with the neurotrophin-3 gene and pretreated with retinoic acid in completely transected spinal cord. Brain Res 1359:256–271
32. Shang AJ, Hong SQ, Xu Q, Wang HY, Yang Y, Wang ZF, Xu BN, Jiang XD, Xu RX (2011) NT-3-secreting human umbilical cord mesenchymal stromal cell transplantation for the treatment of acute spinal cord injury in rats. Brain Res 1391:102–113
33. Urfer R, Tsoulfas P, Soppet D, Escandon E, Parada LF, Presta LG (1994) The binding epitopes of neurotrophin-3 to its receptors trkC and gp75 and the design of a multifunctional human neurotrophin. Embo J 13(24):5896–5909
34. Cao Q, Xu XM, Devries WH, Enzmann GU, Ping P, Tsoulfas P, Wood PM, Bunge MB, Whittemore SR (2005) Functional recovery in traumatic spinal cord injury after transplantation of multineurotrophin-expressing glial-restricted precursor cells. J Neurosci 25(30): 6947–6957
35. Golden KL, Pearse DD, Blits B, Garg MS, Oudega M, Wood PM, Bunge MB (2007) Transduced Schwann cells promote axon growth and myelination after spinal cord injury. Exp Neurol 207(2):203–217
36. Huang EJ, Reichardt LF (2003) Trk receptors: roles in neuronal signal transduction. Annu Rev Biochem 72:609–642
37. Dechant G, Barde YA (2002) The neurotrophin receptor p75(NTR): novel functions and implications for diseases of the nervous system. Nat Neurosci 5(11):1131–1136
38. Teng KK, Felice S, Kim T, Hempstead BL (2010) Understanding proneurotrophin actions: recent advances and challenges. Dev Neurobiol 70(5):350–359
39. Mi S, Lee X, Shao Z, Thill G, Ji B, Relton J, Levesque M, Allaire N, Perrin S, Sands B, Crowell T, Cate RL, McCoy JM, Pepinsky RB (2004) LINGO-1 is a component of the Nogo-66 receptor/p75 signaling complex. Nat Neurosci 7(3):221–228

40. Dubreuil CI, Winton MJ, McKerracher L (2003) Rho activation patterns after spinal cord injury and the role of activated Rho in apoptosis in the central nervous system. J Cell Biol 162(2):233–243
41. Yamashita T, Tucker KL, Barde YA (1999) Neurotrophin binding to the p75 receptor modulates Rho activity and axonal outgrowth. Neuron 24(3):585–593
42. Yamashita T, Higuchi H, Tohyama M (2002) The p75 receptor transduces the signal from myelin-associated glycoprotein to Rho. J Cell Biol 157(4):565–570
43. Dull T, Zufferey R, Kelly M, Mandel RJ, Nguyen M, Trono D, Naldini L (1998) A third-generation lentivirus vector with a conditional packaging system. J Virol 72(11):8463–8471
44. Basso DM, Beattie MS, Bresnahan JC (1995) A sensitive and reliable locomotor rating scale for open field testing in rats. J Neurotrauma 12(1):1–21
45. Pearse DD, Marcillo AE, Oudega M, Lynch MP, Wood PM, Bunge MB (2004) Transplantation of Schwann cells and olfactory ensheathing glia after spinal cord injury: does pretreatment with methylprednisolone and interleukin-10 enhance recovery? J Neurotrauma 21(9):1223–1239
46. Parr AM, Tator CH, Keating A (2007) Bone marrow-derived mesenchymal stromal cells for the repair of central nervous system injury. Bone Marrow Transplant 40(7):609–619
47. Yano S, Kuroda S, Lee JB, Shichinohe H, Seki T, Ikeda J, Nishimura G, Hida K, Tamura M, Iwasaki Y (2005) In vivo fluorescence tracking of bone marrow stromal cells transplanted into a pneumatic injury model of rat spinal cord. J Neurotrauma 22(8):907–918
48. Yoshihara H, Shumsky JS, Neuhuber B, Otsuka T, Fischer I, Murray M (2006) Combining motor training with transplantation of rat bone marrow stromal cells does not improve repair or recovery in rats with thoracic contusion injuries. Brain Res 1119(1):65–75
49. Park HW, Lim MJ, Jung H, Lee SP, Paik KS, Chang MS (2010) Human mesenchymal stem cell-derived Schwann cell-like cells exhibit neurotrophic effects, via distinct growth factor production, in a model of spinal cord injury. Glia 58(9):1118–1132
50. Fehlings MG, Wilcox JT (2011) Spinal cord injury and pain. J Neurosurg Spine 15(6):579–580, discussion 580–581
51. Hama A, Sagen J (2012) Combination drug therapy for pain following chronic spinal cord injury. Pain Res Treat 2012:840486
52. Pezet S, McMahon SB (2006) Neurotrophins: mediators and modulators of pain. Annu Rev Neurosci 29:507–538
53. von Schack D, Casademunt E, Schweigreiter R, Meyer M, Bibel M, Dechant G (2001) Complete ablation of the neurotrophin receptor p75NTR causes defects both in the nervous and the vascular system. Nat Neurosci 4(10):977–978
54. Caporali A, Pani E, Horrevoets AJ, Kraenkel N, Oikawa A, Sala-Newby GB, Meloni M, Cristofaro B, Graiani G, Leroyer AS, Boulanger CM, Spinetti G, Yoon SO, Madeddu P, Emanueli C (2008) Neurotrophin p75 receptor (p75NTR) promotes endothelial cell apoptosis and inhibits angiogenesis: implications for diabetes-induced impaired neovascularization in ischemic limb muscles. Circ Res 103(2):e15–e26

Chapter 22
Axonal Regeneration Across an Artificial Scaffold Combined with Cell Transplantation Applied to the Transected Spinal Cord

Mitsuhiro Enomoto, Madoka Ukegawa, Kazuyuki Fukushima, Kush Bhatt, Yoshiaki Wakabayashi, and Atsushi Okawa

Abstract The effectiveness of cell transplantation therapy for spinal cord injury (SCI) has been increasingly demonstrated in basic and clinical studies. Ethical considerations specific to Japan and a possible immune response justify the use of autologous cells obtained from patients with SCI. Currently available candidates for autologous cells include bone marrow stromal cells (BMSCs), Schwann cells derived from peripheral nerves, olfactory mucosal epithelial cells derived from the olfactory mucosa, and neural stem cells derived from attention-drawing induced pluripotent stem (iPS) cells. Among these, BMSCs have the advantage of being collected relatively easily from bone marrow and maintained in culture, and they are also known to have a protective effect on neural tissue. Studies have been conducted on bridging spinal cord defects with an artificial material known as a scaffold, and scaffolds made of various materials have been applied experimentally to the injured spinal cord. This review provides an overview of the results of studies in which a honeycomb collagen scaffold, as reported by us, or a macroporous scaffold made of

M. Enomoto (✉)
Department of Orthopaedic Surgery, Graduate School, Tokyo Medical and Dental University, 1-5-45 Yushima, Bunkyo, Tokyo, 113-8519, Japan

Hyperbaric Medical Center, Tokyo Medical and Dental University, 1-5-45 Yushima, Bunkyo, Tokyo 113-8519, Japan
e-mail: enomorth@tmd.ac.jp

M. Ukegawa • Y. Wakabayashi • A. Okawa
Department of Orthopaedic Surgery, Graduate School, Tokyo Medical and Dental University, 1-5-45 Yushima, Bunkyo, Tokyo, 113-8519, Japan

K. Fukushima
Department of Orthopaedic Surgery, Saku General Hospital, 197 Usuda, Saku, Nagano 384-0301, Japan

K. Bhatt
Imperial College, Tokyo Medical and Dental University Exchange Program, 1-5-45 Yushima, Bunkyo, Tokyo 113-8519, Japan

K. Uchida et al. (eds.), *Neuroprotection and Regeneration of the Spinal Cord*,
DOI 10.1007/978-4-431-54502-6_22,

D,L-polylactic acid combined with Schwann cells, as reported by Hurtado et al., was transplanted into the spinal cord. We also discuss the results of several studies on cell transplantation with scaffolds.

Keywords Cell transplantation • Regeneration • Scaffold • Spinal cord injury

22.1 Introduction

Regeneration of lost central neural tissue has generally been regarded as inconceivable. However, over the past 20 years, a number of studies have demonstrated the regeneration, repair, and functional recovery of the spinal cord in animal models. Recently, transplantation therapy for spinal cord injury (SCI) using stem or progenitor cells has been extensively reported [1, 2]. We reported in 2003 that embryonic hippocampus/spinal cord-derived neural progenitor cells (NPCs) transplanted into an intact spinal cord can differentiate into glial cells required for the maintenance of spinal cord homeostasis [3]. Subsequently, in 2009, we found that Rho GTPase plays an important role in successful neural stem cell transplantation in the injured spinal cord [4] and in 2010 that NPCs expressing neurotrophic factor-3 (NT-3) promote functional recovery of the injured cord when transplanted around the injured site in rats with chronic SCI [5]. Despite clear evidence of the effectiveness of embryonic brain/spinal cord-derived NPC transplantation for functional recovery of the injured spinal cord, ethical considerations specific to Japan and a possible immune response justify the use of autologous cells obtained from patients with SCI. Currently available candidates for autologous cells include bone marrow-derived mesenchymal stem cells or stromal cells (BMSCs), Schwann cells (SCs) derived from peripheral nerves, olfactory mucosal epithelial cells derived from the olfactory mucosa, and neural stem cells derived from attention-drawing induced pluripotent stem (iPS) cells. Among these, BMSCs can be collected relatively easily from bone marrow and maintained in culture. Another advantage of these cells is their known protective effect on neural tissue [6, 7]. BMSCs have also been injected into the spinal subarachnoid space (intrathecally) in patients with acute to subacute SCI and have demonstrated some favorable outcomes [8, 9]. However, controversy about the effectiveness of BMSC transplantation therapy warrants further basic studies.

Studies have long been conducted on bridging spinal cord defects with an artificial material known as a scaffold. A study in 2002 demonstrated that transplantation of a polymer scaffold seeded with neural stem cells results in the functional recovery of traumatically injured spinal cord [10], while another study reported on the transplantation of a scaffold made of polylactic acid and seeded with SCs genetically engineered to produce neurotrophic factors into a rat model of complete thoracic spinal cord transection [11]. A scaffold with self-assembling properties has also been reported in which materials self-assemble at the site of SCI in response to changes in body temperature and pH [12].

We have produced an atelocollagen-based honeycomb collagen (HC) sponge and performed in vitro experiments using HC sponges with different pore sizes as scaffolds and dorsal root ganglion (DRG) samples. We have also compared the atelocollagen-based HC and random-structure collagen (RC) sponges for spinal cord bridging in a thoracic spinal cord transection model and demonstrated better regeneration of neural fibers and functional recovery with HC than with RC sponges [13]. We have also demonstrated enhanced regeneration of neural fibers and functional recovery after transplantation of a BMSC-seeded HC sponge. Here, we provide an overview of the results of our previous studies and those of a study conducted by Hurtado et al., in which a polylactic acid scaffold seeded with SCs was implanted into the spinal cord [11].

22.2 Honeycomb Collagen Scaffold

22.2.1 Neurite Extension Through Honeycomb Collagen Sponges In Vitro

In 2001, the novel artificial extracellular matrix named HC was created from lyophilized type I atelocollagen and possesses a serial tunnel structure [14]. HC products have a 3-D structure in a unidirectional porous pattern (Fig. 22.1A). We developed collagen scaffolds with three different pore sizes with diameters of 130 μm (HC130), 200 μm (HC200), and 400 μm (HC400). Randomly pored collagen (RPC) was prepared without a unidirectional porous pattern as a control. To stabilize collagen sponges on culture dishes, we established a cubic framework made of 2 % agar in phosphate buffered saline with a center hole of 3 mm diameter and attached it to the bottom of the culture dish before preparing the E16 rat DRGs (Fig. 22.1B). DRGs were carefully placed onto the collagen sponges, which were then fixed after 6 days in vitro and immunostained with anti-neurofilament (NF) 200 antibody. NF-positive neurites were observed along the pore walls inside the HCs in the longitudinal 300 μm sections. To examine the ideal pore size, we cultured DRGs on the HC sponges with different pore sizes (HC130, HC200, and HC400) for 6 days (Fig. 22.1C). The length of the neurites sprouting into HC400 was significantly longer than that in HC130 and RPC (Fig. 22.1C).

22.2.2 Nerve Regeneration After Implantation of a Honeycomb Collagen Sponge into the Transected Spinal Cord

The exposed T8-9 spinal cord of 9-week-old female Sprague Dawley rats was completely transected for 2 mm with an ophthalmic blade. A 2-mm-long scaffold of HC400 or RPC was then implanted between the rostral and caudal spinal cord stumps.

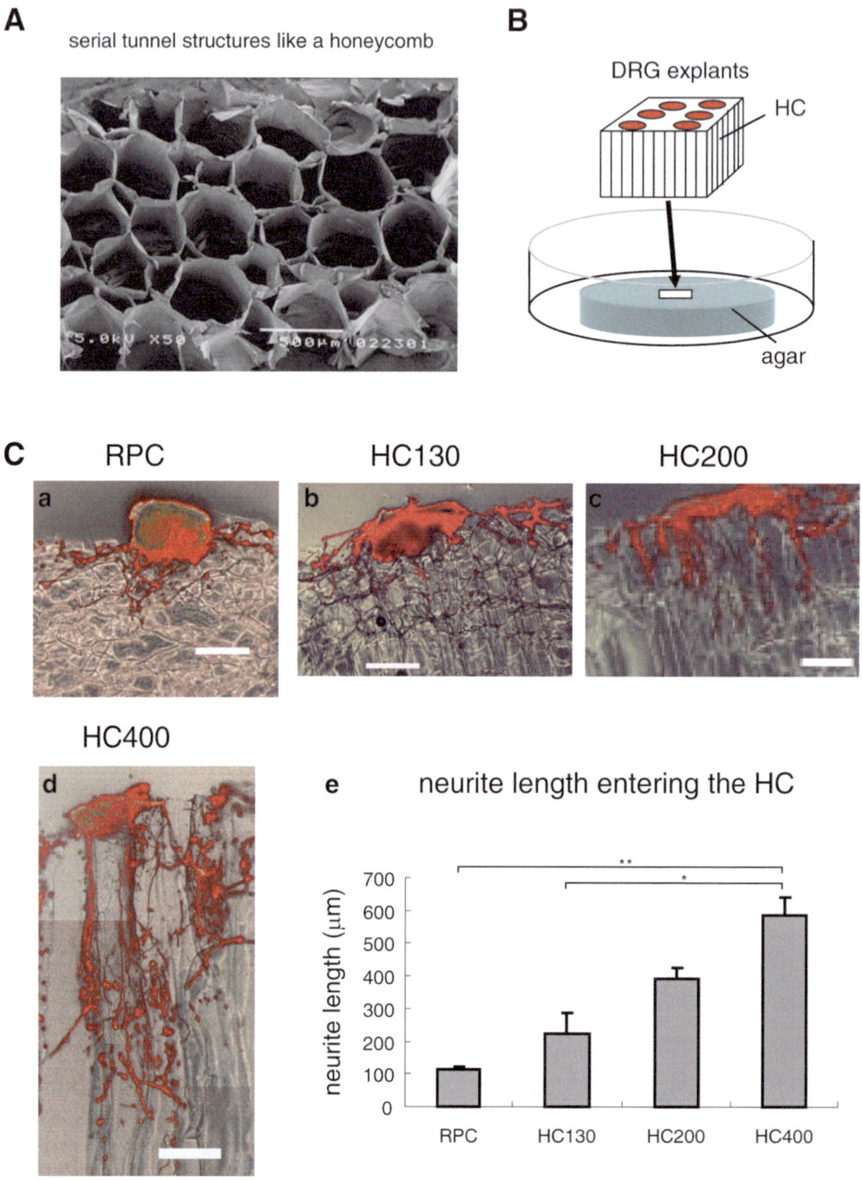

Fig. 22.1 Appearance of honeycomb collagen sponge (HC) and in vitro evaluation of dorsal root ganglions (DRGs) on HC. HC consists of serial tunnel structures resembling a honeycomb (**A**). HC with DRGs explants, indicated by *red circles*, in agarose gel (**B**). Neurofilament (NF)-positive fibers from DRG explants are visible in HC pores of different sizes (**C**, *a–d*). The length of neurites sprouting into HC400 was significantly longer than that of neurites sprouting into HC130 ($*P<0.05$) and RPC ($**P<0.01$). Scale bar: 300 μm (**C**) (Image adapted from Fukushima et al. [13])

Four weeks after implantation, animals were perfused transcardially with 4 % paraformaldehyde in 0.1 M PB, and a 14-mm-long spinal cord section containing the implant was dissected under a microscope. Sagittal sections (30 μm) through the scaffolds were cut on a cryostat and immunostained with NF 200 antibody. In RPCs, NF-positive fibers had penetrated the implanted site, but few fibers had crossed the rostral border (Fig. 22.2a). In contrast, NF-positive fibers were observed beyond the borders between the HCs and the host spinal cords 4 weeks after implantation (Fig. 22.2b). At higher magnification, many NF-positive fibers were observed parallel to the longitudinal midline of the implants (Fig. 22.2d), while several fibers were seen crossing the border between the implanted area and the stumps (Fig. 22.2c, e). These results suggest that the serial tunnel structure of the HCs have a guidance ability which promotes the regeneration of axons across the implanted area.

Several rats were examined by transcranial electrostimulation 10 weeks after HC implantation. Muscle-evoked potentials were observed in the right quadrant muscle with HC implantation. In addition, the spinal cord was re-transected at the distal stump. Both MEPs and contraction of the quadriceps disappeared after the transection. These results indicate that some descending pathways across the HC-implanted area had reconnected.

22.2.3 Neurite Extension Through Honeycomb Collagen Sponges with Bone Marrow Stromal Cells In Vitro and Application to the Hemisected Spinal Cord

BMSCs were prepared from adult Fischer 344 rats as previously described [15]. After one passage, BMSCs were transduced with lentiviral vectors expressing green fluorescent protein. HCs coated with 1 % fibronectin were prepared and mixed with dissociated BMSCs at a concentration of 2×10^5 cells per scaffold. HCs with or without BMSCs were stabilized in the agar filled with DRG medium. Tuj-1-positive neurites and GFP-positive BMSCs were observed in the tubular HC sections after 10 days in vitro (Fig. 22.3a). Quantitatively, neurite length was increased over twofold in the HC combined with BMSCs compared with the control HC, indicating that BMSCs directly support the elongation of neurites into HC in vitro (unpublished data).

For in vivo study, the exposed spinal cord of adult female Fischer 344 rats was hemisected at T9 and a 3-mm hemicord section on the right side was resected. HC or HC combined with BMSCs was implanted between the rostral and caudal spinal cord stumps. Four weeks after implantation, animals were perfused, and a 9-mm-long spinal cord section containing the implant was dissected under a microscope. Horizontal sections of the scaffolds were cut on a cryostat and immunostained with mouse monoclonal anti-SMI31 (a marker for neurofilament M+H) and either rabbit polyclonal anti-GFP antibody or calcitonin gene-related peptide (CGRP) antibody. These antibodies were visualized with appropriate fluorescent secondary antibodies.

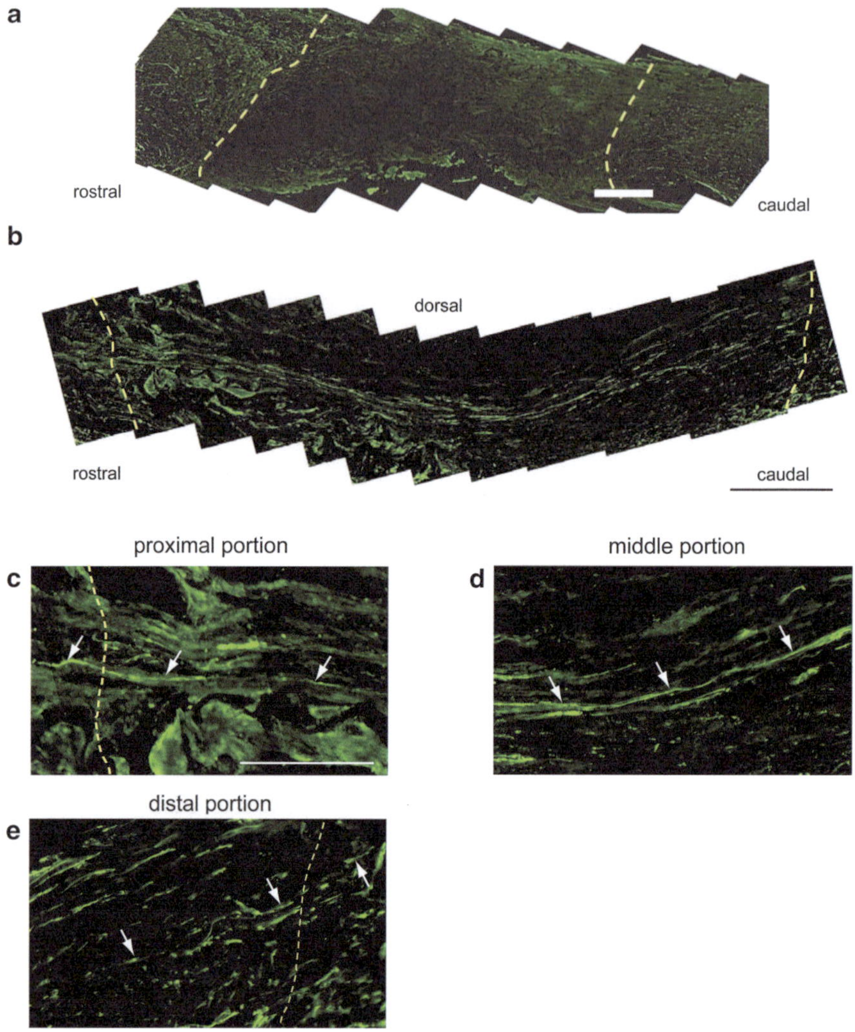

Fig. 22.2 Neurofilament staining of spinal cord-implanted HC. *Yellow dotted lines* indicate the border between the implant and spinal cord (**a**–**c**, **e**). Few NF-positive fibers are visible within the RPC-implanted site (**a**). Many NF-positive fibers are linear and bridge the length of the spinal cord-implanted HC 400 (**b**). In a higher magnification view of the rostral border between the HC and the spinal cord, NF-positive fibers (*arrows*) enter the implanted area across the rostral border between the spinal cord and the HC (**c**). In the middle portion, the NF-positive fibers (*arrows*) run in the sagittal direction (**d**). Some NF-positive fibers (*arrows*) cross the caudal border between the HC and spinal cord (**e**). Scale bar: 250 μm (**a**, **b**); 100 μm (**c**–**e**) (Image adapted from Fukushima et al. [13])

Four weeks after implantation, GFP-positive cells had survived in the implanted area of the HC combined with BMSCs, and SMI31-positive fibers were observed at the site (Fig. 22.3b). Quantitative analysis showed that more SMI31-positive fibers were observed in the HC combined with BMSCs than in the HC only (unpublished

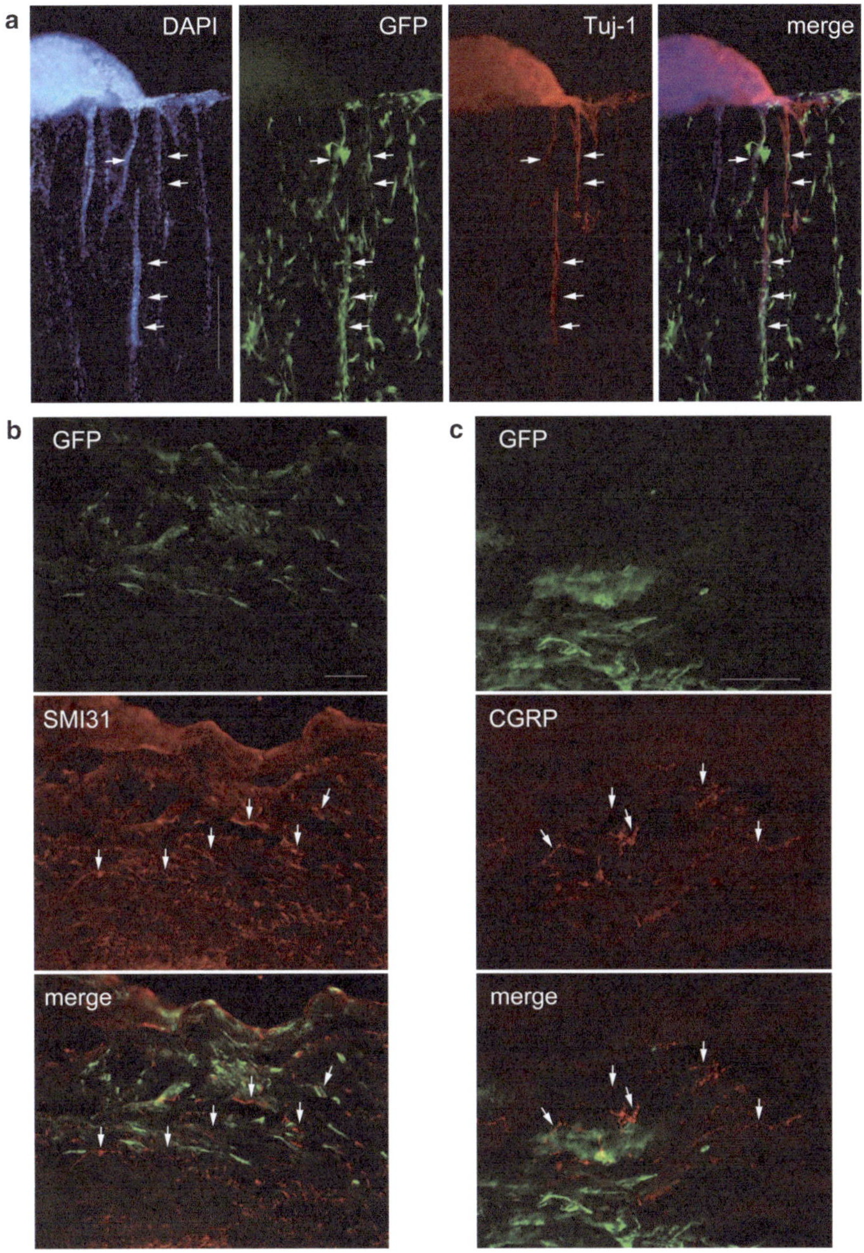

Fig. 22.3 Neurites extending through HC with bone marrow stromal cells in vitro and application to the hemisected spinal cord. The DRG explant is attached to the HC and extends Tuj-1-positive neurites toward and into the porous structure (**a**, *arrows*). Green fluorescent protein (GFP)-labeled BMSCs were distributed in the HC pores (**a**, *green*). GFP-positive cells (**b**, **c**, *green*) are visible at the implantation site. The regenerated nerve fibers are shown as SMI31-positive fibers (**b**, *arrows*). CGRP-positive fibers (**c**, *arrows*) close to the GFP-positive cells. Scale bar: 500 μm (**a**); 200 μm (**b**); 100 μm (**c**)

data). To analyze the growth of sensory fibers, we observed CGRP-positive fibers in the implanted spinal cord. These fibers were observed close to the GFP-positive area (Fig. 22.3c) as regenerated fibers possibly guided by the transplanted BMSCs.

22.3 Poly (D,L-Lactic Acid) Macroporous Scaffold

22.3.1 Implantation of a Poly (D,L-Lactic Acid) Scaffold Combined with Schwann Cells Secreting D15A, a Bifunctional Neurotrophin into the Transected Spinal Cord

The generation and characterization of SC cultures from adult Fischer 344 rat sciatic nerves were described previously [16]. SCs secreting D15A, which has been found to bind and activate TrkB, TrkC, and p75NTR [17], were generated. Freeze-dried poly (D,L-lactic acid) (PLA) macroporous guidance scaffolds have been developed and applied to the transected spinal cord [18]. The scaffolds have longitudinally oriented macropores connected by micropores (Fig. 22.4A), and the diameter of the macropores varies between 75 and 200 μm. Hurtado et al. filled this scaffold with genetically modified rat SCs and analyzed cell survival, scaffold integration, and the axonal regeneration response following implantation into the completely transected thoracic spinal cord of adult rats. The scaffolds were filled with 1 % fibrinogen in DMEM containing 2 % $CaCl_2$, 0.2 % gentamicin, and 2 % aprotinin. A fibrin mixture at a concentration of 1×10^6 cells per scaffold was placed on top of the scaffold, which was drawn gently inside by placing it onto Whatman filter paper. Cells were generally uniformly distributed within the pores of the scaffold, although some small clusters of cells could also be discerned (Fig. 22.4A).

For in vivo study, the exposed T9-10 spinal cord of adult female Fischer 344 rats was transected and 3 mm of tissue which included visible spinal roots was resected. A 4-mm-long scaffold with GFP-SCs or D15A-GFP-SCs, or the 1 % fibrin solution alone as a negative control, was implanted between the rostral and caudal spinal cord stumps. At 1, 2, and 6 weeks after implantation, animals were perfused and a 10-mm-long spinal cord section containing the implant was

→

Fig. 22.4 (continued) (**A**, *upper right*) of the scaffold. Horizontal cryostat sections counterstained with DAPI reveal GFP-positive Schwann cells (SCs) in the scaffold at 1 h (**A**, *lower left*) and 6 h (**A**, *lower right*) after seeding. GFP-positive SCs in the zone between the scaffold (S) and the host spinal cord (H) at 1 week (**B**, *a*), 2 weeks (**B**, *b*), and 6 weeks (**B**, *c*) after implantation. The SCs are mostly elongated and express fluorescent GFP throughout the soma. Axons rapidly extended to the scaffold seeded with D15A-GFP-SCs (**C**). Some axons had grown into the scaffold with either type of SC at 2 weeks (**C**, *left*). RT97-positive axons were associated with GFP-expressing SCs within the scaffold at 6 weeks (**C**, *right*) (Image adapted from Hurtado et al. [11])

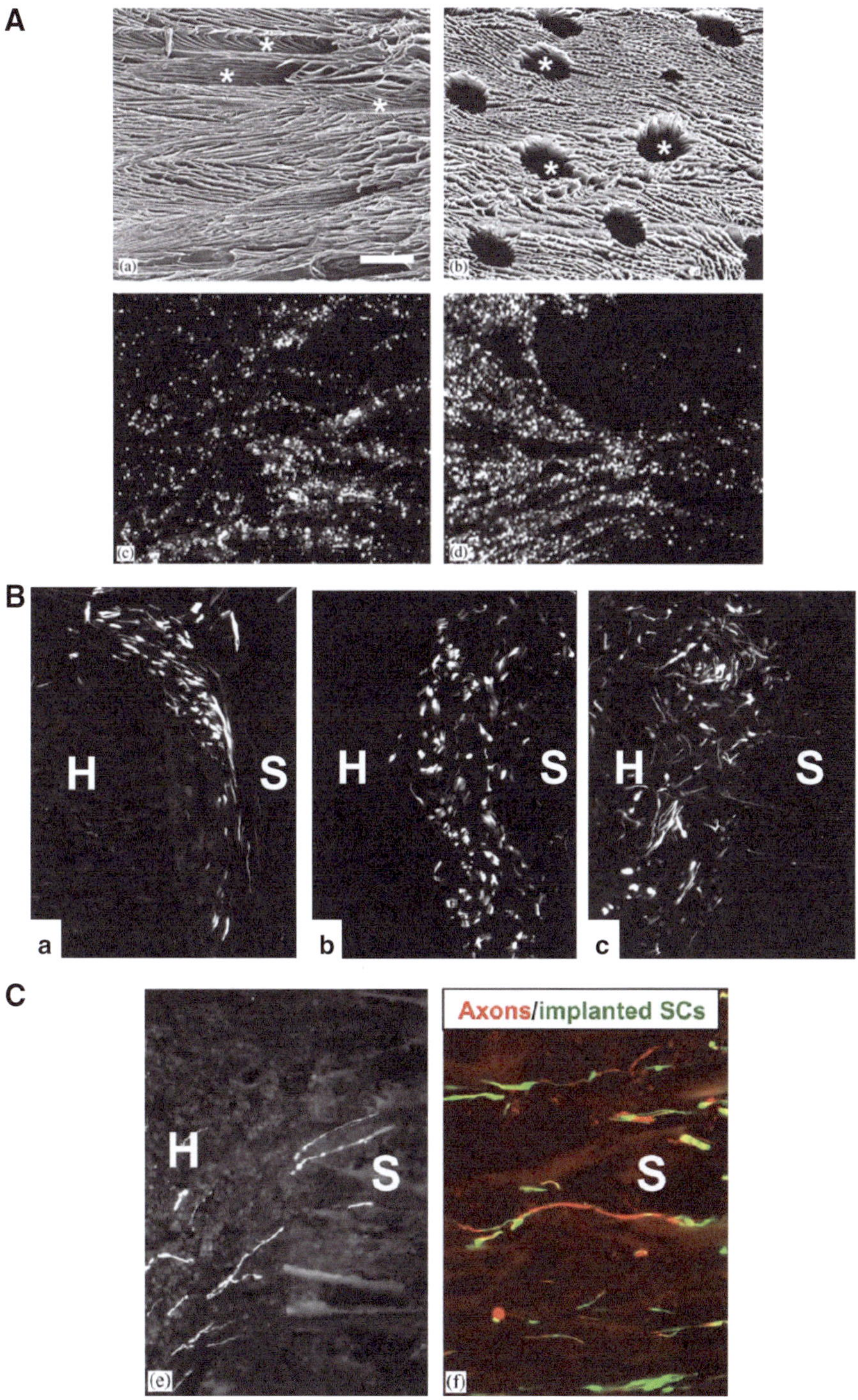

Fig. 22.4 Schwann cell-seeded D,L-polylactic acid scaffolds in the transected spinal cord. Scanning electron micrographs showing a longitudinal section (**A**, *upper left*) and cross section

dissected under a microscope. Horizontal sections of the scaffolds were cut on a cryostat and immunostained with mouse monoclonal antibody against p75, a low-affinity nerve growth factor receptor (192IgG, a marker for SCs), or anti-neurofilament antibody RT97 (a marker for neurofilament H). These antibodies were visualized with appropriate fluorescent secondary antibodies.

Three days after implantation, GFP-positive SCs with elongated processes and expressing bright GFP fluorescence were present within the scaffold and in the region between the scaffold and the host spinal cord. At later time points, a decreasing number of GFP-SCs were observed within the scaffold. Furthermore, at 1 week, 2 weeks (Fig. 22.4B), and 6 weeks (Fig. 22.4B), SCs were found between the scaffold and the cord. The distribution of p75-positive cells was largely similar between rats implanted with a scaffold seeded with fibrin only, GFP-SCs, and D15A-GFP-SCs. At 2 and 6 weeks after grafting, increasing numbers of p75-positive SC were visible in the region between the scaffold and the host cord. Neurofilament-positive axons were also found within the scaffolds seeded with either type of SCs at 2 and 6 weeks (Fig. 22.4C), but not in fibrin-only scaffolds. Often the axons appeared to have penetrated the pores within the scaffold but had not fully extended across the scaffold. The neurofilament-positive axons were associated with implanted SCs (Fig. 22.4C, green) within the scaffold at 6 weeks after implantation.

22.4 Discussion

A scaffold is considered essential for the regeneration of spinal cord tissue in the cavity that forms after SCI. Developments in material engineering have led to the production of scaffolds made of various materials, such as silicone, polyacrylonitrile/polyvinylchloride, collagen, polyglycolic acid, and PLA, and their ability to promote regeneration of the injured spinal cord has been tested [19]. Kuboki et al. proposed “artificial extracellular matrix geometry” by focusing on the importance of the three-dimensional structure of scaffolds and suggested that the geometry of a scaffold significantly influences cellular differentiation into bone, cartilage, or blood vessels and the subsequent growth of these tissues [20]. The HC sponge, developed by Koken Co., Ltd., has a honeycomb structure with uniaxially aligned communicating pores. This material had not been used in neural tissue regeneration studies prior to our studies. An in vitro study using DRG by Fukushima et al. revealed that different HC pore sizes are associated with different neurite outgrowth. Hurtado et al. demonstrated that the use of aligned PLA microfibers resulted in the linear extension of neural fibers from a DRG neurite, yielding greater neurite outgrowth than with a random-structure scaffold [21]. These findings indicate that the geometry of scaffolds also influences in vitro neurite outgrowth, as proposed by Kuboki et al. Fukushima et al. also implanted an HC scaffold into a defect in the rat thoracic spinal cord and found more neural fiber bridges had formed 4 weeks after implantation than with a control collagen sponge with randomly aligned pores. A spinal cord transplantation study conducted by Hurtado et al. showed the extension of more neuronal axons in aligned PLA microfiber scaffolds than in random fiber scaffolds [21]. In addition, implantation of a freeze-dried agarose scaffold with a honeycomb structure into the spinal cord was reported by Stokols and Tuszynski [22]. They noted linear extension of regenerating neural fibers in the scaffold and suggested the honeycomb structure is required for spinal cord regeneration. From these findings, it can be concluded that the geometry of scaffolds has a clear impact on tissue regeneration of the spinal cord.

For further functional reconstruction of the injured spinal cord, implantation of a scaffold alone is unlikely to be sufficient, and the combined use of scaffolds with cell transplantation is essential in both acute and chronic cases of severe crush injury. BMSCs with established safety were allowed to attach to the HC scaffold and were transplanted into an injured spinal cord (Fig. 22.3). BMSCs do not readily differentiate into neural cells and so are not able to survive for long periods in neural tissue after transplantation, but BMSCs have been shown to be capable of producing various neurotrophic factors [23, 24]. We initially evaluated the effect of BMSCs on neurite outgrowth using the in vitro evaluation criteria proposed by Fukushima et al. Enhanced neurite outgrowth was observed in the presence of BMSCs, demonstrating the ability of BMSCs to promote neurite outgrowth. Although the precise mechanism of this effect is unknown, possible mechanisms include the effect of the neurotrophic factors produced by BMSCs or interactions between the cell adhesion factors expressed by BMSCs and neurites. Implantation of HC scaffolds seeded with GFP-labeled BMSCs in a rat model of thoracic spinal cord hemisection resulted in improved motor and sensory functions, with many regenerating neural fibers observed in the HC scaffolds. These findings demonstrate that transplantation of BMSCs with HC scaffolds promotes the bridging of neural fibers at the site of injury, thereby contributing to functional reconstruction of the spinal cord. SC transplantation after SCI provides a favorable environment for axonal regeneration and myelination [25]. Hurtado et al. transplanted D15A-producing SCs (D15A-GFP-SCs) with a scaffold. D15A is a bifunctional neurotrophin with BDNF and NT-3 functions known to promote regeneration of both motor and sensory neurons. In the present study, however, no significant difference was observed in motor function improvement after transplantation of SCs alone or in combination with a scaffold. Although D15A-GFP-SCs were abundant at the host spinal cord-scaffold junction (Fig. 22.4B), only a few regenerating neuronal axons were observed in the macroporous structure. The authors explained that the scaffold contained few viable transplanted SCs and that the 6-week observation period was too short to detect neuronal regeneration. SCs have better ability than BMSCs to remyelinate injured axons after SCI, but to improve functional recovery further, the shape of the scaffolds could be improved to help promote survival of the transplanted cells. Neuronal bridging in the HC and PLA scaffolds was observed in the cranio-caudal direction, given that the normal spinal cord has neural connections in the coronal as well as cranio-caudal direction implies the need to develop these scaffolds with coronally aligned pores.

Furthermore, creating scaffolds appropriate to the severity of injury requires the application of image reconstruction technology that enables accurate assessment of injured areas or cavities, as well as three-dimensional printing technology.

Another promising approach for spinal cord regeneration is the application of iPS cells, a type of pluripotent stem cells derived from adult tissues that is drawing some considerable attention [26]. The combined use of iPS cell-derived neural stem cells with an ideal scaffold could provide an important breakthrough in spinal cord regeneration in the future.

22.5 Conclusion

In this overview of studies on spinal cord regeneration using HC or PLA macroporous scaffolds, we have seen that the geometry of scaffolds has a significant impact on tissue regeneration of the spinal cord and cell transplantation combined with an appropriate scaffold can enhance functional recovery. Among the currently available somatic stem cells derived from autologous tissue, we believe that the use of BMSCs is the most effective option. Further efforts are needed to improve scaffold structure and develop methods for promoting the long-term survival of transplanted cells and thus the regeneration of spinal cord tissue.

Acknowledgements We are grateful to Prof. K. Shinomiya (Yokohama City Minato Red Cross Hospital) and Prof. Y Kuboki (Hokkaido University) for their advice and generous support. We thank Dr. A. Hurtado (Kennedy Krieger/Johns Hopkins University) for advice regarding our animal surgery. This work was supported in part by a Grant-in-Aid for Scientific Research from the Japan Society for the Promotion of Science and a Grant-in-Aid from the General Insurance Association of Japan.

Conflict of Interest None of the authors has any commercial association that might pose or create a conflict of interest with information presented in this article.

References

1. Ruff CA, Wilcox JT, Fehlings MG (2012) Cell-based transplantation strategies to promote plasticity following spinal cord injury. Exp Neurol 235:78–90
2. Mothe AJ, Tator CH (2012) Advances in stem cell therapy for spinal cord injury. J Clin Invest 122:3824–3834
3. Enomoto M, Shinomiya K, Okabe S (2003) Migration and differentiation of neural progenitor cells from two different regions of embryonic central nervous system after transplantation into the intact spinal cord. Eur J Neurosci 17:1223–1232
4. Numano F, Inoue A, Enomoto M, Shinomiya K, Okawa A, Okabe S (2009) Critical involvement of Rho GTPase activity in the efficient transplantation of neural stem cells into the injured spinal cord. Mol Brain 2:37
5. Kusano K, Enomoto M, Hirai T, Tsoulfas P, Sotome S, Shinomiya K, Okawa A (2010) Transplanted neural progenitor cells expressing mutant NT3 promote myelination and partial hindlimb recovery in the chronic phase after spinal cord injury. Biochem Biophys Res Commun 393:812–817
6. Vaquero J, Zurita M (2009) Bone marrow stromal cells for spinal cord repair: a challenge for contemporary neurobiology. Histol Histopathol 24:107–116

7. Vaquero J, Zurita M (2011) Functional recovery after severe CNS trauma: current perspectives for cell therapy with bone marrow stromal cells. Prog Neurobiol 93:341–349
8. Saito F, Nakatani T, Iwase M, Maeda Y, Hirakawa A, Murao Y, Suzuki Y, Onodera R, Fukushima M, Ide C (2008) Spinal cord injury treatment with intrathecal autologous bone marrow stromal cell transplantation: the first clinical trial case report. J Trauma 64:53–59
9. Saito F, Nakatani T, Iwase M, Maeda Y, Murao Y, Suzuki Y, Fukushima M, Ide C (2012) Administration of cultured autologous bone marrow stromal cells into cerebrospinal fluid in spinal injury patients: a pilot study. Restor Neurol Neurosci 30:127–136
10. Teng YD, Lavik EB, Qu X, Park KI, Ourednik J, Zurakowski D, Langer R, Snyder EY (2002) Functional recovery following traumatic spinal cord injury mediated by a unique polymer scaffold seeded with neural stem cells. Proc Natl Acad Sci U S A 99:3024–3029
11. Hurtado A, Moon LD, Maquet V, Blits B, Jérôme R, Oudega M (2006) Poly (D,L-lactic acid) macroporous guidance scaffolds seeded with Schwann cells genetically modified to secrete a bi-functional neurotrophin implanted in the completely transected adult rat thoracic spinal cord. Biomaterials 27:430–442
12. Cigognini D, Satta A, Colleoni B, Silva D, Donegà M, Antonini S, Gelain F (2011) Evaluation of early and late effects into the acute spinal cord injury of an injectable functionalized self-assembling scaffold. PLoS One 6:e19782
13. Fukushima K, Enomoto M, Tomizawa S, Takahashi M, Wakabayashi Y, Itoh S, Kuboki Y, Shinomiya K (2008) The axonal regeneration across a honeycomb collagen sponge applied to the transected spinal cord. J Med Dent Sci 55:71–79
14. Itoh H, Aso Y, Furuse M, Noishiki Y, Miyata T (2001) A honeycomb collagen carrier for cell culture as a tissue engineering scaffold. Artif Organs 25:213–217
15. Woodbury D, Schwarz EJ, Prockop DJ, Black IB (2000) Adult rat and human bone marrow stromal cells differentiate into neurons. J Neurosci Res 61:364–370
16. Morrissey TK, Kleitman N, Bunge RP (1991) Isolation and functional characterization of Schwann cells derived from adult peripheral nerve. J Neurosci 11:2433–2442
17. Urfer R, Tsoulfas P, Soppet D, Escandón E, Parada LF, Presta LG (1994) The binding epitopes of neurotrophin-3 to its receptors trkC and gp75 and the design of a multifunctional human neurotrophin. EMBO J 13:5896–5909
18. Patist CM, Mulder MB, Gautier SE, Maquet V, Jérôme R, Oudega M (2004) Freeze-dried poly(D, L-lactic acid) macroporous guidance scaffolds impregnated with brain-derived neurotrophic factor in the transected adult rat thoracic spinal cord. Biomaterials 25:1569–1582
19. Straley KS, Foo CW, Heilshorn SC (2010) Biomaterial design strategies for the treatment of spinal cord injuries. J Neurotrauma 27:1–19
20. Kuboki Y, Jin Q, Takita H (2001) Geometry of carriers controlling phenotypic expression in BMP-induced osteogenesis and chondrogenesis. J Bone Joint Surg Am 83-A(Suppl 1): S105–115
21. Hurtado A, Cregg JM, Wang HB, Wendell DF, Oudega M, Gilbert RJ, McDonald JW (2011) Robust CNS regeneration after complete spinal cord transection using aligned poly-L-lactic acid microfibers. Biomaterials 32:6068–6079
22. Stokols S, Tuszynski MH (2006) Freeze-dried agarose scaffolds with uniaxial channels stimulate and guide linear axonal growth following spinal cord injury. Biomaterials 27:443–451
23. Nandoe Tewarie RD, Oudega M, Ritfeld GJ (2012) Bone marrow stromal cells for repair of the injured spinal cord. In: Demirer T (ed) New advances in stem cell transplantation, ISBN: 978-953-51-0013-3, InTech, Available from: http://www.intechopen.com/books/new-advances-in-stem-celltransplantation/bone-marrow-stromal-cells-for-repair-of-the-injured-spinal-cord
24. Kim JW, Ha KY, Molon JN, Kim YH (2013) Bone marrow-derived mesenchymal stem cell transplantation for chronic spinal cord injury in rats: comparative study between intralesional and intravenous transplantation. Spine (Phila Pa 1976) 38:E1065–1074
25. Wiliams RR, Bunge MB (2012) Schwann cell transplantation: a repair strategy for spinal cord injury? Prog Brain Res 201:295–312
26. Nakamura M, Okano H (2013) Cell transplantation therapies for spinal cord injury focusing on induced pluripotent stem cells. Cell Res 23:70–80

Chapter 23
Transplantation of Mesenchymal Stem Cells Derived from Bone Marrow in the Injured Spinal Cord

Hideaki Nakajima, Kenzo Uchida, Alexander Rodriguez Guerrero, Shuji Watanabe, Daisuke Sugita, Naoto Takeura, Ai Yoshida, and Hisatoshi Baba

Abstract The present study was designed to investigate the effects of mesenchymal stem cells (MSC) transplantation with a special focus on their effect on macrophage activation after SCI. The transplanted MSC migrated within the injured spinal cord without differentiating into glial or neuronal elements. MSC transplantation was associated with marked changes in the SCI environment, with significant increases in IL-4 and IL-13 levels reductions in TNF-α and IL-6 levels. This was associated simultaneously with increased numbers of alternatively activated macrophages (M2 phenotype: arginase-1 or CD206-positive) and decreased numbers of classically activated macrophages (M1 phenotype: iNOS or CD16/32-positive). These changes were associated with functional locomotor recovery in the MSC-transplanted group, which correlated with preserved axons, less scar tissue formation, and increased myelin sparring. Our results suggested that acute transplantation of MSC after SCI modified the inflammatory environment by shifting the macrophage

H. Nakajima (✉) • K. Uchida • D. Sugita • N. Takeura • A. Yoshida • S. Watanabe • H. Baba
Faculty of Medical Sciences, Department of Orthopaedics and Rehabilitation Medicine, University of Fukui, Matsuoka Shimoaizuki 23-3, Eiheiji, Fukui 910-1193, Japan
e-mail: nhideaki@u-fukui.ac.jp

A.R. Guerrero
Department of Orthopaedics and Rehabilitation Medicine, University of Fukui, 23-3 Matsuoka Shimoaizuki, Eiheiji, Fukui 910-1193, Japan

Service of Neurosurgery, Hospital Nacional Rosales, University of El Salvador, San Salvador, El Salvador

K. Uchida et al. (eds.), *Neuroprotection and Regeneration of the Spinal Cord*, DOI 10.1007/978-4-431-54502-6_23, © Springer Japan 2014

phenotype from M1 to M2 and that this may reduce the effects of the inhibitory scar tissue in the subacute/chronic phase after injury to provide a permissive environment for axonal extension and functional recovery.

Keywords Bone marrow • Macrophage • Mesenchymal stem cell • Spinal cord injury • Transplantation

23.1 Introduction

Mesenchymal stem cells (MSCs) derived from the bone marrow have been shown to promote anatomical and functional recovery in animal models of SCI by promoting tissue sparing [1] and axonal regeneration [2]. The therapeutic benefits of MSC are thought to be primarily related to their secretion of soluble factors and the provision of an extracellular matrix that provides neural protection and support and secondarily to remyelination [3, 4] and neural differentiation [5]. MSCs are attractive candidates for transplantation into patients because they can be easily harvested, expanded and stored, or obtained directly from the patient allowing for autologous transplantation. Evidence suggests that MSCs are immunosuppressive [6], i.e., they possess anti-inflammatory activity and have been used to abrogate graft-versus-host disease [7]. This property, in particular, may contribute to their capacity to reduce the acute inflammatory response to SCI and hence reduce cavity formation as well as decrease astrocyte and microglia/macrophage reactivity [8]. Importantly, MSC transplantation in experimental SCI is reported to enhance tissue preservation after SCI and reduce injury-induced sensitivity to mechanical stimuli, which is functionally indicative of anti-inflammatory activity [9].

Considering the inflammatory response after SCI, different macrophages populations have been found locally, based on their phenotypes and activity, but two subtypes have become of great interest: classically activated macrophages (termed the M1 phenotype) or alternatively activated macrophages (M2 phenotype) [10]. Classically activated macrophages are the product of exposure to T helper 1 (Th1) cytokines, e.g., interferon gamma (IFN-γ) and tumor necrosis factor alpha (TNF-α). Alternatively activated macrophages are the product of T helper 2 (Th2) cytokines, e.g., interleukin (IL)-4 and IL-13 [10].

Alternatively activated macrophages do not only have enhanced phagocytic capacity but also possess anti-inflammatory activity and hence have beneficial effects during the recovery of SCI [11, 12]. MSC transplantation into SCI lesions also attenuates acute inflammation and this is beneficial to functional recovery following SCI. However, the precise mechanisms through which the transplanted MSC attenuate the inflammation after SCI are still unclear. The present study was thus designed to investigate the effects of MSC transplantation in rats with SCI. Specifically, we focused on the potential effects of MSC on alternatively activated macrophages after SCI.

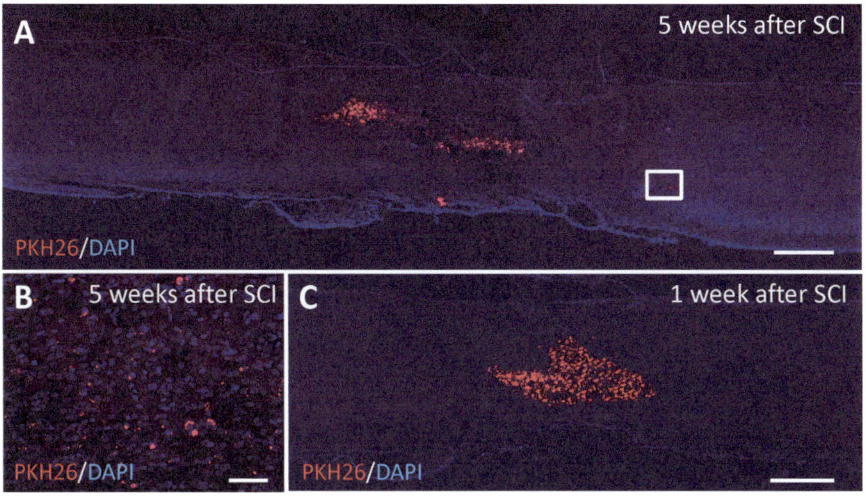

Fig. 23.1 Photomicrograph showing the distribution of PKH26-labeled transplanted MSC counterstained with DAPI staining for nuclei at 1 and 5 weeks after spinal cord injury. Transplanted PKH26-induced fluorescent MSCs survived and appeared only around the injured site at 1 week after spinal cord injury (**c**), whereas a number of PKH-positive cells extended out of the injured lesion at 5 weeks after spinal cord injury (**a**, **b**). (**b**) High-power photomicrograph of the box area of (**a**). Scale bar = 1 mm (**a**, **c**), 50 μm (**b**) (Reprinted, with permission, from [14])

23.1.1 Distribution of Transplanted MSC in Injured Spinal Cord

For in vivo tracing, the human MSC ($CD105^+$, $CD166^+$, $CD29^+$, $CD44^+$, $CD14^-$, $CD34^-$, $CD45^-$) were pre-labeled with the membrane dye PKH26 according to the instructions provided by the manufacturer (Sigma-Aldrich, St. Louis, MO). Three days after the injury (Infinite Horizons Impactor with an impact force of 200 kdyn at T9-10 vertebral level), MSCs were pre-labeled with the membrane dye PKH26, and then 1.0×10^6 MSCs in 5 μL MSCBM were injected into the contusion epicenter using a microsyringe in the treatment group. The control rats were injected with 5 μL of MSCBM alone (no cells) at 3 days after SCI.

The distribution of PKH26-labeled MSC in the injured spinal cord was assessed at 1 and 5 weeks after transplantation in harvested sagittal tissue sections. At 1 week after injury, the transplanted MSCs were distributed only around the injured lesion (Fig. 23.1c). On the other hand, the cells extended out of the injured lesion at 5 weeks (Fig. 23.1a, b). The PKH26-positive area after SCI was 1.23 ± 0.29 mm^2 at 1 week and 0.21 ± 0.06 mm^2 at 5 weeks; those were 72.1 ± 16.8 % and 11.9 ± 3.6 %, respectively, relative to the area at 3 days after SCI.

Immunostaining of spinal cord sections for NeuN, RIP, GFAP, and OX-42 was performed at 5 weeks after transplantation of MSC. There was no obvious colocalization of NeuN, RIP, GFAP, or OX-42 with PKH26-identified MSC. These results indicated that although the MSCs were distributed in areas rich in glial and neuronal processes, there was no evidence that the MSCs themselves had transdifferentiated into glial or neuronal cells.

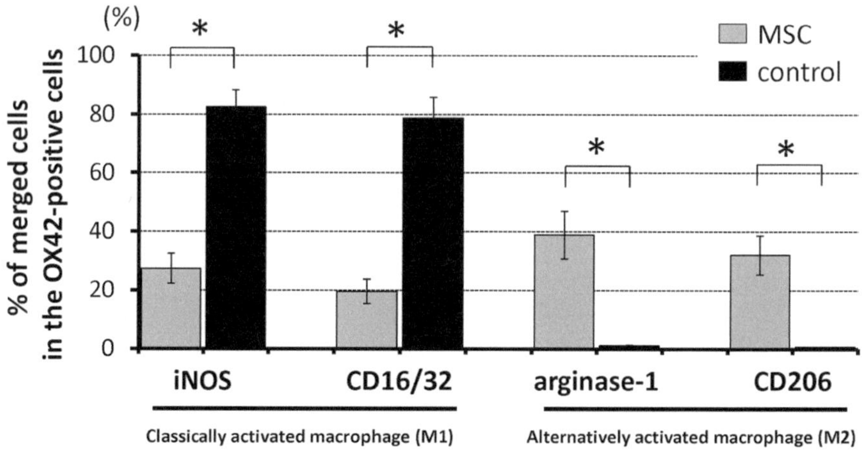

Fig. 23.2 The graph showing differences in the expression of iNOS and CD16/32 for classically activated macrophages (M1 phenotype) and arginase-1 and CD206 for alternatively activated macrophages (M2 phenotype) colocalized OX-42 after MSC transplantation in the injured spinal cord at 1 week after spinal cord injury. Percentage of merged cells of OX42-positive cells in the area 0–1 mm caudal and rostral to the epicenter. Data are mean ± SD. $^*p<0.05$ (Reprinted, in part, with permission, from [14])

23.1.2 *Effects of MSC Transplantation on Phenotype of Infiltrated Macrophages After Spinal Cord Injury*

Higher numbers of classically activated macrophages located mainly in the gray matter around the site of injury, co-expressing iNOS, CD16/32, and OX-42, were found in the control group (82.5 ± 5.8 % and 78.7 ± 7.1 % of OX42-positive cells, respectively) compared with the MSC-transplanted group (27.4 ± 5.1 % and 19.6 ± 4.2 % of the OX42-positive cells, respectively). On the other hand, consistently higher numbers of alternatively activated macrophages, co-expressing arginase-1/CD206 and OX-42, were found in the MSC-transplanted group (38.9 ± 8.1 % and 32.1 ± 6.6 % of the OX42-positive cells, respectively), with a more localized distribution at the site of injury. On the other hand, only a few arginase-1/CD206/OX42-positive cells were seen in the control group (1.2 ± 0.1 % and 0.8 ± 0.05 % of the OX42-positive cells, respectively) (Fig. 23.2).

The profile of the identified macrophages ($CD45^{positive}/CD11b^{high}/GR\text{-}1^{negative}$ cells) was also analyzed quantitatively using flow cytometry. The proportions of $CD45^{positive}/CD11b^{high}/GR\text{-}1^{negative}$ cells (macrophages) within the injured spinal cord were higher in both the MSC (24.5 ± 1.9 %) and control group (30.4 ± 2.1 %) compared with the sham (laminectomy only) group (4.5 ± 1.3 %) at 1 week after SCI. In the control group, at 1 week after SCI, 93.4 ± 5.6 % of these cells were $iNOS^{positive}$ classically activated macrophages (M1 phenotype; 70,984 ± 4,256 cells) whereas no $arginase\text{-}1^{positive}$ alternatively activated macrophages (M2 phenotype) were present. In comparison, in the MSC-transplanted group, only 11.7 ± 1.3 % of these cells were

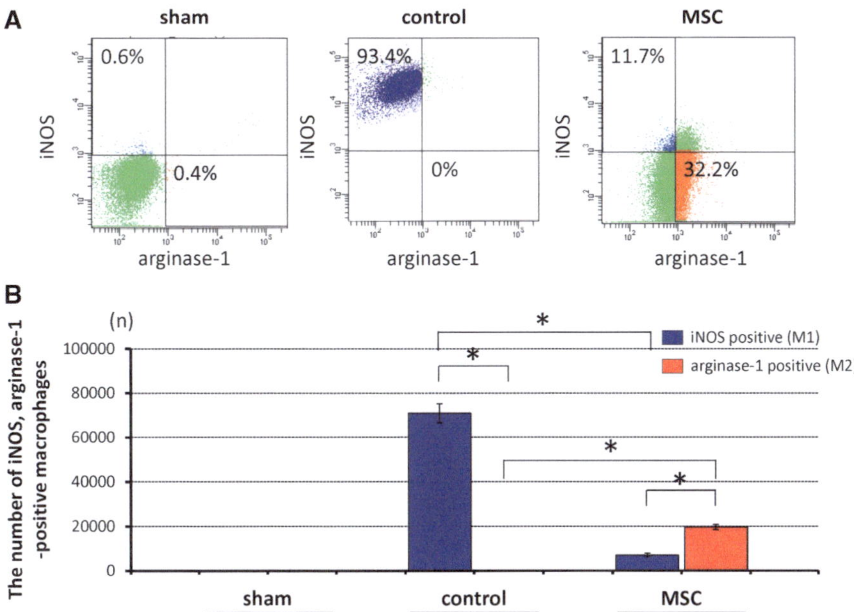

Fig. 23.3 Representative flow cytometry data at 1 week after injury. The number of iNOS^{positive} or arginase-1^{positive} cells within the CD45^{positive}/CD11b^{high}/GR-1^{negative} (macrophages) populations is different between MSC-transplanted and control groups (**a**). Number of iNOS- and arginase-1-positive cells in 250,000 analyzed cells. MSC transplantation reduced the proportion of iNOS^{positive} cells (*blue*, M1 phenotype) and shifted the macrophage phenotype to arginase-1^{positive} cells (*red*, M2 phenotype) at 1 week after spinal cord injury (**b**). Data are mean ± SD. *$p<0.05$ (Reprinted, with permission, from [14])

iNOS^{positive} (7,166 ± 796 cells) and 32.2 ± 1.9 % were arginase-1^{positive} (19,723 ± 1,164 cells) (Fig. 23.3a, b). The difference in the proportions of iNOS^{positive} and arginase-1positive cells between the MSC-transplanted and control group indicated that MSC transplantation seems to reduce the classically activated macrophages (M1 phenotype) and shift the macrophage phenotype to the alternatively activated macrophages (M2 phenotype).

23.1.3 Changes in Cytokine Expression After MSC Transplantation by Immunoblot Analysis and ELISA

Western blotting and ELISA were performed to evaluate the effects of MSC transplantation on TNF-α, IL-6, IL-4, and IL-13 protein levels in the region of the SCI at 1 week after injury. In the MSC-transplanted group, the intensities of the bands for TNF-α and IL-6 were attenuated, whereas those of IL-4 and IL-13 were increased compared with the control group. The amounts of TNF-α and IL-6 proteins were significantly lower (IL-6 dominant) while those of IL-4 and IL-13 were significantly higher (IL-13 dominant) in the MSC-transplanted group compared with the control group.

23.1.4 *Histological Evaluation of Injured Spinal Cord After MSC Transplantation*

In order to examine the beneficial effects of MSC transplantation on spinal cord repair, the severity of trauma at the injury epicenter site was evaluated histopathologically at 5 weeks after SCI. Hematoxylin and eosin staining in the MSC-transplanted group showed a significant decrease in the total cavity areas at epicenter and at 4 mm rostral and caudal to the epicenter compared with the control group (Fig. 23.4a). On LFB-stained samples, images of the MSC-transplanted group demonstrated significantly smaller areas of cystic cavity formation and enhanced staining in both gray and white matters compared with that of the control group. Quantitative analysis of the myelinated areas revealed significant differences between the two groups at the injury epicenter and at 4 mm rostral and caudal to the epicenter (Fig. 23.4b). To determine the effects of MSC transplantation on axonal sparing, we examined sagittal sections of the spinal cords following immunostaining with anti-GAP-43 and anti-RT97 antibodies at 5 weeks after SCI. In the MSC-transplanted group, GAP-43-positive or RT97-positive fibers, embedded within PKH26-labeled MSC, were significantly increased and their neurites were also significantly longer compared with the control group (Fig. 23.4c).

23.1.5 *Changes in Locomotor BBB Score*

The degree of motor disturbance in the hind limbs was assessed between day 3 and 5 weeks after SCI. Significant motor disturbance in the hind limbs was noted in rats of the control group, though some degree of recovery was evident subsequently, which reached a functional plateau (BBB score 9.2 ± 2.1) [13] at 5 weeks after SCI. In contrast, the MSC-transplanted group showed a markedly better functional recovery such that the BBB locomotor score was significantly increased compared to the control group from 1 week after SCI (Fig. 23.5).

23.2 Discussion

The aim of this research was to study the beneficial effects of MSC transplantation in the injured spinal cord, specifically with regard to the effects of MSC on macrophage phenotype and function. The major findings of our research were: (1) MSC-transplanted into the site of spinal cord injury migrated into the adjacent nervous

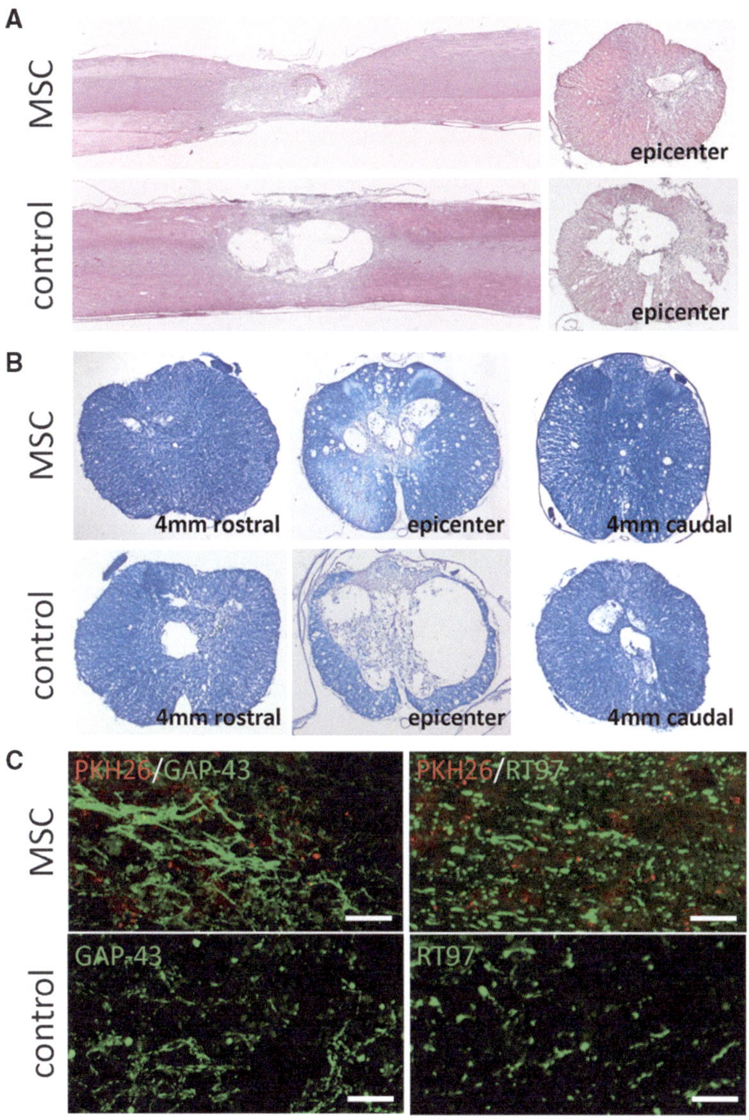

Fig. 23.4 Hematoxylin and eosin staining of midsagittal and axial sections of the lesion epicenter showed a remarkably smaller area of damage and cavity formation in the MSC-transplanted group. The total area of cavitation in the axial sections was significantly different between the two groups (**a**). The axial sections stained with Luxol fast blue (LFB) contained remarkably small area of demyelination in the MSC-transplanted group compared with the control group. Quantification of LFB-positive myelinated area showed a significant difference between the two groups at all examined sites (**b**). Representative images showing greater abundance of GAP-43-positive fibers and RT97-positive fibers in the MSC group compared with that in the control group (5 weeks after injury). Quantification of GAP-43- and RT97-positive fibers areas showed a significant difference between the two groups at all examined sites (**c**). Scale bar = 100 μm (Reprinted, in part, with permission, from [14])

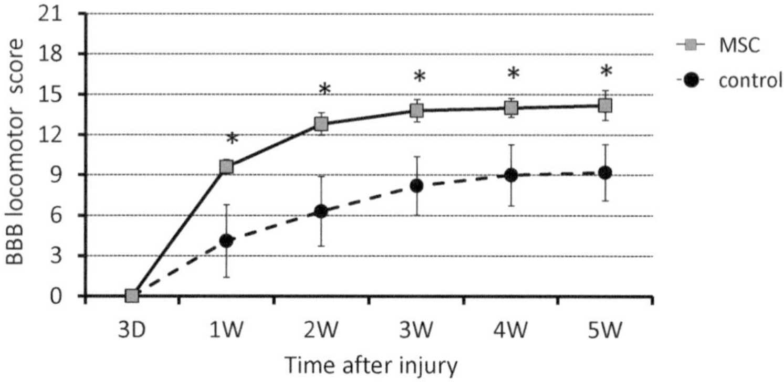

Fig. 23.5 Serial changes in locomotor BBB score after SCI. A significant improvement in hindlimb motor function was observed in the MSC-transplanted group compared with the control group from 1 week and thereafter after the injury. *$p < 0.05$ (Reprinted, with permission, from [14])

tissue to areas rich in glial and neuronal processes, but did not differentiate into glial or neuronal elements; (2) MSC transplantation favored the development of a population of alternatively activated macrophages (M2 phenotype) while preventing the development of a population of classically activated macrophages (M1 phenotype); (3) MSC transplantation was associated with a decrease in TNF-α and IL-6 and an increase in IL-4 and IL-13; (4) MSC transplantation reduced the size of injury site and resulted in less scar tissue formation and increased myelin sparing; and (5) these morphological findings correlated with increased axonal growth and improved locomotor function in the MSC-transplanted group compared with the control group [14].

Several studies reported that MSC can differentiate in vitro into neurons, astrocytes, myocytes, and Schwann cells. In our study, transplanted MSC migrated to the neighborhood of the injured spinal cord, but did not differentiate into glial or neuronal elements. Current thinking is that the potential beneficial effects of MSC in SCI are related to neuronal or glial differentiation of MSC, but rather from their secretion of growth factors and/or cytokines [15], which can provide neuroprotection [16], induction of axonal sprouting [17], neovascularization [18], and immunomodulation [19, 20]. MSC may also promote axonal regeneration or encourage functional plasticity by establishing an environment that supports axonal growth. MSC synthesize a number of neurotrophic cytokines that stimulate nerve growth, such as brain-derived neurotrophic factor (BDNF), nerve growth factor (NGF), and vascular endothelial growth factor (VEGF) [8, 21]. Furthermore, a recent study examined the response of MSC to environmental stimuli in the injured spinal cord tissue and found increased synthesis by these cells of various cytokines, including IL-6, IL-7, and VEGF [22]. Because MSC can alter their gene expression profile in response to the surrounding environment [23, 24], we consider that transplanted MSC do not differentiate into neural cells at least in the injured spinal cord environment, but instead they bring about CNS functional recovery by modifying the SCI environment to directly affect the endogenous cells present in that territory.

Some investigators indicated that hematogenous macrophages are more detrimental, whereas microglia are believed to be relatively beneficial for spinal cord repair due to their higher phagocytic activity and expression of various neurotrophic factors [25]. On the other hand, others indicated that the distinct hematogenous macrophage subset, i.e., alternatively activated macrophages (M2 phenotype), is not only beneficial in spinal cord injury, but also has a distinct role from activated resident microglia. The resident microglia are embedded in the CNS prior to the injury and immediately activated by the insult, whereas alternatively activated macrophages (M2 phenotype) do not encounter the injured CNS tissue prior to their delayed arrival to the damage site [26]. Subsequent studies have correlated such divergent effects to the presence of different macrophage populations with contrasting functions, where classically activated macrophages (M1 phenotype) are the predominant type after SCI, with deleterious effects on the injured tissues, and alternatively activated macrophages (M2 phenotype) have only a short-term response, disappearing within 3 to 7 days after injury [11]. That prevalence of the M1 phenotype over the M2 phenotype may be partially responsible for the lack of functional recovery after SCI.

Previous studies identified TNF-α and IL-6 as the most significant cytokines to generate classically activated macrophage [11], and IL-4 and IL-13 to generate alternatively activated macrophages [27], while identifying microglia as the main source of IL-4 and IL-13. In our study, we found that 3 days after MSC transplantation following a SCI, the local cytokine profile changed into an alternative activating environment, with significant increase in IL-4 and IL-13 levels and simultaneous reduction in TNF-α and IL-6. The increased protein levels of Th2 cytokines (IL-4, IL-13) might activate resident microglia and hematogenous macrophages through the IL-4Rα/Jak1/STAT signaling pathway into alternatively activated macrophages (M2 phenotype), where the reduced levels of Th1 cytokines (TNF-α, IL-6) will prevent the macrophages of shifting back into classically activated macrophages (M1 phenotype) [10, 23].

MSC is thought to act as guiding strands for regenerating axons across the lesion site in the injured cord and along spinal cord tracts by expressing various cell adhesion molecules and receptors [21]. The transplanted MSCs are reported to form bundles that bridged the lesion, which were also populated with immature astrocytes and nerve fiber outgrowths [28]. Alternatively activated macrophages (M2 phenotype) exhibit high phagocytic abilities due to the presence of endosomes/lysosomes and pinocytic structures with digestive enzymes to remove scar tissue and growth inhibitors present in the myelin debris, thus allowing axonal regeneration [11, 12]. In our study, the MSC-transplanted group showed axon preservation and an enhanced spinal cord repair process, based on the increase in NF-H-and GAP-43-positive fibers at 5 weeks after injury, indicating anatomical improvement compared with the control group. The acute or subacute environment of the injured spinal cord may influence the mechanism by which the MSC graft induces tissue protection/repair in a manner that differs from the chronic phase; i.e., in the acute phase, MSC transplantation may have beneficial effect through their anti-inflammatory activity, whereas in the subacute/chronic phase after SCI, the MSC may be used for neurostimulatory and cell bridging effects [7].

23.3 Conclusion

Our results suggested that the transplantation of MSC after SCI shifts the phenotype of macrophages after injury from classically activated macrophages (M1 phenotype) to that of alternatively activated macrophages (M2 phenotype) during the acute phase; this was associated with the presence of relevant cytokine profiles, reduction in inhibitory scar tissue/cavity formation in the subacute/chronic phase, and the provision of a permissive environment for axonal extension and functional recovery.

Acknowledgment This work was supported in part by Grants-in-Aid to HN, KU, and HB for General Scientific Research of the Ministry of Education, Science and Culture of Japan (grants numbers 21591895, 21791389, 22390287, and 23791631). This study was also supported by Grant of Japan Orthopaedics and Traumatology Foundation (No.218).

Conflict of Interest All authors declare that they have no conflict of interest.

References

1. Himes BT, Neuhuber B, Coleman C et al (2006) Recovery of function following grafting of human bone marrow-derived stromal cells into the injured spinal cord. Neurorehabil Neural Repair 20:278–296
2. Wu S, Suzuki Y, Ejiri Y (2003) Bone marrow stromal cells enhance differentiation of cocultured neurosphere cells and promote regeneration of injured spinal cord. J Neurosci Res 72:343–351
3. Akiyama Y, Radtke C, Honmou O et al (2002) Remyelination of the spinal cord following intravenous delivery of bone marrow cells. Glia 39:229–236
4. Akiyama Y, Radtke C, Kocsis JD (2002) Remyelination of the rat spinal cord by transplantation of identified bone marrow stromal cells. J Neurosci 22:6623–6630
5. Zurita M, Vaquero J, Bonilla C et al (2008) Functional recovery of chronic paraplegic pigs after autologous transplantation of bone marrow stromal cells. Transplantation 86:845–85
6. Jiang XX, Zhang Y, Liu B et al (2005) Human mesenchymal stem cells inhibit differentiation and function of monocyte-derived dendritic cells. Blood 105:4120–4126
7. Wright KT, Masri EL, Osman W et al (2011) Bone marrow for the treatment of spinal cord injury: mechanisms and clinical application. Stem Cells 29:169–178
8. Neuhuber B, Timothy Himes B, Shumsky JS et al (2005) Axon growth and recovery of function supported by human bone marrow stromal cells in the injured spinal cord exhibit donor variations. Brain Res 1035:73–85
9. Abrams MB, Dominguez C, Pernold K et al (2009) Multipotent mesenchymal stromal cells attenuate chronic inflammation and injury-induced sensitivity to mechanical stimuli in experimental spinal cord injury. Restor Neurol Neurosci 27:307–321
10. Gordon S (2003) Alternative activation of macrophages. Nat Rev Immunol 3:23–35
11. Kigerl KA, Gensel JC, Ankeny DP et al (2009) Identification of two distinct macrophage subsets with divergent effects causing either neurotoxicity or regeneration in the injured mouse spinal cord. J Neurosci 29:13435–13444
12. Schwartz M (2010) "Tissue-repairing" blood-derived macrophages are essential for healing of the injured spinal cord: from skin-activated macrophages to infiltrating blood-derived cells? Brain Behav. Immun 24:1054–1057
13. Basso DM, Beattie MS, Bresnahan JC (1995) A sensitive and reliable locomotor rating scale for open field testing in rats. J Neurotrauma 12:1–21

14. Nakajima H, Uchida K, Guerrero AR et al (2012) Transplantation of mesenchymal stem cells promotes an alternative pathway of macrophage activation and functional recovery after spinal cord injury. J Neurotrauma 29:1614–1625
15. Sasaki M, Radtke C, Tan AM et al (2009) BDNF-hypersecreting human mesenchymal stem cells promote functional recovery, axonal sprouting, and protection of corticospinal neurons after spinal cord injury. J Neurosci 29:14932–14941
16. Chen X, Li Y, Wang L et al (2002) Ischemic rat brain extracts induce human marrow stromal cell growth factor production. Neuropathology 22:275–279
17. Shen LH, Li Y, Chen J et al (2006) Intracarotid transplantation of bone marrow stromal cells increases axon-myelin remodeling after stroke. Neuroscience 137:393–399
18. Onda T, Honmou O, Harada K et al (2008) Therapeutic benefits by human mesenchymal stem cells (hMSCs) and Ang-1 gene-modified hMSCs after cerebral ischemia. J Cereb Blood Flow Metab 28:329–340
19. Bai L, Lennon DP, Eaton V et al (2009) Human bone marrow-derived mesenchymal stem cells induce Th2-polarized immune response and promote endogenous repair in animal models of multiple sclerosis. Glia 57:1192–1203
20. Ohtaki H, Ylostalo JH, Foraker JE et al (2008) Stem/progenitor cells from bone marrow decrease neuronal death in global ischemia by modulation of inflammatory/immune responses. Proc Natl Acad Sci U S A 105:14638–14643
21. Crigler L, Robey RC, Asawachaicharn A (2006) Human mesenchymal stem cell subpopulations express a variety of neuro-regulatory molecules and promote neuronal cell survival and neuritogenesis. Exp Neurol 198:54–64
22. Zhukareva V, Obrocka M, Houle JD et al (2010) Secretion profile of human bone marrow stromal cells: donor variability and response to inflammatory stimuli. Cytokine 50:317–321
23. Mosser DM, Edwards JP (2008) Exploring the full spectrum of macrophage activation. Nat Rev Immunol 8:958–969
24. Yamaguchi S, Kuroda S, Kobayashi H et al (2006) The effects of neuronal induction on gene expression profile in bone marrow stromal cells (BMSC)–a preliminary study using microarray analysis. Brain Res 1087:15–27
25. Mukaino M, Nakamura M, Yamada O et al (2010) Anti-IL-6-receptor antibody promotes repair of spinal cord injury by inducing microglia-dominant inflammation. Exp Neurol 224:403–414
26. Shechter R, London A, Varol C et al (2009) Infiltrating blood-derived macrophages are vital cells playing an anti-inflammatory role in recovery from spinal cord injury in mice. PLoS Med 6:e1000113
27. Loke P, Nair MG, Parkinson J et al (2002) IL-4 dependent alternatively-activated macrophages have a distinctive in vivo gene expression phenotype. BMC Immunol 3:7
28. Hofstetter CP, Schwarz EJ, Hess D et al (2002) Marrow stromal cells form guiding strands in the injured spinal cord and promote recovery. Proc Natl Acad Sci U S A 99:2199–2204

Chapter 24
Vascular Regeneration Therapies for Spinal Cord Injury

Naosuke Kamei

Abstract As a novel approach for spinal cord regeneration, we focused on the close interaction between the nervous system and blood vessels described as "vascular niche." In our studies, endothelial progenitor cells (EPCs) or cell populations containing EPCs were used for treating spinal cord injury (SCI) in anticipation of causing the formation of vascular niche. Here we introduce the outcomes of following studies: (1) kinetics of endogenous EPCs in SCI, (2) transplantation of Jagged1 deficit EPCs, and (3) transplantation of human $CD133^+$ cells. Bone marrow transplantation (BMT) from Tie2/lacZ transgenic mice into wild-type mice with SCI showed the recruitment of endogenous EPCs from bone marrow into injured spinal cord and the participation of recruited EPCs in angiogenesis and astrogliosis following SCI. Transplantation of EPCs derived from Jagged1 knockout mice revealed the contribution of transplanted EPCs to the enhancement of astrogliosis through Jagged1-Notch signaling. Human cord blood $CD133^+$ cells and ex vivo expanded $CD133^+$ cells promoted functional recovery after SCI.

Keywords Angiogenesis • Astrogliosis • CD133 • Notch

24.1 Introduction

A close relationship between neural stem cells (NSCs) and vascular cells in the adult central nervous system (CNS) have been shown for the "vascular niche" [1–3]. The vascular niche is believed to play a critical role for NSC-driven neurogenesis in

N. Kamei (✉)
Department of Orthopaedic Surgery, Graduate School of Biomedical and Health Sciences, Hiroshima University, 1-2-3 Kasumi, Minami-ku, Hiroshima 734-8551, Japan

Translational Research Medical Center, Hiroshima University Hospital, 1-2-3 Kasumi, Minami-ku, Hiroshima 734-8551, Japan
e-mail: nahkamei@hiroshima-u.ac.jp

K. Uchida et al. (eds.), *Neuroprotection and Regeneration of the Spinal Cord*,
DOI 10.1007/978-4-431-54502-6_24, © Springer Japan 2014

homeostasis as well as during regeneration. In addition, the activation of endogenous NSCs recently came into focus as a critical mechanism involved in the regeneration of the damaged CNS, including spinal cord injury (SCI) [4–6]. We therefore focused on the vascular niche as one of key factors in spinal cord regeneration. Meanwhile, endothelial progenitor cells (EPCs) derived from bone marrow and blood have the potential to differentiate into endothelial cells and to promote neovascularization [7, 8]. In our studies, EPCs were applied for treating SCI in anticipation of causing the formation of vascular niche for spinal cord regeneration. Here we introduce the results of our studies regarding the cell therapy using EPCs for the treatment of SCI.

24.2 Kinetics of Endogenous EPCs in Spinal Cord Injury

We assessed the in vivo kinetics of bone marrow-derived EPCs by EPC colony-forming assay (EPC-CFA) and bone marrow transplantation (BMT) from Tie2 (endothelial-specific receptor tyrosine kinase)/lacZ transgenic mice into wild-type mice with SCI [9].

24.2.1 *Mobilization of Bone Marrow EPCs to Peripheral Blood Following SCI*

EPC-CFA was performed using circulating mononuclear cells for the assessment of circulating EPCs [10]. Peripheral blood mononuclear cells (PB-MNCs) were isolated from non-injured mice (pre SCI) and injured ones at days 0 (immediately after SCI), 3, 7, and 14 after SCI. The EPC-CFA was performed by culturing 1×10^5 PB-MNCs in methyl cellulose-containing medium with stem cell factor (SCF), vascular endothelial growth factor (VEGF), interleukin-3 (IL-3), basic fibroblast growth factor (bFGF), epidermal growth factor (EGF), insulin-like growth factor-1 (IGF-1), and heparin. Colony-forming ability of these cells represents properties as stem/progenitor cells. In addition, these colony-forming cells also have endothelial properties. PB-MNCs slightly decreased immediately after SCI but gradually increased at day 3 or later after SCI. The number of EPC-CFUs peaked at day 3 after SCI but gradually decreased at days 7 and 14. These results suggest that SCI augments mobilization of EPCs especially at day 3 after SCI.

24.2.2 *Recruitment of EPCs into the Damaged Spinal Cord*

To assess the recruitment of bone marrow-derived EPCs into the injured spinal cord, bone marrow from Tie2/lacZ transgenic mice was transplanted to lethally irradiated wild-type mice. SCI was induced in Tie2/lacZ BMT mice. The spinal cord sections were immunostained for β-gal. The β-gal positive cells, which were considered to be bone marrow-derived EPCs recruited into sites of neovascularization, were abundantly observed around the injury site at days 3, 7, 14, and 28 after SCI (Fig. 24.1a–d).

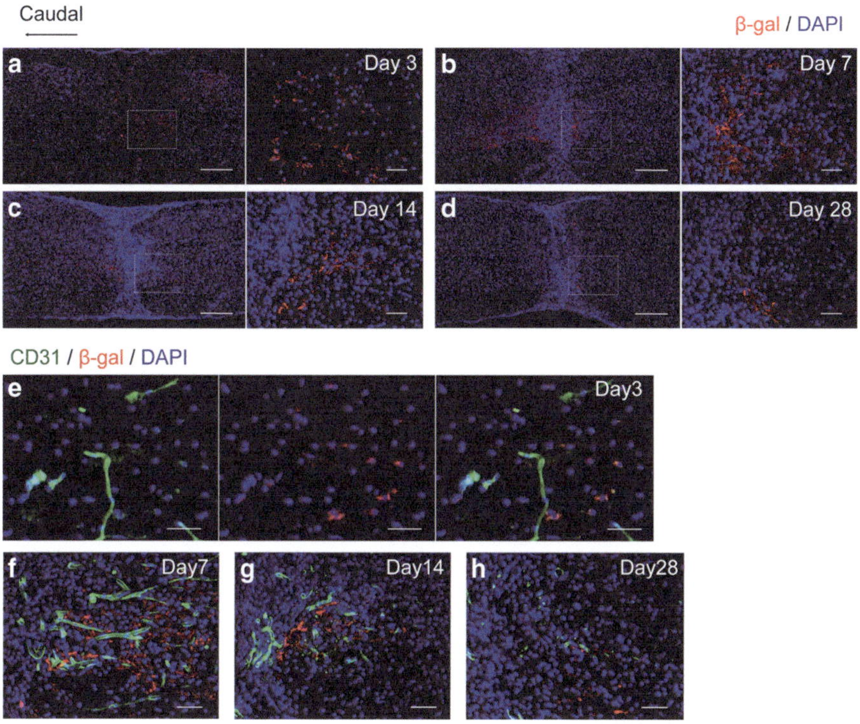

Fig. 24.1 Recruitment of EPCs to injured spinal cord. (**a–d**) Bone marrow (BM)-derived EPCs were serially identified in the spinal cord of wild-type mice with SCI following BM transplantation from Tie2/lacZ transgenic mice. Representative immunohistochemistry for β-gal (*red*) at days 3 (**a**), 7 (**b**), 14 (**c**), and 28 (**d**) after injury. Nuclei were counterstained with DAPI (*blue*). (**e–h**) Immunohistochemical staining for CD31 (*green*) and β-gal (*red*) at days 3 (**e**), 7 (**f**), 14 (**g**), and 28 (**h**) after injury reveals that β-gal positive cells are also labeled with CD31 (**e**). The β-gal positive cells are scattered at day 3, but are distributed along CD31 positive vessels at day 7 or later. Scale bars: *left panel* of (**a–d**), 300 μm; *right panel* of (**a–d**), 50 μm, and (**e–h**), 50 μm

The number of β-gal positive cells markedly increased at day 7 after SCI and then gradually decreased at days 14 and 28. The β-gal positive cells are also labeled with CD31 (endothelial cell marker) at day 3 after injury (Fig. 24.1e). Although the β-gal positive cells were scattered around the injury site at day 3 after SCI, they were aligned along vessels at day 7 or later after SCI (Fig. 24.1f–h). These findings represent that bone marrow-derived EPCs are recruited into spinal cord tissue following SCI, and recruited EPCs are distributed around newly formed blood vessels.

24.2.3 Administration of Exogenous EPCs for Repairing Injured Spinal Cord

To clarify the contribution of EPC recruitment to histological changes in the injured spinal cord, cultured EPCs labeled with DiI-ac-LDL or phosphate buffered saline (PBS) were administered systemically just after SCI. DiI positive cells indicating administered EPCs were observed around the injury site at day 3. Immature reactive astrocytes co-labeled with GFAP and nestin were increased by the administration of EPCs at day 3 after injury. $CD31^+$ blood vessels were also increased by the administration of EPCs at day 3 after injury. These findings suggest that systemically administered EPCs are recruited into the injured spinal cord and enhance neovascularization and astrogliosis following SCI.

24.3 EPCs Enhance Astrogliosis Through Notch Signaling

Although the exact molecular mechanisms underlying the interaction between NSCs and vascular cells still remain elusive, the previous study showed that endothelial cells stimulated the self-renewal of NSCs and enhanced NSC-derived neurogenesis through Notch signaling [11]. We therefore hypothesized that a Notch signaling mediated interaction between NSCs and EPCs might promote the activation of endogenous NSCs and subsequently lead to the enhanced repair of the injured spinal cord. In this study, we used conditional Jagged1 (Jag1) knockout mice (loxP/loxP, Mx-Cre). EPCs were cultured from bone marrow mononuclear cells isolated from $Jag1^{+/+}$ as well as $Jag1^{-/-}$ mice. EPCs (1×10^6 cells in 200 μL of PBS) derived from $Jag1^{+/+}$ mice or $Jag1^{-/-}$ mice were injected to mouse models of SCI intravenously immediately after injury ($Jag1^{+/+}$ EPC group, $Jag1^{-/-}$ EPC group), as well as 200 μL of PBS (PBS group) [12].

24.3.1 Notch Ligands in Cultured EPCs

The levels of expression of Notch ligands, including Jag1 and Delta-like 1 (Dll1), in cultured EPCs were confirmed by quantitative real-time PCR. $Jag1^{-/-}$ EPCs lack expression of Jag1, whereas no significant difference in the expression of Dll1 could be detected between $Jag1^{-/-}$ and corresponding wild-type EPCs.

24.3.2 Functional Recovery After Spinal Cord Injury

The recovery of hindlimb function was assessed using the basso mouse scale (BMS) [13]. The BMS score in the $Jag1^{+/+}$ EPC group was significantly higher than in the PBS and the $Jag1^{-/-}$ EPC group at days 14 or later. Although the average score in the $Jag1^{-/-}$ EPC group was slightly higher than in the PBS group at days 14 or later after SCI, there was no significant difference in the BMS score between these two groups. To assess functionality and recovery of descending pathways from the forebrain to the hindlimb motor neuron pool, motor evoked potentials (MEPs) were monitored in the hamstring muscles. At 6 weeks after SCI, the amplitudes of MEPs in the PBS group, $Jag1^{+/+}$ EPC group, and $Jag1^{-/-}$ EPC group were 13.33 ± 5.16 %, 24.31 ± 7.31 %,

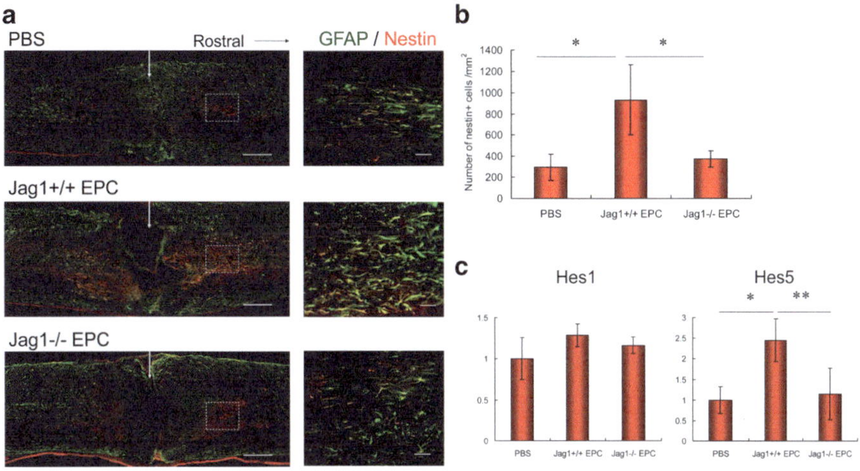

Fig. 24.2 Assessment of astrogliosis. (**a**) Spinal cord tissues at day 3 after injury immunostained with GFAP (*green*) and nestin (*red*). *Arrow* indicates epicenter of injury site. (**b**) Number of nestin$^+$ cells at day 3 after injury ($n=6$). $*P<0.0005$. (**c**) mRNA expressions of Notch effectors Hes1 and Hes5 in spinal cord tissues at day 3 after injury measured by real-time quantitative PCR ($n=6$). Scale bar: (**a**) *large pictures*, 300 μm, and *small pictures*, 50 μm

and 13.73 ± 5.27 % of the pre-injury values, respectively. The amplitude in the Jag1$^{+/+}$ EPC group was significantly higher than in the PBS and the Jag1$^{-/-}$ EPC group. However, there was no significant difference in the amplitudes between the PBS and the Jag1$^{-/-}$ EPC group. These findings suggest that the transplantation of Jag1$^{+/+}$ EPCs but not Jag1$^{-/-}$ EPCs promoted the functional recovery after SCI.

24.3.3 Incorporation of Transplanted EPCs

To assess the incorporation of administered EPCs into injured spinal cord, EPCs were labeled with DiI-acetyl LDL prior to administration. DiI$^+$ cells could be observed around the injury site in both Jag1$^{+/+}$ EPC and Jag1$^{-/-}$ EPC groups; however, no DiI$^+$ cells were detected in the PBS group. No significant difference in the number of incorporated DiI$^+$ cells was detected between these two groups.

24.3.4 Astrogliosis Following Spinal Cord Injury

At day 3 after SCI, reactive astrocytes were stained with antibodies against GFAP and nestin. A large number of reactive astrocytes were observed in the Jag1$^{+/+}$ EPC group, whereas only few could be detected in the PBS and Jag1$^{-/-}$ EPC group (Fig. 24.2a, b). The mRNA expressions of the Notch effectors Hes1 and Hes5 in the injured spinal cord were assessed by real-time quantitative PCR. Although the expression level of Hes1 in the Jag1$^{+/+}$ EPC group was slightly higher than in the PBS and Jag1$^{-/-}$ EPC group, no significant difference in Hes1 expression could be detected. In contrast, the expression level of Hes5 in the Jag1$^{+/+}$ EPC group was significantly higher than in the PBS and the Jag1$^{-/-}$ EPC group, with again no significant difference between the PBS and Jag1$^{-/-}$ EPC group (Fig. 24.2c). At day14 after injury, spinal cord tissues were stained with GFAP for the assessment of astrogliosis. The GFAP negative area in the Jag1$^{+/+}$ EPC group was significantly smaller than in the PBS and Jag1$^{-/-}$ EPC group, the latter showing again no significant difference.

24.3.5 Neovascularization in the Injured Spinal Cord

Spinal cord sections were immunostained with CD31 at days 3 and 14 after injury in order to assess the degree of neovascularization. At day 3 after SCI, although very little or no angiogenesis was observed at the epicenter zone in all groups, CD31^{+} vessels were observed in the border zone. In this area, the mean diameter of vessels in the Jag1$^{+/+}$ EPC group was significantly greater than in the PBS and Jag1$^{-/-}$ EPC group. The number of vessels in the Jag1$^{+/+}$ and Jag1$^{-/-}$ EPC groups was significantly greater than in the PBS group, whereas no significant difference could be observed between both EPC groups. At day14 after injury, a chaotic vascular architecture with large vessels adjacent to small vessels was observed in the PBS and Jag1$^{-/-}$ EPC group, though no morphological abnormalities of the vessels could be observed for the Jag1$^{+/+}$ EPC group. These results suggest that both Jag1$^{+/+}$ EPCs and Jag1$^{-/-}$ EPCs enhanced angiogenesis at day 3 after SCI and that Jag1$^{+/+}$ EPCs but not Jag1$^{-/-}$ EPCs normalized vascular morphology at day 14 after SCI.

24.3.6 Assessment of Axons

To analyze defined subsets of descending axons, immunohistochemistry for TH (a marker for descending noradrenergic and dopaminergic axons as well as sympathetic fibers) and 5HT (a marker for descending serotonergic axons) was performed at day 42 after SCI [14]. To evaluate the axon growth beyond the injury site, quantitative assessment of axons was performed by measuring the area of immunostained axons in the far rostral region (5 mm rostral to the epicenter), the injury site (the caudal region adjacent to the epicenter), and the far caudal region (5 mm caudal to the epicenter). At the injury site, the area of TH^{+} and 5HT^{+} axons in the Jag1$^{+/+}$ EPC group was significantly larger than in the PBS and Jag1$^{-/-}$ group. In addition, the area of 5HT^{+} axons in the Jag1$^{-/-}$ EPC group was significantly larger than in the PBS group. In the far caudal region, TH^{+} and 5HT^{+} axons were clearly observed in the Jag1$^{+/+}$ EPC group, whereas these axons were rare in the PBS and Jag1$^{-/-}$ EPC group. The area of TH^{+} or 5HT^{+} axons in the Jag1$^{+/+}$ EPC group was significantly larger than in the PBS and Jag1$^{-/-}$ group.

24.3.7 Transplantation of Notch Ligand-Overexpressing 3T3 Stromal Cells

To clarify the role of ligand-specific Notch activation for the enhancement of astrogliosis following SCI, 3T3 stromal cells transfected with Jag1, Dll1, or empty vector were transplanted directly into the injury site of spinal cords immediately after SCI (Jag1-3T3 group, Dll1-3T3 group, and empty-3T3 group). At day 3 after injury, spinal cord sections were immunostained with GFAP and nestin. In the assessment of reactive astrocytes stained with GFAP and nestin, a large number of reactive astrocytes were observed in the Jag1-3T3 group, though these cells were rare in the empty-3T3 and Dll1-3T3 groups. The number of nestin^{+} cells in the Jag1-3T3 group was significantly greater than in the empty-3T3 and Dll1-3T3 groups. These findings suggest that Jag1/Notch signaling but not Dll1/Notch signaling enhanced astrogliosis after SCI.

24.4 Transplantation of Human CD133^{+} Cells

The population of CD133^{+} cells in human blood, known to be a subpopulation of CD34^{+} cells, is well characterized as a hematopoietic/endothelial progenitor fraction. CD133^{+} cells in human blood appear to be suited for clinical application as isolation of these cells is relatively safe and raises only limited ethical concerns. However, the acquisition of a sufficient number of cells remains the most important factor limiting clinical application, as the proportion of CD133^{+} cells in respect to the overall number of MNCs in human blood is very small [15]. We developed a serum-free culture system for human cord blood-derived CD133^{+} cells enhancing the cellular function as well as the number of EPCs destined to be used for the revascularization of ischemic organs and tissues [16]. We analyzed and compared ex vivo expanded human cord blood-derived CD133^{+} cells with freshly isolated CD133^{+} cells as well as corresponding CD133^{-} control MNCs in respect to their ability to promote spinal cord repair using in vitro assays and cell transplantation into a mouse SCI model [17].

24.4.1 EPC Colony-Forming Units

One-week expansion culture increased the number of cells 62.8 ± 14.4-fold (Fig. 24.3a). FACS analysis showed that the initial freshly isolated CD133^{+} cell population contained 98 % CD133^{+}/CD34^{+} cells and further confirmed that the expanded cells had a purity of 25 % CD133^{+}/CD34^{+} cells (Fig. 24.3b). To evaluate the content of EPCs in CD133^{-} MNCs, fresh CD133^{+}, and expanded cells, cells were analyzed using EPC-CFA. Colonies consisting of small and round-shaped cells were defined as small EPC colonies, whereas colonies consisting of large and spindle-shaped cells were referred to as large EPC colonies. No EPC colonies were formed by CD133⁻ MNCs. A large portion of the colonies derived from fresh CD133⁺ cells were small EPC colonies. In contrast, approximately two-thirds of the EPC colonies derived from expanded cells were large EPC colonies. The average number of small EPC colonies from expanded cells was significantly less than from fresh CD133⁺ cells. However, the average number of large EPC colonies as well as total EPC colonies from expanded cells was significantly greater than from fresh CD133⁺ cells.

24.4.2 Gene Expression Profiles in CD133⁻ MNCs, Fresh CD133⁺, and Expanded Cells

To clarify the paracrine effects of transplanted cells, we assessed the mRNA expression of various angiogenic or neurotrophic factors and inflammatory cytokines in the CD133⁻ MNCs, fresh CD133⁺, and expanded cells using real-time PCR. Each mRNA expression was normalized to the mRNA expression level of VEGF-A in CD133⁻ MNCs (Fig. 24.3c). In the assessment of growth factors, the mRNA expression levels of VEGF-A, VEGF-B, and IGF-2 in CD133⁻ MNCs were significantly higher than in fresh CD133⁺ and expanded cells. In contrast, the expression levels of angiopoietin 1 (Ang1) and hepatocyte growth factor (HGF) in fresh CD133⁺ and expanded cells were significantly higher than in CD133⁻ MNCs. In addition, the expression level of brain-derived growth factor (BDNF) in expanded cells was significantly higher than in CD133⁻ cells and fresh CD133⁺ cells. In particular, the expression level of Ang1 in fresh CD133⁺ and expanded cells was markedly higher than of the other growth factors (Fig. 24.3c). The expression levels of inflammatory cytokines including tumor necrosis factor-α (TNFα), IL-6, and IL-8 in CD133⁻ MNCs were markedly higher than in fresh CD133⁺ and expanded cells (Fig. 24.3d–f).

24.4.3 Functional Recovery After Spinal Cord Injury

Cell transplantation was performed immediately after SCI. 5×10^4 of CD133⁻ MNCs, fresh CD133⁺ cells, or expanded cells were suspended in 200 μL of PBS and injected intravenously (CD133⁻ group, fresh group and expanded group). 1×10^6 of expanded cells were administered into mice of the high-dose transplantation group (expanded-H group). 200 μL of cell free PBS was injected into control mice (PBS group). The recovery of hindlimb function was assessed by using the BMS. The BMS score in the CD133⁻ group was not significantly different from the PBS group at each time point. At day 7 after injury, the BMS score in the expanded-H group was significantly higher than in the PBS group. The average score in the fresh group and the expanded group was significantly higher than in the PBS group and the CD133⁻ group at days 21 and 28 after SCI. In addition, the average score in the expanded-H

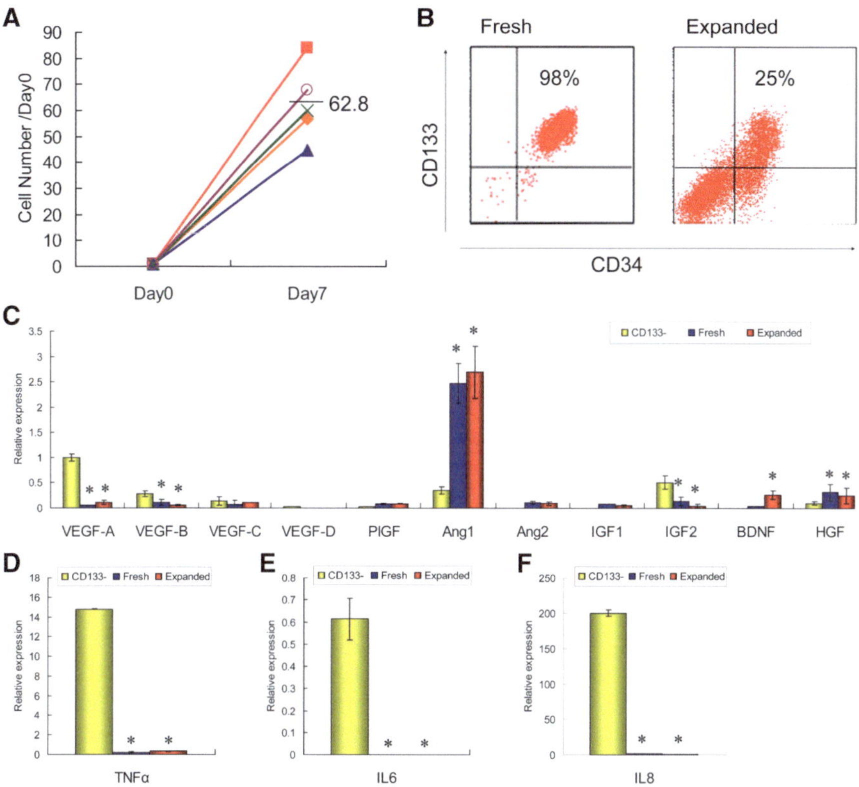

Fig. 24.3 (**a**) Increase in cell number after expansion culture. Cells were expanded on average up to 62.8-fold. (**b**) Flow cytometric analysis of fresh $CD133^+$ and expanded cells. Purity of $CD133^+/CD34^+$ cells was reduced from 98 to 25 % by expansion. (**c–f**) mRNA expression profiles in $CD133^-$ MNCs, fresh $CD133^+$, and expanded cells measured by real-time PCR. *Significantly different from $CD133^-$ MNCs, $p<0.05$

group was significantly higher than in the other groups at day 14 or later. Transcranial electric MEPs were monitored in the hamstring muscles. At 4 weeks after SCI, the amplitude was 14.4 ± 5.0 % of the pre-injury value in the PBS group, while in the $CD133^-$ group, the amplitude was 16.8 ± 9.1 % of the pre-injury value. There was no significant difference in the amplitudes between the PBS and the $CD133^-$ group. In the fresh group, the expanded group, and the expanded-H group, the amplitude was 26.5 ± 4.3 %, 26.7 ± 6.1 %, and 34.8 ± 6.3 % of the pre-injury value, respectively, which was significantly higher than in the PBS and the $CD133^-$ group. Furthermore, the amplitude in the expanded-H group was significantly higher than in the fresh group and the expanded group. These data indicate that the transplantation of fresh $CD133^+$ and expanded cells promoted the improvement of spinal cord function after SCI and that the high-dose transplantation of expanded cells was most effective in promoting functional recovery after SCI.

24.4.4 Incorporation of Transplanted Cells

To assess the incorporation of transplanted cells into injured spinal cord, spinal cord sections were immunostained with the human-specific antibody against mitochondria (hMit). At day 3 after SCI, $hMit^+$ cells were observed around the injury site in the $CD133^-$ group. However, there were no $hMit^+$ cells incorporated into the $CD31^+$ vessels. In contrast, $hMit^+$ cells incorporated into CD31 positive vessels were detected in the fresh group, expanded group, and expanded-H group. The number of $hMit^+$ cells incorporated into the vessels in the expanded-H group was significantly greater than in the fresh or expanded group.

24.4.5 Neovascularization in the Injured Spinal Cord

At day 3 after SCI, the diameter, number, and area of CD31 positive vessels in the spinal cord lesion were analyzed. In the $CD133^-$ group, the number of vessels was significantly greater than in the PBS group, whereas there were no significant differences in the diameter and area of vessels between the $CD133^-$ and PBS group. In the fresh group, expanded group, and expanded-H group, large-diameter vessels were observed in the spinal cord lesion. Mean diameter and the area of vessels in these groups were significantly larger than in the PBS and $CD133^-$ groups. Furthermore, mean diameter and the area of vessels in the expanded-H group were significantly larger than in the fresh and expanded group.

At day 7 after SCI, the diameter and number of CD31 positive vessels in the epicenter of the injury site were analyzed. In the PBS and the $CD133^-$ group, a chaotic vascular architecture with large vessels adjacent to small vessels was observed. In contrast, the diameter of vessels in the fresh group, expanded group, and expanded-H group resembled the values found in the gray matter of normal spinal cord. The mean diameter of vessels in the PBS and $CD133^-$ group was significantly larger than in normal spinal cord and the other groups. Although the number of vessels in all groups was significantly less than in normal spinal cord, the number of vessels in the expanded-H group was significantly greater than in the fresh group and the expanded group. These findings suggest that the transplantation of fresh $CD133^+$ and expanded cells accelerated angiogenesis in the acute phase of SCI and contributed to the morphological normalization of vessels in the subacute phase of SCI.

24.4.6 Astrogliosis in the Injured Spinal Cord

At day 3 after SCI, reactive astrocytes were stained with antibodies against nestin and GFAP and assessed in the damaged area of spinal cord (dotted-line box in Fig. 24.4). Although the average number of reactive astrocytes in the $CD133^-$group was slightly greater than in the PBS group, there was no significant difference in the number of reactive astrocytes between these groups. The number of reactive astrocytes in the

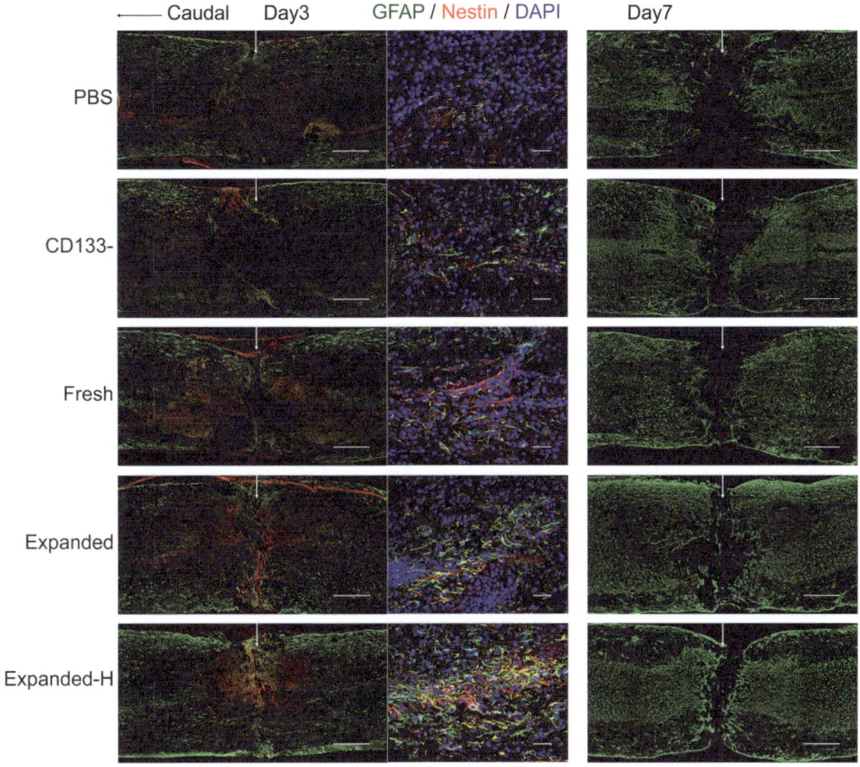

Fig. 24.4 Astrogliosis following spinal cord injury. *Left*: Spinal cord tissues at day 3 after injury immunostained with GFAP (*green*) and nestin (*red*) and additionally stained with DAPI (*blue*). *Right*: Spinal cord tissues at day 7 after injury immunostained with GFAP (*green*). *Arrows* indicate epicenter of injury site. Scale bars: *large pictures*, 300 μm, and *small pictures*, 50 μm

fresh group, expanded group, or expanded-H group was significantly greater than in the PBS group. In particular, the number of reactive astrocytes in the expanded-H group was significantly greater than in the other groups (Fig. 24.4). A large portion of reactive astrocytes were located along the large vessels, which were considered to represent newly formed vessels (Fig. 24.4). At day 7 after SCI, the GFAP negative area in the PBS group was significantly larger than in the other groups, while the GFAP negative area in the expanded-H group was significantly smaller (Fig. 24.4).

24.4.7 Assessment of Axons

To analyze defined subsets of descending axons, immunohistochemistry for TH and 5HT was performed. To evaluate the axon growth into the injury site, the quantitative assessment of axons was performed by measuring the area of immunostained axons in the far rostral region (5 mm rostral to the epicenter), the injury site (the caudal region adjacent to the epicenter), and the far caudal region (5 mm caudal to the epicenter). At the injury site, the area of TH^+ or $5HT^+$ axons in the fresh group, expanded group, and expanded-H group was significantly greater than in the PBS and the $CD133^-$ groups. In addition, the area of TH^+ axons in the expanded-H group was significantly greater than in the fresh group and the expanded group. In the far caudal region, TH^+ or $5HT^+$ axons were observed in the fresh group, expanded group, and expanded-H group, whereas neither TH^+ axons nor $5HT^+$ axons could be detected in the PBS and the $CD133^-$ groups. The area of TH^+ or $5HT^+$ axons in the expanded-H group was significantly greater than in the fresh and expanded groups.

24.5 Discussion

The findings from EPC kinetics study demonstrated that SCI induced the recruitment of EPCs from bone marrow into injured spinal cord and that EPC recruitment enhanced angiogenesis and astrogliosis following SCI. The study using Jag1 knockout mice demonstrated that transplantation of wild-type EPCs promotes astrogliosis and functional recovery following SCI and that Jag1 deletion in EPCs significantly fails to demonstrate these effects. In addition, transplantation of human blood $CD133^+$ and ex vivo expanded $CD133^+$ cells to SCI models demonstrated that the transplantation of fresh $CD133^+$ cells as well as expanded cells from human cord blood promoted neovascularization, astrogliosis, axonal growth, and functional recovery after SCI. Furthermore, high-dose transplantation of expanded cells was highly effective in promoting repair of injured spinal cord. EPCs can be isolated from bone marrow, peripheral blood, and cord blood without ethical and safety problems. In order to apply EPC transplantation in a clinical setting, the appropriate timing and route of administration should be clarified.

24.6 Conclusion

EPC can be one of cell sources of stem cell therapy for SCI.

Conflict of Interest Naosuke Kamei declares that he has no conflict of interest.

References

1. Shen Q, Wang Y, Kokovay E, Lin G, Chuang SM, Goderie SK, Roysam B, Temple S (2008) Adult SVZ stem cells lie in a vascular niche: a quantitative analysis of niche cell-cell interactions. Cell Stem Cell 3(3):289–300
2. Tavazoie M, Van der Veken L, Silva-Vargas V, Louissaint M, Colonna L, Zaidi B, Garcia-Verdugo JM, Doetsch F (2008) A specialized vascular niche for adult neural stem cells. Cell Stem Cell 3(3):279–288

3. Zacchigna S, Lambrechts D, Carmeliet P (2008) Neurovascular signalling defects in neurodegeneration. Nat Rev Neurosci 9(3):169–181
4. Okano H, Sakaguchi M, Ohki K, Suzuki N, Sawamoto K (2007) Regeneration of the central nervous system using endogenous repair mechanisms. J Neurochem 102(5):1459–1465
5. Barnabe-Heider F, Frisen J (2008) Stem cells for spinal cord repair. Cell Stem Cell 3(1):16–24
6. Ohori Y, Yamamoto S, Nagao M, Sugimori M, Yamamoto N, Nakamura K, Nakafuku M (2006) Growth factor treatment and genetic manipulation stimulate neurogenesis and oligodendrogenesis by endogenous neural progenitors in the injured adult spinal cord. J Neurosci 26(46):11948–11960
7. Asahara T, Murohara T, Sullivan A, Silver M, van der Zee R, Li T, Witzenbichler B, Schatteman G, Isner JM (1997) Isolation of putative progenitor endothelial cells for angiogenesis. Science 275(5302):964–967
8. Isner JM, Asahara T (1999) Angiogenesis and vasculogenesis as therapeutic strategies for postnatal neovascularization. J Clin Invest 103(9):1231–1236
9. Kamei N, Kwon SM, Kawamoto A, Ii M, Ishikawa M, Ochi M, Asahara T (2012) Contribution of bone marrow-derived endothelial progenitor cells to neovascularization and astrogliosis following spinal cord injury. J Neurosci Res 90(12):2281–2292
10. Masuda H, Alev C, Akimaru H, Ito R, Shizuno T, Kobori M, Horii M, Ishihara T, Isobe K, Isozaki M, Itoh J, Itoh Y, Okada Y, McIntyre BA, Kato S, Asahara T (2011) Methodological development of a clonogenic assay to determine endothelial progenitor cell potential. Circ Res 109(1):20–37
11. Shen Q, Goderie SK, Jin L, Karanth N, Sun Y, Abramova N, Vincent P, Pumiglia K, Temple S (2004) Endothelial cells stimulate self-renewal and expand neurogenesis of neural stem cells. Science 304(5675):1338–1340
12. Kamei N, Kwon SM, Ishikawa M, Ii M, Nakanishi K, Yamada K, Hozumi K, Kawamoto A, Ochi M, Asahara T (2012) Endothelial progenitor cells promote astrogliosis following spinal cord injury through jagged1-dependent notch signaling. J Neurotrauma 29(9):1758–1769
13. Basso DM, Fisher LC, Anderson AJ, Jakeman LB, McTigue DM, Popovich PG (2006) Basso mouse scale for locomotion detects differences in recovery after spinal cord injury in five common mouse strains. J Neurotrauma 23(5):635–659
14. Kamei N, Kwon SM, Alev C, Ishikawa M, Yokoyama A, Nakanishi K, Yamada K, Horii M, Nishimura H, Takaki S, Kawamoto A, Ii M, Akimaru H, Tanaka N, Nishikawa S, Ochi M, Asahara T (2010) Lnk deletion reinforces the function of bone marrow progenitors in promoting neovascularization and astrogliosis following spinal cord injury. Stem cells 28(2):365–375
15. Yin AH, Miraglia S, Zanjani ED, Almeida-Porada G, Ogawa M, Leary AG, Olweus J, Kearney J, Buck DW (1997) AC133, a novel marker for human hematopoietic stem and progenitor cells. Blood 90(12):5002–5012
16. Masuda H, Iwasaki H, Kawamoto A, Akimaru H, Ishikawa M, Ii M, Shizuno T, Sato A, Ito R, Horii M, Ishida H, Kato S, Asahara T (2012) Development of serum-free quality and quantity control culture of colony-forming endothelial progenitor cell for vasculogenesis. Stem Cells Transl Med 1(2):160–171
17. Kamei N, Kwon SM, Alev C, Nakanishi K, Yamada K, Masuda H, Ishikawa M, Kawamoto A, Ochi M, Asahara T (2013) Ex-vivo expanded human blood-derived CD133+ cells promote repair of injured spinal cord. J Neurol Sci 328(1–2):41–50

Part V
Clinical Relevance

Chapter 25
Stress Distribution of the Spinal Cord and Clinical Relevance in Cervical Spondylotic Myelopathy

Kohei Takahashi, Hiroshi Ozawa, Naoya Sakamoto, Yuka Minegishi, Masaaki Sato, and Eiji Itoi

Abstract Intramedullary stress was analyzed in patients with cervical spondylotic myelopathy (CSM) using a finite element method (FEM). A total of 99 disc levels of 30 patients with CSM were analyzed and divided into two groups: 33 disc levels with high signal intensity (HSI) on T2WI MRI (HSI group) and 66 disc levels without HSI (non-HSI group). Ninety disc levels of 30 patients without myelopathy were set up as a control group. The stress in the HSI group was significantly highest among three groups. The cutoff value to present HSI was 2.30 kPa from a receiver operator characteristics (ROC) analysis. A multiple logistic regression analysis was performed to compare the utility of the three parameters as prognosticators for the onset of myelopathy: intramedullary stress, the cross-sectional area of the spinal

K. Takahashi
Department of Orthopaedic Surgery, Tohoku University School of Medicine, 1-1 Seiryomachi, Aobaku, Sendai 980-8574, Japan

Department of Orthopaedic Surgery, Senboku Kumiai Hospital, 1-30 Toricho Omagari, Daisen, Akita 014-0027, Japan

H. Ozawa (✉) • E. Itoi
Department of Orthopaedic Surgery, Tohoku University School of Medicine, 1-1 Seiryomachi, Aobaku, Sendai 980-8574, Japan
e-mail: hozawa@med.tohoku.ac.jp

N. Sakamoto
Graduate School of Biomedical Engineering, Tohoku University, 6-6-04 Aramaki Aoba, Aobaku, Sendai 980-8578, Japan

Department of Medical Engineering, Kawasaki University of Medical Welfare, 288 Matsushima, Kurashiki, Okayama 701-0193, Japan

Y. Minegishi • M. Sato
Graduate School of Biomedical Engineering, Tohoku University, 6-6-04 Aramaki Aoba, Aobaku, Sendai 980-8578, Japan

K. Uchida et al. (eds.), *Neuroprotection and Regeneration of the Spinal Cord*, DOI 10.1007/978-4-431-54502-6_25, © Springer Japan 2014

cord, and the anteroposterior compression ratio (APCR). Intramedullary stress had the highest odds ratio. The intramedullary stress significantly reduced after surgery. From the analysis of the correlation between the local kyphosis angle and the reduction of the stress after surgery in HSI group, the higher the kyphosis was, the less the reduction of the stress after surgery. In conclusion, intramedullary stress reflected clinical manifestations in patients with CSM.

Keywords Cervical spondylotic myelopathy • Finite element method • Intramedullary stress

25.1 Introduction

In patients with cervical spondylotic myelopathy (CSM), symptoms are attributed to compression of the spinal cord. However, compression of the spinal cord does not always induce symptomatic myelopathy. It is observed in 7.6–26 % of asymptomatic subjects [1, 2].

Numerous factors that contribute to the onset of cervical myelopathy have been reported. However, the degree of spinal cord compression inducing myelopathy remains inadequately understood. The cross-sectional area of the spinal cord and the anteroposterior compression ratio (APCR) of the spinal cord have been reported to be factors indicating the relationship between spinal cord deformities and symptoms of CSM [3–6]. However, it is not easy to evaluate whether the compression is symptomatic in the clinical practice even with those parameters.

Ozawa et al. [7] reported that the distribution of pathological changes in a unilateral spinal cord compression model using rabbits is compatible with the stress distribution drawn from the finite element method (FEM) model. Also, there have been several reports that show the significance of intramedullary stress to the pathogenesis of CSM by biomechanical simulations of cervical spinal cord compression using FEM [8–10]. However, there has been no research that clinically examines the relationship between neurological condition and intramedullary stress distribution in actual patients with CSM.

We considered that intramedullary stress is strongly related to the pathogenesis of cervical myelopathy. To clarify the influence of intramedullary stress on CSM, intramedullary stress distribution of the spinal cord was analyzed in patients with CSM using the FEM, and then the following four issues were investigated.

1. Influence of intramedullary stress on the onset of CSM
2. Comparison of clinical relevance among intramedullary stress, cross-sectional area, and APCR
3. Change of the intramedullary stress after decompression surgery
4. Relationship of intramedullary stress to sagittal alignment of cervical spine

25.2 Material and Methods

25.2.1 *Creating an FEM Model to Analyze Intramedullary Stress*

25.2.1.1 Extracting the Shape of the Spinal Cord

A midsagittal image of T2-weighted magnetic resonance image (T2WI) of the cervical spine was scaled up five times on a tablet (Cintiq 12WX®, Wacom, Japan). The anterior and posterior margins of the spinal cord from the inferior margin of the vertebral body of C2 to the inferior margin of the vertebral body of C7 were marked manually with dots at intervals of approximately 1 mm. The coordinate data of these dots were obtained using ImageJ® software (National Institutes of Health, NIH) (Fig. 25.1). The anterior and posterior margins were approximated by spline curves made from the coordinate data. The shape of the spinal cord was determined by combining the spline curves of the anterior and posterior margins.

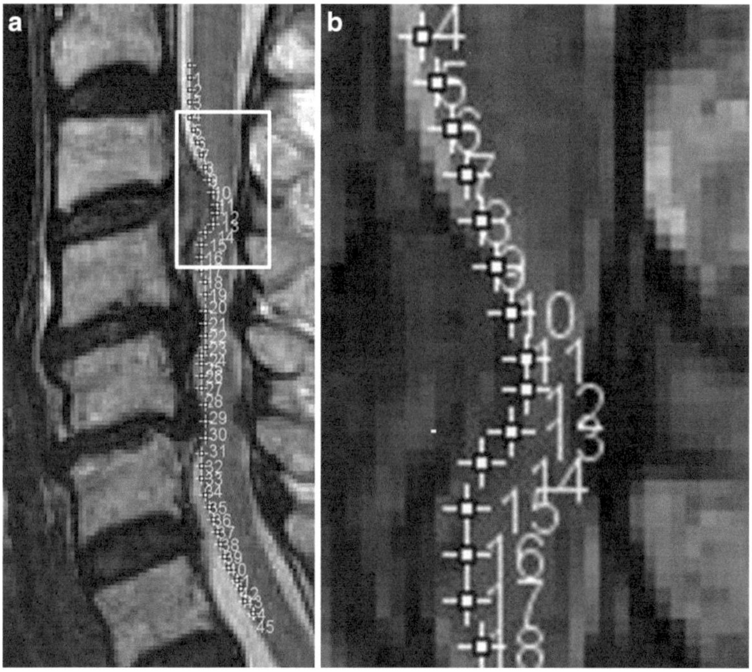

Fig. 25.1 Extracting the shape of the spinal cord. On the midsagittal T2WI images of the cervical spine, the anterior and posterior margins of the spinal cord from the inferior margin of the vertebral body of C2 to the inferior margin of the vertebral body of C7 were marked with dots at intervals of approximately 1 mm (**a**). (**b**) is a magnified figure of the square in (**a**)

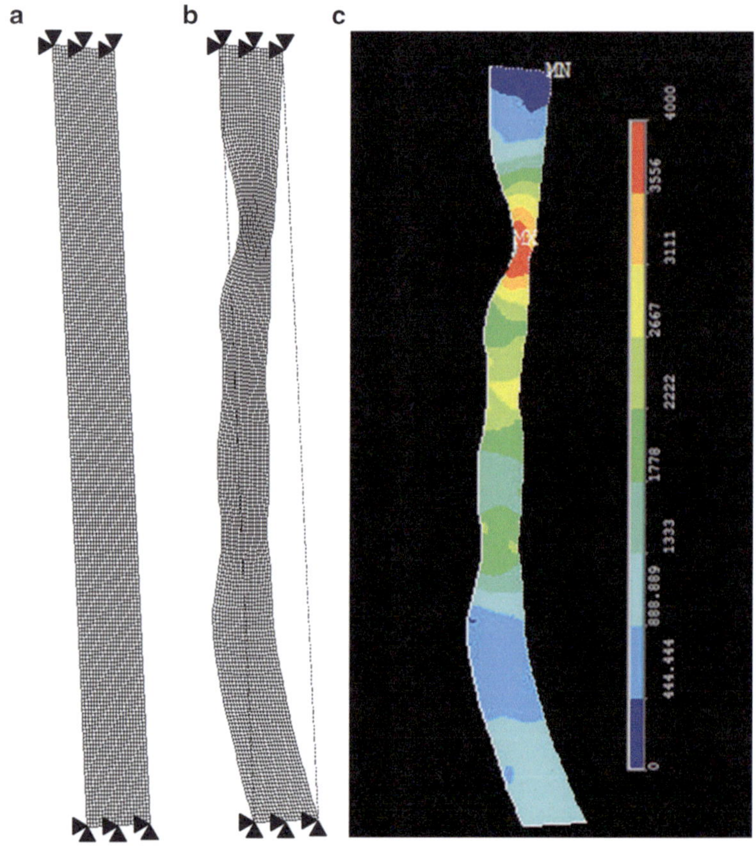

Fig. 25.2 FEM analysis. A straight line model was made by connecting the cranial and caudal corners of the spinal cord approximated by the spline curves (**a**). Then, the fixed displacement obtained from the spinal cord shape was imposed on the straight line model (**b**) and the stress distribution was quantified as the von Mises equivalent stress (**c**)

25.2.1.2 FEM Analysis

A straight line model made by connecting the cranial and caudal corners of the spinal cord approximated by the spline curves was constructed with 4,000 two-dimensional eight-node elements (Fig. 25.2a). Both the cranial (top) and caudal (bottom) edges of the model were constrained in all directions. Then, the fixed displacement obtained from the spinal cord shape was imposed on the straight line model (Fig. 25.2b) and the stress distribution was quantified as the von Mises equivalent stress using Ansys 11.0 software (Ansys Ver. 11, Ansys Inc., USA) (Fig. 25.2c). The initial modulus of elasticity and Poisson's ratio of the spinal cord were applied as 5 kPa and 0.49, respectively, based on a previous study [11]. The area from the middle of the vertebral body of C3 to the middle of the vertebral body of C4 was defined as the C3–4 disc level. The C4–5 and C5–6 disc levels were similarly defined (Fig. 25.3). The maximum stress value at each disc level was defined as the stress at that segment.

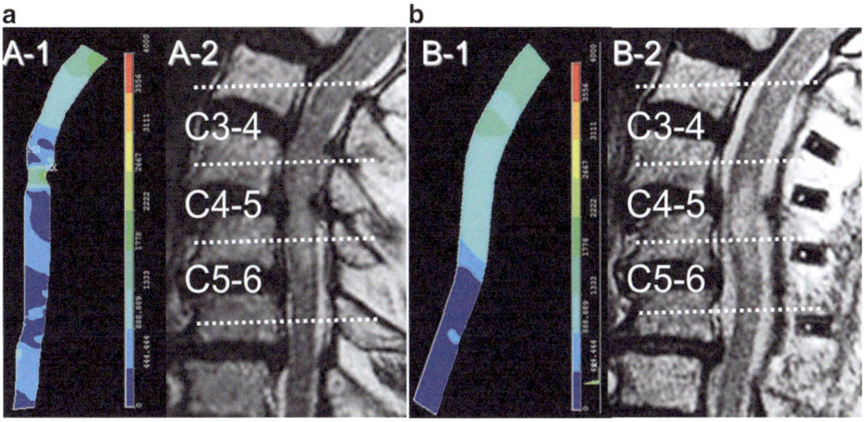

Fig. 25.3 On the preoperative midsagittal T2WI image, the intramedullary stress distribution was analyzed (**a**). The C4-5 disc level presented the highest stress. The postoperative stress was analyzed from midsagittal T2WI image (**b**). The stress at the C4-5 disc level reduced markedly

25.2.2 Patients for Analysis

Thirty-three consecutive patients (21 males and 12 females) with CSM who underwent Kurokawa's laminoplasty at one hospital were evaluated. These patients had been participants of another study designed as a prospective study [12]. All patients with CSM clinically presented transverse lesion syndrome consisting of bilateral motor and sensory deficits of the upper and lower limbs with exaggerated knee and Achilles jerks. These patients underwent preoperative MRI and then postoperative MRI 4 weeks after surgery. The mean age of the patients was 62.1 ± 11.0 (mean±SD) years (95 % confidence interval: 58.2–66.0).

All patients presented high signal intensity (HSI) in any of three disc levels of C3–4, C4–5, and C5–6 on T2WI MRI. The disc levels with HSI were at C3–4 in six cases, at C4–5 in 13 cases, and at C5–6 in 14 cases. A total of 99 disc levels from C3 to C6 in 33 patients were divided into two groups: 33 disc levels with HSI (HSI group) and 66 disc levels without HSI (non-HSI group).

Thirty patients (18 males and 12 females) who underwent cervical MRI for reasons other than myelopathy were enrolled in this study, and 90 disc levels from C3 to C6 were set up as a control group. The mean age of the control patients was 62.1 ± 13.0 (mean±SD) (95 % confidence interval: 57.3–66.9) years. All patients with CSM had spinal cord compression at least in one disc level and some of them had multilevel compression on MRI, while patients in the control group had no obvious spinal cord compression. None of the disc levels in the control group presented HSI on T2WI.

25.3 Illustrative Case

The patient was an 82-year-old male. The disc level presenting HSI was C4–5. The highest intramedullary stress was demonstrated in C4–5 disc level (C3–4: 1.7 kPa, C4–5: 2.9 kPa, and C5–6: 0.7 kPa) (Fig. 25.3a). The intramedullary stress at each disc level was clearly reduced after posterior decompression surgery (C3–4: 1.3 kPa, C4–5: 1.0 kPa, and C5–6: 0.5 kPa) (Fig. 25.3b).

25.4 Influence of Intramedullary Stress on the Onset of Cervical Spondylotic Myelopathy

25.4.1 Relationship Between HSI and Intramedullary Stress

To evaluate the relationship between intramedullary stress and spinal cord degeneration, intramedullary stress was compared among the HSI group, the non-HSI group, and the control group. In all patients with CSM, the disc level with HSI presented the highest stress among the three disc levels evaluated. Intramedullary stress was 3.16 ± 0.86 kPa (mean ± SD) in the HSI group, 1.81 ± 0.72 kPa in the non-HSI group, and 1.01 ± 0.37 kPa in the control group. The stress in the disc level with HSI was significantly highest among three groups ($p < 0.0001$) (Fig. 25.4).

Intramedullary signal change on MRI is generally considered to reflect nerve tissue degeneration [13]. In addition, the level of HSI on T2WI was deemed responsible for symptoms [14, 15]. In the present study, HSI was strongly associated with intramedullary stress. Thus intramedullary high stress due to spinal cord compression was considered to induce nerve tissue damage, resulting in the onset of CSM.

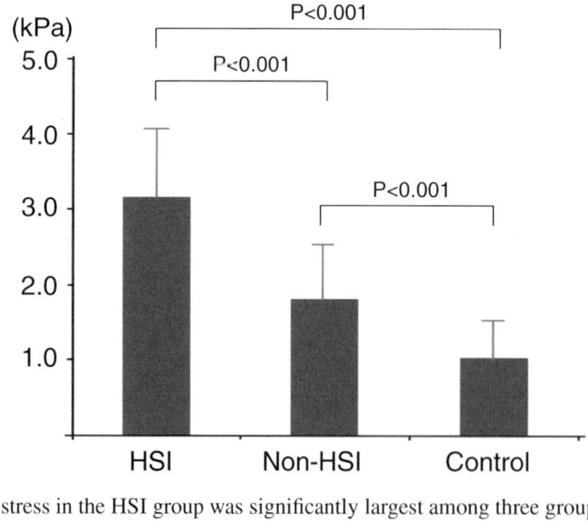

Fig. 25.4 The stress in the HSI group was significantly largest among three groups

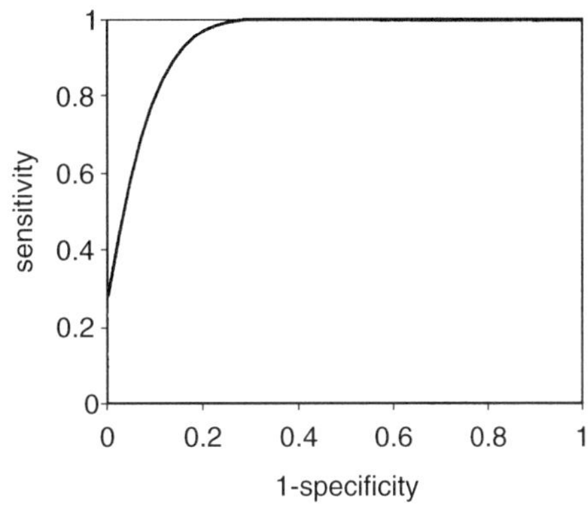

Fig. 25.5 Receiver operator characteristics curve for intramedullary stress. The areas under the curve (AUC) was 0.95. The most qualified cutoff value to cause the HSI was 2.30 kPa (sensitivity 78.8 %, specificity 91.9 %)

25.4.2 *Cutoff Value of Stress to Induce HSI*

The cutoff value of stress to induce HSI was investigated. A total of 189 disc levels in three groups were analyzed from a receiver operator characteristics (ROC) curve, and the cutoff value of stress to present HSI was investigated. The ROC curve is shown in Fig. 25.5. The area under the curve (AUC) was 0.95. The qualified cutoff value to cause the HSI was 2.30 kPa (sensitivity 78.8 %, specificity 91.9 %). There was no disc level presenting high intramedullary stress over 2.3 kPa without spinal cord compression on MRI. None of the disc levels in the control group exceeded 2.30 kPa.

Compression of the spinal cord is observed in 7.6–26 % of asymptomatic subjects [1, 2]. It is not easy to evaluate whether compression of the spinal cord is symptomatic. No disc level in the control group exceeded the cutoff value which was presented in the present study. We considered, therefore, that a threshold of intramedullary stress to present symptoms of myelopathy actually existed. That is, when the intramedullary stress reaches at some extent, neurological dysfunction should become obvious.

25.5 Comparison of Clinical Relevance Among Intramedullary Stress, Cross-Sectional Area, and APCR

A multiple logistic regression analysis was performed to compare the utility of each of these three parameters as prognosticators for the onset of myelopathy. The objective variable was whether the segment presented HSI, while the explanatory variables were stress, cross-sectional area, and APCR. The cutoff values for all the explanatory variables were obtained from the ROC analysis, and explanatory variables were converted to two-valued variables based on the cutoff values. The cutoff values for cross-sectional area and APCR were 57.3 mm^2 (sensitivity 69.7 %, specificity 69.7 %) and 36.2 % (sensitivity 75.8 %, specificity 74.3 %), respectively. The result of the multiple logistic regression analysis was shown in Table 25.1. The odds ratios for stress, cross-sectional area, and APCR were 11.1, 4.1, and 4.3, respectively. Stress showed

Table 25.1 Odds ratio of prognostic parameters

	Odds ratio (95 % CI)	*P* value
Intramedullary stress	11.1 (3.67–38.6)	$p<0.0001$
Area of spinal cord	4.1 (1.30–13.8)	$p=0.016$
APCR	4.3 (1.4–14.1)	$p=0.011$

APCR anteroposterior compression ratio

the largest odds ratio and was found to be the most useful prognosticator for the onset of myelopathy.

In the present study, the disc level with HSI presented the highest stress and the smallest cross-sectional area of the spinal cord among the three disc levels evaluated in all cases. However, in three cases, the disc levels with HSI did not correspond to the disc levels of the lowest APCR. The APCR does not express the severity of spinal cord deformities in some cases, for example, in cases in which the spinal cord is deformed into a boomerang shape or comma shape. We believe that the APCR is not an adequate parameter to express spinal cord deformities since it is calculated only for the transverse and anteroposterior diameters.

Penning et al. [6] reported that long tract signs appear when the cross-sectional area of the spinal cord is reduced by approximately 60 mm^2 or less, based on an analysis of CT myelograms in 80 cases of CSM. Kadanka et al. [5] reported that a cross-sectional area of the spinal cord between 50 and 60 mm^2 is the critical value for significant disability, based on a prospective study of a large cohort of patients with CSM. On the other hand, Golash et al. [16] suggested that the cross-sectional area of the spinal cord is not a prognosticator for the presence of myelopathy since the area overlaps significantly between patients with and those without myelopathy. Kato et al. [17] reported that the cross-sectional area of the spinal cord at any disc level shows a dispersion with a standard deviation of approximately 10 mm^2 based on the cervical MRI images of 1,211 asymptomatic subjects. The absolute value of the cross-sectional area of the spinal cord does not predict the onset of CSM.

We analyzed the intramedullary stress of the patients with CSM from sagittal image. A stress analysis of sagittal MR images reflects both the spinal cord compression and sagittal alignment of the spinal cord, which cannot be expressed on axial images. The sagittal alignment of the cervical spine has a potent effect on the prognosis of CSM [18]. The method of analysis of the sagittal plane implemented in the present study was considered to have an advantage for investigating the pathological conditions of the spinal cord.

25.6 Preoperative and Postoperative Stress Values of the HSI Group

Preoperative and postoperative stress values of the HSI group were compared using paired t-test. The preoperative stress in the HSI group was 3.16 ± 0.86 kPa, and the postoperative stress was down to 1.38 ± 0.43 kPa. It reduced significantly after the surgery ($p<0.0001$) (Fig. 25.6).

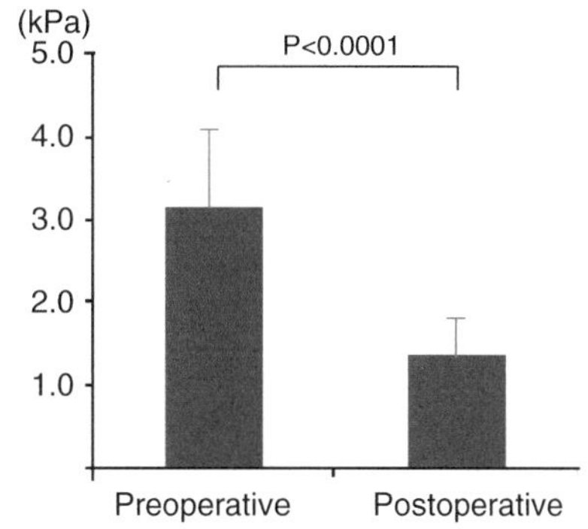

Fig. 25.6 The stress significantly reduced after surgery in the HIS group ($p<0.0001$)

The intramedullary stress of the HSI group significantly reduced after surgery. Reduction of the stress could be attributed to the restoration of spinal cord configuration obtained by surgical decompression. Consequently, reduction of the stress should involve in the decrease of the neuronal tissue damage and improvement of the neurological function.

25.7 Relationship of Intramedullary Stress to Sagittal Alignment of the Cervical Spine

Influence of the sagittal alignment of cervical spine on the postoperative change of intramedullary stress was investigated. The local kyphosis angle was measured on the lateral view of the radiograms. The local kyphosis angle was defined as the angle formed by two lines drawn along the posterior margin of the most cranial and caudal vertebral bodies forming the maximum local kyphosis according to the method described by Suda et al. [18]. Correlation between the local kyphosis angle and the reduction of the stress after surgery was calculated in HSI group. The HSI group were divided into two groups according to the local kyphosis angle: the lordosis group presenting the local kyphosis angle less than 0° (L group) and the kyphosis group presenting the local kyphosis angle exceeding 0° (K group).

The difference between preoperative and postoperative stress in the L group showed a high dispersion independently of the local kyphosis angle. The difference between the preoperative and postoperative stress was not correlated with the local kyphosis angle in the L group ($r=-0.45$, $p=0.07$). In the K group, two variables, however, were negatively correlated ($r=-0.59$, $p=0.02$) (Fig. 25.7). That is, as the kyphosis was severe, the reduction of the stress after surgery was decreased.

It was reported that the sagittal cervical alignment influences on the surgical outcome of CSM. Suda et al. reported that neurological recovery after expansive laminoplasty for CSM was poor in patients with the local kyphosis angle exceeding 13° [18]. Laminoplasty consists of two distinct mechanisms for decompression effect: a direct posterior decompression effect and an indirect anterior decompression effect. Indirect anterior decompression is considered to be attributed to the

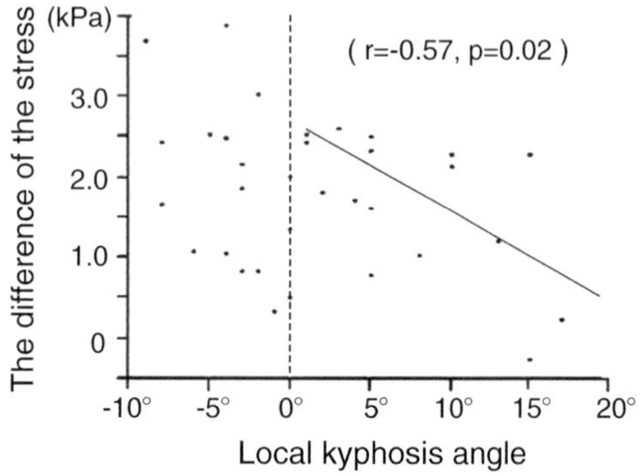

Fig. 25.7 Correlation between local kyphosis angle and the difference of the stress between before and after surgery in HIS group showing significantly negative correlation when the local kyphosis angle exceeded 0°

posterior spinal cord shifting from the anterior compressive lesions, which was demonstrated after posterior decompression surgery [19]. In cases with severe kyphosis, ventral compression after posterior decompression surgery is presumably likely to persist, resulting in poor surgical outcomes. In the present study, the deformity of the spinal cord remained after surgery in K group. It induced the less reduction of stress after surgery. The previous report that the severe kyphotic deformity is a risk factor for poor surgical outcomes was supported from a standpoint of intramedullary stress.

25.8 Conclusion

1. Intramedullary stress should be a highly important factor for the onset of CSM. When the intramedullary stress reaches at some extent, neurological dysfunction should become obvious.
2. Stress was found to be a more important prognosticator for the onset of CSM than the cross-sectional area of the spinal cord and the APCR.
3. Reduction of the stress, which is obtained by posterior decompression surgery, improves the neurological function.
4. The severer the kyphosis was, the less the reduction of the stress was obtained after the posterior decompression surgery.

Conflict of Interest The authors declare that they have no conflict of interest.

References

1. Teresi LM, Lufkin RB, Reicher MA et al (1987) Asymptomatic degenerative disk disease and spondylosis of the cervical spine: MR imaging. Radiology 164:83–88
2. Matsumoto M, Fujimura Y, Suzuki N et al (1998) MRI of cervical intervertebral discs in asymptomatic subjects. J Bone Joint Surg Br 80:19–24

3. Bucciero A, Vizioli L, Tedeschi G (1993) Cord diameters and their significance in prognostication and decisions about management of cervical spondylotic myelopathy. J Neurosurg Sci 37:223–228
4. Fujiwara K, Yonenobu K, Hiroshima K et al (1988) Morphometry of the cervical spinal cord and its relation to pathology in cases with compression myelopathy. Spine 13:1212–1216
5. Kadanka Z, Kerkovsky M, Bednarik J et al (2007) Cross-sectional transverse area and hyperintensities on magnetic resonance imaging in relation to the clinical picture in cervical spondylotic myelopathy. Spine 32:2573–2577
6. Penning L, Wilmink JT, van Woerden HH et al (1986) CT myelographic findings in degenerative disorders of the cervical spine: clinical significance. AJR Am J Roentgenol 146:793–801
7. Ozawa H, Wu ZJ, Tanaka Y et al (2004) Morphologic change and astrocyte response to unilateral spinal cord compression in rabbits. J Neurotrauma 21:944–955
8. Scifert J, Totoribe K, Goel V et al (2002) Spinal cord mechanics during flexion and extension of the cervical spine: a finite element study. Pain Physician 5:394–400
9. Ichihara K, Taguchi T, Sakuramoto I et al (2003) Mechanism of the spinal cord injury and the cervical spondylotic myelopathy: new approach based on the mechanical features of the spinal cord white and gray matter. J Neurosurg 99:278–285
10. Kato Y, Kanchiku T, Imajo Y et al (2010) Biomechanical study of the effect of degree of static compression of the spinal cord in ossification of the posterior longitudinal ligament. J Neurosurg Spine 12:301–305
11. Ozawa H, Matsumoto T, Ohashi T et al (2001) Comparison of spinal cord gray matter and white matter softness: measurement by pipette aspiration method. J Neurosurg (Spine 2) 95:221–224
12. Ozawa H, Sato T, Hyodo H et al (2010) Clinical significance of intramedullary Gd-DTPA enhancement in cervical myelopathy. Spinal Cord 48:415–422
13. Ohshio I, Hatayama A, Kaneda K et al (1993) Correlation between histopathologic features and magnetic resonance images of spinal cord lesions. Spine 18:1140–1149
14. Matsumoto M, Ishikawa M, Ishii K et al (2005) Usefulness of neurological examination for diagnosis of the affected level in patients with cervical compressive myelopathy: prospective comparative study with radiological evaluation. J Neurosurg Spine 2:535–539
15. Seichi A, Takeshita K, Kawaguchi H et al (2006) Neurologic level diagnosis of cervical stenotic myelopathy. Spine 31:1338–1343
16. Golash A, Birchall D, Laitt RD et al (2001) Significance of CSF area measurements in cervical spondylitic myelopathy. Br J Neurosurg 15:17–21
17. Kato F, Yukawa Y, Suda K et al (2012) Normal morphology, age-related changes and abnormal findings of the cervical spine. Part II: magnetic resonance imaging of over 1,200 asymptomatic subjects. Eur Spine J 21:1499–1507
18. Suda K, Abumi K, Ito M et al (2003) Local kyphosis reduces surgical outcomes of expansive open-door laminoplasty for cervical spondylotic myelopathy. Spine 28:1258–1262
19. Hatta Y, Shiraishi T, Hase H et al (2005) Is posterior spinal cord shifting by extensive posterior decompression clinically significant for multisegmental cervical spondylotic myelopathy? Spine 30:2414–2419

Chapter 26
Applications and Limitations of pNF-H, a Novel Biomarker for Spinal Cord Injury: Strategy for the Evaluation of Therapeutic Outcomes

Toru Ogata, Kentaro Hayakawa, and Hirotaka Chikuda

Abstract The development of proper outcome measurements is as important as developing novel therapies. One of the characteristic issues in spinal cord injury (SCI) is the difficulty in severity evaluation at an early time point. In general, the assessment of tissue damage can be achieved by measurement of tissue-specific proteins released into peripheral blood. Phosphorylated neurofilament NF-H (pNF-H) is a cytoskeletal structural protein in neurons. In addition to its physiological function, pNF-H has been reported as a biomarker for axonal damage because of its stability within blood. In both rodent SCI models and human SCI patients, higher pNF-H values in blood correlate with more severe neural tissue damage. It would be possible to determine the severity of SCI by measuring blood pNF-H at either 24 or 96 h after injury. This better prognostic evaluation may reduce the number of required patients in clinical studies and facilitate the development of novel therapies for SCI.

Keywords Biomarker • ELISA • Prognosis

26.1 Introduction

The development of novel therapies for spinal cord injury (SCI) has been attempted in various ways, including surgical, pharmacological, and cellular approaches. Focusing on acute SCI, it is still controversial whether immediate decompression is

T. Ogata (✉)
Research Institute, National Rehabilitation Center for Persons with Disabilities, 4-1 Namiki, Tokorozawa, Saitama 359-8555, Japan
e-mail: ogata-toru@rehab.go.jp

K. Hayakawa • H. Chikuda
Department of Orthopaedic Surgery, The University of Tokyo, 7-3-1, Hongou, Bunkyo-ku, Tokyo 113-0033, Japan

K. Uchida et al. (eds.), *Neuroprotection and Regeneration of the Spinal Cord*, DOI 10.1007/978-4-431-54502-6_26, © Springer Japan 2014

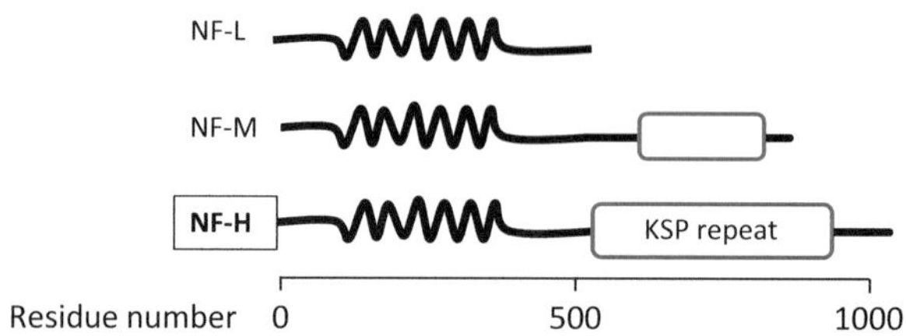

Fig. 26.1 The structure of high molecular weight neurofilament. NF-H is the longest form of neurofilament, having 150 kd as its molecular weight. Near its C-terminus NF-H contains more than 50 repeats of the serine–lysine–proline (KSP) motif, which is phosphorylated by kinases such as CDK5, physiologically

beneficial for SCI without bone lesions [1]. As for pharmacological approach, several drugs are now in clinical trials, such as anti-Nogo drugs [2], minocycline [3], the Rho-inhibitor Cethrin [4], and G-CSF [5], which are intended to either reduce secondary damage or promote neural regeneration and plastic reorganization. Although there are promising preclinical results to support the effectiveness of these therapies, the variability of SCI severity and the difficulty in making an accurate prognostic evaluation make the design of clinical trials impose on including a large number of patients, which is one of the main obstacles in this field.

The proper prognostic evaluation of SCI has been based on clinical findings and radiological results such as magnetic resonance imaging and computed tomography. However, it is sometimes difficult to perform precise neurological evaluation because of damage to other organs and/or the unconsciousness of patients [6]. In addition, spontaneous recovery is frequently observed in acute SCI patients, even in the case of patients manifesting complete paralysis. Therefore, when we observe neurological recovery several months after SCI, we can hardly determine whether the improvement is due to specific therapeutic intervention or the natural course of the patient. Therefore, the development of an objective method to evaluate the severity and prognosis of SCI is necessary.

In other medical fields, blood samples give large amounts of information related to diagnosis and severity. In the field of central nervous system disorders, S100B, a protein expressed in glial cells, and neuron specific enolase (NSE) have been used for the diagnosis of cerebrovascular diseases [7, 8]. These proteins are physiologically expressed within neural cells and thought to be released to peripheral cerebrospinal fluid, and peripheral blood flow, when cells are damaged and the cell membrane is disrupted. Several studies measured these proteins in blood samples from SCI patients, but were of limited usefulness because of their short life in blood and low specificity to the nervous system.

High molecular weight neurofilament (NF-H) is one of the cytoskeletal molecules expressed in neurons (Fig. 26.1). Multiple phosphorylation in its KSP region contributes to the stabilization of the complex with the fiber bundles in axons. In addition to its physiological functions, pNF-H is also known as an accumulating protein in degenerative diseases, such as amyotrophic lateral sclerosis (ALS) [9]. In some types of ALS, the dysfunction of transport systems, which send newly synthesized neurofilaments to axons, causes accumulation of pNF-H at the cell bodies. In 2005, Shaw et al. reported that the phosphorylated form of NF-H (pNF-H) showed resistance to degradation by calpains and is stable in blood [10]. They also insisted that this molecule has the potential to be used as a biomarker to evaluate axonal damage in CNS disorders. In fact, they reported that pNF-H is elevated in both blood samples and cerebrospinal fluid samples from ALS patients [11]. In this chapter, we discuss the usefulness and limitations of this novel biomarker, pNF-H, in the clinical field of SCI.

26.2 Measurement of pNF-H in Rodent Models

To evaluate the sensitivity of blood pNF-H level in discriminating the severity of SCI, we used a mouse SCI model, in which we took daily blood samples from the tail vein. The blood pNF-H values were determined by an enzyme-linked immunosorbent assay (ELISA). The severity of SCI was determined by setting damage force in a spinal cord contusion device. The trend of average pNF-H values showed a single peak pattern regardless of the severity. The values marked their peak value at the third day after injury, returning to the pre-injured level (below minimal detection value) after 2–3 weeks. Although the trends are similar, their peak values differ depending on the severity. The mice who received the most severe injury (90 kdyn) had the highest pNF-H value at 3 days after injury, while mice with less severe SCI show lower pNF-H values. Therefore, blood pNF-H seems to correlate with the degree of trauma in the spinal cord (Fig. 26.2).

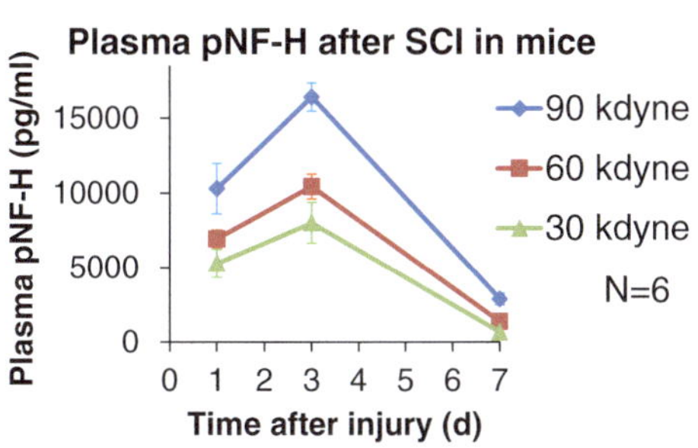

Fig. 26.2 The time course of blood pNF-H levels in rodent SCI model. Mice received various degrees of SCI (impact force: 30, 60, or 90 kdyn). Serial peripheral blood samples were collected to determine pNF-H levels. Regardless of the severity of SCI, the peak pNF-H values were observed at 3 days after injury and higher peak pNF-H values correspond to more severe damage to spinal cord

26.3 Measurement of pNF-H in Humans

To confirm the usability of pNF-H in clinical practice, we collected blood samples from acute SCI patients. In this study, we set inclusion criteria as patients having cervical SCI and not having severe traumatic brain injury. In some cases, blood samples were repeatedly collected until 3 weeks after injury. We recorded clinical symptoms on admission and also at the final examination (average duration of 6 months).

First of all, we confirmed that pNF-H is elevated in SCI patients' blood samples. In most patients who showed complete SCI, pNF-H was initially detected as early as 18 h after injury. Serial samples indicated that the pNF-H level increases gradually for several days after injury (Fig. 26.3). In contrast to the rodent model, in which pNF-H marks its peak value at 3 days after injury, human SCI samples showed sustained elevation of pNF-H even after 3 days. When we plotted the pNF-H values according to the severity of paralysis at end point, we observed higher pNF-H values in complete SCI (AIS A) group compared to incomplete SCI (AIS C and D) group with a statistically significant difference. Thus, the difference was observed at both 24 and 96 h after injury (Fig. 26.4).

In some cases, we continued to measure pNF-H for up to 3 weeks. All four cases (two cases with AIS A and two cases with AIS C) showed sustained elevation of pNF-H even at 3 weeks after injury. At the third week, the difference in pNF-H value between AIS A and C become unclear (data not shown).

26.4 Discussion

We evaluated the usefulness of pNF-H as a biomarker for SCI in both animal models and clinical cases and found that blood pNF-H level in the early phase of SCI is correlated with its overall severity [12, 13].

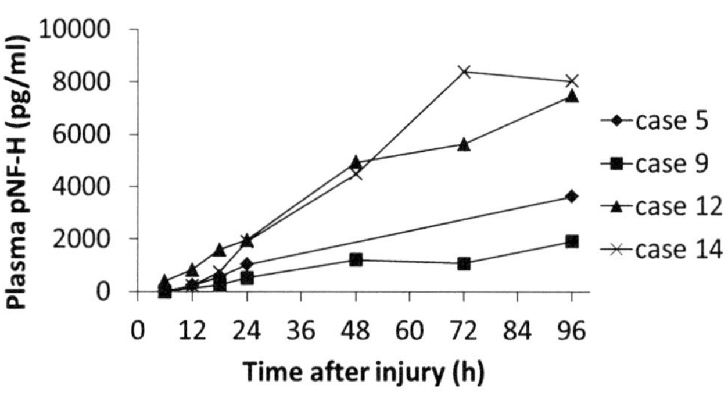

Fig. 26.3 Serial pNF-H measurements in complete SCI patients. The plasma pNF-H levels of four patients who were graded as AIS A at the final follow-up are shown. In those patients, pNF-H was detectable in plasma from 18 h after injury (221–825 pg/ml), and it increased until 96 h after injury (1,919–8,023 pg/ml)

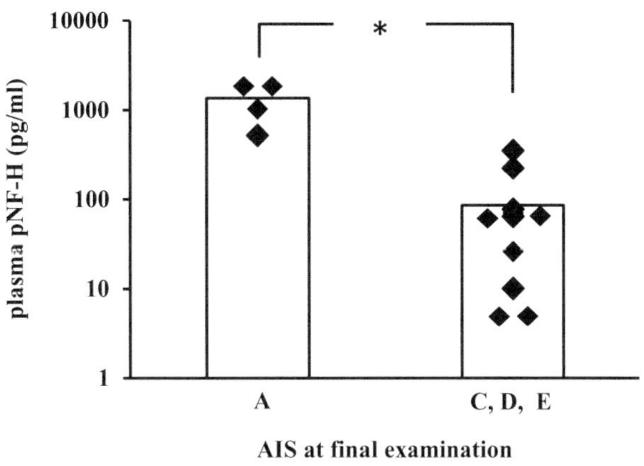

Fig. 26.4 Blood pNF-H level was elevated in accordance with the severity of the injury. There was a marked difference between AIS A patients (complete SCI) and AIS C–E patients (incomplete SCI), with statistical significance at 24 h after injury

Table 26.1 The list of biomarkers for central nervous system disorders

Name	Cell types	Physiological function	Reference
pNF-H	Neurons (axon)	Cytoskeletal molecule	[13]
Tau	Neurons	Microtubule associated protein	[20]
UCHL1	Neurons (cell body)	Deubiquitinating enzyme	[15]
NSE	Neurons	Glycolytic enzyme	[21]
S100B	Astrocytes	Calcium-binding protein	[8]
GFAP	Astrocytes	Intermediate filament	[22]
MBP	Oligodendrocytes	A structural protein of myelin	[23]

26.4.1 Comparison with Other Biomarkers

The characteristics of pNF-H compared to preexisting biomarkers for CNS disorders are (1) it is measureable in blood samples and (2) it remains elevated for several days or even more. The first point enables easy access to samples compared to cerebrospinal fluid, in which most of the biomarkers, including pNF-H, exist at higher concentration than in peripheral blood [14]. Repeated measurement would be useful to achieve more information about the state of injured spinal cord. As for the second point, pNF-H in complete SCI patients remains elevated for more than 1 month. Other biomarkers, such as S100 and NSE, are elevated within blood but their levels return to baseline rapidly (within 24–48 h) [8]. The short duration of the detection time-window makes it difficult to obtain proper samples to evaluate the severity of patients. The gradual increase of pNF-H (detectable at 18 h after injury) may have some disadvantages. Since most of the therapeutic interventions are intended to start as early as possible, the ideal biomarker should be detectable immediately after injury. It would be beneficial to use pNF-H in combination with other biomarkers which become detectable at an early time point, such as S100B or UCHL1 [15]. Table 26.1 shows a list of possible biomarkers in the CNS.

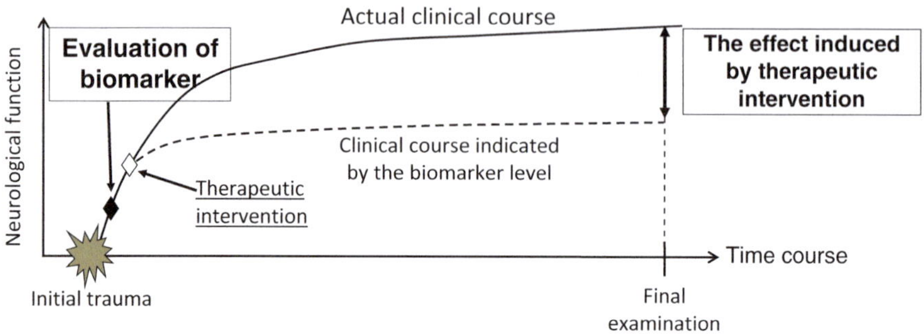

Fig. 26.5 Application of biomarkers for the evaluation of novel therapies for SCI. The evaluation of biomarkers might assist in the precise prediction of prognosis before therapeutic intervention. The effect induced by therapeutic intervention is then estimated by the difference between the actual clinical course and the clinical course indicated by the biomarker level

26.4.2 Possible Applications of pNF-H

One of the possible applications of pNF-H measurement is the prognostic evaluation of acute SCI. A precise prognostic evaluation is helpful to organize rehabilitation programs for each patient. Furthermore, such evaluation may contribute to designing clinical trials of novel therapies for SCI. Several approaches to improve the outcomes of SCI by intervention at an early time point, such as within 1 week after injury, are in the preclinical stage. At the moment, we cannot distinguish patients with "definite complete paralysis," who will remain completely paralyzed after several months, and those with "temporary complete paralysis," who manifest complete paralysis on admission and gradually recover to incomplete paralysis over 1–3 months. If we could set up a definite cutoff line of pNF-H values at 24 h after injury to distinguish these two subgroups at recruitment, we can exclude "temporary paralysis" from clinical trials to improve the specificity of the outcome (schematically shown in Fig. 26.5). To set up such a cutoff value, further clinical studies are required to associate early pNF-H levels with neurological findings in the chronic stage [13].

26.4.3 The Limitation of pNF-H as a Biomarker

Despite its high sensitivity in CNS disorders, the specificity of pNF-H is still controversial. So far, elevation of pNF-H is reported in traumatic brain injury, subarachnoid hemorrhage, ALS, and prolonged febrile seizure [16–19]. We also confirmed that pNF-H is expressed in peripheral nerves and detectable in peripheral nerve injury. Considering that brain trauma is a common comorbidity of cervical SCI, we should be careful in the assessment of blood pNF-H values. In addition, it is possible that patients have elevated pNF-H values prior to their injury, due to other diseases. To exclude such a possibility, it would be recommended to perform sequential measurements of blood pNF-H, in which gradual increases within 7–14 days may represent a newly generated insult to the CNS.

26.4.4 Issues to Be Solved

There remain several unresolved aspects regarding basic knowledge about pNF-H levels. For example, in both rodent and human SCI, blood pNF-H gradually increases for several days, but it is not clear whether the increase represents secondary axonal damage and/or axonal degeneration after a primary injury. As we showed, the time course is different between rodent and human SCI. Considering the large molecular size of pNF-H, its sustained elevation in human SCI implicates certain mechanisms to carry the molecule beyond the blood–brain barrier. At present, we are only able to assess blood-pNF-H levels empirically. The understanding of the mechanisms how pNF-H is released to peripheral blood may give us more insight into the state of the injured spinal cord and enable us to use this biomarker for more theoretical considerations.

26.5 Conclusion

At this moment, we should be careful in using pNF-H values for clinical purposes, including clinical trials; it might be useful in confirming complete paralysis, but its potential to estimate prognosis of incomplete SCI remains unknown. However, in spite of several crucial limitations that have yet to be solved, measurement of blood pNF-H is a novel way to look into the pathological processes after trauma in the spinal cord. Therefore, future studies, both clinical and basic, may provide us with new insight into the pathological processes of the injured spinal cord.

Conflict of Interest Toru Ogata, Kentaro Hayakawa, and Hirotaka Chikuda declare that they have no conflict of interest.

References

1. Chikuda H, Ohtsu H, Ogata T, Sugita S, Sumitani M, Koyama Y, Matsumoto M, Toyama Y (2013) Optimal treatment for spinal cord injury associated with cervical canal stenosis (OSCIS): a study protocol for a randomized controlled trial comparing early versus delayed surgery. Trials 14:245
2. Zorner B, Schwab ME (2010) Anti-nogo on the go: from animal models to a clinical trial. Ann N Y Acad Sci 1198(Suppl 1):E22–E34

3. Casha S, Zygun D, Mcgowan MD, Bains I, Yong VW, Hurlbert RJ (2012) Results of a phase II placebo-controlled randomized trial of minocycline in acute spinal cord injury. Brain J Neurol 135:1224–1236
4. Mckerracher L, Anderson K (2013) Analysis of recruitment and outcomes in the phase I/IIa cethrin clinical trial for acute spinal cord injury. J Neurotrauma 30:1795–804
5. Takahashi H, Yamazaki M, Okawa A, Sakuma T, Kato K, Hashimoto M, Hayashi K, Furuya T, Fujiyoshi T, Kawabe J, Yamauchi T, Mannoji C, Miyashita T, Kadota R, Ito Y, Takahashi K, Koda M (2012) Neuroprotective therapy using granulocyte colony-stimulating factor for acute spinal cord injury: a phase I/IIa clinical trial. Eur Spine J 21:2580–2587
6. Bach-y-Rita P, Illis LS (1993) Spinal shock: possible role of receptor plasticity and non synaptic transmission. Paraplegia 31:82–87
7. Kochanek PM, Berger RP, Bayir H, Wagner AK, Jenkins LW, Clark RS (2008) Biomarkers of primary and evolving damage in traumatic and ischemic brain injury: diagnosis, prognosis, probing mechanisms, and therapeutic decision making. Curr Opin Crit Care 14:135–141
8. Loy DN, Sroufe AE, Pelt JL, Burke DA, Cao QL, Talbott JF, Whittemore SR (2005) Serum biomarkers for experimental acute spinal cord injury: rapid elevation of neuron-specific enolase and S-100beta. Neurosurgery 56:391–397
9. Chou SM, Wang HS, Taniguchi A (1996) Role of SOD-1 and nitric oxide/cyclic GMP cascade on neurofilament aggregation in ALS/MND. J Neurol Sci 139(Suppl):16–26
10. Shaw G, Yang C, Ellis R, Anderson K, Parker Mickle J, Scheff S, Pike B, Anderson DK, Howland DR (2005) Hyperphosphorylated neurofilament NF-H is a serum biomarker of axonal injury. Biochem Biophys Res Commun 336:1268–1277
11. Boylan KB, Glass JD, Crook JE, Yang C, Thomas CS, Desaro P, Johnston A, Overstreet K, Kelly C, Polak M, Shaw G (2013) Phosphorylated neurofilament heavy subunit (pNF-H) in peripheral blood and CSF as a potential prognostic biomarker in amyotrophic lateral sclerosis. J Neurol Neurosurg Psychiatry 84:467–472
12. Ueno T, Ohori Y, Ito J, Hoshikawa S, Yamamoto S, Nakamura K, Tanaka S, Akai M, Tobimatsu Y, Ogata T (2011) Hyperphosphorylated neurofilament NF-H as a biomarker of the efficacy of minocycline therapy for spinal cord injury. Spinal Cord 49:333–336
13. Hayakawa K, Okazaki R, Ishii K, Ueno T, Izawa N, Tanaka Y, Toyooka S, Matsuoka N, Morioka K, Ohori Y, Nakamura K, Akai M, Tobimatsu Y, Hamabe Y, Ogata T (2012) Phosphorylated neurofilament subunit NF-H as a biomarker for evaluating the severity of spinal cord injury patients, a pilot study. Spinal cord 50:493–496
14. Kwon BK, Stammers AM, Belanger LM, Bernardo A, Chan D, Bishop CM, Slobogean GP, Zhang H, Umedaly H, Giffin M, Street J, Boyd MC, Paquette SJ, Fisher CG, Dvorak MF (2010) Cerebrospinal fluid inflammatory cytokines and biomarkers of injury severity in acute human spinal cord injury. J Neurotrauma 27:669–682
15. Blyth BJ, Farahvar A, He H, Nayak A, Yang C, Shaw G, Bazarian JJ (2011) Elevated serum ubiquitin carboxy-terminal hydrolase L1 is associated with abnormal blood–brain barrier function after traumatic brain injury. J Neurotrauma 28:2453–2462
16. Lewis SB, Wolper RA, Miralia L, Yang C, Shaw G (2008) Detection of phosphorylated NF-H in the cerebrospinal fluid and blood of aneurysmal subarachnoid hemorrhage patients. J Cereb Blood Flow Metab 28:1261–1271
17. Boylan K, Yang C, Crook J, Overstreet K, Heckman M, Wang Y, Borchelt D, Shaw G (2009) Immunoreactivity of the phosphorylated axonal neurofilament H subunit (pNF-H) in blood of ALS model rodents and ALS patients: evaluation of blood pNF-H as a potential ALS biomarker. J Neurochem 111:1182–1191
18. Anderson KJ, Scheff SW, Miller KM, Roberts KN, Gilmer LK, Yang C, Shaw G (2008) The phosphorylated axonal form of the neurofilament subunit NF-H (pNF-H) as a blood biomarker of traumatic brain injury. J Neurotrauma 25:1079–1085
19. Matsushige T, Inoue H, Fukunaga S, Hasegawa S, Okuda M, Ichiyama T (2012) Serum neurofilament concentrations in children with prolonged febrile seizures. Journal of the neurological sciences 321:39–42

20. Park D, Joo SS, Lee HJ, Choi KC, Kim SU, Kim YB (2012) Microtubule-associated protein 2, an early blood marker of ischemic brain injury. J Neurosci Res 90:461–467
21. Costine BA, Quebeda-Clerkin PB, Dodge CP, Harris BT, Hillier SC, Duhaime AC (2012) Neuron-specific enolase, but not S100B or myelin basic protein, increases in peripheral blood corresponding to lesion volume after cortical impact in piglets. J Neurotrauma 29:2689–2695
22. Vos PE, Jacobs B, Andriessen TM, Lamers KJ, Borm GF, Beems T, Edwards M, Rosmalen CF, Vissers JL (2010) GFAP and S100B are biomarkers of traumatic brain injury: an observational cohort study. Neurology 75:1786–1793
23. Papa L, Ramia MM, Kelly JM, Burks SS, Pawlowicz A, Berger RP (2013) Systematic review of clinical research on biomarkers for pediatric traumatic brain injury. J Neurotrauma 30:324–338

Chapter 27
Neuroprotective Therapy Using Granulocyte Colony-Stimulating Factor for Acute Spinal Cord Injury: A Multicenter Prospective Controlled Clinical Trial

Masashi Yamazaki, Hiroshi Takahashi, Takeo Furuya, and Masao Koda

Abstract We conducted a multicenter prospective controlled clinical trial to assess the feasibility of neuroprotective therapy using granulocyte colony-stimulating factor (G-CSF) for patients with acute spinal cord injury (SCI). The trial ran from August 2009 to March 2011 and included 45 SCI patients treated within 48 h of onset. Informed consent was obtained from all patients. After providing consent, patients were divided into two groups. In the G-CSF group (19 patients), G-CSF (10 μg/kg/day) was intravenously administered for five consecutive days, and in the control group (26 patients), patients were similarly treated except for the G-CSF administration. We evaluated motor functions using the American Spinal Cord Injury Association (ASIA) score 3 months after onset. The increase in ASIA motor score was significantly higher in the G-CSF group (26.1 ± 18.9) than in the control group (12.2 ± 14.7) (P < 0.01). In cases of incomplete paralysis (18 patients in the G-CSF group and 19 patients in the control group), the increase in motor score was also significantly higher (P < 0.05) in the G-CSF group (27.1 ± 18.9) than in the control group (15.1 ± 15.9). The present results suggest the possibility that G-CSF administration has beneficial effects on neurological recovery in patients with acute SCI. We believe that neuroprotection using G-CSF is an effective therapeutic strategy for acute SCI treatment.

Keywords Clinical trial • G-CSF • Neuroprotective therapy • Spinal cord injury

M. Yamazaki (✉)
Department of Orthopaedic Surgery, University of Tsukuba,
1-1-1 Tennodai, Tsukuba-City, Ibaraki 305-8575, Japan
e-mail: masashiy@md.tsukuba.ac.jp

H. Takahashi • T. Furuya • M. Koda
Department of Orthopaedic Surgery, Chiba University Graduate School
of Medicine, Chiba, Japan

K. Uchida et al. (eds.), *Neuroprotection and Regeneration of the Spinal Cord*,
DOI 10.1007/978-4-431-54502-6_27, © Springer Japan 2014

27.1 Introduction

In Japan, there are currently more than 200,000 people with spinal cord injuries (SCI), and about 50,000 new SCI patients are diagnosed every year. Thus far, however, there has been no treatment to cure SCI, and neurological recovery has been determined according to the degree of injury at the onset. When SCI occurs, the primary injury is mechanical stress to the spinal cord. After that, secondary injury occurs, i.e., an inflammatory reaction caused by the release of pro-inflammatory cytokines [1]. It is conceivable that methylprednisolone sodium succinate (MPSS) relieves secondary injury to the spinal cord [2, 3]. However, many have questioned the efficacy of MPSS [4–7], and the side effects in the respiratory system and digestive organs are often critical for patients [5, 8]. Because of these reports, development of new therapeutic drugs for SCI has been expected.

Granulocyte colony-stimulating factor (G-CSF) is a 19.6-kDa glycoprotein. It is best known as a growth factor for hematopoietic progenitor cells and is commonly used to treat neutropenia and to mobilize peripheral blood-derived hematopoietic stem cells for transplantation [9, 10]. Several recent reports have indicated that G-CSF also has non-hematopoietic functions and can potentially be used for the treatment of neuronal injury, including stroke and neurodegenerative diseases [11–15]. Thus, we hypothesized that administration of G-CSF might have beneficial neuroprotective effects for acute SCI and examined this hypothesis using a compression-induced SCI model in rodents. We previously reported that G-CSF promotes functional recovery after compression-induced SCI and contusive SCI in mice [16–19]. The mechanisms by which G-CSF enhances recovery after SCI are as follows: G-CSF mobilizes bone marrow-derived cells to the injured spinal cord, where it directly suppresses neuronal apoptosis, suppresses the death of oligodendrocytes, protects myelin, suppresses the expression of inflammatory cytokines such as TNF-α and IL-1β, and facilitates arterialization [16–19].

Based on these findings, we conducted a multicenter prospective controlled clinical trial to assess the feasibility of neuroprotective therapy using G-CSF for patients with acute SCI.

27.2 Clinical Trial of G-CSF Neuroprotective Therapy for Acute Spinal Cord Injury

27.2.1 *Study Design and Population*

This clinical trial was an open-label, multicenter, prospective controlled study and was performed with the approval of the Institutional Review Board of each institute. Starting in August 2009, we recruited SCI patients within 48 h of onset. We restricted the age of the study patients to 16–85 years old. We excluded patients in the following categories: (1) those with intracranial pathologies (e.g., tumors, infection, or ischemia); (2) those having a history of major bleeding requiring blood transfusion or a history of leukopenia, thrombocytopenia, or hepatic or renal dysfunction, severe heart failure, or splenomegaly; and (3) those with evidence of malignant disease within the last 5 years. We also excluded patients who were pregnant or nursing. Eligible patients provided informed consent for participation in the trial.

We assigned patients to a G-CSF group or a control group. The G-CSF group was given G-CSF (Gran®, Kyowa Hakko Kirin, Tokyo) intravenously at 10 μg/kg/day for five consecutive days. The control group received similar treatments as the G-CSF group except for the G-CSF administration. Regarding patient selection, G-CSF therapy was performed only at Chiba University Hospital. At the institution, all SCI patients fulfilling the inclusion criteria described above underwent G-CSF administration during the study period. At the other institutes, patients were treated without G-CSF administration. No patient in either the G-CSF or control group was given MPSS in the follow-up period. Surgeries for spinal decompression and stabilization were performed as soon as possible after injury in both groups.

27.2.2 Evaluation of Safety and Feasibility

We evaluated motor and sensory functions of the patients using the American Spinal Cord Injury Association (ASIA) score (motor score; range, 0–100) [20] and ASIA impairment scale (AIS grade; range, A to E). In the present study, two orthopedic spine surgeons specializing in cervical spine surgery evaluated patients' neurological status independently at 1 week and 3 months after onset and calculated the mean data. The administration of G-CSF was kept unknown to the investigators until the end of the study. In addition, we analyzed hematological data from the treated patients. We also evaluated adverse events related to G-CSF therapy. Patients were asked daily to describe their responses regarding common G-CSF side effects.

Results are presented as means ± standard deviation of the mean. Statistical analysis was performed using the Mann–Whitney U test for the improvement of ASIA scores, Fisher's exact probability test for the improvement of AIS grade, and Student's t-test for the blood data. A P value less than 0.05 was considered statistically significant.

27.2.3 Patient Data

From August 2009 to March 2011, a total of 56 patients were enrolled in this trial. Among them, 45 patients were followed up after G-CSF administration or initial treatment for 3 months and were evaluated. Twenty-six patients were enrolled in the G-CSF group. In one patient, however, fever developed the day after initiation of G-CSF administration, so administration was discontinued. Five cases dropped out during follow-up, and one case demonstrated postoperative paralysis. Thus, we excluded these seven patients from the study. Finally, 19 patients who received

Table 27.1 Patient data for G-CSF and control groups

	G-CSF	Control	*P*
Number of cases	19	26	
Gender			
Male	13	20	
Female	6	6	
Age (years)			
	57.7 ± 9.34 (38–68)	58.5 ± 18.0 (23–85)	0.871
Cause of injury			
Fall	11	16	
Road trauma	6	8	
Sports	1	1	
Falling object	1	0	
Others	0	1	
Level of injury			
C2/3	0	2	
C3/4	5	7	
C4/5	8	7	
C5/6	4	8	
C6/7	2	2	
ASIA impairment scale (AIS)			
A	1	7	
B	2	2	
C	5	5	
D	11	12	
Time of first examination after injury (h)	3.95 ± 2.74 (1–12)	10.3 ± 14.6 (1–48)	0.068
Time of G-CSF administration after injury (h)	32.4 ± 16.6 (6–48)		

G-CSF were evaluated (Table 27.1). Thirty patients were enrolled in the control group. Among them, three cases dropped out during follow-up. In one additional case, no motor paralysis was present. Thus, we excluded these four cases, leaving 26 patients in the control group for evaluation (Table 27.1).

27.2.4 AIS

The change of AIS grade between the first examination and 3 months after onset is shown in Table 27.2. In the analysis of total cases, AIS grade improved at least one step in 11 of 19 (57.9 %) patients in the G-CSF group and in 9 of 26 (34.6 %) patients in the control group (Table 27.3). In cases of incomplete paralysis (AIS grade at first examination: B, C, or D), AIS grade improved at least one step in 11 of 18 (61.1 %) patients in the G-CSF group and in 6 of 15 (31.6 %) patients in the control group (Table 27.3). Furthermore, when we restricted the subjects to incomplete paralysis cases with severe and moderate symptoms (AIS grade at first

Table 27.2 ASIA impairment scale (AIS)

G-CSF group						Control group					
Grade at first examination	Grade at 3 months after onset					Grade at first examination	Grade at 3 months after onset				
	A	B	C	D	E		A	B	C	D	E
A	1					A	4	2	1		
B			1	1		B		1	1		
C				4	1	C		1	2	2	
D				7	4	D				9	3

AIS grade
A: complete paralysis
B: sensory incomplete paralysis, motor complete paralysis
C: motor incomplete paralysis (muscle grading <3/5)
D: motor incomplete paralysis (muscle grading >3/5)
E: normal

Table 27.3 Improvement of AIS

	G-CSF (%)	Control (%)	*P*
Total cases	11/19 (57.9)	9/26 (34.6)	0.106
Incomplete paralysis cases (AIS: B, C, D)	11/18 (61.1)	6/15 (31.6)	0.07
Incomplete paralysis cases (AIS: B, C)	7/7 (100)	3/7 (42.9)	0.035*

*$P<0.05$
Data are expressed as number of neurologically improved patients/number of examined patients (neurological improvement was defined as an increase in at least one clinical grade)

examination: B or C), AIS grade improved at least one step in all 7 patients in the G-CSF group and in 3 of 7 (42.9 %) patients in the control group ($P<0.05$) (Table 27.3).

27.2.5 ASIA Motor Score

In the analysis of total cases, the ASIA motor score at the first examination was 61.6±27.3 in the G-CSF group and 51.3±36.6 in the control group; thus, scores were higher in the G-CSF group, although this difference was not statistically significant (Table 27.4). At 1 week after onset, the improvement in motor score was greater in the G-CSF group (increased points: 13.6±11.3) than in the control group (increased points: 2.69±7.9) ($P<0.01$). Still greater improvement in scores was observed at the three-month follow-up in the G-CSF group (increased points: 26.1±18.9) compared to the control group (increased points: 12.2±14.7) ($P<0.01$) (Table 27.4).

In cases of incomplete paralysis (AIS grade at first examination: B, C, or D), the ASIA motor score at the first examination was 63.6±26.8 in the G-CSF group and 65.0±32.6 in the control group; the difference between groups was not statistically significant (Table 27.5). At 1 week after onset, greater improvement in motor score

Table 27.4 ASIA motor score (total cases)

	G-CSF ($n=19$)	Control ($n=26$)	P
At first examination	61.6±27.3 (14–98)	51.3±36.6 (0–97)	0.497
1 week after onset	75.2±23.4 (27–100)	54.0±37.3 (0–100)	0.075
Increased points for 1 week	13.6±11.3 (1–50)	2.69±7.9 (−11–24)	0.0011*
3 months after onset	87.7±17.5 (35–100)	63.7±36.5 (0–100)	0.052
Increased points for 3 months	26.1±18.9 (1–73)	12.2±14.7 (−7–48)	0.0067*

Patients whose AIS grade at the first examination was A, B, C, or D were analyzed
*$P<0.01$

Table 27.5 ASIA motor score (incomplete paralysis cases)

	G-CSF ($n=18$)	Control ($n=19$)	p
At first examination	63.6±26.8 (14–98)	65.1±32.6 (7–97)	0.475
1 week after onset	77.4±21.9 (27–100)	68.7±31.9 (6–100)	0.574
Increased points for 1 week	13.9±11.6 (1–50)	3.58±9.0 (−11–24)	0.0049*
3 months after onset	90.6±12.3 (51–100)	80.2±26.3 (19–100)	0.417
Increased points for 3 months	27.1±18.9	15.1±15.9	0.044**

Patients whose AIS grade at the first examination was B, C, or D were analyzed
*$P<0.01$
**$P<0.05$

was observed in the G-CSF group (increased points: 13.9±11.6) than in the control group (increased points: 3.58±9.0) ($P<0.01$). The improvement was still observed at the three-month follow-up in the G-CSF group (increased points: 27.1±18.9) compared with the control group (increased points: 15.1±15.9) ($P<0.05$) (Table 27.5).

27.2.6 Blood Data

In the G-CSF group, white blood cell (WBC) counts immediately before G-CSF administration averaged 9.55±3.58 ($\times 10^3/mm^3$). During the administration, WBC counts increased to 34.2±10.9 ($\times 10^3/mm^3$), ranging from 12.4 to 56.9 ($\times 10^3/mm^3$) (Table 27.6). G-CSF mobilized cells of the neutrophil lineage, while lymphocytes were unaffected (Table 27.6). G-CSF also increased the level of circulating monocytes and basophils. There was no significant change in inflammation during G-CSF administration, as indicated by C-reactive protein levels (Table 27.6).

27.2.7 Adverse Events

In one patient in the G-CSF group, fever >40 °C developed the day after the start of G-CSF administration, and administration was discontinued. The cause of the fever proved to be from a urinary tract infection, and the infection was relieved by administration of antibiotics. No relationship was found between the infection and G-CSF

Table 27.6 Blood data before and after G-CSF administration

	Baseline	Peak value after G-CSF administration	*P*
White blood cell (×10³/mm³)	9.55 ± 3.58 (4.0–16.7)	34.2 ± 10.9 (12.4–56.9)	<0.01
Granulocytes (×10³/mm³)	7.39 ± 3.20 (2.79–14.3)	29.3 ± 10.3 (10.2–49.5)	<0.01
Eosinophils (×10³/mm³)	0.11 ± 0.16 (0–0.73)	0.27 ± 0.37 (0–1.22)	0.061
Basophils (×10³/mm³)	0.023 ± 0.029 (0–0.14)	0.079 ± 0.10 (0–0.32)	0.017
Monocytes (×10³/mm³)	0.58 ± 0.26 (0.25–1.38)	1.30 ± 0.71 (0.12–3.10)	<0.01
Lymphocytes (×10³/mm³)	1.45 ± 0.40 (0.84–2.51)	1.45 ± 0.98 (0.13–3.93)	0.99
CRP (mg/dl)	3.30 ± 6.86 (0–25.6)	4.93 ± 6.55 (0.2–28.0)	0.41

Peak value after G-CSF administration: highest value between the first day and the seventh day after G-CSF administration
CRP = C-reactive protein

administration. In one case, mild hepatic dysfunction (GOT: 91 U/L [normal range: 13–33 U/L], GPT: 99 U/L [normal range: 8–42 U/L]) was seen on the fifth day after the start of G-CSF administration, but it spontaneously resolved. No other severe adverse events occurred during or after G-CSF administration.

27.3 Discussion

27.3.1 Non-hematopoietic Effects of G-CSF

Experimental studies on acute myocardial infarction (AMI) have shown that stem cell mobilization by G-CSF protects the myocardium and that the mobilized cells are found in the myocardium [21]. In ischemic stroke models, G-CSF suppresses neuronal apoptosis as well as the expression of inflammatory cytokines, showing neuroprotective effects [11–15]. We made similar observations in acute SCI [16–19]. Based on these results, clinical trials have been initiated for patients with AMI [22–27] and neurological disorders such as cerebral infarction [28] and amyotrophic lateral sclerosis (ALS) [29, 30]. Many clinical trials in AMI have reported the safety and feasibility of G-CSF administration [22–27]. A clinical trial of G-CSF administration for cerebral infarction showed that neurological symptoms were significantly improved by G-CSF administration, although only seven patients received treatment [28]. In ALS, stem cell mobilization by G-CSF delays ALS progression and improves the quality of life [30]. In the present study, we first conducted a clinical trial with G-CSF for patients with acute SCI.

27.3.2 G-CSF Neuroprotective Therapy for Acute SCI

In our previous phase I/IIa clinical trials of G-CSF neuroprotective therapy for acute SCI and worsening symptoms of compression myelopathy, we determined that the appropriate dose, route, and duration of G-CSF administration was 10 μg/kg/day by intravenous injection over five consecutive days [31, 32]. We also performed a phase IIb controlled clinical trial of G-CSF neuroprotective therapy for patients with worsening symptoms of thoracic myelopathy and obtained data that G-CSF administration caused their neurological recovery [33]. Based on these results, we conducted the present clinical trial as a multicenter prospective controlled study to verify the efficacy of G-CSF neuroprotective therapy in patients with acute SCI. In these patients, the pathophysiology of the injured spinal cord and symptoms differed depending on the site of vertebral injury (cervical, thoracic, and thoracolumbar) and the severity of the injury. Therefore, to increase the reliability of the data in the present study, we restricted the subjects to those with cervical injury and excluded thoracic and thoracolumbar injury patients.

We analyzed whether G-CSF administration improved muscle power in the upper and lower extremities using the ASIA motor score. One week and three months after injury, the motor score significantly increased in the G-CSF group compared with the control group. Notably, the increase in motor score in the G-CSF group was more prominent at 1 week after onset compared with that at the three-month follow-up. This result indicated that G-CSF administration had a neuroprotective effect in cells in the descending tracts in the white matter and cells at the injured spinal segments in the gray matter. We suggest that such effects resulted in earlier and better improvement of motor function of patients.

Among the seven patients in the G-CSF group whose AIS grade was B or C at first examination, AIS grade improved at least one step in each case. When the analysis was restricted to subjects with incomplete paralysis and moderate to severe symptoms (AIS grade, B or C), the improvement of AIS grade in the G-CSF group was statistically superior to that in the control group. This finding suggests that G-CSF neuroprotective therapy is most effective for patients whose paralysis is moderate to severe. Future analyses of G-CSF neuroprotective therapy for acute SCI should target subjects with moderate to severe incomplete paralysis.

27.3.3 Side Effects of G-CSF

Previous reports have described the side effects of G-CSF administration. Mild symptoms included low back and pelvic pain, fever, listeriosis, headache, nausea, and vomiting [34–36]. Symptoms were transient and disappeared two or three days after cessation of the drug. In the present trial, one patient developed fever one day after starting G-CSF administration. However, this proved to be due to a urinary tract infection and was resolved following administration of antibiotics. One patient demonstrated mild hepatic dysfunction, which spontaneously resolved.

In contrast, severe symptoms can include cerebral infarction, AMI, and rupture of the spleen [35, 37]. At high G-CSF doses (20 μg/kg/day), the risk of such events grows. Above all, if WBC counts remain $>50\times10^3/mm^3$, the risk of rupture of the spleen increases [35]. In the present trial, moderate doses of G-CSF (10 μg/kg/day) were administered, and no severe side effects were observed. Thus, we suggest that the G-CSF dose (10 μg/kg/day), duration (five consecutive days), and route (intravenous administration) employed herein are generally safe for the treatment of acute SCI patients.

To date, MPSS has been clinically used for treatment of acute SCI patients to relieve secondary injury to the spinal cord [2, 3]. However, the side effects related to MPSS treatment, such as pneumonia and gastric ulcer, cannot be ignored [3–7]. Considering this aspect, we believe that G-CSF neuroprotective therapy is much safer than MPSS treatment.

27.3.4 Future Investigation

In the present study, G-CSF administration was performed at one institution, while the control group consisted of patients from other institutions. Thus, we suggest that the homogeneity between the G-CSF group and the control group was insufficient. Furthermore, the number of patients analyzed was small, and the follow-up period was short. The biggest limitations of the present study were that it was an open-label study and assignment of patients to the G-CSF and control groups was not randomized. We therefore cannot deny the possibility that a placebo effect of injection may have helped improve neurological symptoms. In addition, we cannot ignore the bias that the evaluator knew which patients received drug.

To increase the reliability of the data, the next study should be designed as a randomized, double-blind placebo-controlled study. Indeed, we plan to perform a phase IIb clinical trial with a large number of patients and longer follow-up periods. By conducting such a study, we will be able to reach a firmer conclusion about the effectiveness of G-CSF neuroprotective therapy for patients with acute SCI.

27.4 Conclusion

Despite the limitation that patient selection was not randomized, the present results suggest the possibility that G-CSF administration has beneficial effects on neurological recovery in patients with acute SCI. We believe that neuroprotection using G-CSF is an effective therapeutic strategy for acute SCI treatment.

Acknowledgment The authors thank Drs. Takayuki Fujiyoshi, Tsuyoshi Sakuma, Kei Kato, Mitsuhiro Hashimoto, Koichi Hayashi, Junko Kawabe, Chikato Mannoji, Tomohiro Miyashita, Ryo Kadota, Yukio Someya, Osamu Ikeda, Masayuki Hashimoto, Akihiko Okawa, and Kazuhisa Takahashi (Department of Orthopaedic Surgery, Chiba University Graduate School of Medicine), Drs. Kota Suda, Tomomichi Kajino, and Haruki Ueda (Spinal Cord Injury Center, Hokkaido Chuo Rosai Hospital), Dr. Yasuo Ito (Department of Orthopaedic Surgery, Kobe Red Cross Hospital), Dr. Takayoshi Ueta (Department of Orthopaedic Surgery, Japan LHWO Spinal Injuries Center), and Dr. Hideki Hanaoka (Department of Clinical Research, Chiba University Hospital) for their kind support in the present study. This work was supported by a Health Labor Science Research Grant of Japan.

Conflict of Interest Authors (Masashi Yamazaki, Hiroshi Takahashi, Takeo Furuya, and Masao Koda) declare that we have no conflict of interest.

References

1. Pannu R, Barbosa E, Singh AK, Singh I (2005) Attenuation of acute inflammatory response by atorvastatin after spinal cord injury in rats. J Neurosci Res 79(3):340–350
2. Bracken MB, Shepard MJ, Collins WF, Holford TR, Young W, Baskin DS et al (1990) A randomized controlled trial of methylprednisolone or naloxone in the treatment of acute spinal cord injury: results of the second national acute spinal cord injury study. N Engl J Med 322(20):1405–1411
3. Bracken MB, Shepard MF, Holford TR, Leo Summers L, Aldrich EF, Fazl M et al (1997) Administration of methylprednisolone for 24 or 48 hours or tirilazad mesylate for 48 hours in the treatment of acute spinal cord injury: results of the third national acute spinal injury randomized controlled trial. JAMA 277(20):1597–1604
4. Hurlbert RJ (2000) Methylprednisolone for acute spinal cord injury: an inappropriate standard of care. J Neurosurg 93(1 Suppl):1–7
5. Ito Y, Sugimoto Y, Tomioka M, Kai N, Tanaka M (2009) Does high dose methylprednisolone sodium succinate really improve neurological status in patient with acute cervical cord injury?: a prospective study about neurological recovery and early complications. Spine 34(20): 2121–2124
6. Pointillart V, Petitjean ME, Wiart L, Vital JM, Lassie P, Thicoipe M et al (2000) Pharmacological therapy of spinal cord injury during the acute phase. Spinal Cord 38(2):71–76
7. Polland ME, Apple DF (2003) Factors associated with improved neurologic outcomes in patients with incomplete tetraplegia. Spine 28(1):33–39
8. Matsumoto T, Tamaki T, Kawakami M, Yoshida M, Ando M, Yamada H (2001) Early complications of high-dose methyl-prednisolone sodium succinate treatment in the follow-up of acute cervical spinal cord injury. Spine 26(4):426–430
9. Nicola NA, Metcalf D, Matsumoto M, Johnson GR (1983) Purification of a factor inducing differentiation in murine myelomonocytic leukemia cells. Identification as granulocyte colony-stimulating factor J Biol Chem 258(14):9017–9023
10. Roberts AW (2005) G-CSF: a key regulator of neutrophil production, but that's not all! Growth Factors 23(1):33–41
11. Gibson CL, Jones NC, Prior MJ, Bath PM, Murphy SP (2005) G-CSF suppresses edema formation and reduces interleukin-1β expression after cerebral ischemia in mice. J Neuropathol Exp Neurol 64(9):763–769
12. Kawada H, Takizawa S, Takanashi T, Morita Y, Fujita J, Fukuda K et al (2006) Administration of hematopoietic cytokines in the subacute phase after cerebral infarction is effective for functional recovery facilitating proliferation of intrinsic neural stem/progenitor cells and transition of bone marrow-derived neuronal cells. Circulation 113(5):701–710
13. Komine-Kobayashi M, Zhang N, Liu M, Tanaka R, Hara H, Osaka A et al (2006) Neuroprotective effect of recombinant human granulocyte colony-stimulating factor in transient focal ischemia of mice. J Cereb Blood Flow Metab 26(3):402–413
14. Schäbitz WR, Kollmar R, Schwaninger M, Juettler E, Bardutzky J, Schölzke MN et al (2003) Neuroprotective effect of granulocyte colony-stimulating factor after focal cerebral ischemia. Stroke 34(3):745–751
15. Schneider A, Kuhn HG, Schäbitz WR (2005) A role for G-CSF (granulocyte-colony stimulating factor) in the central nervous system. Cell Cycle 4(12):1753–1757
16. Koda M, Nishio Y, Kamada T, Someya Y, Okawa A, Mori C et al (2007) Granulocyte colony-stimulating factor (G-CSF) mobilizes bone marrow-derived cells into injured spinal cord and promotes functional recovery after compression-induced spinal cord injury in mice. Brain Res 1149:223–231
17. Nishio Y, Koda M, Kamada T, Someya Y, Kadota R, Mannoji C et al (2007) Granulocyte colony-stimulating factor attenuates neuronal death and promotes functional recovery after spinal cord injury in mice. J Neuropathol Exp Neurol 66(8):724–731

18. Kawabe J, Koda M, Hashimoto M, Fujiyoshi T, Furuya T, Endo T et al (2011) Neuroprotective effects of granulocyte colony-stimulating factor and relationship to promotion of angiogenesis after spinal cord injury in rats: laboratory investigation. J Neurosurg Spine 15(4):414–421
19. Kadota R, Koda M, Kawabe J, Hashimoto M, Nishio Y, Mannoji C et al (2012) Granulocyte colony-stimulating factor (G-CSF) protects oligodendrocyte and promotes hindlimb functional recovery after spinal cord injury in rats. PLoS One 7(11):e50391
20. Maynard FM Jr, Bracken MB, Creasey G, Ditunno JF Jr, Donovan WH, Ducker TB et al (1997) International standards for neurological and functional classification of spinal cord injury. Am Spinal Inj Assoc Spinal Cord 35(5):266–274
21. Iwasaki H, Kawamoto A, Ishikawa M, Oyamada A, Nakamori S, Nishimura H et al (2006) Dose-dependent contribution of CD34-positive cell transplantation to concurrent vasculogenesis and cardiomyogenesis for functional regenerative recovery after myocardial infarction. Circulation 113(10):1311–1325
22. Engelmann MG, Theiss HD, Hennig-Theiss C, Huber A, Wintersperger BJ, Werle-Ruedinger AE et al (2006) Autologous bone marrow stem cell mobilization induced by granulocyte colony-stimulating factor after subacute ST-segment elevation myocardial infarction undergoing late revascularization: final results from the G-CSF-STMI (Granulocyte Colony-Stimulating Factor ST-Segment Elevation Myocardial Infarction) trial. J Am Coll Cardiol 48(8):1712–1721
23. Ince H, Petzsch M, Kleine HD, Eckard H, Rehders T, Burska D et al (2005) Prevention of left ventricular remodeling with granulocyte colony-stimulating factor after acute myocardial infarction: final 1-year results of the front-integrated revascularization and stem cell liberation in evolving acute myocardial infarction by granulocyte colony-stimulating factor (FIRSTLINE-AMI) trial. Circulation 112(9 suppl):173–180
24. Ripa RS, Jorgensen E, Wang Y, Thune JJ, Nilsson JC, Sondergaard L et al (2006) Stem cell mobilization induced by subcutaneous granulocyte colony-stimulating factor to improve cardiac regeneration after acute ST-elevation myocardial infarction: result of the double-blind, randomized, placebo-controlled stem cells in myocardial infarction (STEMMI) trial. Circulation 113(16):1983–1992
25. Takano H, Hasegawa H, Kuwabara Y, Nakayama T, Matsuno K, Miyazaki Y et al (2007) Feasibility and safety of granulocyte colony-stimulating factor treatment in patients with acute myocardial infarction. Int J Cardiol 122(1):41–47
26. Valgimigli M, Rigolin GM, Cittanti C, Malagutti P, Curello S, Percoco G et al (2005) Use of granulocyte-colony stimulating factor during acute myocardial infarction to enhance bone marrow stem cell mobilization in humans: clinical and angiographic safety profile. Eur Heart J 26(18):1838–1845
27. Zohlnhofer D, Ott I, Mehilli J, Schomig K, Michalk F, Ibrahim T et al (2006) REVIVAL-2 investigators: stem cell mobilization by granulocyte colony-stimulating factor in patients with acute myocardial infarction: a randomized controlled trial. JAMA 295(9):1003–1010
28. Shyu WC, Lin SZ, Lee CC, Liu DD, Li H (2006) Granulocyte colony-stimulating factor for acute ischemic stroke: a randomized controlled trial. CMAJ 174(7):927–933
29. Nefussy B, Artamonov I, Deutsch V, Naparstek E, Nagler A, Drory VE (2010) Recombinant human granulocyte-colony stimulating factor administration for treating amyotrophic lateral sclerosis: A pilot study. Amyotroph Lateral Scler 11(1–2):187–193
30. Zhang Y, Wang L, Fu Y, Song H, Zhao H, Deng M et al (2009) Preliminary investigation of effect of granulocyte colony stimulating factor on amyotrophic lateral sclerosis. Amyotroph Lateral Scler 10(5–6):430–431
31. Takahashi H, Yamazaki M, Okawa A, Sakuma T, Kato K, Hashimoto M et al (2012) Neuroprotective therapy using granulocyte colony-stimulating factor for acute spinal cord injury: a phase I/IIa clinical trial. Eur Spine J 21(12):2580–2587
32. Sakuma T, Yamazaki M, Okawa A, Takahashi H, Kato K, Hashimoto M et al (2012) Neuroprotective therapy using granulocyte-colony stimulating factor for patients with worsening symptoms of compression myelopathy, part 1: a phase I and IIa clinical trial. Eur Spine J 21(3):482–489

33. Sakuma T, Yamazaki M, Okawa A, Takahashi H, Kato K, Hashimoto M et al (2012) Neuroprotective therapy using granulocyte-colony stimulating factor for patients with worsening symptoms of thoracic myelopathy, a multicenter prospective controlled trial. Spine 37(17):1475–1478
34. Anderlini P, Przepiorka D, Seong D, Miller P, Sundberg J, Lichtiger B et al (1996) Clinical toxicity and laboratory effects of granulocyte colony-stimulating factor (filgrastim) mobilization and blood stem cell apheresis from normal donors and analysis of charge for procedures. Transfusion 36(7):590–595
35. Becker PS, Wagle M, Matous S, Swanson RS, Pihan G, Lowry PA et al (1997) Spontaneous splenic rupture following administration of granulocyte colony-stimulating factor (G-CSF) occurrence in an allogeneic donor of peripheral blood stem cells. Biol Blood Marrow Transplant 3(1):45–49
36. Murata M, Harada M, Kato S, Takahashi S, Ogawa H, Okamoto S et al (1999) Peripheral blood stem cell mobilization and apheresis: analysis of adverse events in 94 normal donors. Bone Marrow Transplant 24(10):1065–1071
37. Falzetti F, Aversa F, Minelli O, Tabilio A (1999) Spontaneous rupture of spleen during peripheral blood stem cell mobilization in a healthy donor. Lancet 353(9152):555

Chapter 28
Assessment of Injured Spinal Cord Using Diffusion Tensor Tractography

Kanehiro Fujiyoshi, Tsunehiko Konomi, Osahiko Tsuji, Masayuki Yamada, Keigo Hikishima, Suketaka Momoshima, Hideyuki Okano, Yoshiaki Toyama, and Masaya Nakamura

Abstract In spinal cord injury (SCI), the evaluation of axonal fibers is important to assess the severity of injury and efficacy of any treatment protocol, but conventional methods such as tracer injection in the brain parenchyma are highly invasive and require histological evaluation, precluding clinical applications. Magnetic resonance imaging (MRI) is essential for predicting prognosis and planning treatment of patients with SCI noninvasively. However, the information provided by conventional T1- and T2-weighted MRI of the spinal cord is essentially limited to the differentiation of the white matter from the gray matter. By contrast, diffusion-weighted magnetic resonance imaging (DWI) provides much information about biological structures. In particular, diffusion tensor imaging (DTI) and diffusion tensor tractography (DTT) are powerful tools for evaluating white matter fibers in the central nervous system. We previously established a reproducible SCI model in adult common

K. Fujiyoshi • T. Konomi
Department of Orthopaedic Surgery, Keio University School of Medicine, 35 Shinanomachi, Shinjuku, Tokyo 160-8582, Japan

Department of Physiology, Keio University School of Medicine, 35 Shinanomachi, Shinjuku, Tokyo 160-8582, Japan

Department of Orthopedic Surgery, National Hospital Organization, Murayama Medical Center, 2-37-1 Gakuen, Musashimurayama, Tokyo 208-0011, Japan

O. Tsuji
Department of Orthopaedic Surgery, Keio University School of Medicine, 35 Shinanomachi, Shinjuku, Tokyo 160-8582, Japan

Department of Physiology, Keio University School of Medicine, 35 Shinanomachi, Shinjuku, Tokyo 160-8582, Japan

Department of Orthopedic Surgery, Saitama Social Insurance Hospital, 4-9-3 Kitaurawa, Urawa, Saitama-city, Saitama 330-0074, Japan

M. Yamada
Fujita Health University, School of Health Sciences, Faculty of Radiological Technology, 1-98 Dengakugakubo, Kutsukake-cho, Toyoake, Aichi 470-1192, Japan

K. Uchida et al. (eds.), *Neuroprotection and Regeneration of the Spinal Cord*, DOI 10.1007/978-4-431-54502-6_28, © Springer Japan 2014

marmosets and demonstrated that DTT could be used to trace the neural tracts in the intact and injured spinal cord of these animals in vivo. Recently, many reports using DTT to analyze the spinal cord area have been published. Based on the findings from our experimental studies, we are now routinely performing DTT of the human spinal cord clinically. In this chapter, we outline the basic principles of DTT and describe the characteristics, limitations, and clinical application of DTT in the spinal cord.

Keywords DTI (diffusion tensor imaging) • DTT (diffusion tensor tractography) • DWI (diffusion-weighted MR imaging) • MRI (magnetic resonance imaging) • SCI (spinal cord injury)

Abbreviations

MRI	Magnetic resonance imaging
DWI	Diffusion-weighted MR imaging
DTI	Diffusion tensor imaging
DTT	Diffusion tensor tractography
FA	Fractional anisotropy
ADC	Apparent diffusion coefficient

28.1 Introduction

We previously established a reproducible spinal cord injury (SCI) model in adult common marmosets and demonstrated that transplantation of human neural stem/progenitor cells into the injured spinal cord promoted functional recovery [1].

K. Hikishima
Department of Physiology, Keio University School of Medicine,
35 Shinanomachi, Shinjuku, Tokyo 160-8582, Japan

Central Institute for Experimental Animals, 3-25-12 Tonomachi,
Kawasaki, Kanagawa 210-0821, Japan

S. Momoshima
Department of Radiology, Keio University School of Medicine,
35 Shinanomachi, Shinjuku, Tokyo 160-8582, Japan

H. Okano
Department of Physiology, Keio University School of Medicine,
35 Shinanomachi, Shinjuku, Tokyo 160-8582, Japan

Y. Toyama • M. Nakamura (✉)
Department of Orthopaedic Surgery, Keio University School of Medicine,
35 Shinanomachi, Shinjuku, Tokyo 160-8582, Japan
e-mail: masa@a8.keio.jp

An increase of axonal fibers, evaluated through histological methods, was observed near the transplanted neural stem/progenitor cells and was interpreted to be involved in the functional improvement. Such evaluation of axonal fibers is essential to assess the severity of SCI and efficacy of any treatment protocol [2, 3], but conventional methods such as tracer injection in brain parenchyma are technically demanding and highly invasive [4, 5]. Since histological examinations are required to evaluate tracer studies, it has been impossible to evaluate axonal fibers in vivo and follow the sequential growth of axonal fibers in the same animal. Understanding the value of such an examination method, we therefore sought to establish a noninvasive method to evaluate axonal fibers in vivo.

Magnetic resonance imaging (MRI) is essential for predicting prognosis and planning treatment of patients with SCI [6, 7]. Our previous study using common marmosets also demonstrated that MRI could detect pathological changes after SCI [8]. However, the information provided by conventional T1- and T2-weighted MRI of the spinal cord is essentially limited to the differentiation of the white matter from the gray matter. Conventional MRI depicts the white matter as a uniform tissue although it actually contains a complex array of directionally oriented nerve fibers. Methods to visualize the pathways of the white matter in vivo have been long sought, and recently diffusion tensor tractography (DTT) has demonstrated this ability [9–11].

Diffusion tensor imaging (DTI) is a new imaging technique that takes advantage of the anisotropic nature of water diffusion in biological tissue to obtain detailed microstructural information [12–15]. By analyzing and reconstructing that data obtained by DTI, DTT can follow the orientation of nerve fibers to trace specific neural pathways such as the corticospinal tract (CST) in the brain [10, 16–18]. Compared to the brain, however, DTT of the spinal cord is more difficult due to its smaller size and in vivo bulk motion [19–21]. Several researchers have recently reported on successful DTT of the human spinal cord [22–25]. However, since these DTT images were not confirmed with detailed histological studies, whether DTT actually reflects the anatomical axonal fibers remains unclear. Therefore, we performed DTT of both intact and injured spinal cords in common marmosets and confirmed the accuracy of DTT through histology.

28.2 Diffusion MRI and Diffusion Tensor

The usefulness of "Diffusion MRI," which exploits the diffusion of water molecules, has also recently become widely recognized. Reports on diffusion MRI of the brain were first published in the 1980s [12, 26], and after its use to examine acute stroke in the 1990s [27, 28] was reported, this technique became known worldwide. It is expected to become even more useful, due to the recent development of diffusion-weighted whole-body imaging with background body signal suppression (DWIBS), which can be used to evaluate the metastases of malignant tumors three dimensionally [29]. In these techniques, "diffusion" refers to the Brownian motion of water molecules, and it is strictly differentiated from their "flow." Thus, diffusion-weighted

MR imaging (DWI)[1] is a method for detecting and visualizing water molecule diffusion information in tissues by adding a gradient magnetic field called a motion proving gradient (MPG). The MRI scans that clinicians regularly use are acquired by DWI, which differs from conventional MRI methods in that it provides high-contrast resolution based on diffusion, which allows new information on lesions to be obtained.

The direction of water molecule diffusion in living tissues is always limited to some degree. The property by which the rate of diffusion varies with direction is called diffusion anisotropy or anisotropic diffusion [30]. To detect lesions by DWI, the anisotropy is deliberately reduced by using imaging techniques or processing, to avoid detecting the signals from normal white matter. The diffusion-weighted images from which the effect of anisotropic diffusion has been eliminated are sometimes called isotropic diffusion-weighted images (isotropic DWI). Anisotropic diffusion is represented as an ellipsoid, and isotropic diffusion is represented as a sphere [31].

The white matter of the spinal cord is composed of nerve fiber bundles that course in a craniocaudal direction in a relatively ordered manner, and the water within them diffuses along the course of the axons. Thus, white matter has high anisotropy, and the nerve fibers can be tracked and visualized based on their anisotropy information by DTT. To conduct DTT, parameters such as the apparent diffusion coefficient (ADC), which is an expression of the magnitude of the diffusion, and the fractional anisotropy (FA), which is an expression of the anisotropy of the diffusion, must be calculated. Tensor analysis is used in calculating these parameters [15, 19, 32], which gives rise to the name, "tensor diffusion."[2]

28.3 Diffusion Anisotropy and Tensor Analysis

FA and FA Maps: Because information about diffusion in various directions is needed to measure anisotropy, it is necessary to acquire MR images to which MPG has been applied in at least 6 axes and to acquire T2-weighted images to which MPG has not been applied. Eigen values ($\lambda_1, \lambda_2, \lambda_3$), which determine the magnitude of the diffusion, and Eigen vectors (v_1, v_2, v_3), which determine their direction, are calculated by tensor analysis of the data obtained in this way. The collected anisotropy information in each voxel is approximated as a "diffusion ellipsoid" (Fig. 28.1). This information is depicted in two dimensions as an FA (fractional anisotropy) map (Fig. 28.2). (FA is a commonly used anisotropy index.) FA takes on values between 0 (perfectly isotropic diffusion) and 1 (the hypothetical case of an infinite cylinder) and is thus directly comparable between subjects. FA is calculated by the formula:

[1] According to textbooks, DWI "includes all MRI images weighted with proton diffusion motion by some method," but in practice it is more narrowly defined as meaning the original images acquired by adding a diffusion-weighted gradient magnetic field [33].

[2] Tensor is a function of a vector variable that possesses multilinearity, and when multiplied by the vector (on the left), it forms a matrix that yields vectors, with each component of the matrix being closely related to the coordinate system [30]. In actuality, a 3×3, 2-step matrix operation is necessary.

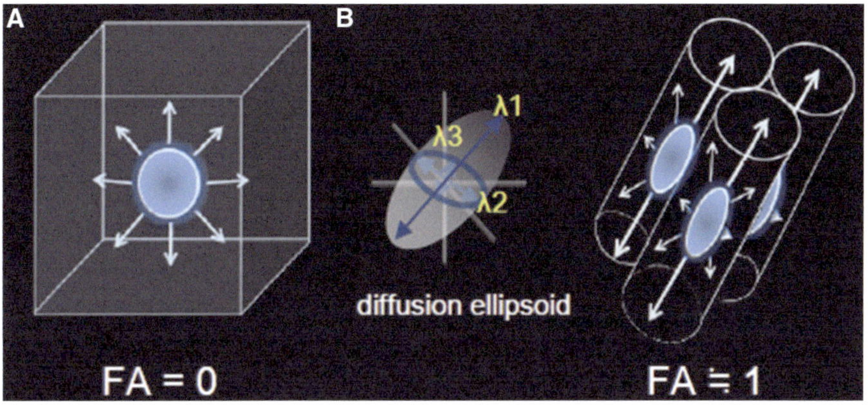

Fig. 28.1 Diffusion of water molecules. (**a**) Isotropic diffusion is represented as a sphere. (**b**) Anisotropic diffusion is approximated by a diffusion ellipsoid. The diffusion ellipsoid is calculated from an eigenvalues (λ_1, λ_2, λ_3) and eigenvectors (v_1, v_2, v_3)

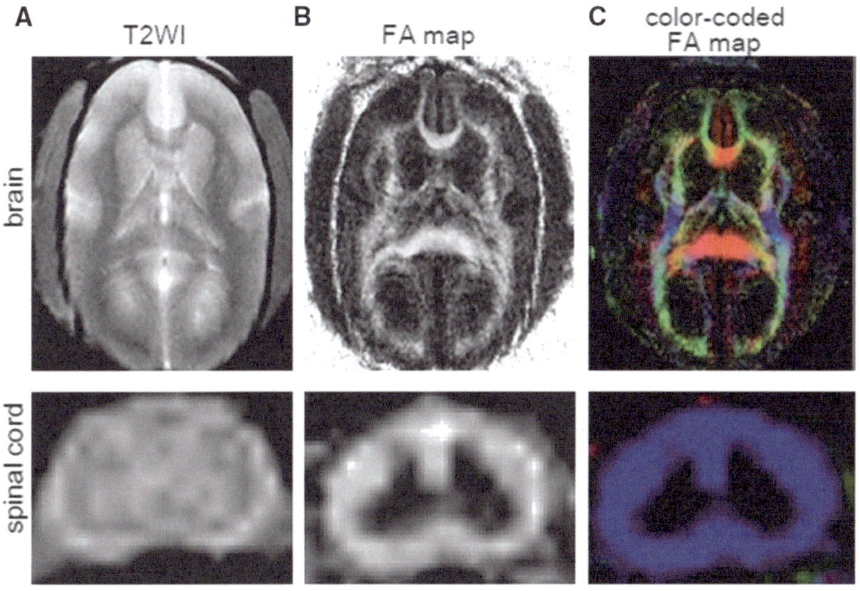

Fig. 28.2 Conventional MRI and diffusion tensor imaging in the brain and spinal cord of a living common marmoset. (**a**) T2-weighted MR images. (**b**) FA maps. (**c**) Color-coded FA maps. (Reprinted from Fujiyoshi et al. [31])

$$ADC = \frac{\lambda 1 + \lambda 2 + \lambda 3}{3} = D$$

$$FA = \sqrt{\frac{3}{2}} \frac{\sqrt{(\lambda 1 - <D>)^2 + (\lambda 2 - <D>)^2 + (\lambda 3 - <D>)^2}}{\sqrt{\lambda 1^2 + \lambda 2^2 + \lambda 3^2}}$$

In isotropy, λ_1, λ_2, and $\lambda_3 = <D>$, and FA becomes 0.

As anisotropy increases, $\lambda_1 >> \lambda_2 = \lambda_3$, and FA approaches 1.

The strength of the signal in an FA maps represents the magnitude of the FA, and unlike conventional DWI, it is quantitative. FA is known to decrease at lesion sites, such as those of cerebral infarction and hemorrhages, and we have reported that FA also decreases in Wallerian degeneration [34]. Diffusion tensor analysis has the novel feature of not only quantifying anisotropy by FA and other parameters but also analyzing directionality. In contrast to FA, the ADC is an index that expresses the magnitude of the diffusion irrespective of its direction.

Color-Coded FA Maps and RBG Color: FA maps that show anisotropy in different colors according to its axis are called color-coded FA maps (or “color maps”). Color maps make it possible to differentiate fibers based on the direction in which they run. The colors are arbitrary, but red (*R*ed) is often assigned to the left-right, blue (*Bl*ue) to the superior-inferior, and green (*G*reen) to the anterior-posterior orientation, and this system is referred to as RBG color [35]. Figure 28.2 shows a color map of an axial section of the common marmoset spinal cord, in which the white matter fibers can be seen as blue tracts in the craniocaudal direction.

Diffusion Tensor Tractography: MRIs that make use of tensor analysis, such as FA maps and color maps, are collectively called DTI. In the broadest sense DTT can be considered a subtype of DTI, but DTT is often deliberately differentiated from DTI. DTT reveals the course of fibers, such as those in the white matter, by tracking the direction of the major axis of the ellipsoid of every voxel, i.e., by tracking the predominant directions of anisotropy and reconstructing it in three dimensions. Numerous algorithms for tracking anisotropy exist, but the fiber assignment by continuous tracking (FACT) algorithm [36] is the best known. Simply stated, the fiber tracts are reconstructed by tracking the major axis of the largest diffusion ellipsoid for every neighboring pixel (voxel). DTT can clearly depict white matter fibers, such as the CST and corpus callosum in the brain, which have been difficult to distinguish by conventional MRI, and there is even a report of it being used for neurosurgical navigation [37]. An advantage of DTT is that the researcher or clinician can selectively choose the information to be depicted any number of times, by setting a region of interest (ROI).

Several software programs have been developed for DTT analysis, but we use the free software dTV for DTI analysis developed by the Image Computing and Analysis Laboratory, Department of Radiology, University of Tokyo Hospital, Japan. The dTV software is available at http://www.ut-radiology.umin.jp/people/masutani/dTV.htm [10]. The steps for performing DTI and DTT are shown in Fig. 28.3.

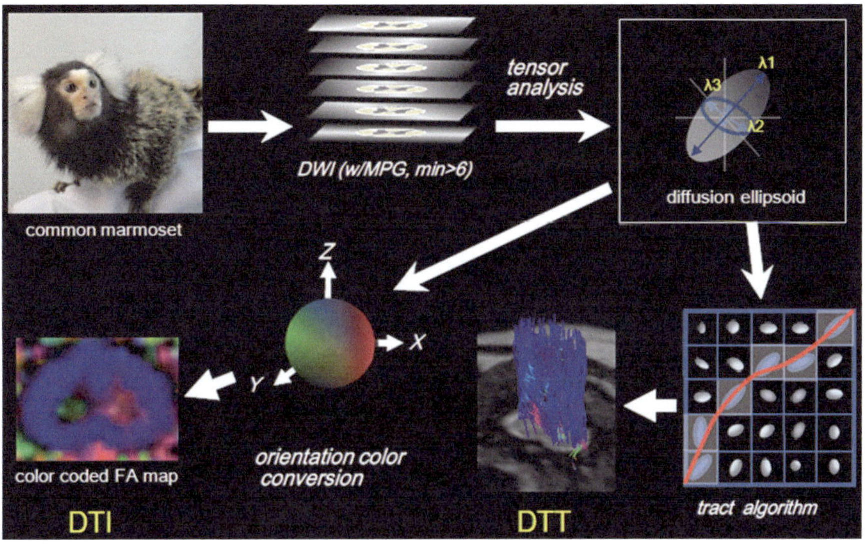

Fig. 28.3 Flow charts for performing DTI and DTT. (Reprinted from Fujiyoshi et al. [31])

28.4 DTT of the Spinal Cord

Clinical Need for DTT of the Spinal Cord: The spinal cord white matter is composed of many nerve fiber bundles, but tissue specimens appear uniform, and it is impossible to observe the individual projections unless a special dye is used. Moreover, because proton relaxation times are very similar for different fiber bundles, it is impossible to tell them apart by DTI, even using the black and white contrast provided by T1- or T2-weighted MR imaging (T1WI or T2WI). Thus, although information about fiber tracts and the integrity of axons in the spinal cord is extremely important, it has been difficult to obtain in vivo. Even when the latest artifact-reducing imaging sequences and high-magnetic-field MRI scanners are used, the fiber bundles comprising individual tracts in the spinal cord white matter cannot be distinguished. To make a prognosis or select the appropriate treatments for the spinal cord injuries that we have discussed here, it is extremely important to know where axons have been destroyed or demyelinated and to what extent axons have been spared. Until now however, even using the best imaging technology available, T1WI and T2WI, only the location of the injury and the degree of compression have been detectable.

In the last decade or so, many reports have described the use of DTT to depict neuronal fibers in the white matter of the brain. High-resolution data for the spinal cord, in contrast, has been difficult to obtain, because the spinal cord is smaller than the brain, it is located deep in the body, and imaging it requires discriminating among tissues and materials with different magnetic properties, such as the spinal cord white matter, cerebrospinal fluid, vertebrae, muscle, and air that are intermingled within a small space [19, 20]. Thus, although occasional reports on the use of DTT to depict the spinal cord in humans have been published, their precision has been low, and few have included histological studies [23–25]. To apply DTT of the spinal cord clinically, this method must be verified by conducting a detailed comparison between the DTT and histological findings. We therefore performed DTT imaging of the spinal cord in a primate, the common marmoset, and examined its accuracy by conducting comparative tissue studies.

DTT of the Cervical Cord of a Primate, the Common Marmoset: We created a reproducible model of SCI in the common marmoset, which is a primate and therefore more closely related than rodents to humans, and found that the transplantation of human neural stem cells contributed to functional recovery in this model [1, 8]. Unfortunately, there are still no reports of curing complete spinal cord injuries in humans, although functional recovery can be anticipated if approximately 5–10 % of the axons are spared from injury. At the animal experiment level, injured axons can be evaluated histologically by injecting a tracer, such as biotinylated dextran amine (BDA), into the primary motor cortex of the cerebrum, but such an analysis obviously cannot be used in the clinic.

To examine whether DTT might be used to assess injured axons in humans, we first used it to examine common marmosets with spinal cord injuries. In these animal experiments, the images and spin-echo sequence were acquired by a 7-Tesla MRI, and we obtained the first clear DTT depiction of the primate spinal cord [37]. To determine whether the DTT results accurately reflected the condition of the axons, we created a simpler cervical cord (C5/6) hemisection injury model and performed DTT 2 weeks later after sacrificing the animal (postmortem model). In a reconstruction of the nerve fiber interruption, DTT clearly depicted the hemisection injury, which was detectable by conventional MRI only in the form of T1 and T2 contrast (Fig. 28.4). Moreover, the DTI and DTT results reflected the histological results obtained with Luxol fast blue (LFB) and other staining methods.

Next, by optimizing the depth of anesthesia to minimize artifacts from respiratory movements and cerebrospinal fluid pulsation, and by making various modifications based on the findings in the postmortem model, we were able to use DTT to reproducibly depict the different fiber tracts of the spinal cord in living common marmosets (Fig. 28.5). Moreover, we were able to depict the pyramidal decussation with DTT, which has been difficult to depict by other methods (Fig. 28.6), and demonstrated that DTT was could be used as a tool for fiber tracking instead of conventional tracers.

We also performed longitudinal DTT, behavioral, and histological analyses before and after contusive SCI in common marmosets. By comparing the tract fiber estimate depicted by DTT with neuronal fibers labeled with anti-neurofilament antibodies, we determined the optimal fractional anisotropy (FA) threshold for fiber tracking to be 0.40. The ratio of the number of tract fiber estimate at the lesion site to the number before SCI was significantly correlated with the functional recovery after SCI. Moreover, comparison of the longitudinal pre- and post-SCI FA and axial diffusivity ($\lambda_{\parallel}$) values revealed that they decreased after injury at the sites caudal to the lesion epicenter in the CST and rostral to the lesion epicenter in the dorsal column [39] (Figs. 28.7 and 28.8). In summary, diffusion imaging is more sensitive

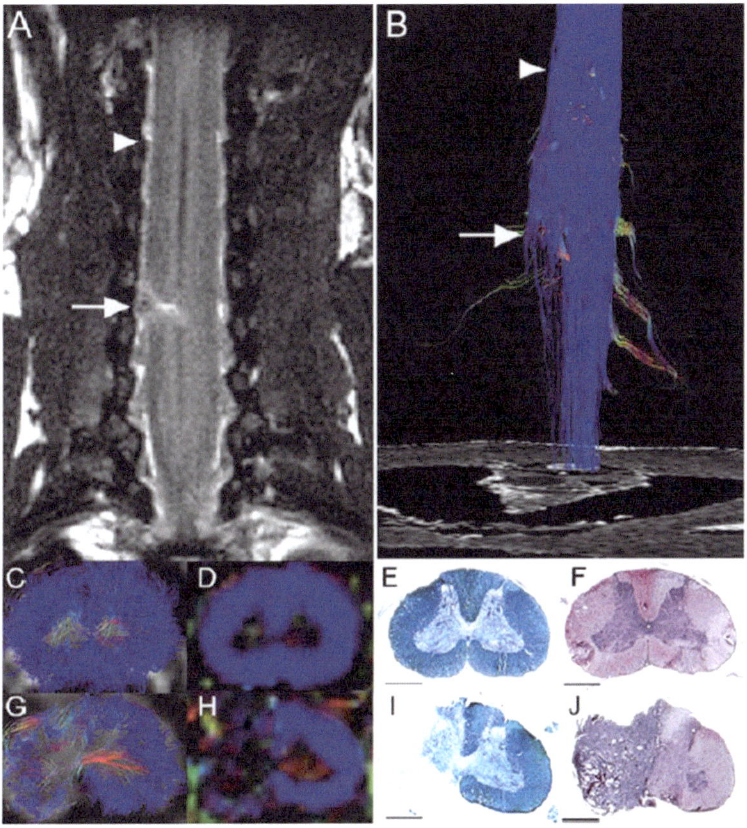

Fig. 28.4 DTT of the hemisected spinal cord at 2 weeks after injury in a postmortem common marmoset. (**a**) Coronal T2-weighted MRI depicted the hemisection injury as a low-intensity area with no change in the cord caudal to the injury. (**b**) DTT of the hemisected spinal cord. The ROI was placed in the upper cervical spinal cord and DTT was traced in the caudal direction revealing disruption of white matter fibers on the hemisected side. The traced tracts became untraceable at the injury site while tracts on the contralateral side continued caudally. *Arrows* indicate the hemisection site and *arrowheads* indicate the point 8 mm cranial to the injury site in (**a**) and (**b**). DTT (**c**, **g**), FA map (**d**, **h**), LFB staining (**e**, **i**), and HE staining (**f**, **j**) of the spinal cord 8 mm cranial to the injury site (**c**–**f**) and at the hemisection site (**g**–**j**). While normal FA and anatomy of the spinal cord was confirmed cranial to the hemisection site, there was a significant decrease in FA of the white matter fibers at the hemisection site (**g** and **h**). Consistent with these changes in DTT (**g**) and color-coded FA map (**h**), demyelination was seen at the hemisection site (**i**). (Scale bars: 1 mm). (Reprinted from Fujiyoshi et al. [38])

than conventional MRI for precisely determining the extent of spinal disorders via noninvasive, longitudinal examinations, in both human patients and animal models. Moreover, FA analysis may prove more useful than other diffusional indices, because of its simplicity, accuracy, and ability to reveal diverse spinal cord disorders especially in the clinical situation.

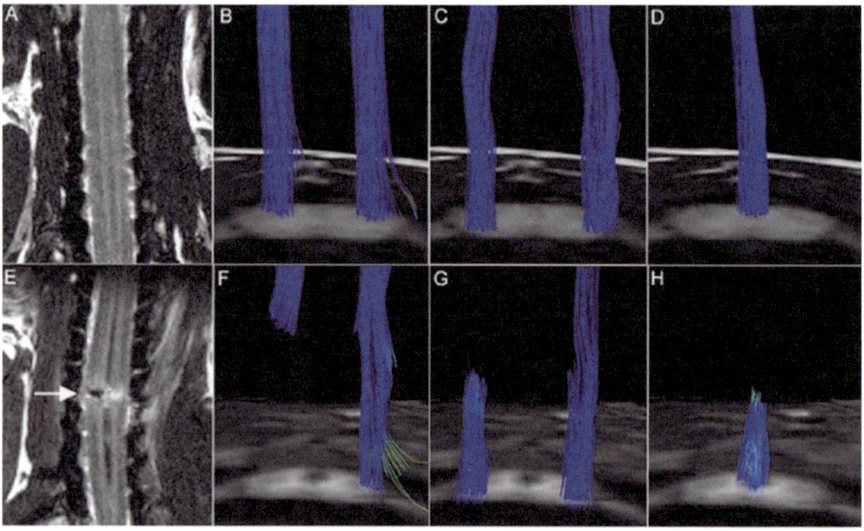

Fig. 28.5 In vivo pathway-specific DTT of intact and injured spinal cords in live common marmosets. (**a**–**d**) T2WI and tract-specific DTT of the intact spinal cord. (**e**–**h**) Hemisected spinal cord 2 weeks after injury. DTT of the CST (**b**, **f**), spinothalamic tract (**c**, **g**), and dorsal column-medial lemniscus pathway (**d**, **h**) in both groups revealed tract disruption at the hemisection site (C5/6 level) in all pathways. Although there are some limitations, pathway-specific DTT conducted in live animals yielded results similar to those observed in postmortem animals, especially with respect to major tract morphology. (Reprinted from Fujiyoshi et al. [38])

28.5 DTI of the Spinal Cord

As the performance of MRI devices improves, the number of DTI studies of the spinal cord should increase. There are two categories of such studies. One involves visualizing the spinal cord disorders by tractography, including the visualization of inflammatory and degenerative disorders [40, 41], the localization and characterization of spinal cord tumors [25, 42], and characterization of the deformation and interruption of local fibers caused by arteriovenous malformations [43] and Brown-Sequard syndrome [44].

The other category involves the quantitative analysis and examination of correlations between diffusion and both functional and histological conditions. Budde et al. revealed that axial diffusion in the ventrolateral white matter in the experimental autoimmune encephalomyelitis (EAE) mouse model was significantly negatively correlated with the EAE clinical score and was significantly lower in mice with severe EAE than in mice with moderate EAE [45]. In the ventral white matter tracts of the spinal cord of ALS-affected mice, the diffusion values altered with disease progression [46, 47]. In an SCI study, Kim et al. identified the spared, normal ventrolateral white matter by the hyperacute axial diffusion 3 h after injury, and a histological analysis performed 14 days later showed a good correlation with the spinal contusion injury [48]. Loy et al. demonstrated that axial diffusion in ventral white matter differentiated mild, moderate, and severe contusive SCI, with good histological correlation [49].

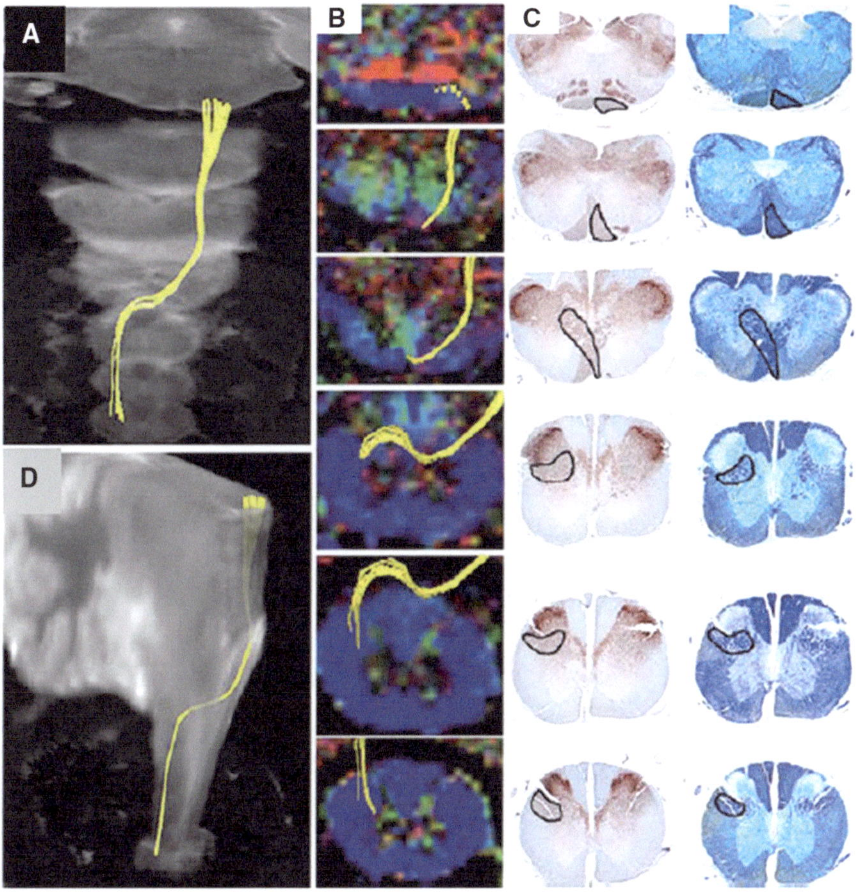

Fig. 28.6 Pathway-specific DTT in a postmortem common marmoset revealing the course of the corticospinal tract with pyramidal decussation. (**a**, **b**) DTT of the pyramidal decussation superimposed on three dimensional MR images to macroscopically confirm that the pyramidal decussation was depicted in the proper height in the medulla and the upper cervical cord, using the cerebellum as a reference point. (**c**) DTT of the pyramidal decussation superimposed on axial color-coded FA maps. (**I**) Axial histological slices of the same points in (**c**) stained for CaMKII-α to reveal the location of CST fibers (**d**) and LFB to delineate the configuration of the white matter (**e**). In each slice, the area through which the DTT CST tract passes was positive for CaMKII-α and LFB, confirming the accuracy of DTT. (Scale bars: 1 mm) (Partial modification of Fujiyoshi et al. [38])

In summary, these recent studies indicate that the quantitative DTI parameters are sensitive and specific biomarkers for spinal cord white matter integrity.

Several clinical studies suggest that the increased sensitivity of DTI makes it appropriate for the early detection of myelopathic changes in patients with cervical myelopathy. A significant positive correlation between the FA at the compressed level and the clinical assessment has been demonstrated [50, 51]. This correlation was also seen in patients with SCI [23, 52]. Chang et al. revealed that quantitative fiber tract results correlate to some extent with the severity of cervical SCI in patients [53].

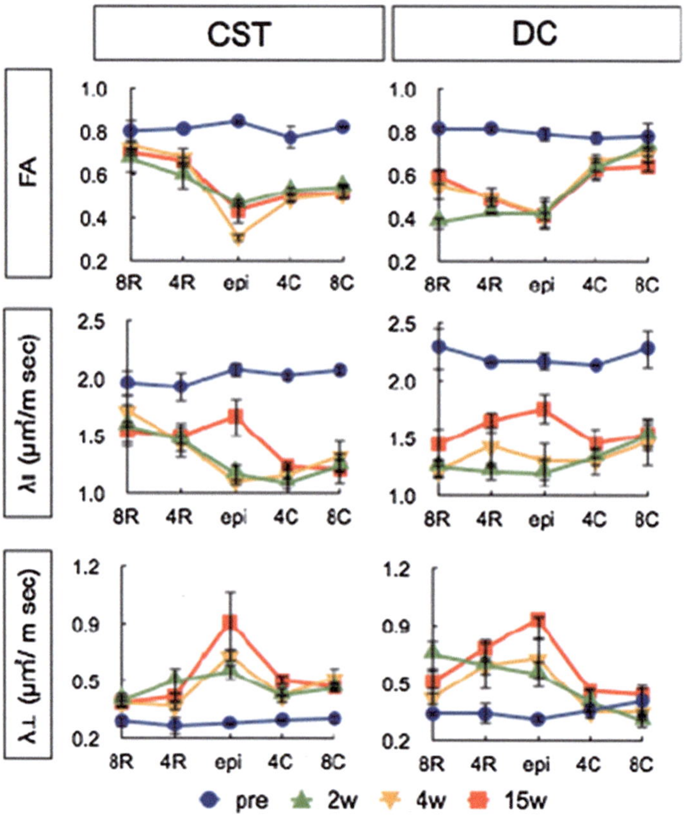

Fig. 28.7 Alteration in FA values in corticospinal tract- and dorsal column-specific ROIs. Changes in the FA, $\lambda_{\parallel}$, and $\lambda_{\perp}$ values for the CST- and DC-specific ROIs at sites epicenter (epi), 4 and 8 mm rostral away from the lesion epicenter (4R, 8R), 4 and 8 mm caudal away from the lesion epicenter (4C, 8C). FA and $\lambda_{\parallel}$ values of the CST at epi, 4C and 8C were significantly lower than the pre-injury values after the injury. In contrast, the FA and $\lambda_{\parallel}$ values of the DC at epi, 4R and 8R were significantly decreased after the injury and gradually recovery in FA was shown. $\lambda_{\parallel}$ and $\lambda_{\perp}$ values were increasing in epicenter of both DC and CST in chronic phase. (Reprinted from [39])

28.6 Limitations of DTT and Future Prospects

Resolution: DTT does not depict the axons themselves, although this is frequently misunderstood. The voxel size required for analyzing anisotropy is far greater than the diameter of an axon, so the diffusion anisotropy of fiber bundles composed of 10^2–10^3 axons or more is what is actually depicted.

Depiction of Complicated Axonal Pathways: Closely related to the resolution problem, the anisotropies of fibers oriented in different directions within the same voxel sometimes cancel each other out. This is the result of a partial volume effect that stops the tracking. Conversely, if the anisotropy is not cancelled out, the sum of the

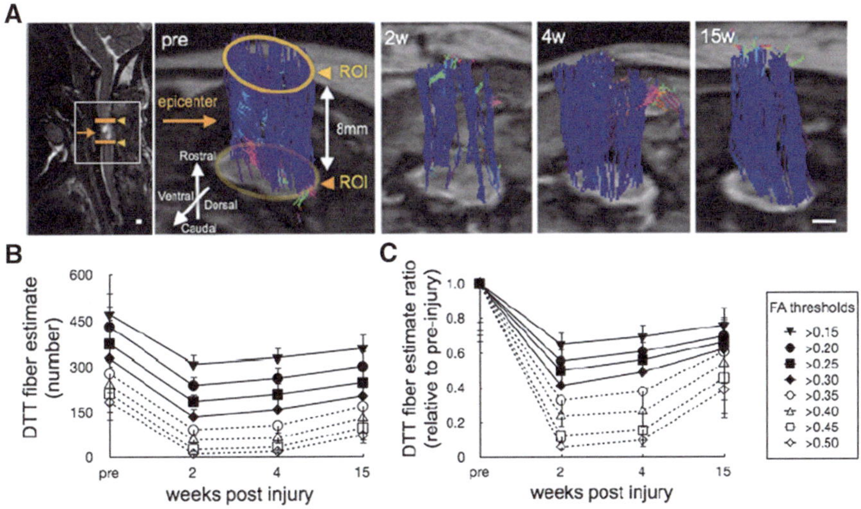

Fig. 28.8 Change in DTT fiber estimate over time after SCI with different FA thresholds. (**a**) Time-dependent changes in DTT fibers estimate after contusive SCI shown by two ROI-based fiber tracking (FA threshold >0.20; 50° angle of deflection threshold; 8 mm distance between the two ROIs). The *yellow arrow* indicates the lesion epicenter and *yellow arrowheads* indicate the rostral and caudal ROIs. Quantitative analysis of the number of two-ROI DTT fiber estimate (**b**) and its value relative to the pre-injury fiber estimate (**c**) using different FA thresholds. (**b**) The number was lower 2 weeks after injury compared with their pre-injury number and gradually increased. The number of DTT fiber detected decreased as the FA threshold increased. (**c**) The pattern of change in the DTT fiber estimate ratio was similar to that in the number of DTT fiber estimate. The DTT fiber estimate ratio decreased as the FA threshold increased. Scale bar indicates 0.5 mm. (Partial modification of [39])

conflicting information allows tracking, but sometimes leads to the depiction of a structure that cannot actually exist. Therefore, DTT images do not always reflect actual anatomical structures. We have addressed this issue by setting a threshold value for FA that reduces the likelihood of depicting an erroneous tract and setting a threshold value for anisotropy tracking that prevents sharp changes in direction. At present, we consider it necessary to interpret DTT results cautiously, drawing on all of the anatomical and histological information available, just as when reading ordinary MRI scans. Complicated, multiaxial neural pathways can be analyzed by using a high *b* value[3] [54, 55]. By increasing the *b* value, we have succeeded in clearly depicting the optic chiasm (Fig. 28.9), brain stem, and cervical nerve roots (Fig. 28.10), but because these analyses require an enormous amount of time, they have not reached the point of clinical application.

[3] The "*b* value" is related to the diffusion setting in DWI. It is calculated by the following formula, in which γ (MHz) is the gyromagnetic ratio, G (mT/m) is the size of the MPG, δ (ms) is the MPG application time, and Δ (ms) is the starting time of each pair of gradient magnetic fields.

$$b = \gamma^2 G_x^{\,2} \delta^2 \left(\Delta - \delta / 3 \right)$$

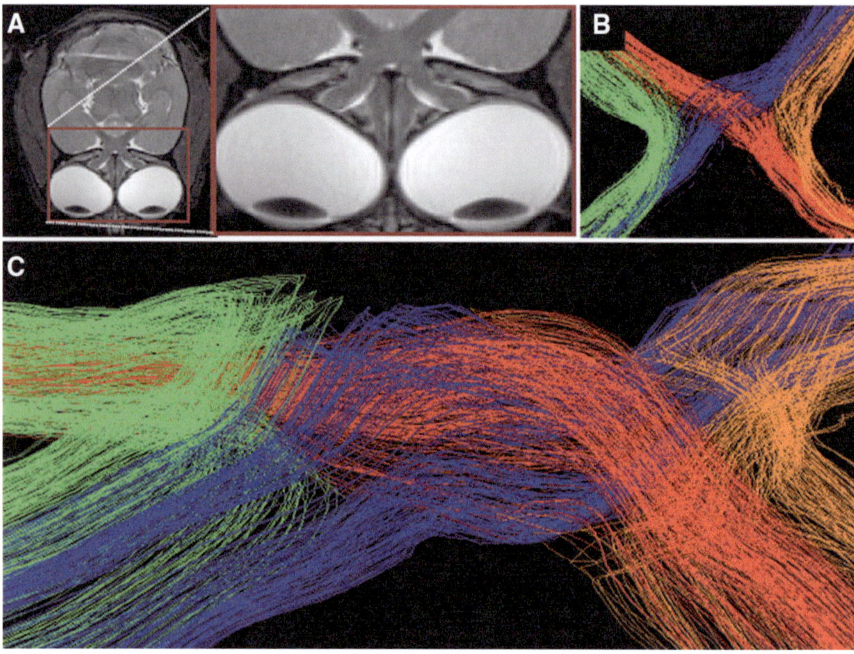

Fig. 28.9 HARDI (high angular resolution diffusion imaging) of the optic chiasma in the common marmoset. (**a**) T2-weighted MR images (axial) of the common marmoset brain. (**b**, **c**) Overview (**b**) and frontal view (**c**) of HARDI in the optic chiasma. HARDI was found to depict the path of the optic nerve in a more anatomically and histologically correct manner

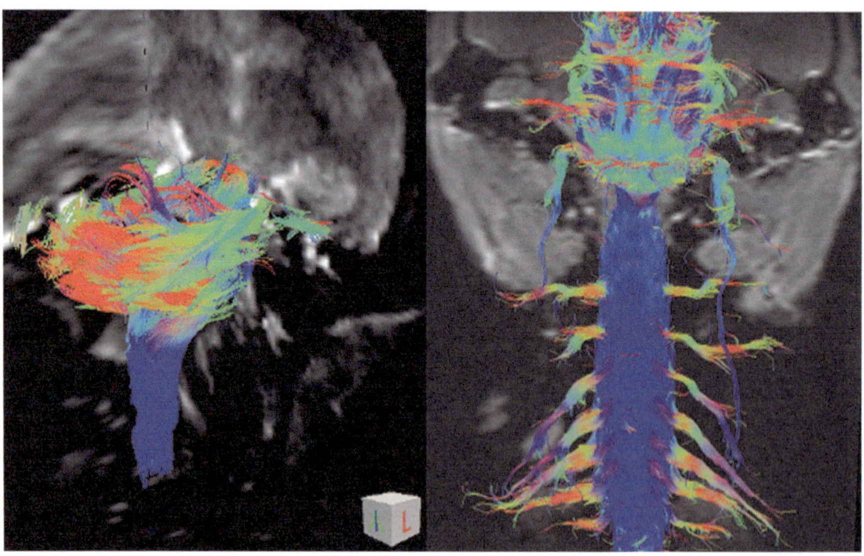

Fig. 28.10 HARDI (high angular resolution diffusion imaging) of spinal cord, the brain stem, cervical nerve roots, and cranial nerves in the common marmoset

Thus, the *b* value is an index that indicates the degree of diffusion, and higher *b* values mean greater diffusion. For the DTT images that we obtained in this study, we used $b = 1{,}000$. By contrast, a "high" *b* value is 2,500 or more, which makes it possible to detect intracellular diffusion and the diffusion of more complicated nerve pathways that cannot be perceived by conventional DWI.

28.7 Clinical Application of DTT

By exploiting our DTT findings from the spinal cords of marmosets, we have already applied this method clinically to a fairly large number of cases. We are currently assessing the usefulness of DTT for examining cervical spondylotic myelopathy [56] (Fig. 28.11), ossification of the posterior longitudinal ligament (OPLL), and spinal cord tumors, as well as SCI [31] (Fig. 28.12). The application of DTT is restricted to diseases of the cervical region, because it is difficult to obtain high-resolution images in the trunk, which currently prevents detailed analysis.

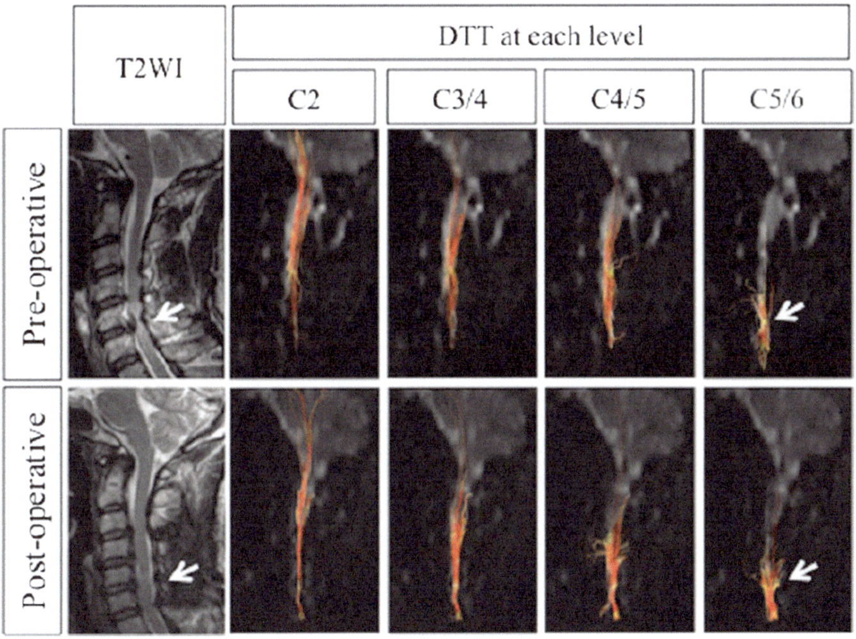

Fig. 28.11 Representative case. A 54-year-old man with cervical spondylotic myelopathy. Preoperative T2-weighted MRI (T2WI) showed spinal cord compression at the level of C5–C6, where the fiber tracts (FTs) were disrupted (*arrow*). The preoperative FT ratio 68 % (219 fibers at the C5–C6 level/322 fibers at the C2 level) (*upper row*). Consistent with the recovery of the FTs after laminoplasty, the FT ratio was increased to 86 % (265 fibers at the C5–C6 level/308 fibers at the C2 level) (*lower row*). (Reprinted from [56])

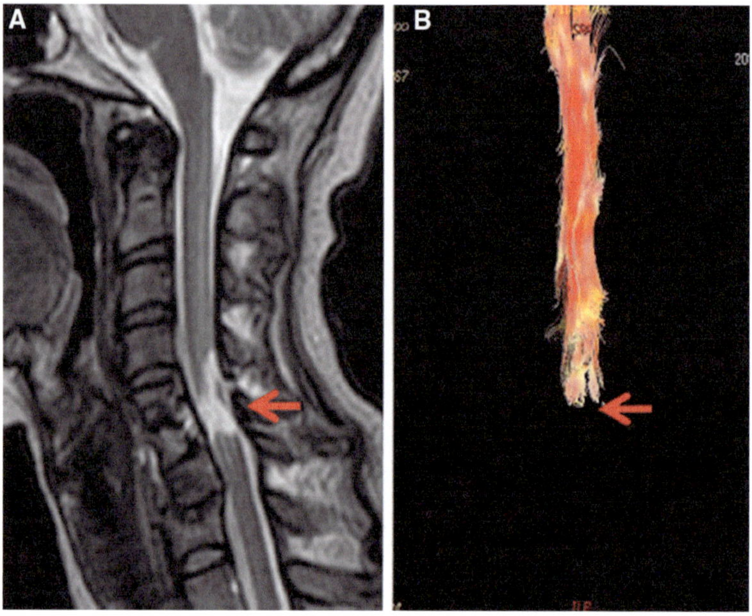

Fig. 28.12 Diffusion tensor tractography (DTT) images from a human patient. T2-weighted MR images (sagittal; **a**) and DTT (**b**) images of a complete spinal transection in a human patient. This patient suffered from complete paraplegia due to fracture-dislocation at C6 level. By setting the region of interest at C1 level, DTT was traced in the caudal direction revealing the disruption of white matter fibers at the lesion epicenter. *Arrows* indicate the lesion epicenter. (Reprinted from Fujiyoshi et al. [31])

We hope that future advances in the development of MRI hardware and software will enable researchers to overcome the problems of long image acquisition time and resolution. Moreover, we believe that by revealing more anatomical structural information about the tracts, it will be possible to detect and evaluate the lesions of even more spinal cord diseases.

28.8 DTI and Statistical Analysis: Combination with Functional MRI

Although manual or semi-automated-guided ROI measurements are needed to assess diffusional changes in the spinal cord, questions arise about the validity of the investigator-determined ROI, given interindividual variability, even though the ROI can be defined so that the measurement is highly reliable. Moreover, it is difficult to decide on the ROI in cases where the location and/or type of abnormality is unknown [57, 58].

To resolve these problems, a voxelwise statistical analysis can be used to evaluate the structural MRI, to identify differences in anatomical structures between a control and experimental group, or to detect longitudinal changes within groups in brain studies [59, 60]. Voxelwise statistical analyses of FA data are carried out using tract-based spatial statistics (TBSS) [61], which is part of the Oxford Centre for Functional MRI of the Brain's Software Library [62]. TBSS projects all of the each subject's FA data onto a mean FA tract skeleton, before applying voxelwise cross-subject statistics. Another technique, voxel-based morphometry (VBM), allows the investigation of focal differences in brain anatomy using a statistical approach, called statistical parametric mapping [60, 63, 64]. Unlike diffusion tensor analysis, these methods permit the spatial detection of structural differences within the entire brain.

Some authors have suggested that voxel-based and ROI-based methods provide different types of information and that a voxel-based analysis can be used as an exploratory whole-brain approach to identify abnormal brain regions, which should then be validated using ROI-based analyses. These methods may be complementary to each other in terms of DTI analysis [57, 65]. Furthermore, brain templates are currently available for use in applying voxel-based analysis across a variety of animal species to detect subtle anatomical differences [59, 66–70].

Endo et al. recently measured the BOLD-functional MRI (fMRI) signal in rats with thoracic transection injury and found that hind limb stimulation results in significant lumbar dorsal horn (spinothalamic) activation in the dorsal horn caudal to the injury [71–73]. However, it is difficult to distinguish the BOLD signal of white matter from that of the cell bodies or gray matter. Therefore, the structural tract anatomy revealed by DTI-MRI needs to be further improved, and the data obtained from BOLD and DTI need to be better integrated, to address this question. A combination of BOLD-fMRI and DTI should be able to track the regrowth of damaged tracts connecting functional neurons [72]

28.9 Conclusion

Beyond the utility of this technique to monitor the extent of spinal cord lesions, this technique may prove instrumental in evaluating chronic plastic changes associated with spontaneous functional recovery, as well as the ability of therapeutic interventions such as cell transplantation [74, 75] and growth factor infusion [76] to enhance this "remodeling process." DTT of the spinal cord is a powerful tool with tremendous potential if its properties and limitations are fully understood and correctly applied.

Acknowledgements This work was supported by grants from MEXT, CREST, JST in Japan, from the General Insurance Association of Japan, from the "Funding Program for World-leading Innovative R&D on Science and Technology," and by a grant-in-aid from the 21st Century and Global COE Programs of MEXT, Japan, to Keio University.

Animal Preparation: All interventions and animal care procedures were performed in accordance with the Laboratory Animal Welfare Act, Guide for the Care and Use of Laboratory Animals (National Institutes of Health), and Guidelines and Policies for Animal Surgery provided by the Animal Study Committee of the Central Institute for Experimental Animals, and they were approved by the ethics committee of Keio University.

Informed Consent: We obt`ained adequate informed consent from both the healthy volunteer and the patients with cervical spondylotic myelopathy and SCI.

Conflict of Interest: The authors declare that they have no competing financial interests.

References

1. Iwanami A, Yamane J, Katoh H, Nakamura M, Momoshima S, Ishii H, Tanioka Y, Tamaoki N, Nomura T, Toyama Y, Okano H (2005) Establishment of graded spinal cord injury model in a nonhuman primate: the common marmoset. J Neurosci Res 80:172–181
2. Olson L (2002) Medicine: clearing a path for nerve growth. Nature 416:589–590
3. Kaneko S, Iwanami A, Nakamura M, Kishino A, Kikuchi K, Shibata S, Okano HJ, Ikegami T, Moriya A, Konishi O, Nakayama C, Kumagai K, Kimura T, Sato Y, Goshima Y, Taniguchi M, Ito M, He Z, Toyama Y, Okano H (2007) A selective Sema3A inhibitor enhances regenerative responses and functional recovery of the injured spinal cord. Nat Med 12:1380–1389
4. Ralston DD, Ralston HJ 3rd (1985) The terminations of corticospinal tract axons in the macaque monkey. J Comp Neurol 242:325–337
5. Lacroix S, Havton LA, McKay H, Yang H, Brant A, Roberts J, Tuszynski MH (2004) Bilateral corticospinal projections arise from each motor cortex in the macaque monkey: a quantitative study. J Comp Neurol 473:147–161
6. Kulkarni MV, Williams JC, Yeakley JW, Andrews JL, McArdle CB, Narayana PA, Howell RR, Jonas AJ (1987) Magnetic resonance imaging in the diagnosis of the cranio-cervical manifestations of the mucopolysaccharidoses. Magn Reson Imaging 5:317–323
7. Yamashita Y, Takahashi M, Matsuno Y, Sakamoto Y, Oguni T, Sakae T, Yoshizumi K, Kim EE (1990) Chronic injuries of the spinal cord: assessment with MR imaging. Radiology 175: 849–854
8. Iwanami A, Kaneko S, Nakamura M, Kanemura Y, Mori H, Kobayashi S, Yamasaki M, Momoshima S, Ishii H, Ando K, Tanioka Y, Tamaoki N, Nomura T, Toyama Y, Okano H (2005) Transplantation of human neural stem cells for spinal cord injury in primates. J Neurosci Res 80:182–190
9. Ito R, Mori S, Melhem ER (2002) Diffusion tensor brain imaging and tractography. Neuroimaging Clin N Am 12:1–19
10. Masutani Y, Aoki S, Abe O, Hayashi N, Otomo K (2003) MR diffusion tensor imaging: recent advance and new techniques for diffusion tensor visualization. Eur J Radiol 46:53–66
11. Mori H, Masutani Y, Aoki S, Abe O, Hayashi N, Masumoto T, Yamada H, Yoshikawa T, Kunimatsu A, Ohtomo K, Kabasawa H (2003) [Simple visualization of the corticospinal pathway using tractography: one-ROI and two-ROI methods]. Nippon Igaku Hoshasen Gakkai Zasshi 63:51–53
12. Le Bihan D, Breton E, Lallemand D, Grenier P, Cabanis E, Laval-Jeantet M (1986) MR imaging of intravoxel incoherent motions: application to diffusion and perfusion in neurologic disorders. Radiology 161:401–407
13. Moseley ME, Cohen Y, Kucharczyk J, Mintorovitch J, Asgari HS, Wendland MF, Tsuruda J, Norman D (1990) Diffusion-weighted MR imaging of anisotropic water diffusion in cat central nervous system. Radiology 176:439–445
14. Basser PJ, Mattiello J, LeBihan D (1994) MR diffusion tensor spectroscopy and imaging. Biophys J 66:259–267
15. Mori S, Zhang J (2006) Principles of diffusion tensor imaging and its applications to basic neuroscience research. Neuron 51:527–539
16. Conturo TE, Lori NF, Cull TS, Akbudak E, Snyder AZ, Shimony JS, McKinstry RC, Burton H, Raichle ME (1999) Tracking neuronal fiber pathways in the living human brain. Proc Natl Acad Sci U S A 96:10422–10427
17. Kamada K, Todo T, Morita A, Masutani Y, Aoki S, Ino K, Kawai K, Kirino T (2005) Functional monitoring for visual pathway using real-time visual evoked potentials and optic-radiation tractography. Neurosurgery 57:121–127, discussion 121–127

18. Lee JS, Han MK, Kim SH, Kwon OK, Kim JH (2005) Fiber tracking by diffusion tensor imaging in corticospinal tract stroke: topographical correlation with clinical symptoms. NeuroImage 26:771–776
19. Basser PJ, Jones DK (2002) Diffusion-tensor MRI: theory, experimental design and data analysis—a technical review. NMR Biomed 15:456–467
20. Maier SE, Mamata H (2005) Diffusion tensor imaging of the spinal cord. Ann N Y Acad Sci 1064:50–60
21. Kharbanda HS, Alsop DC, Anderson AW, Filardo G, Hackney DB (2006) Effects of cord motion on diffusion imaging of the spinal cord. Magn Reson Med 56:334–339
22. Holder CA, Muthupillai R, Mukundan S Jr, Eastwood JD, Hudgins PA (2000) Diffusion-weighted MR imaging of the normal human spinal cord in vivo. AJNR Am J Neuroradiol 21:1799–1806
23. Facon D, Ozanne A, Fillard P, Lepeintre JF, Tournoux-Facon C, Ducreux D (2005) MR diffusion tensor imaging and fiber tracking in spinal cord compression. AJNR Am J Neuroradiol 26:1587–1594
24. Tsuchiya K, Fujikawa A, Suzuki Y (2005) Diffusion tractography of the cervical spinal cord by using parallel imaging. AJNR Am J Neuroradiol 26:398–400
25. Ducreux D, Lepeintre JF, Fillard P, Loureiro C, Tadie M, Lasjaunias P (2006) MR diffusion tensor imaging and fiber tracking in 5 spinal cord astrocytomas. AJNR Am J Neuroradiol 27:214–216
26. Le Bihan D, Breton E, Lallemand D, Aubin ML, Vignaud J, Laval-Jeantet M (1988) Separation of diffusion and perfusion in intravoxel incoherent motion MR imaging. Radiology 168: 497–505
27. Burdette JH, Elster AD, Ricci PE (1999) Acute cerebral infarction: quantification of spin-density and T2 shine-through phenomena on diffusion-weighted MR images. Radiology 212: 333–339
28. Burdette JH, Ricci PE, Petitti N, Elster AD (1998) Cerebral infarction: time course of signal intensity changes on diffusion-weighted MR images. AJR Am J Roentgenol 171:791–795
29. Yamashita T, Kwee TC, Takahara T (2009) Whole-body magnetic resonance neurography. N Engl J Med 361:538–539
30. Le Bihan D, Mangin JF, Poupon C, Clark CA, Pappata S, Molko N, Chabriat H (2001) Diffusion tensor imaging: concepts and applications. J Magn Reson Imaging 13:534–546
31. Fujiyoshi K, Konomi T et al (2013) Diffusion tensor imaging and tractography of the spinal cord from experimental studies to clinical application. Exp Neurol 242:74–82
32. Le Bihan D, van Zijl P (2002) From the diffusion coefficient to the diffusion tensor. NMR Biomed 15:431–434
33. Aoki S, Abe O, Masutani Y (eds) (2005) New edition: making sense of diffusion MRI (Japanese). Shujunsha, Tokyo
34. Takagi T, Nakamura M, Yamada M, Hikishima K, Momoshima S, Fujiyoshi K, Shibata S, Okano H, Toyama Y, Okano H (2009) Visualization of peripheral nerve degeneration and regeneration: monitoring with diffusion tensor tractography. NeuroImage 44:884–892
35. Pajevic S, Pierpaoli C (2000) Color schemes to represent the orientation of anisotropic tissues from diffusion tensor data: application to white matter fiber tract mapping in the human brain. Magn Reson Med 43:921
36. Mori S, van Zijl PCM (2002) Fiber tracking: principles and strategies - a technical review. NMR Biomed 15:468–480
37. Kamada K, Todo T, Masutani Y, Aoki S, Ino K, Takano T, Kirino T, Kawahara N, Morita A (2005) Combined use of tractography-integrated functional neuronavigation and direct fiber stimulation. J Neurosurg 102:664–672
38. Fujiyoshi K, Yamada M, Nakamura M, Yamane J, Katoh H, Kitamura K, Kawai K, Okada S, Momoshima S, Toyama Y, Okano H (2007) In vivo tracing of neural tracts in the intact and injured spinal cord of marmosets by diffusion tensor tractography. J Neurosci 27:11991–11998
39. Konomi T, Fujiyoshi K et al (2012) Conditions for quantitative evaluation of injured spinal cord by in vivo diffusion tensor imaging and tractography: preclinical longitudinal study in common marmosets. NeuroImage 63:1841–1853

40. Cruz LC Jr, Domingues RC, Gasparetto EL (2009) Diffusion tensor imaging of the cervical spinal cord of patients with relapsing-remising multiple sclerosis: a study of 41 cases. Arq Neuropsiquiatr 67:391–395
41. Renoux J, Facon D, Fillard P, Huynh I, Lasjaunias P, Ducreux D (2006) MR diffusion tensor imaging and fiber tracking in inflammatory diseases of the spinal cord. AJNR Am J Neuroradiol 27:1947–1951
42. Setzer M, Murtagh RD, Murtagh FR, Eleraky M, Jain S, Marquardt G, Seifert V, Vrionis FD (2010) Diffusion tensor imaging tractography in patients with intramedullary tumors: comparison with intraoperative findings and value for prediction of tumor resectability. J Neurosurg Spine 13:371–380
43. Ozanne A, Krings T, Facon D, Fillard P, Dumas JL, Alvarez H, Ducreux D, Lasjaunias P (2007) MR diffusion tensor imaging and fiber tracking in spinal cord arteriovenous malformations: a preliminary study. AJNR Am J Neuroradiol 28:1271–1279
44. Rajasekaran S, Kanna RM, Karunanithi R, Shetty AP (2010) Diffusion tensor tractography demonstration of partially injured spinal cord tracts in a patient with posttraumatic brown sequard syndrome. J Magn Reson Imaging 32:978–981
45. Budde MD, Kim JH, Liang HF, Russell JH, Cross AH, Song SK (2008) Axonal injury detected by in vivo diffusion tensor imaging correlates with neurological disability in a mouse model of multiple sclerosis. NMR Biomed 21:589–597
46. Kim JH, Wu T-H, Budde MD, Lee J-M, Song S-K (2011) Noninvasive detection of brainstem and spinal cord axonal degeneration in an amyotrophic lateral sclerosis mouse model. NMR in Biomedicine 24(2):163–169
47. Underwood CK, Kurniawan ND, Butler TJ, Cowin GJ, Wallace RH (2010) Non-invasive diffusion tensor imaging detects white matter degeneration in the spinal cord of a mouse model of amyotrophic lateral sclerosis. NeuroImage 1–28
48. Kim JH, Loy DN, Wang Q, Budde MD, Schmidt RE, Trinkaus K, Song S-K (2010) Diffusion tensor imaging at 3 hours after traumatic spinal cord injury predicts long-term locomotor recovery. J Neurotrauma 27:587–598
49. Loy DN, Kim JH, Xie M, Schmidt RE, Trinkaus K, Song S-K (2007) Diffusion tensor imaging predicts hyperacute spinal cord injury severity. J Neurotrauma 24:979–990
50. Budzik J-F, Balbi V, Thuc V, Duhamel A, Assaker R, Cotten A (2010) Diffusion tensor imaging and fibre tracking in cervical spondylotic myelopathy. Eur Radiol 1–8
51. Xiangshui M, Xiangjun C, Xiaoming Z, Qingshi Z, Yi C, Chuanqiang Q, Xiangxing M, Chuanfu L, Jinwen H (2010) 3T magnetic resonance diffusion tensor imaging and fibre tracking in cervical myelopathy. Clin Radiol 65:465–473
52. Shanmuganathan K, Gullapalli RP, Zhuo J, Mirvis SE (2008) Diffusion tensor MR imaging in cervical spine trauma. AJNR Am J Neuroradiol 29:655–659
53. Chang Y, Jung T-D, Yoo DS, Hyun JK (2010) Diffusion tensor imaging and fiber tractography of patients with cervical spinal cord injury. J Neurotrauma 27:2033–2040
54. Schmahmann JD, Pandya DN, Wang R, Dai G, D'Arceuil HE, de Crespigny AJ, Wedeen VJ (2007) Association fibre pathways of the brain: parallel observations from diffusion spectrum imaging and autoradiography. Brain 130:630–653
55. Tuch DS, Reese TG, Wiegell MR, Wedeen VJ (2003) Diffusion MRI of complex neural architecture. Neuron 40:885–895
56. Nakamura M, Fujiyosi K et al (2012) Clinical significance of diffusion tensor tractography as a predictor of functional recovery after laminoplasty in patients with cervical compression myelopathy. J Neurosurg Spine 17:147–152
57. Abe O, Takao H, Gonoi W, Sasaki H, Murakami M, Kabasawa H, Kawaguchi H, Goto M, Yamada H, Yamasue H, Kasai K, Aoki S, Ohtomo K (2010) Voxel-based analysis of the diffusion tensor. Neuroradiology 52:699–710
58. Ciccarelli O, Catani M, Johansen-Berg H, Clark C, Thompson A (2008) Diffusion-based tractography in neurological disorders: concepts, applications, and future developments. Lancet Neurol 7:715–727

59. Hikishima K, Quallo MM, Komaki Y, Yamada M, Kawai K, Momoshima S, Okano HJ, Sasaki E, Tamaoki N, Lemon RN, Iriki A, Okano H (2010) Population-averaged standard template brain atlas for the common marmoset (*Callithrix jacchus*). NeuroImage 1–9
60. Wright IC, McGuire PK, Poline JB, Travere JM, Murray RM, Frith CD, Frackowiak RS, Friston KJ (1995) A voxel-based method for the statistical analysis of gray and white matter density applied to schizophrenia. NeuroImage 2:244–252
61. Smith SM, Jenkinson M, Johansen-Berg H, Rueckert D, Nichols TE, Mackay CE, Watkins KE, Ciccarelli O, Cader MZ, Matthews PM, Behrens TE (2006) Tract-based spatial statistics: voxelwise analysis of multi-subject diffusion data. NeuroImage 31:1487–1505
62. Smith SM, Jenkinson M, Woolrich MW, Beckmann CF, Behrens TE, Johansen-Berg H, Bannister PR, De Luca M, Drobnjak I, Flitney DE, Niazy RK, Saunders J, Vickers J, Zhang Y, De Stefano N, Brady JM, Matthews PM (2004) Advances in functional and structural MR image analysis and implementation as FSL. NeuroImage 23(suppl 1):S208–219
63. Ashburner J, Friston KJ (2000) Voxel-based morphometry-the methods. NeuroImage 11: 805–821
64. De Laat KF, Tuladhar AM, Van Norden AGW, Norris DG, Zwiers MP, De Leeuw F-E (2011) Loss of white matter integrity is associated with gait disorders in cerebral small vessel disease. Brain 134:73–83
65. Giuliani N, Calhoun V, Pearlson G, Francis A, Buchanan R (2005) Voxel-based morphometry versus region of interest: a comparison of two methods for analyzing gray matter differences in schizophrenia. Schizophrenia Res 74:135–148
66. Black KJ, Koller JM, Snyder AZ, Perlmutter JS (2001) Template images for nonhuman primate neuroimaging: 2. Macaque. NeuroImage 14:744–748
67. Black KJ, Snyder AZ, Koller JM, Gado MH, Perlmutter JS (2001) Template images for nonhuman primate neuroimaging: 1. Baboon. NeuroImage 14:736–743
68. McLaren DG, Kosmatka KJ, Oakes TR, Kroenke CD, Kohama SG, Matochik JA, Ingram DK, Johnson SC (2009) A population-average MRI-based atlas collection of the rhesus macaque. NeuroImage 45:52–59
69. Quallo MM, Price CJ, Ueno K, Asamizuya T, Cheng K, Lemon RN, Iriki A (2010) Creating a population-averaged standard brain template for Japanese macaques (*M. fuscata*). NeuroImage 52:1328–1333
70. Rilling JK, Barks SK, Parr LA, Preuss TM, Faber TL, Pagnoni G, Bremner JD, Votaw JR (2007) A comparison of resting-state brain activity in humans and chimpanzees. Proc Natl Acad Sci U S A 104:17146–17151
71. Endo T, Spenger C, Westman E, Tominaga T, Olson L (2008) Reorganization of sensory processing below the level of spinal cord injury as revealed by fMRI. Exp Neurol 209:155–160
72. Harel N, Strittmatter S (2008) Functional MRI and other non-invasive imaging technologies: providing visual biomarkers for spinal cord structure and function after injury. Exp Neurol 211:324–328
73. Lilja J (2006) Blood oxygenation level-dependent visualization of synaptic relay stations of sensory pathways along the neuroaxis in response to graded sensory stimulation of a limb. J Neurosci 26:6330–6336
74. Tsuji O, Miura K et al (2010) Therapeutic potential of appropriately evaluated 'safe' induced pluripotent stem cells for spinal cord injury. Proc Natl Acad Sci U S A 107:12704–12709
75. Nori S, Okada S et al (2011) Grafted human-induced pluripotent stem cell–derived neurospheres promote motor functional recovery after spinal cord injury in mice. Proc Natl Acad Sci U S A 108:16825–16830
76. Kitamura K et al (2011) Human hepatocyte growth factor promotes functional recovery in primates after spinal cord injury. PLos One 6:e27706

Chapter 29
Clinical Significance of 3D-MRI/^{18}F-FDG PET Fusion Imaging of Patients with Cervical Compressive Myelopathy

Kenzo Uchida, Hideaki Nakajima, Hidehiko Okazawa, Hirohiko Kimura, Ai Yoshida, and Hisatoshi Baba

Abstract The present study was designed to evaluate the use of three-dimensional (3D)-MRI/^{18}F-FDG PET fusion imaging to define intramedullary signal changes on MRIs and local glucose metabolic rate measured on ^{18}F-FDG PET in relation to clinical outcome and prognosis. Quantitative analysis of intramedullary signal changes on MRIs included calculation of the signal intensity ratio (SIR). On fusion images, the maximal count at the lesion was adopted as the standardized uptake value (SUV_{max}). The SUV ratio (SUVR) was also calculated. Neurological assessment was conducted using the Japanese Orthopaedic Association (JOA) scoring system. The SIR on T1-weighted images (WIs), but not SIR on T2-WIs, correlated with preoperative JOA score and postoperative neurological improvement. Lesion-SUVmax correlated with SIR on T1-WIs, but not with SIR on T2-WIs, and also with postoperative neurological outcome. The SUVR correlated better than SIR on T1-WIs and lesion-SUV_{max} with neurological improvement. Longer symptom duration correlated negatively with SIR on T1-WIs, positively with SIR on T2-WIs, and negatively with SUV_{max}. Our results suggest that low-intensity signal on the T1-WIs correlates with poor postoperative neurological outcome. SUV_{max} measured at lesions with increased signal intensity and SUVR measured on fusion MRI/PET are sensitive parameters for prediction of clinical outcome.

K. Uchida (✉) • H. Nakajima • H. Baba • A. Yoshida
Faculty of Medical Sciences, Department of Orthopaedics and Rehabilitation Medicine, University of Fukui, Matsuoka Shimoaizuki 23-3, Eiheiji, Fukui 910-1193, Japan
e-mail: kuchida@u-fukui.ac.jp

H. Okazawa
Biomedical Imaging Research Center, University of Fukui, Matsuoka Shimoaizuki 23, Eiheiji, Fukui 910-1193, Japan

H. Kimura
Department of Radiology, Faculty of Medical Sciences, University of Fukui, Matsuoka Shimoaizuki 23, Eiheiji, Fukui 910-1193, Japan

K. Uchida et al. (eds.), *Neuroprotection and Regeneration of the Spinal Cord*,
DOI 10.1007/978-4-431-54502-6_29,

Keywords [^{18}F]-fluorodeoxyglucose (FDG) positron emission tomography (PET) • Cervical myelopathy • Fusion imaging • MRI • Spinal cord

29.1 Introduction

It is important to assess spinal cord function in patients amenable to neurosurgical treatment for cervical compressive myelopathy. The majority of the conventional tests focus on evaluation of neural conductivity across the damaged spinal cord [1] or morphological and pathological changes at the compressed cord that can be identified on magnetic resonance imaging (MRI). MRI is a valuable tool before surgical decompression because it visualizes not only the magnitude of spinal cord compression but also the intramedullary signal intensity. Many authors have reported changes in intramedullary high-signal intensity on T2-weighted MR imaging in patients with compressive spondylotic lesions of the cervical spinal cord [2–5]. Such abnormality in intramedullary high-signal intensity is considered to represent myelomalacia or cord gliosis secondary to a long-standing compression of the spinal cord [4]. Therefore, the presence of intramedullary high-signal intensity in patients with compressive myelopathy indicates the existence of a chronic spinal cord compressive lesion. However, the prognostic capacity of these imaging parameters remains controversial, especially with regard to the change in signal intensity of the spinal cord on T2-weighted MRI. The cause of controversy is thought to be the lack of quantitative assessment of these changes in signal intensity.

[^{18}F]-fluorodeoxyglucose (FDG) positron emission tomography (PET) has been used to investigate neural tissue metabolic activity including that of the spinal cord [6]. We used high-resolution ^{18}F-FDG PET to visualize the cervical spinal cord and quantify its metabolic activity [7] and also reported that patients with cervical myelopathy have a variable degree of glucose utilization rate in the whole cervical spinal cord [8] and that impaired glucose metabolic activity in these patients correlated closely with the severity of preoperative neurological dysfunction [9]. Recent studies by another group demonstrated that spinal cord regional changes in ^{18}F-FDG uptake have prognostic significance in cervical myelopathy [10, 11]. Thus, it is possible that the combination of MRI and ^{18}F-FDG PET could uncover new features of cervical compressive myelopathy with respect to prognosis.

The present study was designed to evaluate the utility of three-dimensional (3D)-MRI/^{18}F-FDG PET fusion imaging in the detection of spinal cord lesions and define intramedullary signal changes on MRI and local glucose metabolic rate measured on ^{18}F-FDG PET in relation to clinical outcome and the prognosis.

29.1.1 *MRI/^{18}F-FDG PET Image Fusion and Assessment*

Our study included 24 patients with diagnosis of cervical compressive myelopathy (cervical spondylotic myelopathy: CSM 20 cases; ossification of posterior longitudinal ligament: OPLL 4 cases). Their neurological statuses were evaluated using the

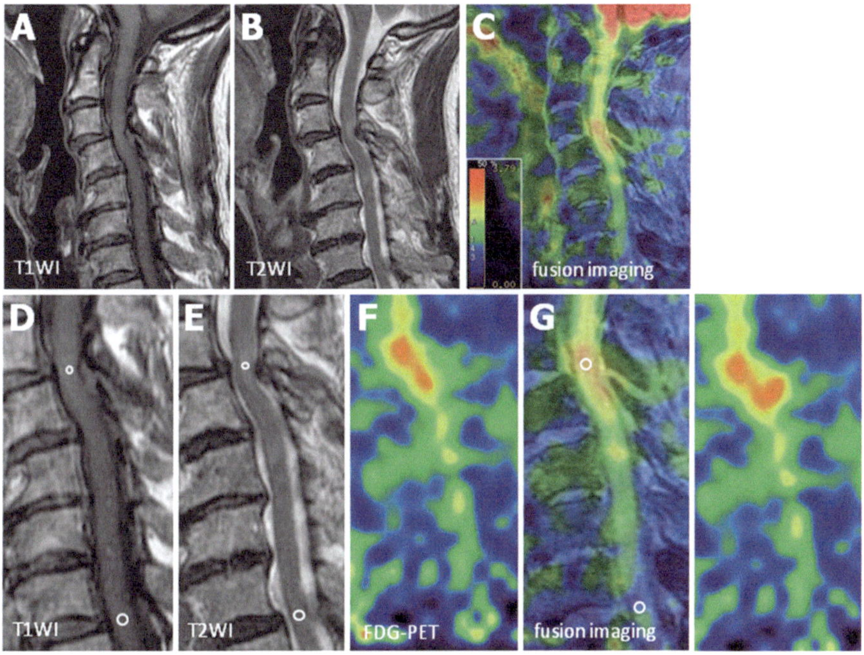

Fig. 29.1 An 80-year-old woman with cervical spondylotic myelopathy was treated surgically and showed a neurological improvement rate of 75.0 % at follow-up. (**a**) Midsagittal T1-weighted MRI, (**b**) midsagittal T2-weighted MRI, (**c**) MRI/PET fusion imaging (**d**, **e**), (**f**) ^{18}F-FDG PET sagittal image, and (**g**) MRI/PET fusion sagittal slice demonstrate a focal increase in ^{18}F-FDG uptake at the level of increased signal intensity lesion (Reprinted, with permission, from [29])

Japanese Orthopaedic Association (JOA) scoring system and the involved levels of compression were assessed using 3T MRI and ^{18}FDG-PET fusion imaging. Signal intensity change in the cord was qualitatively assessed on both T1- and T2-weighted images. In quantitative analysis of the signal change, the signal intensity ratio (SIR) on both T1-WIs and T2-WIs was calculated by the following equation:

$$SIR = \left[\frac{mid\text{–}sagittal\ cervical\ spinal\ cord\ on\ signal\ intensity\ at\ lesions\left(0.05\,cm^2\right)}{mid\text{–}sagittal\ normal\ cord\ signal\ intensity\ on\ the\ cervical\ disc\ levels\ between\ \mathrm{C7}\ and\ \mathrm{T1}\left(0.3\,cm^2\right)} \right]$$

Using the Advantage Workstation (GE Healthcare), the same slices of cervical 3D-MRI using 3.0 Tesla (T) Signa system and ^{18}F-FDG PET images were fused automatically. On fusion images, the maximal count at the lesion was adopted as the standardized uptake value (SUV_{max}). The SUV ratio, similar to SIR, (SUVR) was also calculated.

Examples are shown in Figs. 29.1 and 29.2. Figure 29.1 shows a significant increase in ^{18}F-FDG uptake (SUV_{max} =2.50, SUVR = 1.84) at the level of the lesion

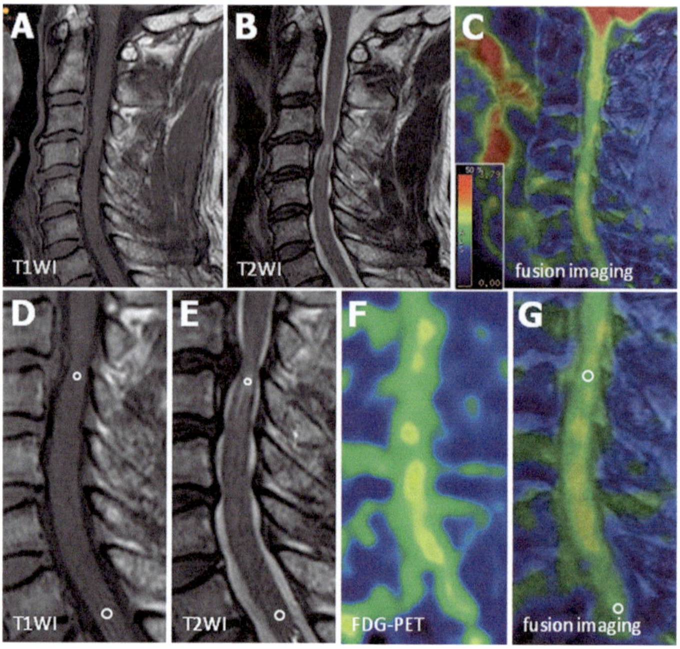

Fig. 29.2 A 62-year-old man with cervical spondylotic myelopathy was treated surgically and showed a poor neurological improvement rate of 28.6 % at follow-up. (**a**) Midsagittal T1-weighted MRI, (**b**) midsagittal T2-weighted MRI, (**c**) MRI/PET fusion imaging (**d**, **e**), (**f**) ^{18}F-FDG PET sagittal image, and (**g**) MRI/PET fusion sagittal slice demonstrate inconspicuous ^{18}F-FDG uptake at the level of lesion with increased signal intensity (Reprinted, with permission, from [29])

(SIR on T1-WI = 1.29, SIR on T2-WI = 1.55). The neurological improvement rate was considered good (75.0 %) at follow-up. On the other hand, Fig. 29.2 demonstrates the no increase in ^{18}F-FDG uptake (SUV_{max} = 1.60, SUVR = 0.87) at the level of the lesion (SIR on T1-WI = 0.99, SIR on T2-WI = 1.48). The neurological improvement rate at follow-up was poor (28.6 %).

29.1.2 *Relationship Between Signal Intensity Ratio on MRI and Clinical Outcome*

The SIR on T1-WIs correlated significantly with preoperative JOA score ($R = 0.430$; $p < 0.05$) and postoperative neurological improvement ($R = 0.617$; $p < 0.01$). However, there were no correlation between high change in intramedullary signal intensity on T2-WIs and preoperative JOA score ($R = 0.174$) or postoperative neurological improvement ($R = 0.256$).

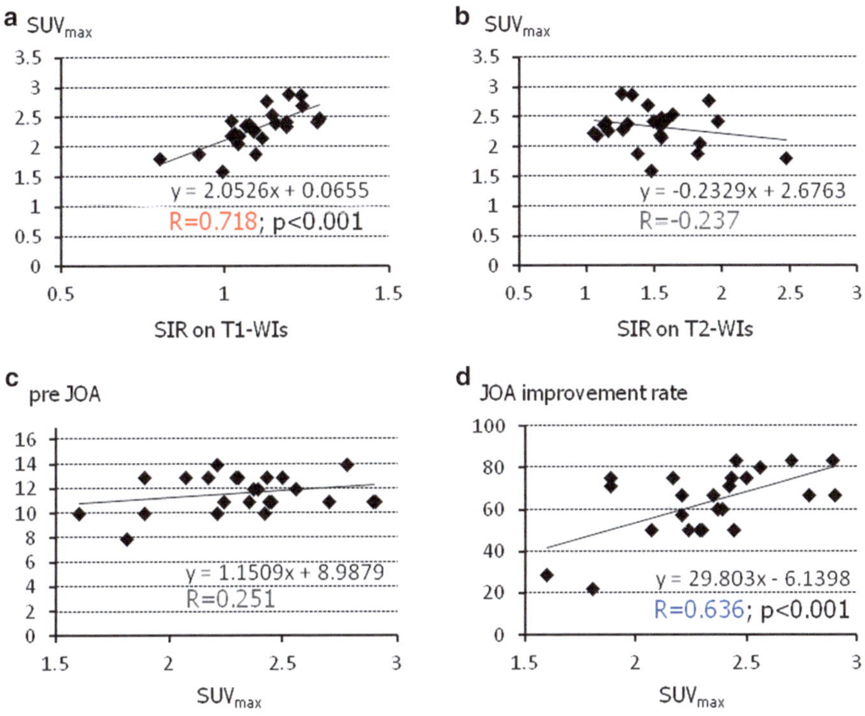

Fig. 29.3 Relationship between SUV measured at the lesion with increased signal intensity on MRI/PET fusion image and signal intensity ratio (SIR) and neurological scores. SUV_{max} at the sagittal lesion with increased cord intensity correlated strongly with the SIR on T1-WIs (**a**) but not on T2-WIs (**b**). SUV_{max} did not correlate with preoperative JOA score (**c**), but correlated with postoperative neurological improvement (**d**) (Reprinted, with permission, from [29])

29.1.3 Clinical Significance of SUV_{max} for Lesions with Increased Signal Intensity

Figure 29.3 shows the relationship between SUV_{max} for lesions with increased signal intensity on the sagittal plane and SIR on T1-WIs and T2-WIs as well as neurological scores. SUV_{max} for such lesions correlated significantly with SIR on T1-WIs ($R=0.718$; $p<0.001$, Fig. 29.3a) but not on T2-WIs ($R=0.237$, Fig. 29.3b). Furthermore, SUV_{max} correlated with postoperative neurological improvement ($R=0.636$; $p<0.001$, Fig. 29.3d) but not with preoperative JOA score ($R=0.251$, Fig. 29.3c).

29.1.4 Clinical Significance of the SUV Ratio

Figure 29.4 shows the relationship between SUVR and SIR on T1-WIs and T2-WIs as well as neurological score. SUVR correlated significantly with SIR on T1-WIs ($R=0.704$; $p<0.001$, Fig. 29.4a) but not on T2-WIs ($R=0.210$, Fig. 29.4b).

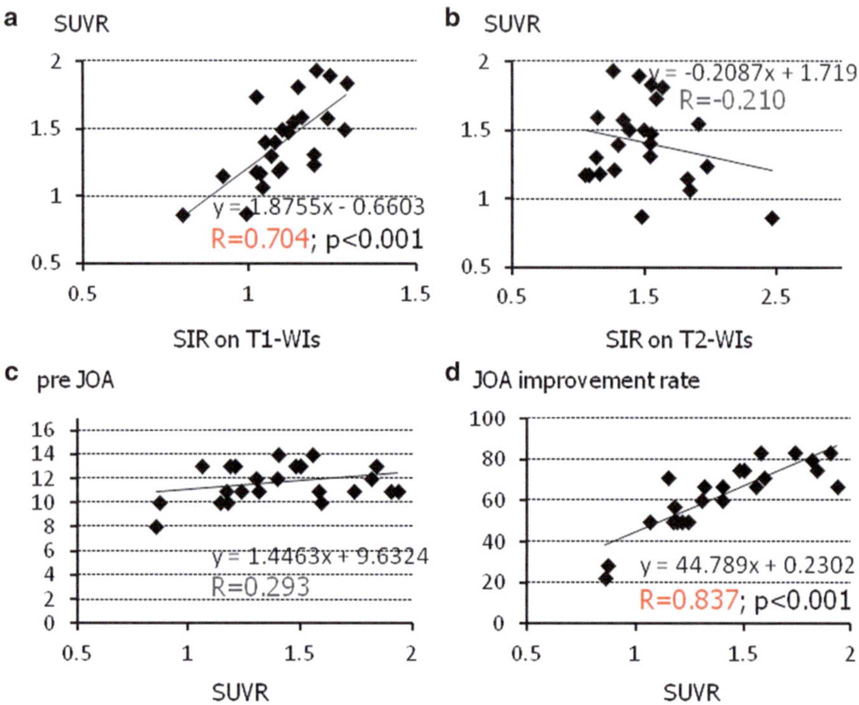

Fig. 29.4 Relationship between SUV ratio (SUVR) on MRI/PET fusion image and signal intensity ratio (SIR) and neurological scores. SUVR correlated strongly with SIR on T1-WIs (**a**) but not on T2-WIs (**b**). SUVR did not correlate with preoperative JOA score (**c**), but correlated with post-operative neurological improvement (**d**) (Reprinted, with permission, from [29])

Furthermore, SUV_{max} correlated significantly with postoperative neurological improvement, and the correlation coefficient was much higher than that of SUV_{max} for lesions with increased signal intensity on the sagittal plane ($R=0.837$; $p<0.001$, Fig. 29.4d), but not with preoperative JOA score ($R=0.293$, Fig. 29.4c).

29.2 Discussion

Elucidation of the factors that contribute to prognosis of patients with CSM and OPLL has been investigated by several groups [5, 12–15]. It is important to know those factors that determine neurological improvement after surgery. Age at surgery [16], duration of neurological symptoms [5, 13, 14, 16–18], and existence of signal changes on preoperative MRI [2–4, 19, 20] have been considered key predictors of surgical outcome. These factors could also have a significant impact on the surgical outcome of the patients in the present study as well, although we focused herein on the signal intensity changes on MRI and local glucose metabolism at the affected mono-segmental spinal cord lesion on PET using high-resolution MRI/PET fusion imaging.

While the MRI provides the highest specificity in the assessment of morphological changes and intramedullary state of the spinal cord, it is almost impossible to estimate the potential recovery of the spinal cord on preoperative MRI without quantitative analysis. Furthermore, the signal intensity on the MRI is irregular in each scan because different sequence parameters are set for each individual patient. On the other hand, ^{18}F-FDG PEt allows visualization of the metabolic activity of the spinal cord neural tissue in the same condition in each scan, and this parameter correlates closely with neurological prognosis. We quantified previously glucose utilization in the cervical spinal cord of patients with myelopathy [8]. Furthermore, Kamoto et al. [7] reported that the normal metabolic rate of glucose utilization in the cervical spinal cord (SUV) in healthy Japanese subjects (age, 40–70 years) was 1.93 ± 0.23, although this value was found to be 2.12 ± 0.48 and 1.84 ± 0.23 by Nakamoto et al. [21] and Floeth et al. [11], respectively. In another study, we reported that patients with mild to moderate myelopathy have significantly high SUV of the entire cervical spinal cord, while those with marked and profound tetraparesis had significantly low SUV [9]. Thus, a high SUV seems to reflect hyperactive neuronal activity within the spinal cord. In our latest study, patients with poor neurological improvement rate were found to have low preoperative SUV and significantly low postoperative neurological improvement [22]. Unfortunately, our results showed that preoperative SUV was not significantly different among patients with increased signal intensity on MRI.

The combination of the same slice 2 highest-end modalities (3D-MRI using 3T MRI and ^{18}F-FDG PET) in near real-time simultaneous scan has enabled us to image the metabolic function with detectable accuracy at the cervical spinal cord level. Our results showed that ^{18}F-FDG PET is more suitable and sensitive for the detection of changes in low-signal intensity on T1-weighted images on MRI/PET fusion imaging. Our results also suggested that SUV_{max} for lesions with increased signal intensity correlates with the SIR on T1-WIs and postoperative neurological outcome, but not with SIR on T2-WIs. Additionally, the SUVR is more sensitive to predict neurological improvement than SIR on T1-WIs or SUV_{max} in signal intensity lesions. Floeth et al. [10] demonstrated a significant decrease in ^{18}F-FDG uptake in the area of the lower cervical cord in patients with myelopathy than the control group. This could be the reason that made SUVR a more sensitive factor than SUV_{max} at the signal intensity lesion.

The present quantitative study based on MRI/PET fusion also showed no correlation with SIR on T2-WIs, while SIR on T1-WIs correlated with preoperative JOA score and postoperative neurological improvement. Theoretically, progressive changes should be observed as a high-signal intensity in the intramedullary lesion in patients with cervical compressive myelopathy. High-signal intensity is observed on T2-weighted MRI in patients with early-stage myelomalacia. Some patients at an intermediate stage display a variable degree of cystic necrosis of the central gray matter, which is better visualized on T2-weighted MRI. Finally, central cystic degeneration, syrinx formation, and atrophy are the main features of late-stage myelomalacia [23, 24]. On the other hand, the significance of decreased signal intensity on T1-weighted MRI has also been studied. Several groups have confirmed that a low-signal intensity on preoperative T1-weighted MRI is a predictor of poor prognosis [20, 25]. Based on the results reported in the literature, changes in high-signal intensity on T2-weighted images at early stages of compressive myelopathy are indicative of edema and gliosis (which may be reversible), whereas changes in low-intensity signal on T1-weighted images could reflect myelomalacia and necrosis (which are considered irreversible). Decompression of the spinal cord by surgery can restore blood circulation in the spinal cord, reduce swelling, and enhance regeneration of nerve fibers, thus reducing or normalizing the high-signal intensity in the intramedullary region. In the late stage, necrosis and syrinx become irreversible, making surgery ineffective.

Spinal cord autopsy findings of patients with cervical myelopathy include demyelination, white matter axonal loss, and gray matter neuronal loss [26, 27]. In contrast, other studies [28] have shown the presence of neurogenic progenitor cells within the spinal cord and that these cells can differentiate into neurons and glial cells. The observed changes in glucose metabolism on ^{18}F-FDG PET in cervical myelopathy could reflect neuronal plasticity in the compressed spinal cord; neural activity, deterioration of synaptic function, loss of neurons and neural tissue, changes in blood flow, and the magnitude of mechanical compression. We believe that glucose metabolism (SUV) measured by MRI/PET fusion is suitable for visualization of neural tissue metabolic activity and that ^{18}F-FDG PET is a more sensitive tool for assessment of the clinical outcome and prognosis of patients with cervical compressive myelopathy [29].

29.3 Conclusion

This is the first study of measurement of regional glucose metabolism in the affected spinal cord of patients with cervical compressive myelopathy using MRI/PET fusion imaging. 3D-MRI/^{18}F-FDG PET fusion imaging is useful for mapping the exact level of cervical spinal cord lesion on ^{18}F-FDG PET. Assessment of neurological function by ^{18}F-FDG PET may be equal or better than that by signal intensity on T1-WIs. Preoperative glucose utilization rate on ^{18}F-FDG PET seems suitable for prediction of postoperative neurological outcome.

Acknowledgment This work was supported in part by grants from the Japanese Governmental Investigation Committee on Ossification of the Spinal Ligaments (2000–2012).

Conflict of Interest All authors declare that they have no conflict of interest.

Informed Consent All procedures followed were in accordance with the ethical standards of the responsible committee on human experimentation (institutional and national) and with the Helsinki Declaration of 1975, as revised in 2000 (5). Informed consent was obtained from all patients for being included in the study.

References

1. Baba H, Maezawa Y, Imura S et al (1996) Spinal cord evoked potential monitoring for cervical and thoracic compressive myelopathy. Paraplegia 34:100–106
2. Mehalic TF, Pezzuti RT, Applebaum BI (1990) Magnetic resonance imaging and cervical spondylotic myelopathy. Neurosurgery 26:217–227
3. Takahashi M, Sakamoto Y, Miyawaki M et al (1987) Increased MR signal intensity secondary to chronic cervical cord compression. Neuroradiology 29:550–556
4. Takahashi M, Yamashita Y, Sakamoto Y et al (1989) Chronic cervical cord compression: clinical significance of increased signal intensity on MR images. Radiology 173:219–224
5. Wada E, Yonenobu K, Suzuki S et al (1999) Can intramedullary signal change on magnetic resonance imaging predict surgical outcome in cervical spondylotic myelopathy? Spine 24: 455–462
6. Di Chiro G, Oldfield E, Bairamian D et al (1983) Metabolic imaging of the brain stem and spinal cord: studies with positron emission tomography using 18F-2-deoxyglucose in normal and pathological cases. J Comput Assist Tomogr 7:937–945
7. Kamoto Y, Sadato N, Yonekura Y et al (1998) Visualization of the cervical spinal cord with FDG and high-resolution PET. J Comput Assist Tomogr 22:487–491
8. Baba H, Uchida K, Sadato N et al (1999) Potential usefulness of 18F-2-fluoro-deoxy-D-glucose positron emission tomography in cervical compressive myelopathy. Spine 24: 1449–1454
9. Uchida K, Kobayashi S, Yayama T et al (2004) Metabolic neuroimaging of the cervical spinal cord in patients with compressive myelopathy: a high-resolution positron emission tomography study. J Neurosurg Spine 1:72–79
10. Floeth FW, Stoffels G, Herdmann J et al (2011) Prognostic value of 18F-FDG PET in monosegmental stenosis and myelopathy of the cervical spinal cord. J Nucl Med 52:1385–1391
11. Floeth FW, Stoffels G, Herdmann J et al (2010) Regional impairment of 18F-FDG uptake in the cervical spinal cord in patients with monosegmental chronic cervical myelopathy. Eur Radiol 20:2925–2932
12. Uchida K, Nakajima H, Sato R et al (2005) Multivariate analysis of the neurological outcome of surgery for cervical compressive myelopathy. J Orthop Sci 10:564–573
13. Fujiwara K, Yonenobu K, Ebara S et al (1989) The prognosis of surgery for cervical compression myelopathy. An analysis of the factors involved. J Bone Joint Surg Br 71:393–398
14. Koyanagi T, Hirabayashi K, Satomi K et al (1993) Predictability of operative results of cervical compression myelopathy based on preoperative computed tomographic myelography. Spine 18:1958–1963
15. Singh A, Crockard HA, Platts A et al (2001) Clinical and radiological correlates of severity and surgery-related outcome in cervical spondylosis. J Neurosurg 94(2 Suppl):189–198
16. Okada Y, Ikata T, Yamada H et al (1993) Magnetic resonance imaging study on the results of surgery for cervical compression myelopathy. Spine 18:2024–2029
17. Ebersold MJ, Pare MC, Quast LM (1995) Surgical treatment for cervical spondylitic myelopathy. J Neurosurg 82:745–751
18. Matsuyama Y, Kawakami N, Mimatsu K (1995) Spinal cord expansion after decompression in cervical myelopathy. Investigation by computed tomography myelography and ultrasonography. Spine 20:1657–1663
19. Matsuda Y, Miyazaki K, Tada K et al (1991) Increased MR signal intensity due to cervical myelopathy. Analysis of 29 surgical cases. J Neurosurg 74:887–892
20. Morio Y, Teshima R, Nagashima H et al (2001) Correlation between operative outcomes of cervical compression myelopathy and mri of the spinal cord. Spine 26:1238–1245
21. Nakamoto Y, Tatsumi M, Hammoud D et al (2005) Normal FDG distribution patterns in the head and neck: PET/CT evaluation. Radiology 234:879–885

22. Uchida K, Nakajima H, Yayama T et al (2009) High-resolution magnetic resonance imaging and 18FDG-PET findings of the cervical spinal cord before and after decompressive surgery in patients with compressive myelopathy. Spine 34:1185–1191
23. Ohshio I, Hatayama A, Kaneda K et al (1993) Correlation between histopathologic features and magnetic resonance images of spinal cord lesions. Spine 18:1140–1149
24. Ito T, Oyanagi K, Takahashi H et al (1996) Cervical spondylotic myelopathy. Clinicopathologic study on the progression pattern and thin myelinated fibers of the lesions of seven patients examined during complete autopsy. Spine 21:827–833
25. Suri A, Chabbra RP, Mehta VS et al (2003) Effect of intramedullary signal changes on the surgical outcome of patients with cervical spondylotic myelopathy. Spine J 3:33–45
26. Kameyama T, Hashizume Y, Ando T et al (1995) Spinal cord morphology and pathology in ossification of the posterior longitudinal ligament. Brain 118(Pt 1):263–278
27. Mizuno J, Nakagawa H, Chang HS et al (2005) Postmortem study of the spinal cord showing snake-eyes appearance due to damage by ossification of the posterior longitudinal ligament and kyphotic deformity. Spinal Cord 43:503–507
28. Yamamoto S, Yamamoto N, Kitamura T et al (2001) Proliferation of parenchymal neural progenitors in response to injury in the adult rat spinal cord. Exp Neurol 172:115–127
29. Uchida K, Nakajima H, Okazawa H et al (2012) Clinical significance of MRI/^{18}F-FDG PET fusion imaging of the spinal cord in patients with cervical compressive myelopathy. Eur J Nucl Med Mol Imaging 39:1528–1537

Chapter 30
Visualization of Electrophysiological Activity in the Spinal Cord Using Magnetospinography

Shigenori Kawabata

Abstract Magnetospinography is a promising noninvasive imaging technique that can estimate the magnitude and spatiotemporal spread of currents derived from activities of the spinal cord or nerves by measuring magnetic fields (spinal cord evoked magnetic fields, SCEMFs) over the skin surface. Visualization of electrophysiological activity in different spinal tracts and segments holds great potential for preclinical studies in animals with experimental lesions or mutations affecting spinal cord development and function. Moreover, improvements in magnetic sensors and analytic techniques now allow for SCEMF measurements from humans and may soon be used for clinical diagnosis. In the near future, magnetospinography is expected to contribute greatly to clinical practice for the diagnosis and treatment of spinal cord disorders.

Keywords Electrophysiology • Magnetoneurography • Magnetospinography • Spinal cord function

30.1 Introduction

Minimally invasive methods to evaluate spinal cord function are required for the elucidation of pathogenic mechanisms and the development of novel treatments for spinal cord disorders. Among the several electrophysiological methods available for examining spinal cord electrical activity, measurement of spinal cord evoked potentials affords high spatial and temporal resolution [1, 2]. Because electrical currents generated by the spinal cord are altered by the surrounding tissue such as bone and

S. Kawabata (✉)
Department of Orthopaedic Surgery, Tokyo Medical and Dental University,
1-5-45 Yushima, Bunkyo-ku, Tokyo 113-8510, Japan
e-mail: kawabata.orth@tmd.ac.jp

K. Uchida et al. (eds.), *Neuroprotection and Regeneration of the Spinal Cord*,
DOI 10.1007/978-4-431-54502-6_30,

soft tissue, surface measurements are impeded and precise evaluation of spinal cord activity requires the insertion of electrodes into the vertebral column near the spinal cord. Accordingly, current techniques for measuring spinal cord evoked potentials are not amenable to repeated examinations and have not been widely used for clinical diagnosis or study.

Magnetic fields, on the other hand, which are generated by neuronal currents (according to Ampère's circuital law), are less affected by the surrounding tissues. This gives neuromagnetic recordings a theoretical advantage for high spatial resolution [3]. Indeed, magnetoencephalography has already been applied in clinical medicine and basic research. However, the magnetic fields produced by spinal cord activity are smaller and propagate faster than magnetic fields generated by the cerebral cortex, so applications for cortical physiology and pathology are more advanced. However, magnetospinography is gradually approaching clinical feasibility with the development of biomagnetometers specialized for the spinal cord.

30.2 Animal Studies

Magnetic fields produced by the spinal cord are only about one-hundred-millionth the size of geomagnetism, so magnetically shielded rooms are needed to prevent interference from both geomagnetism and magnetic noise from the environment. Highly sensitive superconducting quantum interference device (SQUID) sensors are required to detect the biomagnetic fields from the spinal cord.

Earlier animal studies required laminectomy to place the sensors close enough to the epidural surface for a sufficient signal-to-noise ratio. Due to progress in multichannel sensor systems and signal processing techniques, however, magnetic fields have recently been detected at the skin surface as discussed below.

30.2.1 Visualization of Spinal Tract Activities

Kawabata and colleagues successfully recorded ascending spinal cord evoked magnetic fields (SCEMFs) in laminectomized animals following thoracic stimulation using a single channel SQUID biomagnetometer [4]. Briefly, cervical laminectomy was performed under intravenous anesthesia with muscle relaxants and the dura exposed. Electrical stimuli were applied to the lower thoracic spinal cord by a catheter epidural electrode. SCEMFs were measured at 35 different points (7 rows × 5 lines, points 10 mm apart) over the cervical spine. The measured magnetic fields exhibited a clear quadrupolar pattern that propagated at 80–120 m/s, consistent with action potential transmission in spinal cord axons. After spinal cord transection, propagation of SCEMFs stopped at the transection site.

Magnetospinography was also used to visualize descending electrical activity in the corticospinal tract in response to stimulation of the motor cortex by measuring

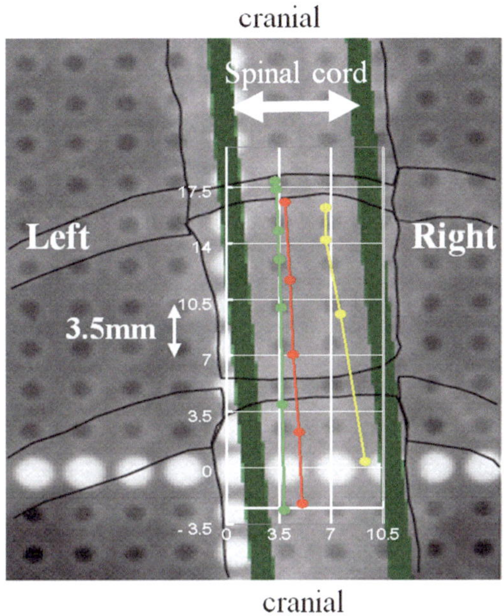

Fig. 30.1 Sequential positions of estimated current dipoles superimposed on an anterior–posterior X-ray image and a schematic representation (*black lines*) of the spine at the thoracic level. *Thick green lines* were drawn on pedicles of spines to indicate the lateral boundaries. *Left green line* traces the sequential movement of the estimated dipoles after stimulation of the right motor cortex. *Right yellow line* traces the sequential movement of the estimated dipoles after stimulation of the left motor cortex. *Middle red line* traces the ascending current dipoles after stimulation of the left sciatic nerve

SCEMFs over the thoracic dural tube [5]. Furthermore, ascending neural activity likely originating in the posterior funiculus was detected between the right and left corticospinal tracts in response to stimulation of the sciatic nerve (Fig. 30.1).

30.2.2 Visualization of Spinal Segment Activity

Tomizawa and colleagues recorded segmental SCEMFs from the dura of the rabbit lumbar spinal cord in response to sciatic nerve stimulation [6]. The distribution of SCEMFs exhibited a quadrupolar pattern propagating from caudal to rostral with short latency. After the conductive magnetic fields passed, stationary dipolar fields appeared and were sustained at several vertebral levels. Thus, in addition to action potential propagation through the fiber tracts, SCEMFs can reveal somal and synaptic activity at multiple spinal cord levels.

30.2.3 Electrophysiological Diagnosis of Conduction Blocks After Spinal Cord Stimulation

In a significant technical leap, Tomori and colleagues visualized spinal cord electrophysiological activity using magnetospinography from the skin surface [7]. They established an incomplete conduction block model using a Fogarty balloon catheter inserted into the epidural space of the cervical spine. Electrical stimuli were applied to the lower thoracic spinal cord with an epidural catheter electrode and SCEMFs were recorded over the skin surface of the neck.

Decreases in conduction velocity and amplitude at the compression site were first detected by spinal cord evoked potentials from the epidural space, confirming the spinal cord lesion. The distribution of magnetic fields showed a characteristic quadrupolar pattern propagating from caudal to rostral. After compression, the amplitude and the conduction velocity of the magnetic fields decreased near the lesion, especially the trailing magnetic fields. These results demonstrate that non-invasive diagnosis of an incomplete conduction block is possible in experimental animals.

Also in their study, reconstructed electrical current sources were estimated by a novel spatial filter technique. While conventional dipole estimation methods express the electrical currents from nerve activity by one or two representative current dipoles, this special filter technique is able to estimate and visualize electrical activity over the whole measurement area. Using this analytic method, estimated currents were successfully imaged over the cervical spine in response to stimulation of the lower thoracic spine. Moreover, thorough investigation of changes in estimated currents around the lesions showed that current components perpendicular to the long axis of the spinal cord, which correspond to depolarization, and the rostral peak of the trailing component parallel to the long axis stopped and decreased in amplitude at the incomplete block lesion (Fig. 30.2).

30.2.4 Electrophysiological Diagnosis of Conduction Block by Peripheral Nerve Stimulation

Sakaki and colleagues measured SCEMFs from the lumbar spinal cord of the incomplete conduction block model in response to sciatic nerve stimulation in rabbits [8]. Again, SCEMFs were attenuated at the lesion. Thus, lesion sites may be localized by peripheral nerve stimulation.

30.3 Visualization of Spinal Cord Electrophysiological Activity in Humans

All procedures followed were in accordance with the ethical standards of the responsible committee on human experimentation and with the Helsinki Declaration of 1975, as revised in 2000 (5). Informed consent was obtained from all patients for being included in the study.

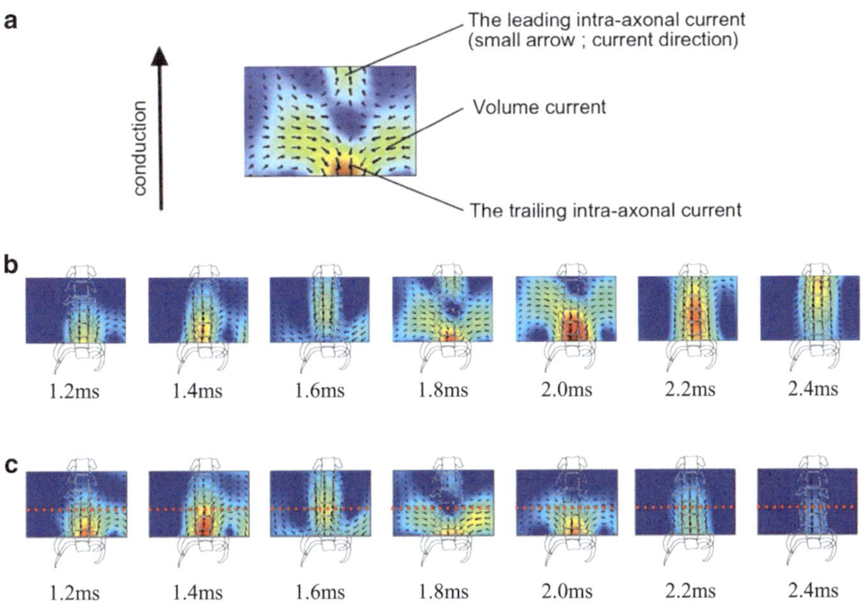

Fig. 30.2 (**a**) Distribution of estimated current sources reconstructed using the spatial filter technique. *Small arrows* indicate the current direction, and colors represent the current intensity (*red* > *blue*). Intra-axonal currents and volume currents are mapped within the measurement area. (**b**) Distribution of estimated current sources superimposed on a schematic representation of the spine (*gray lines*) before compression. Electrophysiological activity in the spinal tract, including intra-axonal currents with upward and downward directions and volume currents perpendicular to the spinal cord, propagates from caudal to rostral. (**c**) Reconstructed currents after compression. The intensity of the leading and trailing intra-axonal currents gradually decreases (2.0 ms) around the compression site (*red dots*). The decrease in the trailing intra-axonal and volume currents (which correspond to depolarization) is larger than the decrease in the leading intra-axonal current

30.3.1 Systems for Magnetospinography

Human SCEMFs must also be measured in a magnetically shielded room. My colleagues and I have developed and evaluated several types of biomagnetometers optimized for human SCEMF recording, including those for measurement in the prone position or sitting position, and have continued to improve them. Our newest SQUID biomagnetometer is a supine position type and its measuring surface is curved to conform to cervical lordosis [9, 10]. A sensor array composed of 40 vector gradiometers positioned in an 8×5 matrix covers a 90 mm × 140 mm measurement area. In situ X-ray images of the cervical spine are used to reveal the position of the subject's spine relative to the SQUID sensors (Fig. 30.3).

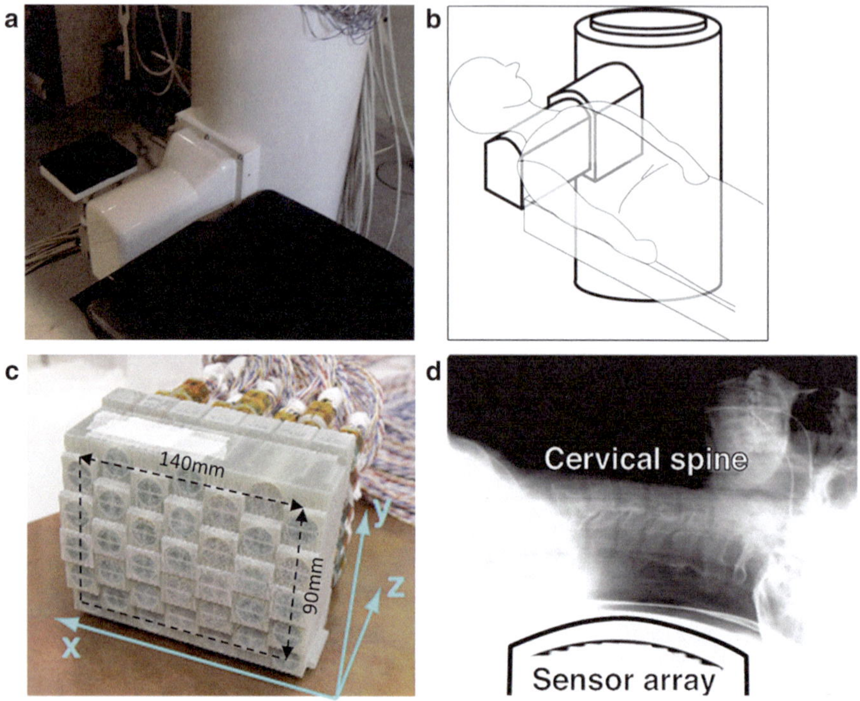

Fig. 30.3 (**a**) The SQUID biomagnetometer for magnetospinography, (**b**) schematic representation of a biomagnetometer and a subject in the supine position, (**c**) sensor array, and (**d**) In situ lateral X-ray image showing the sensor position relative to the cervical spine

30.3.2 Spinal Cord Evoked Magnetic Fields in Healthy Subjects

Cervical SCEMFs from healthy subjects can be obtained from the skin surface in response to stimulation of the thoracic spinal cord or peripheral nerves in the upper extremities [10, 11] (Fig. 30.4).

30.3.3 Neuromagnetic Fields in the Lumbar Spinal Canal

Ishii and colleagues successfully measured neuromagnetic fields from the skin over the lumbar spine in response to stimulation of the tibial nerve at the ankles and visualized propagation of neuromagnetic fields from the intervertebral foramina into the spinal canal [12].

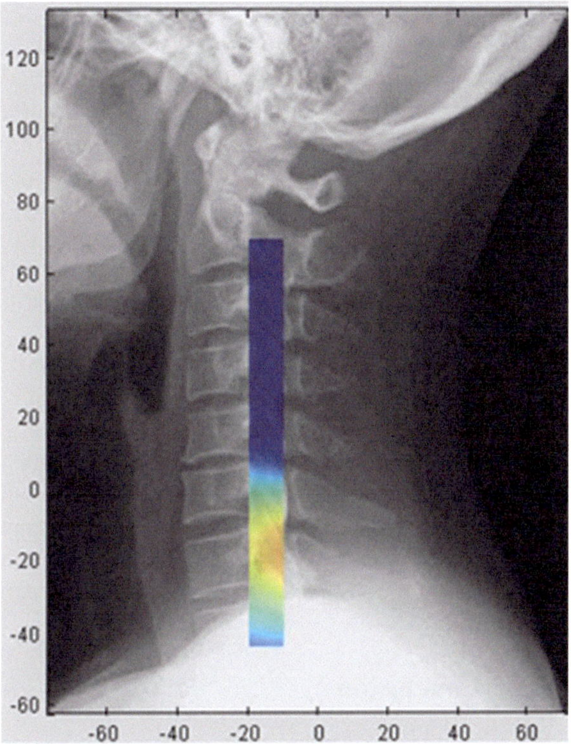

Fig. 30.4 Estimated ascending currents superimposed on an X-ray image 6.3 ms after thoracic spinal cord stimulation

30.3.4 Clinical Application

Using our current measurement system, we are able to detect cervical SCEMFs from the majority of patients with cervical myelopathy (data not shown). Future studies will investigate methods for the diagnosis of spinal cord lesions using the obtained SCEMFs.

30.4 Discussion

The studies presented here confirm that magnetospinography is a promising electrophysiological tool for exploring spinal physiology because it allows for noninvasive mapping of estimated electrical currents from spinal cord activities with high spatial and temporal resolution, even when measured from the skin surface. Continued improvements could lead to routine use in clinical medicine for pathogenic studies, diagnosis, and treatment monitoring.

There are, however, several technical challenges that limit the fidelity of current estimates by biomagnetometry. One is that electrical currents perpendicular to the skin surface produce very small magnetic fields. For example, measurements over the dorsal neck are not able to estimate electrical currents in the anteroposterior direction. When electrical currents oblique to the measuring surface are measured, only vector components parallel to the measuring surface are estimated. If we could measure from the lateral plane, SCEMFs derived from electrical currents in the anteroposterior direction could be detected in theory. However, this limitation can be used to advantage for separating electrical currents according to direction.

Another limitation is specificity. The electrical currents giving rise to the magnetic fields measured by magnetospinography may be flowing in the spinal canal or around the spine from extraspinal sources. Users of this technology should always be cognizant of this fact.

Current magnetospinography techniques use the SQUID sensor, which consumes expensive liquid helium for refrigeration and also requires a magnetically shielded room, so the costs of this methodology may be prohibitive. At present, alterative lower-cost sensors with sensitivities sufficient for magnetospinography are being developed and should greatly expand the application of this technology. These developments in magnetospinography systems may lead to broad clinical application, contribute to the elucidation of spinal disease pathogenesis, and facilitate the development of treatments for spinal cord disorders.

30.5 Conclusion

Measurement of SCEMFs using magnetospinography allows for the noninvasive estimation of electrical currents from neural activities with high spatial and temporal resolution. Magnetospinography is a feasible and promising electrophysiological mapping technique both for research and clinical diagnosis and treatment of spinal disorders.

Acknowledgements This work was supported in part by a Grant-in-Aid for Scientific Research from the Japan Society for the Promotion of Science and Secom Science and Technology Foundation.

Conflict of Interest None of the authors have any commercial association that might pose or create a conflict of interest with information presented in this article.

References

1. Shinomiya K, Furuya K, Sato R, Okamoto A, Kurosa Y, Fuchioka M (1988) Electrophysiologic diagnosis of cervical OPLL myelopathy using evoked spinal cord potentials. Spine 13(11): 1225–1233
2. Shinomiya K, Okamoto A, Komori H, Matsuoka T, Yoshida H, Muto N, Furuya K (1990) Prognosticating study for cervical myelopathy using evoked spinal cord potentials. Spine 15(10):1053–1057
3. Okada YC, Lahteenmaki A, Xu C (1999) Experimental analysis of distortion of magnetoencephalography signals by the skull. Clin Neurophysiol 110(2):230–238

4. Kawabata S, Komori H, Mochida K, Harunobu O, Shinomiya K (2002) Visualization of conductive spinal cord activity using a biomagnetometer. Spine 27(5):475–479
5. Ohkubo H, Komori H, Kawabata S, Fukuoka Y, Shinomiya K (2003) Estimation of localization of neural activity in the spinal cord using a biomagnetometer. J Med Dent Sci 50(2):177–182
6. Tomizawa S, Kawabata S, Komori H, Hoshino Fukuoka Y, Shinomiya K (2008) Evaluation of segmental spinal cord evoked magnetic fields after sciatic nerve stimulation. Clin Neurophysiol 119(5):1111–1118
7. Tomori M, Kawabata S, Tomizawa S, Ishii S, Enomoto M, Adachi Y, Sato T, Shinomiya K, Okawa A (2010) Diagnosis of incomplete conduction block of spinal cord from skin surface using spinal cord evoked magnetic fields. J Orthop Sci 15(3):371–380
8. Sakaki K, Kawabata S, Tomori M, Ishii S, Tomizawa S, Okawa A, Shinomiya K (2011) Diagnosis of incomplete spinal cord injury using spinal cord evoked magnetic fields after peripheral nerve stimulation. J Spine Res 2(2):206–211
9. Adachi Y, Miyamoto M, Kawai J, Uehara G, Ogata H, Kawabata S, Sekihara K, Kado H (2011) Improvement of SQUID magnetometer system for extending application of spinal cord evoked magnetic field measurement. IEEE Trans Appl Superconductivity 21(3):485–488
10. Adachi Y, Kawai J, Miyamoto M, Ogata H, Tomori M, Kawabata S, Sato T, Uehara G (2009) A SQUID system for measurement of spinal cord evoked field of supine subjects. IEEE Trans Appl Superconductivity 19(3):861–866
11. Sato T, Adachi Y, Tomori M, Ishii S, Kawabata S, Sekihara K (2009) Functional imaging of spinal cord electrical activity from its evoked magnetic field. IEEE Trans Biomed Eng 56(10):2452–2460
12. Ishii S, Kawabata S, Tomizawa S, Tomori M, Sakaki K, Shinomiya K, Sekihara K, Sato T, Adachi Y, Okawa A (2012) Conductive neuromagnetic fields in the lumbar spinal canal. Clin Neurophysiol 123(8):1656–1661

Chapter 31
Spinal Synaptic Plasticity in Chronic Pain

Wataru Taniguchi and Terumasa Nakatsuka

Abstract Spinal synaptic plasticity induces pathological chronic pain such as neuropathic pain. However, little is known about the mechanism of spinal synaptic plasticity in chronic pain. Although there are many causes for and various forms of spinal synaptic plasticity, several mechanisms have been revealed in recent years. Spinal synaptic plasticity consists of (1) a change in excitatory synaptic transmission efficiency (e.g., LTP, windup), (2) a change of synaptic network in the dorsal horn (e.g., Aβ-fiber sprouting into lamina II), (3) neurotrophic factors, (4) activation of ion channels (e.g., P2X receptors, TRPV1, TRPA1), and (5) activation of microglia in the spinal cord. In this chapter we review these mechanisms of spinal synaptic plasticity, which induce chronic pain. As we have investigated the activation of P2X receptors, TRPV1, and TRPA1 in the dorsal horn using whole-cell patch-clamp methods, we have discussed these studies in detail.

Keywords Chronic pain • Microglia • Neuropathic pain • Spinal cord • Synaptic plasticity

31.1 Introduction

Nociceptive pain is an important defensive mechanism that warns an individual of imminent damage to the body. However, it only becomes harmful when the alarm is allowed to persist. This pathological pain is a clinical condition termed chronic pain and may be insidious to the life of the individual who is suffering from it. It deviates

W. Taniguchi (✉) • T. Nakatsuka
Pain Research Center, Kansai University of Health Sciences,
2-11-1 Wakaba, Kumatori, Osaka 590-0482, Japan
e-mail: wtaniguchi@kansai.ac.jp

K. Uchida et al. (eds.), *Neuroprotection and Regeneration of the Spinal Cord*,
DOI 10.1007/978-4-431-54502-6_31, © Springer Japan 2014

from the role of biophylaxis, and pain itself becomes a target to treat. Although chronic pain is induced by various factors, synaptic plasticity in the spinal cord is recognized as a main cause [1, 2]. Recent studies have shed some light on the mechanisms involved in spinal synaptic plasticity. In this chapter, we introduce several critical molecular mechanisms related to the relationship between spinal synaptic plasticity and chronic pain.

31.2 The Mechanism of Pain Transmission in the Spinal Cord

31.2.1 Excitatory Synaptic Transmission in the Spinal Cord

The dorsal horn neurons in the spinal cord receive nociceptive pain information from primary sensory afferents and relay it to the central nervous system. The impulse (action potential) through Aδ-fibers or C-fibers does not reach dorsal horn neurons directly as an electrical signal, because the dorsal horn neurons in the spinal cord are separated from the central terminals of Aδ-fibers or C-fibers by a synaptic cleft (a distance of approximately 20 nm). The dorsal horn neurons connect C-fibers or Aδ-fibers via chemical synapses, which mediate the excitation of dorsal horn neurons by glutamate released from presynaptic terminals. Glutamate release produces an excitatory postsynaptic potential (EPSP) in dorsal horn neurons [3] (Fig. 31.1). EPSPs evoked by low-frequency action potential discharge of primary afferents are mediated principally by the activation of α-amino-3-hydroxyl-5-methyl-4-isoxazole-propionate (AMPA) receptors, which are a subtype of glutamate receptors. N-methyl-D-aspartate (NMDA) receptors, another subtype of glutamate receptors, contribute little to the postsynaptic responses to glutamate release under basal conditions because of tonic inhibition of current flow by extracellular Mg^{2+} pore blockade at the resting membrane potential. However, NMDA receptors are important for spinal neuroplasticity, because they contribute to the generation of EPSP and action potentials during chronic pain following activation via kinase-mediated phosphorylation of the receptor (see Sect. 31.2.1). Moreover, nociceptive pain information is modulated by many interneurons and various endogenous neurotransmitters and neuromodulators at the presynapse or the postsynapse in the dorsal horn. For example, when substance P, a neuropeptide, is released from the central terminal of some C-fibers to the synaptic cleft and binds to the neurokinin 1 (NK1) receptor at the cell membrane of dorsal horn neurons, slow EPSP is induced in dorsal horn neurons [4] (Fig. 31.1). This slow EPSP is induced by closing the potassium channel via activation of G proteins in the cell membrane. Similarly, excitatory neuropeptides such as substance P contribute to slow excitatory synaptic transmission through G proteins.

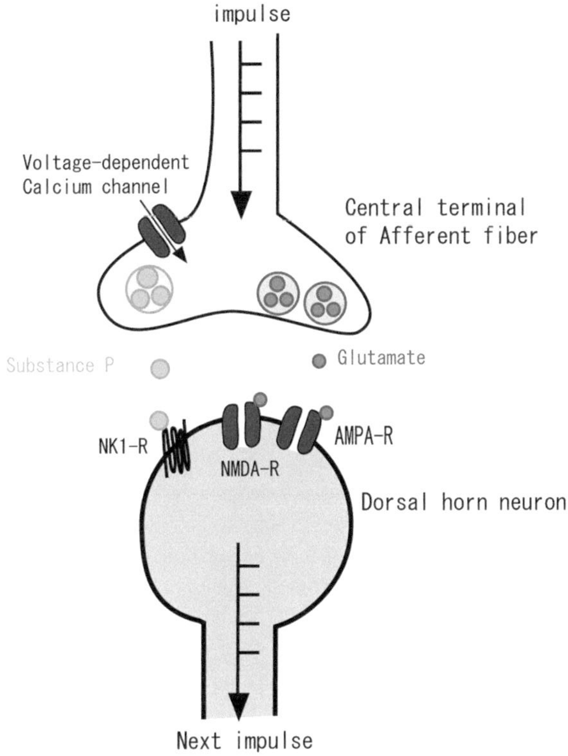

Fig. 31.1 Excitatory synaptic transmission in the dorsal horn. When an impulse is transmitted to central terminals of afferent fibers, excitatory neurotransmitters are released. Glutamate and substance P act at each receptor on the dorsal horn neuron and induce an impulse

Activation of ion channels such as the TRP channel and P2X (ATP receptor) in presynaptic terminals enhances glutamate release, which in turn enhances fast EPSP [5–9] (see Sects. 31.3.4 and 31.3.5).

31.2.2 Inhibitory Synaptic Transmission in the Spinal Cord

Although dorsal horn neuron action potential discharge is driven by glutamatergic EPSPs, the activity of these neurons is powerfully suppressed by inhibitory inputs in both the pre- and postsynapse. The inhibitory effect is mainly produced by γ-aminobutyric acid (GABA) and/or glycine postsynaptically, which are released from the terminals of inhibitory interneurons (Fig. 31.2). These interneurons induce fast inhibitory postsynaptic potentials (IPSPs) on dorsal horn neurons to mediate the activation of $GABA_A$ and glycine receptors. $GABA_A$ and glycine receptors are ligand-gated Cl^- channels. Channel opening inhibits action potentials by

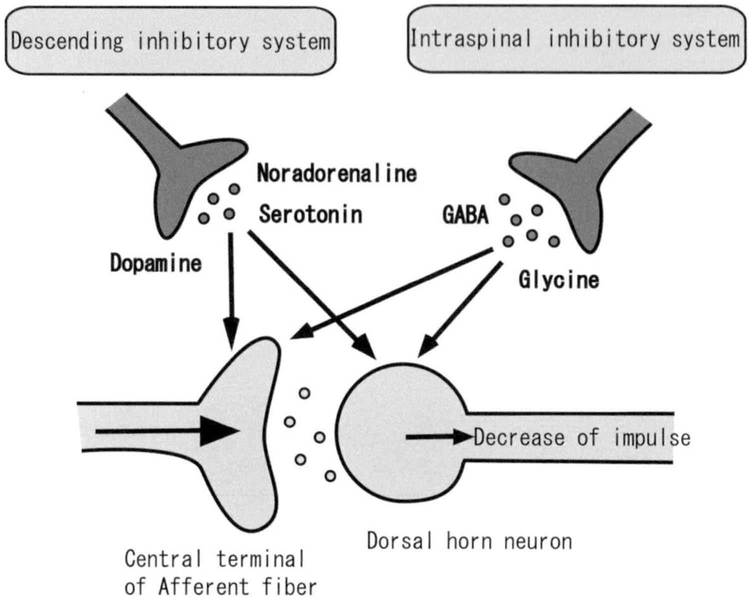

Fig. 31.2 The endogenous inhibitory system. The endogenous inhibitory system consists of the descending inhibitory system and the intraspinal inhibitory system

hyperpolarizing the cell membrane. Activation of G-protein-coupled receptors produces postsynaptic inhibition of excitatory synaptic transmission to hyperpolarize cell membranes by activating K^+ channels. This type of channel includes receptors such as the $GABA_B$ receptor, adenosine receptor, and opioid μ-receptor. Moreover, some endogenous substances suppress the release of glutamate from primary afferent terminals, therefore inhibiting discharge of dorsal horn neurons presynaptically. This presynaptic inhibition involves many of the same chemical mediators that cause postsynaptic inhibition, with receptors localized on the presynaptic terminals of primary afferents. There are not only networks within the spinal cord but also inhibitory projections to the dorsal horn from the brainstem, which is known as the descending inhibitory system. Serotonin [10] from the raphe nucleus, noradrenaline [10, 11] from the locus ceruleus, and dopamine [12, 13] from the hypothalamus A11 act on 5-HT1A receptors, α2 receptors, and D2-like receptors in dorsal horn neurons pre- and postsynaptically, respectively.

31.3 Spinal Synaptic Plasticity Induces Pathological Chronic Pain

There are two types of plasticity in the nervous system: one is central nervous sensitization, and the other is peripheral sensitization. In particular, central sensitization in the spinal cord has much to do with chronic pain. Although spinal synaptic

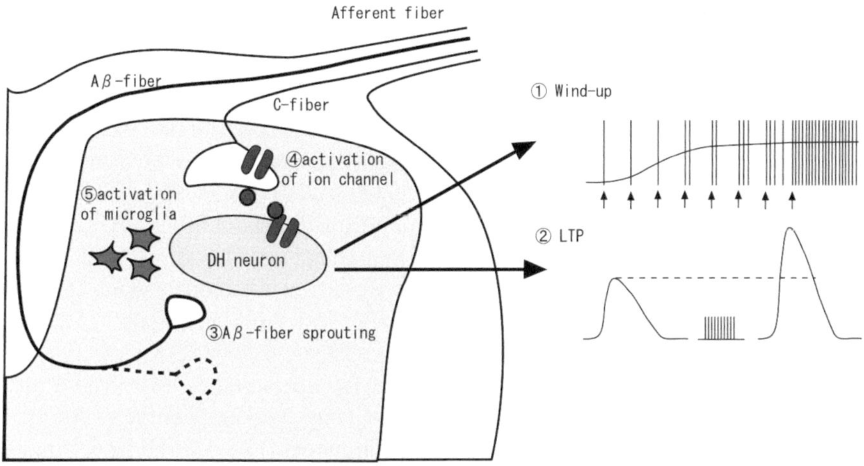

Fig. 31.3 Spinal synaptic plasticity. Spinal synaptic plasticity is induced by various causes. For example, ① windup, ② LTP, ③ Aβ-fiber sprouting into laminaII, ④ activation of ion channels on the central terminal of afferent fibers, and ⑤ activation of microglia

plasticity induces pathological chronic pain, there are many causes and various forms of spinal synaptic plasticity. In recent years, the influential mechanisms involved in spinal synaptic plasticity have become clear. We describe some convincing mechanisms in the following explanation.

31.3.1 Change in Efficiency of Excitatory Synaptic Transmission

The change in efficiency of excitatory synaptic transmission by nervous activation plays an important role in the enhancement of pain, as well as memory and learning in the hippocampus. With respect to electrophysiological phenomena, the enhancement of efficiency in excitatory synaptic transmission occurs by windup and long-term potentiation (LTP). Windup is when noxious peripheral stimulation that is more intense or sustained induces primary afferent nociceptors to discharge at higher frequencies (Fig. 31.3①). LTP refers to high-frequency primary afferent stimulation that induces the potentiation of glutamate receptor-mediated responses at synapses onto dorsal horn neurons (Fig. 31.3②). Windup and LTP are considered to be involved in the release of peptide neuromodulators such as substance P, together with glutamate, from central terminal C-fibers. These peptides act on their G-protein-coupled receptors to produce depolarizing synaptic potentials lasting up to tens of seconds. Moreover, both phenomena are also considered to be related to the activation of NMDA receptors by phosphorylation via kinase, and the subsequent current flow through NMDA receptors leads to a rise in intracellular Ca^{2+} levels.

31.3.2 Alterations to the Synaptic Network in the Dorsal Horn

The synaptic network changes dynamically according to neural activity, for example, growth or regression of axons, the appearance of new synapses, or the disappearance of existing synapses. Alterations to the synaptic network (synaptic morphology change) in the dorsal horn have been suggested to lead to pain in chronic inflammation [14] or peripheral nerve injury. Under normal conditions, noxious information is transmitted through Aδ- and C-fibers to the superficial dorsal horn, especially substantia gelatinosa (SG) neurons (lamina II of Rexed), while innocuous mechanical information is transmitted through Aβ-fibers to the deep dorsal horn (lamina III–IV). In past studies, it was shown that C-fibers were missing in the sciatic nerve amputation pain model, and approximately 10 % of Aβ-fibers started to extend axons (sprouting), with input into lamina II [15, 16] (Fig. 31.3③). Moreover, Aβ-fiber sprouting was observed in the inflammation pain model [17]. Aβ-fiber sprouting in these pain models plays an important role in brain-derived neurotrophic factor (BDNF), which is released from C-fibers into the spinal cord. The mechanism of allodynia has been suggested to occur when innocuous mechanical information is converted to noxious information. This process occurs when Aβ-fibers connect to SG neurons, which project noxious information to the more central nervous system during pathological conditions such as chronic inflammation and neuropathic pain.

31.3.3 Neurotrophic Factors

Neurotrophic factors are supplied to nerve cells by many kinds of cells (e.g., glia cells, dorsal root ganglion (DRG) neurons, Schwann cells, keratinocytes, and fibroblasts) and have various influences on the transmission of noxious information. During inflammation, the production of nerve growth factor (NGF) increases and causes hyperalgesia. NGF interacts with the TrkA receptor at the peripheral terminals of nociceptive fibers and is carried to DRG neurons by a retrograde axial. The NGF-TrkA complex controls gene expression in DRG neurons and promotes the production of neuropeptides, excitatory ion channels, and BDNF. BDNF is transferred to the central terminal of nociceptive fibers, which are projected to the spinal cord, where it acts upon its receptor, TrkB, on dorsal horn neurons. The subsequent activation of TrkB receptors on dorsal horn neurons modulates pain information [18]. Furthermore, BDNF also contributes to the change in the synaptic network in the dorsal horn, as mentioned above, during inflammation and neuropathic pain.

31.3.4 Activation of P2X Receptors

Much attention has been given to ion channels in the central terminals of Aδ- and C-fibers, which enhance nociceptive pain information by increasing glutamate release when these channels are activated by endogenous mediators (Fig. 31.4).

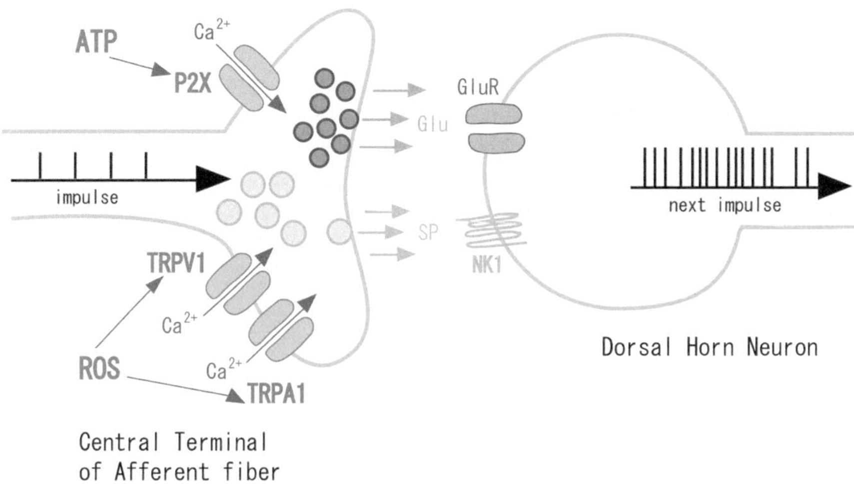

Fig. 31.4 Activation of ion channels. When ion channels in the central terminals of afferent fibers are activated, excitatory neurotransmitters are released. The P2X receptor is activated by ATP. TRPV1 and TRPA1 are activated by ROS and so on

For example, these ion channels include the ATP-dependent P2X receptor, the transient receptor potential (TRP) receptor family, voltage-dependent Na^+ channels, and acid-sensing ion channel 3 (ASIC3). In particular, we focused our attention on the P2X receptor in the dorsal horn. The P2X receptor family consists of at least seven P2X subunits ($P2X_1$–$P2X_7$). Each functional P2X receptor is composed of three or more P2X subunits, forming a pore structure that is permeable to cations including Ca^{2+}. Therefore, the P2X receptor family is a ligand-gated ion channel family. We examined the role of P2X receptors in modulating excitatory synaptic transmission by using patch-clamp recordings from dorsal horn neurons of the rat spinal cord [6, 7, 19, 20]. Distinct subtypes of P2X receptors were located at central terminals of primary afferents that innervate onto lamina II and lamina V neurons. On activation, these P2X receptors enhanced the release of glutamate in various ways. In lamina II neurons, the modulation of glutamate release by presynaptic P2X receptors was mainly transient. In contrast, the P2X receptor-mediated modulation of glutamate release was relatively long lasting in lamina V neurons [20]. Pharmacological studies suggested that lamina II neurons were involved in homomeric $P2X_3$ receptors, while lamina V neurons were involved in non-$P2X_3$ receptors [20]. Differences among P2X-expressing afferent fibers innervating lamina II and lamina V neurons were also seen in terms of capsaicin sensitivity [19]. P2X-expressing afferent central terminals in lamina II were derived from capsaicin-sensitive primary afferents, while those in lamina V were from capsaicin-insensitive primary afferents [19]. Because $P2X_3$-expressing afferent central terminals directly make synapses with lamina II neurons, the inputs from these afferent terminals could forward excitatory synaptic activities. On the contrary, the activities conveyed to lamina V neurons from $P2X_3$-expressing primary afferents were polysynaptic; these inputs together with monosynaptic inputs from P2X-expressing and capsaicin-insensitive afferents were shown to converge on lamina V neurons. These results indicate that distinct subtypes of P2X receptors are expressed in central terminals of primary afferents innervating onto superficial and deep dorsal horn neurons and modulate glutamate release in a different manner. Furthermore, P2X receptors were localized at lamina V neurons to mediate postsynaptic sensory transmissions [21]. Using the whole-cell patch-clamp technique, we investigated whether the activation of postsynaptic P2X receptors can modulate synaptic transmission in lamina V neurons. The ATP analogue generated an inward current in lamina V neurons. These pre- and postsynaptic actions may serve to understand P2X receptor-mediated modulation of various sensations.

31.3.5 Activation of TRPV1 and TRPA1 in the Central Terminals of Afferent Fibers

We have also focused on and examined the role of TRP receptors in modulating excitatory synaptic transmission. TRP channels belong to a family of ion channels that are activated by temperature and which are expressed in primary sensory nerve terminals where they provide information about thermal changes in the environment. There are six thermosensitive ion channels in mammals (TRPV1, TRPV2, TRPV3, TRPV4, TRPM8, and TRPA1), all of which belong to the TRP superfamily [22]. These channels are involved in chemical, mechanical, and thermal nociception. TRP channels are drug targets for the relief of pain, including neuropathic pain. In particular, TRPV1 (TRP vanilloid 1) and TRPA1 (TRP ankyrin 1) have been a major focus of research into the mechanisms of inflammatory and neuropathic pain. In addition to their expression at peripheral nerve endings, we revealed that TRPV1 and TRPA1 are expressed at the central terminals of primary afferent fibers and that their activation facilitates excitatory synaptic transmission in SG neurons by increasing glutamate release by whole-cell patch-clamp recording [5, 8, 9]. Therefore, activation of TRPV1 and TRPA1 at the central terminals of primary afferent fibers results in the enhancement of glutamate release (Figs. 31.3④ and 31.4). This enhancement leads to central sensitization and spinal synaptic plasticity. However, it is unclear which endogenous mediators act on TRPV1 or TRPA1 in the spinal cord. Reactive oxygen species (ROS) have been recognized to play an important role in the central neuropathic pain of the spinal cord. Spinal cord injury (SCI) increases levels of highly toxic ROS, which can damage neural, glial, and microvascular elements, resulting in sensory and motor neuron apoptosis. We investigated the effect of ROS on glutamatergic excitatory synaptic transmission in SG neurons [23], using the whole-cell patch-clamp technique. We showed that ROS enhances the spontaneous release of glutamate from presynaptic terminals onto SG neurons through TRPA1 and TRPV1 channel activation [23] (Fig. 31.4). Therefore, excessive activation of these ion channels by ROS may induce central sensitization in the spinal cord and result in chronic pain such as that following SCI. Thus, ROS may be one of the mediators which activate TRPV1 or TRPA1.

31.3.6 *Activated Microglia in the Spinal Cord Induce Neuropathic Pain*

Glia cells consist of astrocytes, oligodendrocytes, and microglia. The number of glial cells is several times greater than neurons in the spinal cord. Glial cells are considered to have no electrical activity and mainly play a role in the maintenance and supplementation of neuron function. Microglia were thought to play a role in immunity; however, recent studies revealed that glia cells are also involved in the adjustment of nervous activity. In particular, microglia in the spinal cord contributes to the mechanism of neuropathic pain after peripheral nerve injury [24, 25]. Recently, we showed that the number of activated microglia in the SG correlated to the frequency and amplitude of spontaneous excitatory postsynaptic current (sEPSC) using in vivo patch-clamp methods [26]. Under normal conditions, microglia are in their "resting" state, but following injury, such as peripheral nerve injury, they become "activated" (Fig. 31.3⑤). The activated microglia causes morphologic changes such as cell soma enlargement and shrinkage. Moreover, it was reported that the $P2X_4$ receptor specifically increases on activated microglia in the neuropathic pain model. The $P2X_4$ receptor is one subtype of the P2X receptor family and is found to be expressed in only microglia. When ATP stimulates the $P2X_4$ receptor on activated microglia, mechanical hypersensitivity in the neuropathic pain model is induced [25]. With respect to this mechanism, it becomes clear that BDNF, which is released from activated microglia in the spinal cord, acts on dorsal horn neurons [27]. BDNF involves the reduction of expression of the K^+-Cl^- cotransporter KCC2 in SG neurons. KCC2 normally plays a role in the extrusion of Cl^- from cells. As a consequence, there is a rise in intracellular Cl^- in SG neurons, resulting in a depolarizing shift in the anion reversal potential and hyperexcitability by means of dramatically reducing $GABA_A$-ergic and glycinergic inhibition (Fig. 31.5). This is recognized as one mechanism of allodynia. It is also becoming clear that intermediates, such as interferon γ [28] and interferon regulatory factor 8 [29], activate "resting" microglia.

31.4 Conclusion

Pain itself plays an important role as a warning signal; however, chronic pain is known to be pathological and hazardous to the body and goes beyond the warning signals. Chronic pain is therefore refractory because disease-developing mechanisms are complex, limiting the selection of effective treatments. However, in the world of fundamental research, we are on the verge of discovering the mechanism of chronic pain once and for all, which will allow us to improve treatments dramatically.

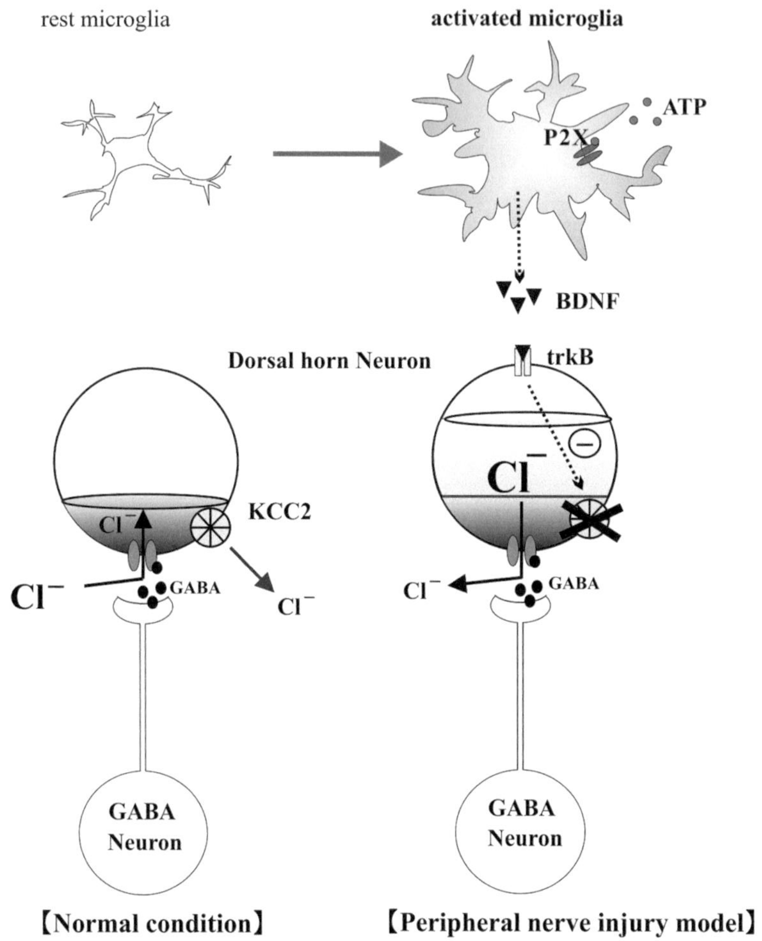

Fig. 31.5 Mechanism of activated microglia-induced allodynia. In the peripheral nerve injury model, resting microglia are activated and release BDNF. BDNF acts on TrkB receptors and causes downregulation of KCC2. Because intracellular Cl^- concentrations are increased, dorsal horn neurons are depolarized when GABA acts on $GABA_A$ receptors

Conflict of Interest The authors declare that they have no conflict of interest.

References

1. Salter MW (2010) Dorsal horn plasticity and neuron–microglia interactions. In: Mogil J (ed) Pain 2010 an updated review refresher course syllabus. IASP, Seattle, pp 12–23
2. Sandkühler J (2013) Spinal cord plasticity and pain. In: McMahon SB (ed) Wall and Melzack's textbook of pain, 6th edn. Elsevier Churchill Livingstone, London, pp 94–110

3. Yoshimura M, Jessell T (1990) Amino acid-mediated EPSPs at primary afferent synapses with substantia gelatinosa neurons in the rat spinal cord. J Physiol 430:315–335
4. De Koninck Y, Henry JL (1991) Substance P-mediated slow excitatory postsynaptic potential elicited in dorsal horn neurons in vivo by noxious stimulation. Proc Natl Acad Sci U S A 88:11344–11348
5. Kosugi M, Nakatsuka T, Fujita T et al (2007) Activation of TRPA1 channel facilitates excitatory synaptic transmission in substantia gelatinosa neurons of the adult rat spinal cord. J Neurosci 27:4443–4451
6. Nakatsuka T, Gu JG (2001) ATP P2X receptor-mediated enhancement of glutamate release and evoked EPSCs in dorsal horn neurons of the rat spinal cord. J Neurosci 21:6522–6531
7. Nakatsuka T, Gu JG (2006) P2X purinoceptors and sensory transmission. Pflugers Arch 452:598–607
8. Uta D, Furue H, Pickering AE et al (2010) TRPA1-expressing primary afferents synapse with a morphologically identified subclass of substantia gelatinosa neurons in the adult rat spinal cord. Eur J Neurosci 31:1960–1973
9. Yang K, Kumamoto E, Furue H et al (1998) Capsaicin facilitates excitatory but not inhibitory synaptic transmission in substantia gelatinosa of the rat spinal cord. Neurosci Lett 255:135–138
10. Yoshimura M, Furue H (2006) Mechanisms for the anti-nociceptive actions of the descending noradrenergic and serotonergic systems in the spinal cord. J Pharmacol Sci 101:107–117
11. Sonohata M, Furue H, Katafuchi T et al (2004) Actions of noradrenaline on substantia gelatinosa neurones in the rat spinal cord revealed by in vivo patch recording. J Physiol 555:515–526
12. Tamae A, Nakatsuka T, Koga K et al (2005) Direct inhibition of substantia gelatinosa neurones in the rat spinal cord by activation of dopamine D2-like receptors. J Physiol 568:243–253
13. Taniguchi W, Nakatsuka T, Miyazaki N et al (2011) In vivo patch-clamp analysis of dopaminergic antinociceptive actions on substantia gelatinosa neurons in the spinal cord. Pain 152:95–105
14. Nakatsuka T, Park JS, Kumamoto E et al (1999) Plastic changes in sensory inputs to rat substantia gelatinosa neurons following peripheral inflammation. Pain 82(1):39–47
15. Okamoto M, Baba H, Goldstein PA et al (2010) Functional reorganization of sensory pathways in the rat spinal dorsal horn following peripheral nerve injury. J Physiol 532:241–250
16. Woolf CJ, Shortland P, Coggeshall RE (1992) Peripheral nerve injury triggers central sprouting of myelinated afferents. Nature 355:75–78
17. Matayoshi S, Jiang N, Katafuchi T et al (2005) Actions of brain-derived neurotrophic factor on spinal nociceptive transmission during inflammation in the rat. J Physiol 569:685–695
18. Malcangio M, Lessmann V (2003) A common thread for pain and memory synapses? Brain-derived neurotrophic factor and trkB receptors. Trends Pharmacol Sci 24:116–121
19. Nakatsuka T, Furue H, Yoshimura M et al (2002) Activation of central terminal vanilloid receptor-1 receptors and alpha beta-methylene-ATP-sensitive P2X receptors reveals a converged synaptic activity onto the deep dorsal horn neurons of the spinal cord. J Neurosci 22:1228–1237
20. Nakatsuka T, Tsuzuki K, Ling JX et al (2003) Distinct roles of P2X receptors in modulating glutamate release at different primary sensory synapses in rat spinal cord. J Neurophysiol 89:3243–3252
21. Shiokawa H, Nakatsuka T, Furue H et al (2006) Direct excitation of deep dorsal horn neurones in the rat spinal cord by the activation of postsynaptic P2X receptors. J Physiol 573:753–763
22. Tominaga M (2007) Nociception and TRP channels. Handb Exp Pharmacol 489–505
23. Nishio N, Taniguchi W, Sugimura YK et al (2013) Reactive oxygen species enhance excitatory synaptic transmission in rat spinal dorsal horn neurons by activating TRPA1 and TRPV1 channels. Neuroscience 247:201–212
24. Inoue K, Tsuda M (2012) Purinergic systems, neuropathic pain and the role of microglia. Exp Neurol 234:293–301
25. Tsuda M, Shigemoto-Mogami Y, Koizumi S et al (2003) P2X4 receptors induced in spinal microglia gate tactile allodynia after nerve injury. Nature 424:778–783
26. Takiguchi N, Yoshida M, Taniguchi W et al (2012) Distinct degree of radiculopathy at different levels of peripheral nerve injury. Mol Pain 8:31

27. Coull JA, Beggs S, Boudreau D et al (2005) BDNF from microglia causes the shift in neuronal anion gradient underlying neuropathic pain. Nature 438:1017–1021
28. Tsuda M, Masuda T, Kitano J et al (2009) IFN-γ receptor signaling mediates spinal microglia activation driving neuropathic pain. Proc Natl Acad Sci U S A 106:8032–8037
29. Masuda T, Tsuda M, Yoshinaga R et al (2012) IRF8 is a critical transcription factor for transforming microglia into a reactive phenotype. Cell Rep 1:334–340

Chapter 32
Evaluation of Pain with Functional Neuroimaging

Takahiro Ushida, Kazuhiro Shimo, and Tatsunori Ikemoto

Abstract Pain is generally caused by peripheral events, and patients and medical professionals therefore tend to focus locally on those parts of the body where patients complain of pain. However, pain modulation occurs in patients who suffer pain not only due to localized factors but also due to various causes such as repeating memories of pain, environmental/social problems, and the mental/psychological state of the patient.

According to the International Association for the Study of Pain, pain is defined as "an unpleasant sensory and emotional experience associated with actual or potential tissue damage, or described in terms of such damage," and indeed, these types of incidents that are encountered clinically indicate that pain is a subjective experience of the brain. In recent years, functional neuroimaging techniques have frequently been applied to depict pain and its attendant sensory and emotional experiences as an image or to quantify these factors from the perspective that pain is perceived in the brain.

We conducted a review of the current state of functional neuroimaging in the brain and spinal cord based on recent research findings.

Keywords Brain • Functional neuroimaging • Spinal cord

T. Ushida (✉) • K. Shimo • T. Ikemoto
Multidisciplinary Pain Center, School of Medicine, Aichi Medical University, Nagakute, Aichi 480-1195, Japan

Institute of Physical Fitness, Sports Medicine and Rehabilitation, School of Medicine, Aichi Medical University, Nagakute, Aichi, Japan
e-mail: ushidat-koc@umin.ac.jp

K. Uchida et al. (eds.), *Neuroprotection and Regeneration of the Spinal Cord*,
DOI 10.1007/978-4-431-54502-6_32, © Springer Japan 2014

32.1 Introduction

Pain is generally caused by peripheral stimulation, and patients and medical professionals therefore tend to focus locally on those parts of the body where patients complain of pain, such as the "leg," "hip," and "neck." However, pain modulation occurs in patients who suffer pain not only due to local factors, but also due to various causes such as repeating memories of pain, environmental/social problems, and the mental/psychological state of the patient. As this modulation becomes stronger or weaker, the severity of the primary pain and the accompanying discomfort can vary greatly.

According to the International Association for the Study of Pain, pain is defined as "an unpleasant sensory and emotional experience associated with actual or potential tissue damage, or described in terms of such damage," and indeed, these types of incidents that are encountered clinically indicate that pain is a subjective experience of the brain. Traditionally, questionnaires such as the visual analogue scale (VAS), numeric rating scale (NRS), and McGill Pain Questionnaire have been used to assess pain. However, in recent years, functional neuroimaging techniques (Table 32.1) such as functional magnetic resonance imaging (fMRI), positron emission tomography (PET), and single photon emission computed tomography (SPECT) have frequently been applied to depict pain and its attendant sensory and emotional experiences as an image or to quantify these factors from the perspective that pain is perceived in the brain. We introduce herein the endeavors using these methods to evaluate pain involving the musculoskeletal system, focusing primarily on research progress to date.

32.2 Transmission of Pain Signals at the Spinal Cord Level and Efforts to Visualize This Phenomenon

Pain impulses traveling to the spinal cord from the periphery via primary afferent fibers are transmitted to spinothalamic tract cells, which are a type of cell in the spinal dorsal horn, and subsequently transmitted as pain signals to the brain via the

Table 32.1 Types of functional Imaging Technologies

	Target	Spatial resolution (mm)	Temporal resolution (S)
EEG/MEG	Neuronal current	10	0.001
fMRI	Regional changes in blood flow	4–5	1–10
PET	Oxygen consumption, glucose metabolism etc.	5–10	30–1,000
SPECT	Changes in blood flow change	10	60–1,000
NIRS (near-infrared spectroscopy)	Changes in blood flow change	8–	0.01–

ventrolateral pathway on the opposite side. In contrast to the brain, which ultimately experiences pain through various modulations, the spinal cord receives fewer of these modulations and tends to directly reflect nerve response to outside stimulation. For this reason, a method of inserting an electrode directly into the dorsal horn of the spinal cord to record neural activities of spinothalamic tract cells has been widely applied in animal studies, and this particular method has been used to elucidate mechanisms of pain exacerbation such as spinal cord sensitization and to evaluate drug treatments. However, direct insertion of a needle into the spinal cord can be difficult in humans, so studies using fMRI and PET have been progressing as an alternative.

32.2.1 Spinal fMRI Studies in Healthy Subjects

Although research to evaluate spinal cord function has only just scratched the surface, our group has been proceeding with the analysis of spinal cord activity induced by a mechanical pain stimulation device, using the blood oxygen level-dependent (BOLD) method. Functional tasks to elicit spinal cord activity are conducted using our original plastic mechanical pain stimulation device. Functional MRI using echo planar imaging (EPI) was conducted on healthy subjects administered painful stimuli, BOLD signal changes were recorded with a 3-T MRI scanner, and analysis was undertaken using statistical parametric mapping (SPM) (www.fil.ion.ucl.ac.uk/spm/). Since large mechanical movements occur in the cervical vertebrae due to breathing and swallowing, we created and utilized a cervical collar to suppress these movements during imaging. As a result, we were able to visualize the inner spinal cord area that was activated in response to the nociceptive stimuli applied in the study (Fig. 32.1). However, variations in activation were seen between subjects. Before clinical application can be achieved, the function of a spinal cord that has flattened and shrunk in size due to spinal cord compression will need to be assessed in the future. We therefore believe that further technical improvements in the method are essential [1].

32.2.2 Spinal PET Imaging in Patients with Neuropathic Pain in the Spinal Cord

PET and SPECT are imaging modalities that detect gamma-ray distributions emitted from drugs administered to the body, allowing the creation of tomographic images. PET is a method in which radioisotopes that emit positrons are injected into the body to produce gamma-rays that arise during pair annihilation between positron and electrons in the body and is performed with a sensor set up to enclose the body. Uchida et al. investigated glucose metabolism in the cervical spinal cord using fusion

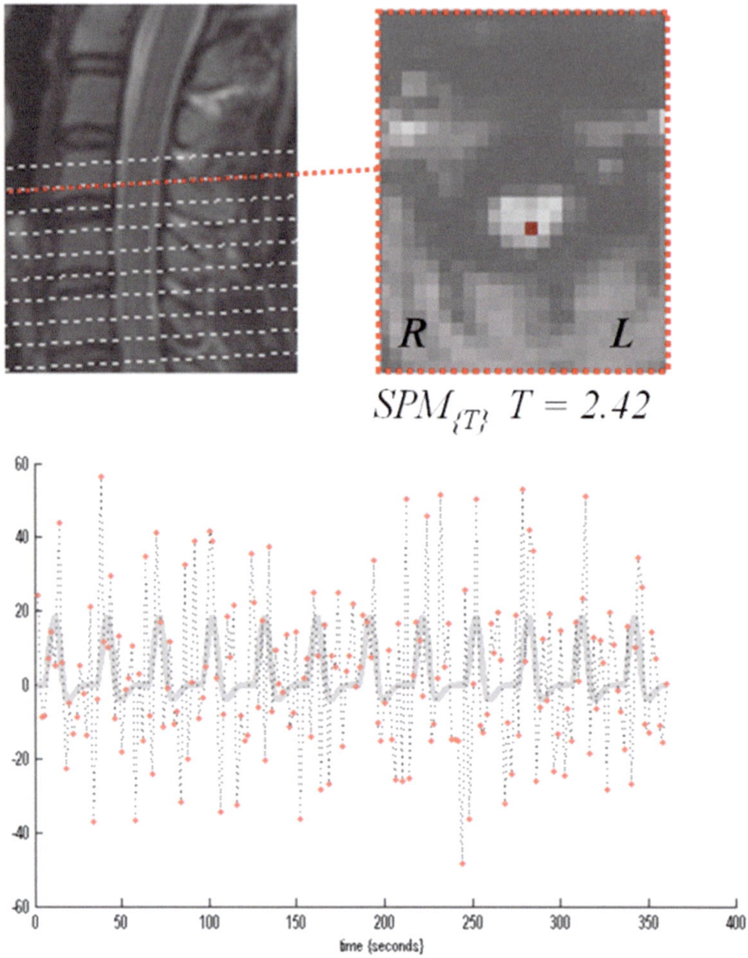

Fig. 32.1 Time-dependent changes in BOLD signal and site of spinal cord activity

images of 3-T MRI and 18 fludeoxyglucose (FDG)-PET in patients with compressive cervical myelopathy [2]. We applied this PET technology to assess whether functional changes in the spinal cord occur in patients with neuropathic pain in the spinal cord. We observed sites of FDG uptake in the spinal cord and were able to obtain an image that suggests enhanced neural activity due to pain. However, some aspects of the results, such as resolution, remain to be optimized in the future (Fig. 32.2).

Previous findings from functional neuroimaging of the spinal cord suggest that both fMRI and PET will be able to be applied to humans in the future as methods to evaluate pain. However, further investigations are necessary before these approaches can be used in clinical cases such as cervical myelopathy.

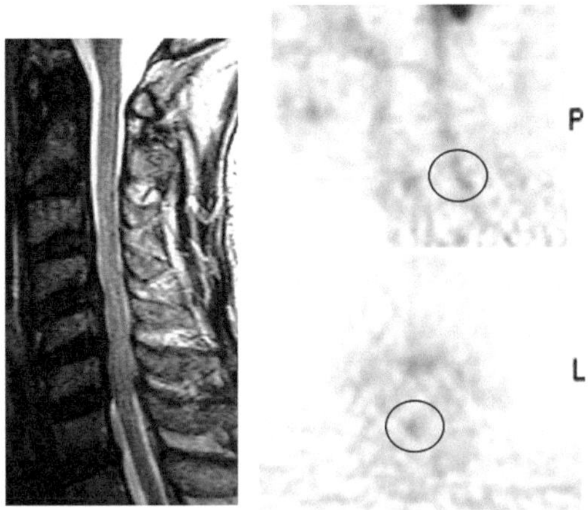

Fig. 32.2 Cervical spinal FDG PET (left cervical radiculopathy, 60's years, male). In collaboration with the Department of Orthopedic Surgery at the University of Fukui

32.3 Functional Brain Imaging and Musculoskeletal Pain

Previous studies of functional brain imaging in healthy subjects have revealed that the pain signals that ascend through the spinal cord are primarily projected to the region of cerebral cortex called the "pain matrix," an area related to pain. This region includes the first and second somatosensory areas (S1 and S2), insular cortex, anterior cingulate gyrus, and medial prefrontal cortex via the thalamus. However, in clinical settings where patients with chronic pain require pain evaluation, plastic changes and sensitization of the nervous system may be induced, and a transmission pathway may not necessarily be experienced in a similar manner to that in healthy subjects with acute pain. Here, we show functional neuroimaging findings from previous studies of chronic musculoskeletal pain, focusing on the latest research outcomes.

32.3.1 Brain Activity in the Thalamus and Acute and Chronic Pain

The thalamus is said to be the center of senses and is where pain transmission from the aforementioned spinothalamic tract terminates. The thalamus has therefore been a major focus in pain research for many years, and many detailed analyses have been conducted.

In studies that have investigated neural activity in the thalamus using PET or SPECT, neural activity in the thalamus is known to be enhanced in acute pain pathology. However, several reports on chronic pain have indicated a decrease in thalamic activity on the side contralateral to where the transmission of stimulation primarily occurs in pain conditions [3, 4]. Such decreases in contralateral thalamic activity are also known to be exacerbated with longer disease staging, and this is thought to imply plastic changes in the central nervous system [5]. Several causes have been postulated for such changes: (1) persistent and chronic pain activates the inhibitory system to suppress thalamic function; (2) the cortical sensory area has fallen into a persistently and easily excitable state due to chronic input from the thalamus, and even small pain signal inputs from the thalamus equate to the recognition of pain; or (3) enhancement of blood flow is not required because synaptic transmission at the thalamus has become extremely efficient. However, several reports on chronic pain have indicated enhancement of thalamic activity on the contralateral side, so further mechanistic clarification is necessary.

32.3.2 *Evaluation of Induced Pain in the Brain Using fMRI*

Functional MRI offers not only good spatial resolution but also moderate temporal resolution and is appropriate for the evaluation of brain activity when and where pain is inflicted.

32.3.2.1 Brain Activity when Pain Stimulation Is Inflicted (Comparison Between Healthy Subjects and Patients with Neuropathic Pain)

With the objective of investigating brain activity in patients with allodynia who experience pain from stimuli that would not normally provoke pain, Ikemoto et al. captured the brain activity of such patients using fMRI following mechanical stimulation (non-nociceptive stimulation) that would not normally provoke pain at the site in which they experience pain and compared these results to when healthy subjects were provoked with mechanical nociceptive and non-nociceptive stimulation [6]. Results indicated that when healthy subjects were provoked with mechanical nociceptive stimulation, enhancement of activity in the thalamus, somatosensory areas (S1 and S2), cingulate gyrus, and cerebellum was detected. On the other hand, even though stronger pain was observed in patients on the VAS compared to healthy subjects, activity in the thalamus, which is the center for pain from the periphery, was not detected. Activities are now known to arise in S1, S2, cingulate gyrus (primarily anterior cingulate gyrus), as well as the motor cortex and supplementary motor cortex (Fig. 32.3) [7]. Peyron et al. [8] conducted a study of brain activity upon inflicting mechanical stimulation that would not normally provoke pain on the affected side as well as the unaffected side in patients with allodynia and reported results similar to those reported by Ikemoto et al.

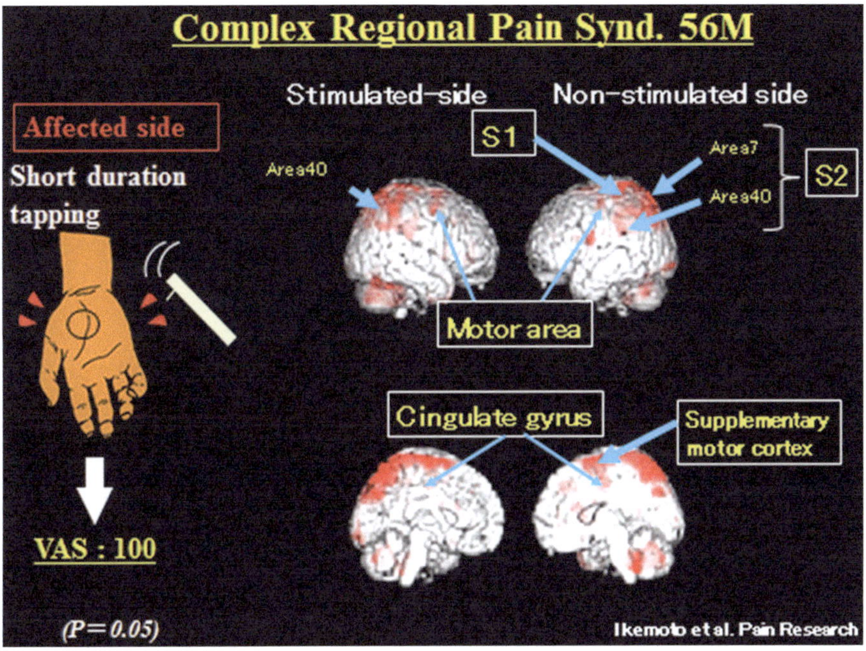

Fig. 32.3 In CRPS patient, even though stronger pain was observed on the VAS , activity in the thalamus, which is the center for pain from the periphery, was not detected. Activities are now known to arise in S1, S2, cingulate gyrus (primarily anterior cingulate gyrus), as well as the motor cortex and supplementary motor cortex

32.3.2.2 Brain Activity Sites During Reproduction of Joint Pain and Low Back Pain Induced by External Stimulation

Even in chronic pain that is generally considered to represent a repetition of acute pain in conditions such as osteoarthritis of the knee, pain while walking and localized tenderness are observed. Since pain is confined in these patients, attempts have been made to stimulate the tender sites with a special device. As a result, fMRI revealed that patients with osteoarthritis of the knee exhibit significant neural activity in areas of the pain matrix such as bilateral thalami, S2, insula, supplementary motor cortex, and anterior cingulate gyrus, as well as pain when pressure stimulation is applied to tender sites [9].

In addition, low back pain due to external stimulation has been reproduced, and the associated brain activity has been examined. Kobayashi et al. [10] reproduced low back pain by applying pressure stimuli to the lumbar area in patients with chronic low back pain and reported the brain activity during such reproduction. In patients with low back pain, significant brain activity was observed in the prefrontal cortex, supplementary motor cortex, premotor cortex, thalamus, insula, and posterior cingulate gyrus compared to healthy subjects. This cerebral network associated with low back pain is termed the "LBP matrix." Neural activities in the prefrontal cortex, which are known to be deeply associated with cognitive function, and in the posterior cingulate gyrus where unpleasant emotions are known to be reflected when chronic pain patients experience pain have been clarified to occur in a different area than the "pain matrix," which is a pain-related region that is observed in acute pain experienced by healthy subjects.

32.3.2.3 Cranial Nerve Activity and Virtual Pain Stimulation Induced by Image Presentation

In patients with neuropathic pain, thalamic activity had not been detected even when patients experienced strong pain with pain stimulation. Similarly to the findings of PET and SPECT studies, plastic changes to the nerves in the brain are considered to be a possible cause of this phenomenon. In addition, this indicated that even when thalamic activity is decreased, pain is thought to be provoked in patients with neuropathic pain.

A virtual experiment on pain was therefore conducted by having subjects view videos [11]. Patients with neuropathic pain who suffer allodynia were shown a video where a palm was being touched by a brush and subsequently demonstrated that, compared to healthy subjects, activity in the prefrontal cortex and anterior cingulate gyrus was enhanced. The anterior cingulate gyrus had previously been shown to be activated in healthy subjects when they watched "a painful image" [12] (Fig. 32.4), so the video of a brush touching the palm may have unconsciously induced a "painful" emotion in patients with neuropathic pain. In addition, the possibility was suggested that some kind of obstacle to the integration of cognitive and emotional aspects of pain is caused in the medial prefrontal area.

It was postulated that similar results may ensue when patients with low back pain experience virtual pain in the brain as to when patients with neuropathic pain receive similar treatment. Brain activity was therefore investigated when an image of "a man carrying luggage in a half-crouching position" was shown to patients [6]. The group of patients who had previously experienced low back pain showed significant brain activity in regions such as the supplementary motor cortex, premotor cortex, visual association cortex, thalamus, insula, posterior cingulate gyrus, fusiform gyrus, hippocampus, and posterior parietal lobe compared to those who had not previously experienced low back pain. Furthermore, the visual information of "a man carrying luggage in a half-crouching position" induced all subjects in the low back pain group to complain of unpleasantness, and some even complained of pain. In contrast, in the non-low back pain group, no one complained of pain or unpleasantness. Supplementary motor cortex, premotor cortex, thalamus, insula, and posterior cingulate gyrus are all common to the "LBP matrix," which is activated when pain is actually inflicted. As a result, patients who have previously experienced low back pain, even without actual nociceptive stimulation, were suggested to experience unpleasant emotions that can be described as virtual low back pain from visual information (Fig. 32.5).

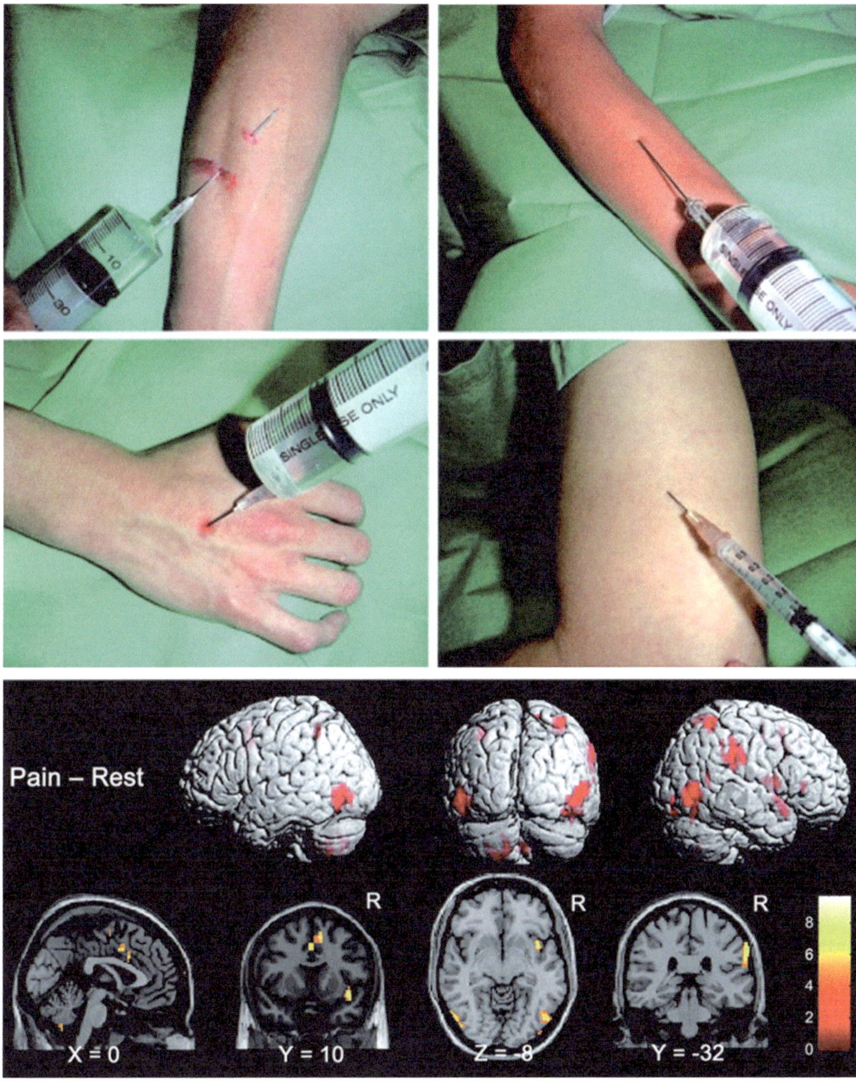

Fig. 32.4 Ogino et al. [12]

32.3.3 *Evaluation of Resting Brain Activity (Default Mode Network)*

Previous studies of the evaluation of brain function related to pain were structured based on the principle of determining sites at which brain activity develops on external stimulus. Our studies that we have described thus far have also focused on the pain matrix activity of sites such as the thalamus and cingulate gyrus.

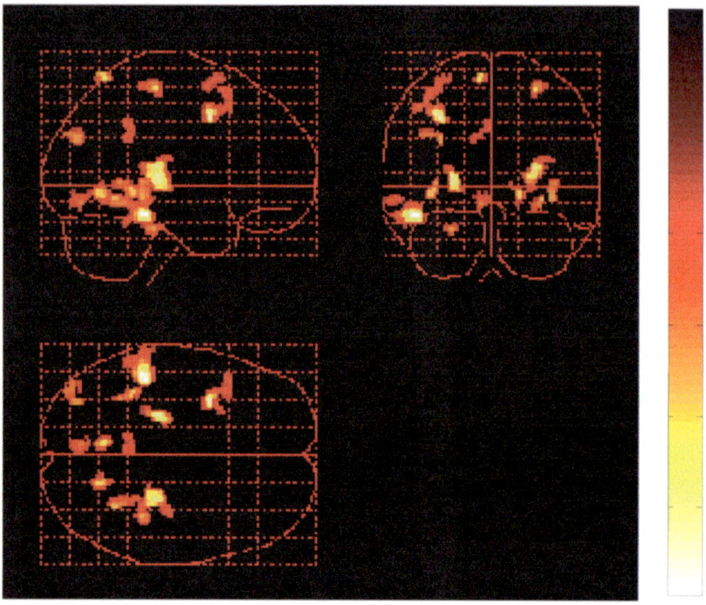

Fig. 32.5 Areas of cortical activation in the LBP group compared with the non-LBP group in response to virtual LBP stimuli (task-control condition) detected by fMRI ($p<0.0005$, Z score>3.4, uncorrected threshold)

Meanwhile, Raichle et al. indicated while researching brain activity that, in a control state of not doing anything, there are parts of the brain that show higher activity compared to when subjects are not on psychological tasks, and this has been termed the "default network" or "resting state" [13].

Baliki et al. conducted finger exercise tasks and compared healthy subjects and patients with chronic low back pain in terms of the parts of the brain showing decreased activity and subsequently found that enhanced activity is observed at rest in the prefrontal cortex and cingulate and posterior cingulate gyrus, indicating that abnormality in the default mode network may have occurred in patients with low back pain [14] (Fig. 32.6). Patients who complain of a chronic pain often state that they "don't do anything all day and stay still because it is painful" or that their "pain is alleviated when carrying out other activities." This suggests that brain activity at rest is associated with the development and maintenance of chronic pain, and future development in this area of research is therefore anticipated.

32.3.4 Potential for Clinical Application of Brain Function Evaluation

Compared to healthy subjects, the volume of grey matter is known to be decreased in the dorsolateral prefrontal cortex, thalamus, brainstem, and SI in patients with

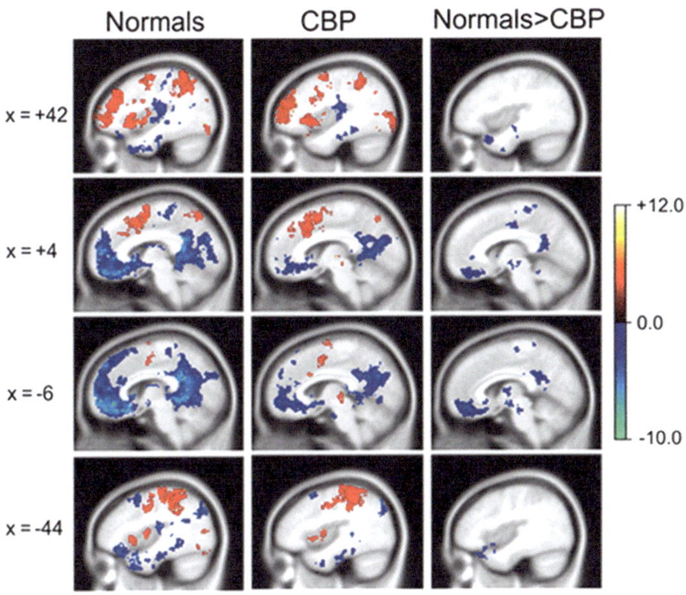

Fig. 32.6 Baliki et al. [14]

chronic low back pain [15–17]. Seminowicz et al. [18] investigated changes in the brain before and after treatment in patients with chronic low back pain and reported a significant increase in the volume of the left dorsolateral prefrontal cortex after treatment. Furthermore, increases in dorsolateral prefrontal cortex volume caused by treatment appear to be related to the severity of pain and improvement in ADL due to treatment (Fig. 32.7). In addition, a distortion in cognitive function is known to occur in patients with chronic low back pain [19–21], but brain activity while performing tasks related to cognitive function is indicated to broaden in the activated regions and conversely to become narrower in the suppressed brain regions compared to healthy subjects. These findings indicate that cognitive information processing in the brain differs between patients with chronic low back pain and healthy subjects. In a study of older patients with chronic low back pain, Buckalew et al. [22] compared brain images between those with disabling (hindered ADL, activities of daily life) low back pain and those with non-disabling (maintained ADL) low back pain. No differences in brain volume were seen between groups, but diffusion tensor analysis showed that anisotropy of the corpus callosum ampulla was decreased in the disabling group and that a correlation existed between decreased anisotropy and duration of low back pain ailment. Interestingly, even within patients with chronic low back pain who have similar durations of illness or degree of pain, brain images sometimes reflect the differences in how pain affects daily life.

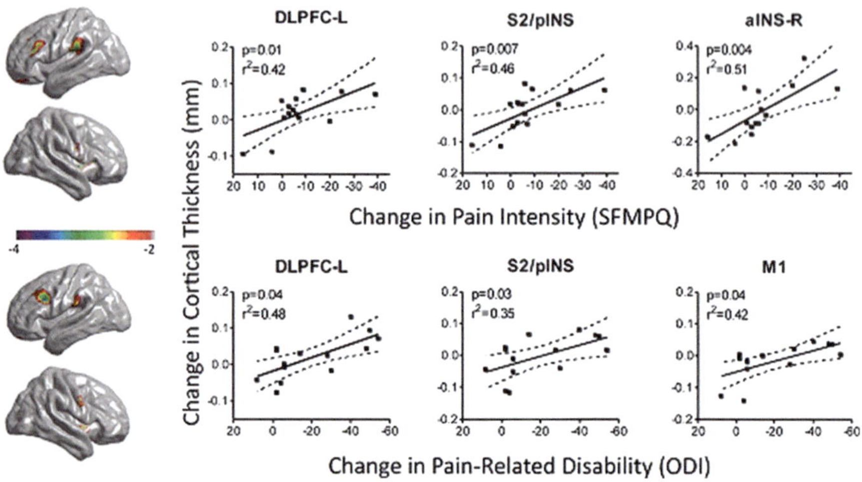

Fig. 32.7 Parts of the brain where volume change occurred in association with improved pain and ADL due to treatment (modification of [18])

32.3.5 *Significance of Functional Neuroimaging as a Method to Evaluate Individual Patients with Pain*

Since pain largely involves subjective elements, determining the degree of pain from the outside with standard procedures is difficult. Functional neuroimaging techniques, including fMRI, are considered to play an essential role in the evaluation of pain. Pain in the musculoskeletal system has also been revealed to be associated with activity of the "pain matrix" and it is therefore necessary to consider the changes in the central nervous system and not only the periphery where pain is inflicted. For example, comparing and studying the "pain matrix" brain activity in patients before and after intervention can lead to objective determination of the degree to which subjective and emotional pain is decreased. To conduct pain evaluation in each patient, the reproducibility and reliability of fMRI data are required for every individual patient. However, several problems (as shown below) have been encountered and clinical application has yet to be achieved. For example, in a group study, pain was found to be largely influenced by memory, awareness, and emotion, which counterbalance each other. Pain is therefore difficult to evaluate and study reproduction is problematic, as the above problems change day by day. To overcome these issues, future studies will need to determine what type of pain-related task targets which part of the brain to recognize and reflect pain and related unpleasantness and where to focus evaluations for chronic situations. In particular, pain-related tasks that adequately reflect the actual patient image have yet to be developed for pain in the musculoskeletal system, and we believe that further investigations and research in this field are essential.

32.4 Summary

We conducted a review of the current state of functional neuroimaging in the brain and spinal cord based on recent research findings. For patients with chronic pain in whom objective diagnosis is difficult, diagnosis and appropriate treatment will require elucidation of the mechanisms of pain development and maintenance in the spinal cord and brain, and establishment of imaging techniques to evaluate subjective and emotional aspects of pain in individual patients will also be indispensable.

Conflict of Interest The authors declare that they have no conflict of interest.

References

1. Ikemoto T, Ushida T, Ueno T (2011) Neuronal activity of cervical spinal cord to palm pain using functional magnetic resonance imaging. J Spine Res 2(2):223–226
2. Uchida K, Nakajima H, Yayama T, Kobayashi S, Shimada S, Tsuchida T, Okazawa H, Mwaka E, Baba H (2009) High-resolution magnetic resonance imaging and 18FDG-PET findings of the cervical spinal cord before and after decompressive surgery in patients with compressive myelopathy. Spine (Phila Pa 1976) 34(11):1185–1191
3. Iadarola MJ, Max MB, Berman KF, Byas-Smith MG, Coghill RC, Gracely RH, Bennett GJ (1995 Oct) Unilateral decrease in thalamic activity observed with positron emission tomography in patients with chronic neuropathic pain. Pain 63(1):55–64
4. Usui C, Doi N, Nishioka M, Komatsu H, Yamamoto R, Ohkubo T, Ishizuka T, Shibata N, Hatta K, Miyazaki H, Nishioka K, Arai H (2006 Apr) Electroconvulsive therapy improves severe pain associated with fibromyalgia. Pain 121(3):276–280
5. Fukumoto M, Ushida T, Zinchuk VS, Yamamoto H, Yoshida S (1999 Nov 20) Contralateral thalamic perfusion in patients with reflex sympathetic dystrophy syndrome. Lancet 354(9192):1790–1791
6. Shimo K, Ueno T, Younger J, Nishihara M, Inoue S, Ikemoto T, Taniguchi S, Ushida T (2011) Visualization of painful experiences believed to trigger the activation of affective and emotional brain regions in subjects with low back pain. PLoS One (Research Support, Non-US Gov't) 6(11):e26681
7. Ikemoto T, Ushida T, Tanaka S, Morio K, Zinchuk VS, Tani T, Taniguchi S, Ushida A (2003) Painful mechanical stimulation evokes activation of distinct functional areas in the brain: comparison of normal subjects and two patients with neuropathic pain. Pain Res 18:137–144
8. Peyron R, Schneider F, Faillenot I, Convers P, Barral FG, Garcia-Larrea L, Laurent B (2004 Nov 23) An fMRI study of cortical representation of mechanical allodynia in patients with neuropathic pain. Neurology 63(10):1838–1846
9. Baliki MN, Geha PY, Jabakhanji R, Harden N, Schnitzer TJ, Apkarian AV (2008) A preliminary fMRI study of analgesic treatment in chronic back pain and knee osteoarthritis. Mol Pain 4:47
10. Kobayashi Y, Kurata J, Sekiguchi M, Kokubun M, Akaishizawa T, Chiba Y, Konno S, Kikuchi S (2009) Augmented cerebral activation by lumbar mechanical stimulus in chronic low back pain patients: an FMRI study. Spine (Phila Pa 1976) 34(22):2431–2436
11. Ushida T, Ikemoto T, Taniguchi S, Ishida K, Murata Y, Ueda W, Tanaka S, Ushida A, Tani T (2005 Fall) Virtual pain stimulation of allodynia patients activates cortical representation of pain and emotions: a functional MRI study. Brain Topogr 18(1):27–35
12. Ogino Y, Nemoto H, Inui K, Saito S, Kakigi R, Goto F (2007 May) Inner experience of pain: imagination of pain while viewing images showing painful events forms subjective pain representation in human brain. Cereb Cortex 17(5):1139–1146

13. Raichle ME, Snyder AZ (2007) A default mode of brain function: a brief history of an evolving idea. Neuroimage 37(4):1083–1090
14. Baliki MN, Geha PY, Apkarian AV, Chialvo DR (2008) Beyond feeling: chronic pain hurts the brain, disrupting the default-mode network dynamics. J Neurosci (Comparative Study Research Support, NIH, Extramural) 28(6):1398–1403
15. Apkarian AV, Sosa Y, Sonty S et al (2004) Chronic back pain is associated with decreased prefrontal and thalamic gray matter density. J Neurosci 24(46):10410–10415
16. Buckalew N, Haut MW, Morrow L et al (2008) Chronic pain is associated with brain volume loss in older adults: preliminary evidence. Pain Med 9(2):240–248
17. Schmidt-Wilcke T, Leinisch E, Gänssbauer S et al (2006) Affective components and intensity of pain correlate with structural differences in gray matter in chronic back pain patients. Pain 25(1–2):89–97
18. Seminowicz DA, Wideman TH, Naso L et al (2011) Effective treatment of chronic low back pain in humans reverses abnormal brain anatomy and function. J Neurosci 31(20):7540–7550
19. Apkarian AV, Sosa Y, Krauss BR et al (2004) Chronic pain patients are impaired on an emotional decision-making task. Pain 108(1–2):129–136
20. Kewman DG, Vaishampayan N, Zald D et al (1991) Cognitive impairment in musculoskeletal pain patients. Int J Psychiatry Med 21(3):253–262
21. Lee DM, Pendleton N, Tajar A et al (2010) Chronic widespread pain is associated with slower cognitive processing speed in middle-aged and older European men. Pain 151(1):30–36
22. Buckalew N, Haut MW, Aizenstein H et al (2010) Differences in brain structure and function in older adults with self-reported disabling and nondisabling chronic low back pain. Pain Med 11(8):1183–1197

Index

K. Uchida et al. (eds.), *Neuroprotection and Regeneration of the Spinal Cord*, DOI 10.1007/978-4-431-54502-6, © Springer Japan 2014

MIX
Papier aus verantwortungsvollen Quellen
Paper from responsible sources
FSC® C105338

If you have any concerns about our products,
you can contact us on
ProductSafety@springernature.com

In case Publisher is established outside the EU,
the EU authorized representative is:
Springer Nature Customer Service Center GmbH
Europaplatz 3, 69115 Heidelberg, Germany

Printed by Libri Plureos GmbH
in Hamburg, Germany